This is a medical and social history of Italy's largest city during the cholera epidemics of 1884 and 1910–11. It also is the first extended study of cholera in modern Italy, which sets Naples in a comparative international framework.

The book explores the factors that exposed Naples to risk; it examines such popular responses as social hysteria, riots and religiosity; and it traces therapeutic strategies. The disease is also related to larger historical issues, such as the nature of liberal statecraft, the 'Southern Question', mass emigration, organized crime, urban renewal and the medical profession.

Cholera in Naples became a metaphor for discontent with the regime: the 1884 outbreak was a national issue which led to the rebuilding of the city amidst widespread corruption. Despite rebuilding, the city suffered a major epidemic in 1910–11. Stunned, the Italian state launched a campaign of silence. The authorities suppressed the truth, lied to the international community and fabricated statistics. This work thus extends the historiography of cholera in Europe into the twentieth century and analyses the only known case in which a major epidemic was systematically concealed.

NAPLES IN THE TIME OF CHOLERA, 1884–1911

NAPLES
IN THE
TIME OF CHOLERA,
1884–1911

FRANK M. SNOWDEN

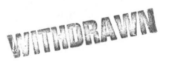

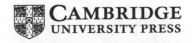
CAMBRIDGE
UNIVERSITY PRESS

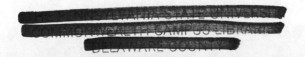

Published by the Press Syndicate of the University of Cambridge
The Pitt Building, Trumpington Street, Cambridge CB2 1RP
40 West 20th Street, New York, NY 10011–4211, USA
10 Stamford Road, Oakleigh, Melbourne 3166, Australia

First published 1995

Printed in Great Britain at the University Press, Cambridge

A catalogue record for this book is available from the British Library

Library of Congress cataloguing in publication data

Snowden, Frank M. (Frank Martin), 1946–
Naples in the time of cholera, 1884–1911 / Frank M. Snowden.
p.   cm.
Includes bibliographical references.
ISBN 0 521 48310 7
1. Cholera – Italy – Naples – History.
I. Title.
RC133.I9N386   1995
614.5′14′094573 – dc20   94-43875   CIP

ISBN 0 521 48310 7 hardback

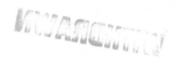

For Judith

Contents

List of figures   *page* xi
List of tables   xii
Preface   xiv
Glossary of Italian and Neapolitan terms   xv

Introduction   1

PART I: SANITARY ANXIETIES

1   A city at risk   11

PART II: THE PUBLIC EPIDEMIC OF 1884

2   From Provence to the Bay of Naples   59
3   Death in Naples, 1884   99
4   Survival and recovery   155

PART III: *RISANAMENTO* AND MIASMA

5   Rebuilding: medicine and politics   181

PART IV: THE SECRET EPIDEMIC OF 1910–1911

6   The return of cholera: 1910   233
7   Concealment and crisis: 1911   297

Conclusion: Neapolitan cholera and Italian politics   360

APPENDIX

Appendix   371

Notes   380
Select bibliography   448
Index   463

Figures

Map 1.1	The Bay of Naples	*page* 12
Map 1.2	The *sezioni* of Naples	13
Map 2.1	Italy and Provence	60
Map 5.1	The renewal and expansion of Naples	182
Map 5.2	*Risanamento*	183
Map 6.1	Apulia	234

Tables

1.1 European capital cities: average annual deaths per 1,000 inhabitants, 1878–83   14
1.2 Naples: annual deaths per 1,000 inhabitants, 1878–83   16
1.3 Cholera in Naples, 1836–73   16
1.4 Population of the ten largest Italian cities, 1884   18
1.5 Naples: population per square kilometer, 1884   18
1.6 Average industrial salaries and wages in Naples, 1884   33
1.7 Prevailing prices in Naples, 1884   34
1.8 Male wages in selected trades in Europe, 1884 (expressed in 1884 US dollars)   35
1.9 Naples: average rent per room (1806 = 100)   39
1.10 Eligible voters in Naples for the municipal elections of 1875   48
3.1 Causes of death in Naples in 1884   105
3.2 Cholera in the *sezioni* of Naples, 1884   107
3.3 Success of treatment in the Neapolitan cholera hospitals, 1884   112
3.4 Age at death of cholera victims in the *sezione* Mercato in 1884   118
3.5 Rates of death from cholera by age group: Italy, 1884   119
3.6 Cholera in Paris, 1832–92   152
4.1 Deaths from cholera in Naples, 1886–94   176
5.1 Expenses of phase one of *risanamento*   203
5.2 Assets available to complete phase one of *risanamento*   203
5.3 Flow of the population evicted by *risanamento*, 1889–1900   214
5.4 Naples: residents per square decametre, 1912   222
5.5 Daily food budget of an average Neapolitan family, 1910   223
5.6 Leading causes of death in Naples, 1909   223
5.7 Expenditure on hospitals per 1,000 inhabitants in 1910   224
6.1 Deaths from cholera in Naples, 1884 and 1910   252
6.2 Cases of gastro-enteritis in Naples, 18–24 September, 1910   260
6.3 Annual average number of trans-oceanic emigrants, 1876–1910   270
6.4 Shipping tonnage in 1910   270

6.5 Passengers handled by leading European seaports in 1908 271
6.6 Emigrants detained at the *Casa degli emigranti* 288
6.7 Monthly emigration from Naples, 1909–10 289
7.1 Cases of cholera among Italian immigrants at Ellis
   Island, 1911 319
7.2 Cholera carriers among Italian immigrants at Ellis Island, 1911 320
7.3 Cholera deaths in Naples, 1911 329
7.4 Summer mortality in Naples, 1908–11 330
7.5 Italian emigration to North and South America, 1910 339
7.6 Italian emigration to Argentina, 1910–13 343
7.7 Patient statistics: Cotugno Lazaretto, 3 May to 31 August 1911 357
A1 Male deaths from cholera classified by occupational group: Italy, 1884 372
A2 Deaths from cholera by province: Italy, 1884 373
A3 Deaths from gastro-enteritis in Naples, 1911 375
A4 Daily wages of farm workers in Italy, 1905 376
A5 Steerage fares from Naples to New York, 1905 11 376
A6 Deaths from cholera in Italy in 1911 377
A7 Reported deaths and bacteriologically confirmed deaths, Italy 1911 379
A8 Monthly departures of emigrants from Naples and Genoa, 1909 379

Preface

History is a collective enterprise, and one of my chief pleasures as an author is to express my appreciation to the many people who have contributed to this project. Professors Francesco Barbagallo and Paolo Frascani generously provided me with helpful advice on archives in Naples. Dr M. Soscia, Medical Director of the Cotugno Hospital, was a kind host, and he graciously assisted me in locating materials in the Hospital library and archive. The staffs at the National Library of Medicine at Bethesda, Maryland; the National Archives in Washington; the National Library at Naples; the Archive of the Bank of Naples; the State Archive at Naples; and the Sterling Library at Yale University provided endless and invaluable assistance in locating sources.

Colleagues at Royal Holloway, University of London and at Yale University have given helpful advice and support. Professors Henry Turner, Jr and John Harley Warner read the first draft of the manuscript, and made wise and valuable suggestions. The anonymous readers at Cambridge University Press offered helpful and informed criticism. Naturally, I alone am responsible for any errors that remain.

Research also requires financial support, and the Wellcome Trust made possible numerous field trips to Naples and to Washington, and enthusiastically encouraged my early research proposal. Sabbatical leave from Yale University and a grant from the Griswold Humanities Fund enabled me to bring the work to completion.

Most of all, however, I would like to express thanks to my wife, Judith. She was an inexhaustible source of enthusiasm, advice and humour. It is more than a rhetorical flourish to state that this book would not have appeared without her. The original idea for this project began in our discussions; she encouraged me to continue when I considered abandoning it after first learning of the wholesale wartime destruction of documents relating to the city of Naples in the Giolittian era; and she had the idea that material on the Neapolitan epidemic of 1911 must have survived in American archives.

Glossary of Italian and Neapolitan terms used in the text

ampliamento	expansion
asilo degli emigranti	quarantine station for emigrants
banchista	unofficial emigrant banker
basso (pl. *bassi)*	ground-floor slum dwelling
basso ceto	lower classes
caionzari	makers of catgut
carabiniere (pl. *carabinieri*)	military police
Casa degli emigranti	state-run emigrant hostel
colmate	landfills
colonna infame	column of infamny
comune	municipality
Consiglio superiore di sanità	Superior Health Council
dazio consumo	consumption levy
decimi di alea	builders' contingency fund
Direzione generale della sanità	Department of Public Health
duce	leader
fondaco (pl. *fondaci*)	slum tenement
gioco piccolo	underground lottery
giunta	executive committee of city hall
insipienza	stupidity
locanda	boarding house
locandiere	boarding-house proprietor
medico condotto	public health doctor
opere pie	Catholic benevolent associations
ottobrate	October harvest festival
padulano	market gardener
plebe	common people
popolino	lower classes
popolaglia	rabble
popolo minuto	lower classes

questore	chief of police
risanamento	urban renewal
scirocco	South-East wind
sevaioli	makers of tallow
sezione	borough of the city of Naples
signore	gentleman
squarciare	to rip out
stralci	cuts
sventramento	disembowelment
sventrare	to disembowel
untore	poisoner
vanella	skylight
vico	lane
zingaro	gypsy

Introduction

This book, perhaps like many works of history, began as much by accident as by design. The idea for it originated through research on an entirely unrelated topic – the violent political history of the anarcho-syndicalist movement among the farm workers of the South of Italy during the height of the Liberal regime between 1900 and the First World War. Field work for that purpose revealed frequent references to Asiatic cholera during the summer of 1910 and the social responses it provoked, which included riots, assaults on physicians, a xenophobic fury against gypsies, mass flight and the revival of religiosity and superstition. These events were intriguing and unexpected in a modern industrial state in the twentieth century.[1] Furthermore, it rapidly began to appear that the disease offered as illuminating a means of examining the structure of southern Italian society as the original political history on which I had embarked. My interest grew further with the realization that, despite the tumults that marked its passage, the epidemic had never been the subject of study by a modern historian, and was almost totally ignored in general histories of the period. The intention of writing a history of the epidemic of 1910 in Italy began to take firmer shape.

Recent writings on Asiatic cholera made the idea of a study of a twentieth-century epidemic still more appealing. There is an extensive international literature on cholera, with monographs on Britain, France, Spain, Germany, Canada, Russia, Sweden and the United States. But there is a serious imbalance in the field with an overwhelming emphasis on the dramatic first European experiences with the disease, and almost nothing at all on Italy. Only the study by Richard Evans of Hamburg in 1892 addresses the problem of the later epidemics in any of its aspects. Indeed, ignoring the Italian experience entirely, leading authorities argue that the last pandemic to affect Europe was the fifth in the 1880s and 1890s and that the sixth pandemic spared the industrial world entirely. My sense was that it was possible to fill a substantial gap by considering the sixth pandemic, which struck Italy even later – after the discoveries of Robert Koch and the germ theory of disease had unravelled the mysteries of the aetiology of cholera. In what ways was the later history of the disease different from the more familiar

1

experience of Europeans in the 1830s? Did the availability of adequate scientific explanations radically alter the nature of popular reactions and government policy?

My interest in the sixth pandemic grew with the discovery that unexpected reasons were partly responsible for the almost total amnesia into which the final significant episode of cholera in Italy has fallen. The disease ravaged the nation in 1911 as well as 1910, but the state succeeded to a very large extent in concealing the epidemic from its own citizens, from the larger international community, and from historians. At the initiative of the Prime Minister, Giovanni Giolitti, the Italian public health authorities systematically lied about the real sanitary condition of the kingdom; they censured the press and muzzled the medical profession; and they comprehensively violated the Paris Sanitary Convention to which Italy was a signatory. Here was a novel episode in the history of cholera which had no counterpart in the literature on other nations. The temptation to delay announcing the truth and to minimize the extent and intensity of an outbreak were commonplace, but there was no precedent for a policy of total secrecy as a comprehensive national policy for confronting an epidemic of cholera. What were the reasons for such a course? Were there sinister conclusions to be drawn about the nature of statecraft in an ostensibly Liberal regime? How was Giolitti so successful in such a venture?

After the decision to examine the epidemic of 1910 and 1911 in Italy, it proved natural to single out Naples because it stood at the centre of the events of those years. One of the most important seaports on the Continent with a reputation for fearful insalubrity, the great metropolis of the South had a pre-eminently important role in the history of cholera as the most frequently and seriously devastated of all Italian cities. Furthermore, in 1911, Naples was the key element in the conspiracy of silence. Although the city once again experienced the greatest mortality in the kingdom, the 'official' version of events has always been that Naples was entirely spared. To understand the disease and public policy towards it in the former capital was to go a long way toward unravelling the conspiracy and explaining the reasons for the strategy of secrecy.

Research in Naples revealed still more compelling reasons to justify a monograph on the modern Neapolitan experience of cholera, but in ways that altered the original chronology with which the project began. For a study of the impact of cholera on society, Naples formed a particularly important case study because the earlier epidemic of 1884 led to the renewal and rebuilding of the city in accordance with the dominant medical theory of the aetiology of the disease. Furthermore, the renewal project left a powerful legacy for the future course of political life in the city. Such vast sums were devoted to the scheme, such enormous expectations were aroused, and so many tens of thousands of people were forcibly evicted from their homes that the success of the venture in terms of making the city permanently immune to the disease after 1884 became a test of legitimacy for the governors of the city. When the disease reappeared in 1910, it threatened to undermine the authority of the ruling Catholic party and to catapult the opposition republicans and socialists into power. So explosive was the issue that it led to threats of an industrial lockout, a general strike and the erection of barricades in the city centre. It also played an important part in the downfall of the national government in the spring of 1911. Cholera remained at the centre of Neapolitan political life in a way that has not been considered elsewhere.

For this reason, the epidemic of 1910–11 could not be understood on its own. The reaction to the disease in the tumultuous course of the sixth pandemic depended absolutely on the events of the fifth, which affected Naples in 1884, and on the vicissitudes of renewal and rebuilding in the intervening years. The period 1884 to 1911 emerged as an indivisible whole in the epidemic history of Naples.

This point is worth stressing because of a major controversy in the field. Modern historians of Asiatic cholera have been torn between two conflicting poles with respect to the nature and status of their enterprise. On the one side there is the claim enunciated by Asa Briggs and Louis Chevalier. Two of the founding figures of the field over three decades ago, they took an expansive view of the capacity of epidemic diseases to provide a revealing shaft of light by means of which to explore the structure and workings of modern European society. No less than wars and revolutions, they argued, the sudden crises of cholera invasions laid bare hidden layers of popular belief and superstition, exposed living standards and housing conditions, demonstrated the nature of social and class relations, and clarified the priorities of statecraft. They therefore urged scholars to respond to the challenge of producing a comparative history of the five successive waves of the disease that afflicted the continent after 1830. With regard to the significance of Asiatic cholera, Briggs wrote that,

> Whenever it threatened European countries, it quickened social apprehensions. Wherever it appeared, it tested the efficiency and resilience of local administrative structures. It exposed relentlessly political, social and moral shortcomings. It prompted rumours, suspicions and at times violent social conflicts. It inspired not only sermons but novels and works of art. For all these reasons a study of the history of cholera is something far more than an exercise in medical epidemiology, fascinating in themselves though such exercises are; it is an important and neglected chapter in social history.[2]

And this call has found a fruitful response in the labours of historians, who in the following thirty years have produced a range of excellent monographs on the impact of Asiatic cholera on western societies.

The suggestion of Briggs, the example of Chevalier's work, and the research that they inspired, have not gone without challenge and re-examination from an opposing perspective on the capacity of the subject to provide illumination. Charles Rosenberg, one of the earliest scholars to enter the discipline and the historian of cholera in the United States, concluded as early as the 1960s that the disease had limited lasting impact.[3] More recently, Margaret Pelling has argued that the attention lavished on the dramatic emergencies of cholera has been misplaced, with distorting effect on the understanding of nineteenth-century society. Epidemic cholera was an exotic disease imported from outside that caused sporadic and unrepresentative crises and left little permanent trace. In her view, the proper task of the historian is to examine conditions that are long-term and typical of the society. For the medical historian of industrializing Europe, the important task, Pelling reasons, is to examine the 'fevers' – chronic maladies that were the everyday, enduring concerns of society and of the medical profession.[4] The medical impact of cholera, she argues, has been exaggerated because of the high drama that accompanied epidemic invasions and the extensive records they left in their wake. As she explains with specific reference to Britain,

> As a cause of death and debility in mid-nineteenth-century England, cholera was surpassed among epidemic diseases by 'common continued fever' (chiefly typhoid, relapsing fever, and some typhus), scarlet fever, smallpox, and measles, and accounted for only a very small proportion of the area of highest mortality, which occurred among infants and young children. All the known epidemic diseases were exceeded in incidence and effect by the many forms of tuberculosis ... Cholera has, however, attracted some of the kind of attention from historians that other diseases, excepting plague, have conspicuously lacked. There are many reasons for this: the shock value of cholera, abundantly recorded at the times of its appearance; its coincidence with other dramatic and disturbing forces, particularly the social and the political; its assumed relation to innovation in institutional and administrative structures; the comparative superiority of the records of its appearances; and the abundance of its literature.[5]

In Pelling's opinion, a more balanced and revisionist assessment is in order.

Naples is an ideal case with which to test these opposing positions and to place the debate in a different perspective. The epidemics of 1884 and 1910–11 confirm the insight of Briggs and Chevalier that the sudden emergencies of Asiatic cholera provide valuable opportunities to explore the texture of life in a community. The emergency of 1884 in particular produced a great outpouring of reports by doctors, officials and journalists on all aspects of housing, diet, wages and illness. These sources provide a highly informative and telling means of exploring living conditions in Liberal Italy. More than material circumstances alone, however, the vast literature on the cholera epidemic of 1884 – and the events that literature describes – documents the attitudes of contemporaries. The epidemic demonstrates the distrust between doctors and patients, class and social tensions, the divergence of popular and official religion, the relations between municipal officials and the people they governed, the sense of injustice felt by broad swathes of public opinion in Naples at the inequality they suffered as southerners. The emergency inspired a great flood of reflections on the disaster that overwhelmed the city. Since both conditions and mentalities were lasting phenomena embedded in the physical structures and social relationships of the city, they were essential aspects of Neapolitan life, and not, as Pelling and Rosenberg imply, atypical ephemera. Cholera was one of the great enduring preoccupations of the city and its governors.

But the chief interest of Naples for the debate between Briggs and Pelling is a different one. The epidemic of 1884 was a major transformative event in the history of the city with consequences that helped to shape and define the whole period to the end of the Giolittian era and beyond. Cholera crystallized the political and cultural current known as the 'Southern Question' and the 'Problem of Naples', producing a clear and fully articulated perception that the travails of the city were not a misfortune but a social injustice due to the policies of the Liberal state and its neglect of the South and its leading city. It also inaugurated the renewal of the city and created the expectation of effective and decisive action to prevent a recurrence, placing public health at the centre of political life in the city. In addition, through the renewal scheme, cholera initiated the practice of major public-works schemes as a means of overcoming the disabilities of the South, tapping a rich vein of clientage and patronage in the Mezzogiorno that has continued down to the era of Tangentopoli. Finally, the disease marked a major stage in the emergence of the medical profession as a powerful interest in the inner councils of municipal politics. The intention of this book is to examine the proposition that in all of these respects Naples makes a significant case study in the social, political and medical impact of the most dreaded disease of the nineteenth century.

The work that follows is divided into four parts. Part I is an analysis of the vulnerability of Naples to epidemic cholera. Here the important issue of the proper use of hindsight in medical history arises. Since an essential purpose of the discussion is to explain the devastating outbreak of 1884, it would be antiquarian not to make use of the greatly extended understanding of the mechanisms of the disease that epidemiologists and historians have acquired during the intervening century. To neglect these insights would be to fail to explain the events that followed. Nevertheless, it should be made explicit that the intention of Chapter 1 is not to indict a nineteenth-century city for not possessing twentieth-century hygienic understanding. More interesting is the fact that Neapolitans on the eve of the fifth pandemic were strikingly aware of the danger to which the city was exposed. Chapter 1, therefore, is also an exploration of a deeply rooted contemporary anxiety and of the reasons that the authorities responsible for public health failed to take remedial action within the context of the medical knowledge available to them.

Part II, consisting of Chapters 2 to 4, is an examination of the epidemic of 1884. It begins in Chapter 2 with a consideration of the arrival of cholera in Europe at Toulon and Marseilles in June; the desperate attempt of the Italian authorities, who had long neglected sanitary reform, to keep the disease from reaching Italy by resorting to military means of public health in the form of lazarettos, quarantine and sanitary cordons; and the transmission of cholera to Naples by returning emigrants escaping Provence. Chapter 3 explores the epidemic itself, concentrating on such themes as the anti-cholera campaign of the municipal authorities; the popular response to the disease in the form of mass flight, a poisoning hysteria, concealment, an outburst of religious fervour and violent riots; and the therapeutic strategies of the medical profession. Part II then concludes in Chapter 4 with an examination of the mechanisms that enabled the population and the authorities to cope with so overwhelming a disaster.

Since the campaign against cholera was conceived by contemporaries in terms of the military metaphors of battle, Part III deals with what might be termed the 'inter-war years' between the invasion of 1884 and the return of the enemy in 1910. These years were dominated by the attempt, through a vast programme of renewal and rebuilding, to construct an impregnable line of sanitary defences. This period also marked the emergence of the medical profession as a powerful force in the life of the city.

Part IV analyses the return of cholera in 1910–11. The importance of this early twentieth-century epidemic, however, was very different from that of 1884. By 1910 the relations between patients and doctors had changed; the sanitary policy of the state had fundamentally altered; and the scale of the autumn outbreak was severely limited in scale. It would be idle, therefore, to expect the outburst to have produced a literature or a popular response commensurate with that of the disaster of 1884. The interest of 1910 and of Chapter 6 lies in the challenge that the return of the disease posed to the rule of the dominant party in Neapolitan politics, to the economic interests of the city, and to the rule of the weak ministry of Luigi Luzzatti. So severe were the economic and political consequences of cholera in 1910 that in the following year Luzzatti's successor, Giovanni Giolitti, opted for a policy of total concealment. Chapter 6 attempts, first, to establish that a major epidemic did in fact occur, and then to explain the success of the state in keeping it secret. Chapter 7 explores the conspiracy of silence.

For the historian of the last major cholera epidemic in Neapolitan history, the available sources pose severe problems that merit explicit recognition. Part of the difficulty was the direct result of the state's policy of concealment. Inevitably, the effect of such a strategy was that the epidemic was virtually never discussed or even mentioned in the press, in parliamentary debates, in the patient records of the city's hospital for infectious diseases, in the cemetery register, in the proceedings of the city council and its executive committee, or in municipal or government reports. Official statistics for these months, moreover, were systematically falsified to support the public posture ordered by the Prime Minister. Chance greatly compounded the already serious problem of sources. In normal circumstances, the policy of suppressing a major medical emergency in the largest city in the kingdom would have left a substantial record in the secret archives of the city and the prefecture. Unfortunately, these archives, deposited for safekeeping outside Naples during the Second World War, were destroyed by fire by retreating German soldiers. It is impossible, therefore, to reconstruct the events of 1911 in the same manner and detail that is possible for the nineteenth century because critical sources were either intentionally silenced at the time or subsequently destroyed by misadventure. To demonstrate the nature and extent of the disease, I have relied instead on the archive of the United States Public Health and Marine Hospital Service. Because of the mass emigration of Italians to the United States from the port of Naples, the American authorities kept a vigilant watch on sanitary conditions in the city, and their reports constitute the most important means of demonstrating the scale and importance of the epidemic. Against that background, the silences in municipal and national records in Naples acquire a new eloquence as a vast record of the systematic nature of the cover-up ordered by the Prime Minister and of its overwhelming success.

The Conclusion returns to the challenge posed by the debate between Briggs and Pelling as seen from the vantage point of modern Naples. What lessons did the final major cholera epidemics in its history provide concerning Italian society and the Liberal regime? In what ways does the epidemic experience of a single city illuminate larger themes in the political history of modern Italy?

PART I

Sanitary anxieties

1

A city at risk

With a population of nearly half a million people occupying an area of 8 square kilometers, Naples in 1884 was the largest city in Italy.[1] A great Mediterranean seaport famous for evil smells and foul water, it provided perfect conditions for an epidemic of Asiatic cholera. So well known were the pernicious effects of even a visit to the city that in the final decades of the nineteenth century the Neapolitan economy suffered severely as frightened tourists avoided Naples entirely or made fleeting visits to the ancient sights, where they drank only wine and covered their noses.[2] The press, complained Alderman Vincenzo Pizzuti in 1873, 'writes of us as if we were semi-barbarian Africans'.[3]

The city faced south onto the Bay of Naples, stretching for three miles in an arc along the coast. To the traveller arriving by sea, Naples rose above the harbour in the shape of an amphitheatre. The Lower City, built on land reclaimed from the Mediterranean, formed the stage. It was enclosed to the north and west by a semicircle of hills; to the east by swamps; and to the south by the waters of the Bay. The stage was divided into two unequal crescents by the spur of the Pizzofalcone hill. To the west stood the small and salubrious neighbourhood of Chiaia; to the east, the teeming slums of the Old City. The slopes of the encircling hills were graced by the elegant homes of the Upper City.

The medical histories of Upper and Lower Naples were sharply divergent, and it was common for local doctors to write of the great metropolis as consisting of two separate cities. Epidemic diseases primarily afflicted the Lower City. Lower Naples encompassed four of the twelve administrative boroughs or *sezioni* of the city – Mercato, Pendino, Porto and Vicaria – as well as portions of the adjacent *sezioni* of San Giuseppe and San Lorenzo. Lying at an average altitude of 4.09 metres above sea-level, the Lower City occupied an area of 511,873 square metres bounded by the Via della Marina to the south, the Corso Garibaldi to the east, and the Via Medina to the north and west. Here in the heart of the Old City stood 4,567 buildings housing approximately 300,000 people and intersected by a dense maze of 598 streets. The only broad thoroughfare was the Via del Duomo at its centre, and the only large open space was the Piazza del Mercato.[4]

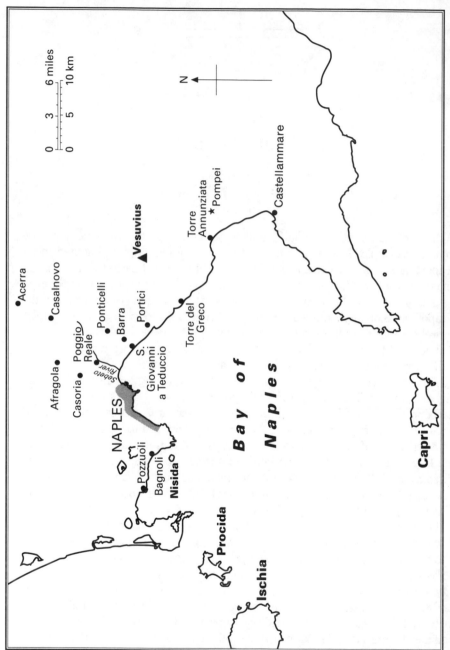

Map 1.1   The Bay of Naples

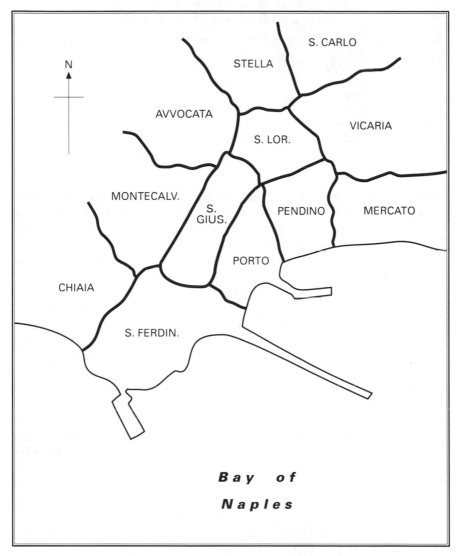

Map 1.2 The *sezioni* of Naples

Mortality figures for the five years 1878–83 establish both the insalubrity of the city as a whole and the medical primacy of Old Naples in particular. Neapolitan officials, of course, had their own polemical agenda in publishing such information. The gloomy sanitary statistics of the city were an important means of justifying the public-works programmes that were the chief emphasis of the administrations led by Mayors San Donato, Girolamo Giusso and Nicola Amore. Medicine was a means to legitimate mayoral campaign promises, fiscal

Sanitary anxieties

Table 1.1. *European capital cities: average annual
deaths per 1,000 inhabitants, 1878–83*

Vienna	20.6
Brussels	23.1
London	23.2
Paris	24.6
Athens	24.7
Berlin	29.7
Naples	31.8

decisions and patronage. Even after due allowance is made for the political purposes for which statistics were kept, however, the rate of death for the city as a whole – 31.84 deaths for every 1,000 inhabitants – was indisputably high by the international standards of the time. The metropolis of the former Kingdom of the Two Sicilies compared unfavourably with the major capital cities of western Europe as Table 1.1 demonstrates.[5]

The reputation of the city for infection and death even produced a 'demographic panic' among its informed residents analogous to the more famous anxiety in *fin de siècle* France. The population of France in the closing decades of the nineteenth century lagged behind the upward surge in the major nations of western Europe, giving rise to fears of racial degeneration and national decline.[6]

So too demography was a source of concern among Neapolitans. The population of the ex-capital multiplied far more slowly than that of other major cities in the kingdom. In the forty years after unification, the population of Naples increased by only 26 per cent while other Italian cities expanded at double, triple and even quadruple that rate. Turin grew 63 per cent in the same period from 205,000 inhabitants to 336,000, and Milan 103 per cent from 242,000 to 491,000.[7] For many Neapolitans, the explanation for the relative decline of their city was simple. They conceived of Naples as a great mortuary. Therefore, argued Councillor Salvatore Trinchese in 1890, public health was the great issue that would determine the life or death of the city.[8] Francesco Saverio Nitti, the most authoritative of all observers of Neapolitan conditions, concluded that the former capital 'lay dying on the shores of the Tyrrhenean Sea'.[9]

The endemic maladies that caused the gravest apprehension were the 'fevers' – 'miasmatic', 'pernicious', 'typhoidal' and 'petecchial', according to the medical terminology of the day.[10] Scurvy, rickets, syphilis, tuberculosis and anaemia were rife.[11] Physicians were also perplexed by a new illness peculiar to the city. Defying diagnosis, the malady was deemed to have originated in the sewers and polluted subsoil of the southern metropolis. This newly recognized disease caused Naples to be shunned by outsiders, and it came to be known as the 'Naples fever'.[12] So serious was the morbidity of these various threats to public health that the city council resolved on several occasions that all discussion of them be conducted in secret in order not to spread alarm.[13] In 1876 Mayor Gennaro Di San Donato applied this policy of censure, interrupting a discussion of epidemic disease and rebuking the speaker for his 'regrettable analysis' that would only cause rumours to spread.[14]

The depth of the anxiety surrounding public health can be readily appreciated by recalling the epidemic history of the city. In the half century ending in 1885, Naples had experienced twelve epidemics, four of typhoid and eight of cholera. These two diseases had caused the loss of 48,000 lives, of whom 42,000 were attributed to cholera alone.[15] These official estimates, moreover, are probably too low, given the desire of the authorities to minimize public awareness of the extent of the health problem. For good reason, then, Mark Twain, during a hurried visit in 1867, worried deeply about the meaning of the tourist's cliché, 'See Naples and die'. His conclusion was not entirely reassuring: 'I do not know that one would necessarily die after merely seeing it, but to attempt to live there might turn out a little differently.'[16] Such fear was shared by Eugenio Fazio, Professor of Hygiene at the University of Naples. In a curious but telling image, he described his native city as 'a living cemetery'.[17]

Aggregate mortality figures, however, mask a systematic pattern of inequality between the Upper City and the Lower. During the 'normal' quinquennium 1878–83 when the metropolis was free of epidemic diseases, the mortality rates for the four boroughs of the Lower City were all above the average for the city (see Table 1.2). By contrast, wealthy San Ferdinando established the municipal record with a low of 21.8 deaths per thousand, closely followed by the other privileged *sezioni*, where rates of death well below 30 per 1,000 were the norm.[18]

If one moves from general mortality to the specific issue of death by cholera, a similar pattern emerges. With seven epidemics of Asiatic cholera before 1884, Naples was one of the most frequently and severely stricken cities in Europe. The record of cholera in the 'City of the Sirens' prior to 1884 is shown in Table 1.3.[19] Comparative rates of death from cholera show a striking divergence in fortune between the Upper and Lower Cities. In every outbreak in Naples there was a frightful overrepresentation of the inhabitants of the boroughs of Mercato, Pendino, Porto, and Vicaria among the dead, as Chapters 3, 4, 6 and 7 demonstrate for the last two major epidemics of Asiatic cholera to strike the city – those of 1884 and 1910-11. The Naples Deputy Rocco De Zerbi stressed this point in a speech to parliament in 1884. In each outburst, De Zerbi explained, the disease had concentrated its fury in what he designated the 'deadly zone' of the Lower City. In 1837, for example, the aggregate rate of death from cholera was eight for every thousand inhabitants of the city. Pendino, Mercato and Porto, however, suffered rates of 17.7, 18.9 and 30.6 respectively. An identical pattern recurred in 1854, 1865–66 and 1873.[20] Unlike such diseases as tuberculosis, influenza and smallpox that strike at all social classes without distinction, cholera exhibited a strong preference for the poor.

Cholera does not strike its victims at random. It is spread in only one way – the

Table 1.2. *Naples: annual deaths per 1,000 inhabitants, 1878–83*

Porto	33.7
Pendino	33.3
Mercato	32.9
Vicaria	32.0

Table 1.3. *Cholera in Naples, 1836–73*

Year	Population of Naples	Duration (in Days)	Deaths	% to die of Cholera
1836	437,563	91	5,963	1.36
1837	432,720	154	11,714	2.71
1854	442,505	71	9,600	2.17
1855	434,050	107	1,300	0.31
1865	444,880	70	2,200	0.49
1866	442,804	85	3,470	0.78
1873	457,530	116	1,280	0.28

ingestion of food and water contaminated by human excrement. With such a particular means of propagation, cholera is an infallible indicator of destitution and squalor, of overcrowded dwellings and sanitary neglect, of defective sewers and unwashed hands, of suspect produce and recycled clothing. Even if swallowed, the bacillus that causes the disease – the *Vibrio cholerae* – is usually killed by the digestive processes of a healthy and well-nourished person. The vibrio succumbs rapidly to the acidic gastric juices of a robust stomach.

A deficient or defective diet, however, allows the cholera germ to breach the defensive ramparts of the body. Malnutrition, gastro-intestinal illness, alcohol, and unripe or over-ripe fruit upset the normal acidity of the stomach, rendering the subject vulnerable to infection. Similarly, indigestion resulting from dietary excesses or unsuitable food allows the germ a safe passage through the stomach by reducing the time of digestion and allowing the vibrio to shelter in a protecting mass of undigested matter. Cholera, therefore, selects its victims disproportionately among the poor, the under-nourished, and the ill.

In all of these respects, the Lower City of Naples proved a gracious host to the disease. Cholera is a disease of the gut, and the impoverished boroughs of the Old City were – in the celebrated phrase of the writer Matilde Serao – the 'bowels of Naples'.[21] It is important, therefore, to examine the specific conditions of the Lower City that predisposed it to infection when cholera approached in 1884. Of particular concern are six high-risk factors that exposed the population to danger – housing, sanitation, the water supply, sewage, poverty and public health. Each must be examined in turn.

HOUSING

An ancient city hemmed in on all sides by hills, marsh and sea, Lower Naples had no space for expansion. By the nineteenth century its population had far out-grown its narrow confines, so that its most striking characteristic was a fearful overcrowding. A first indication of the press of people is the sheer size of the population of Naples in comparison with other Italian cities. The ten largest cities in Italy in June 1884 are shown in Table 1.4.[22]

Overpopulation was a precondition for many of the problems of the city. Size, however, combined with a long history of *laissez-faire*. Modern Naples suffered all the consequences of unregulated and unplanned urbanization. With no housing or sanitary code and no municipal plan, buildings sprang up and extended upwards in a total anarchy of stone. Gardens, parks and green spaces had vanished long ago in a furious building mania. Mercato, Pendino, Porto and Vicaria were configured as a labyrinth of alleys on either side of which towered giant tenements built around cramped, airless courtyards. Some were in such an advanced state of disrepair that they resembled heaps of broken masonry. Buildings of four to eight storeys nearly touched at their summits, casting a perpetual shadow over the winding, unpaved passageways at their base. These dark lanes were sometimes so narrow that three people walking abreast could barely make their way and no vehicle could pass. A typical example was the Vico Fico in the borough of Mercato. Permanently festooned with drying linen that dripped on pedestrians below, it measured 50 metres in length and 3 in breadth, with buildings 30 metres tall.[23] Even in mid-summer mud and moisture were omnipresent, and an evil black stream wound its way slowly down the centre of a lane that no official of the city ever visited.

Here on the sea-level plain had been erected the most shocking city of nineteenth-century Europe – a city of such height that Mark Twain wrote that it resembled three American cities superimposed one on top of another. 'If there is an eighth wonder in the world,' he noted, 'it must be the dwelling-houses of Naples. I honestly believe a good majority of them are a hundred feet high!'[24] But the living conditions within were still more dramatic than their striking external appearance. The slums of Naples, commented the *British Medical Journal*, were the worst in Europe. According to the journal's correspondent, the nearest comparison could be found only in the worst slums of Cairo. 'Barbarous', 'squalid' and 'obscene' were the epithets he reserved for the place.[25] Reaching a similar conclusion, the French Consul Marcellin Pellet argued that the frightful slums of Paris described by Victor Hugo, Eugène Sue and Emile Zola paled before the gruesome reality of contemporary Lower Naples.[26] The Manchester known to Friedrich Engels and the East End of London portrayed by Charles Dickens and Henry Mayhew were far less menacing. Such were the results of 'incredible negligence'.[27]

A population greater than that of Milan and Venice combined lived in a crush that the city council described as 'incredible, greater than that of any other city in the world!'[28] Every street, alley and courtyard struck Mark Twain as resembling

Table 1.4. *Population of the ten largest Italian cities, 1884*

City	Population
Naples	496,499
Milan	324,193
Rome	301,188
Turin	252,832
Palermo	252,033
Genoa	181,075
Florence	168,167
Venice	134,658
Messina	130,367
Bologna	122,488

Table 1.5. *Naples: population per square kilometer, 1884*

City or Borough	Population
London	13,000
Rome	28,000
Paris	29,000
Turin	34,000
Naples	64,000
Naples: *sezioni* of Porto, Pendino and Mercato	130,000

the bustle of Broadway in New York City. At every turn the impression was the same – 'swarms', 'throngs', 'masses' and 'multitudes'.[29] The French visitor Ameury Duval pictured the city as a 'human anthill' that, by comparison, made Paris and London seem like desert landscapes.[30] Confirming these impressions, a survey of 1883 comparing Naples and its three most populous boroughs with other European cities revealed the densities per square kilometer shown in Table 1.5.[31]

In the Lower City the total urban space available per person was less than eight square metres – a figure which compared, at the other extreme among European capitals, with 344 square metres in London.[32] Such was the prodigious demand for space in Lower Naples that the population squeezed into vertical rookeries at the rate of seven or eight people, often of more than one family, in a single windowless room that served at once as kitchen, sittingroom, bedroom and latrine. For many, the same room doubled by day as a workshop and by night as a store-room. In time of illness, it also served as the sick-room. In the Vico Fico the average size of a room occupied by seven people was five square metres with ceilings so low that they seemed about to crush the inhabitants. A double mattress where five people slept occupied half of the space in these lairs, leaving just enough room for a single straw mattress for the remaining two tenants.[33]

The savage overcrowding of the Vico Fico, however, was not extreme by Neapolitan standards. Frequently in the Lower City, Mayor Nicola Amore reported, there was less than half a square metre of floor space per inhabitant.[34] These dismal dwellings were universally described as 'animal dens', 'pigsties', 'caves' and 'rabbit warrens' – terms that were all the more appropriate because the occupants commonly shared their room with the hens and chickens that helped to provide their subsistence.

Accommodation of any sort was desperately sought. Such was the limitless supply of humanity to be housed in the Old City that buildings could be let in a state of total disrepair. The unplastered walls were crumbling with age, blackened with filth and encrusted with mould. Dark streaks of damp were just visible in the half-light. Since there was no plumbing, the inhabitants disposed of household waste by throwing it onto the stairway, into the courtyard, onto the alley below. The stagnant air was nauseating with the stench of rotting organic waste; the streets swarmed with flies; and every dwelling was infested with armies of rats, vermin and 'all the bloodsucking insects known to man'.[35] Describing the Via Funneco Verde in the borough of Porto – a lane so foul that it filled passers-by with nausea – the poet Salvatore Di Giacomo wrote, 'This is not a street at all, but a cockroach-run.'[36]

Most notorious of all were the dwellings known as *fondaci*, which transformed their tenants into urban troglodytes. They were built like the inside of a dovecote: tiers of one-room caves rose above a tiny, damp courtyard that was shrouded even at noon in semi-darkness. Examining the health of the city in 1910, a correspondent of the local paper, *Il Mattino*, visited the *fondaci* of the Vico Guardia in the borough of Mercato. Here he found conditions that had not changed, he wrote, in a hundred years. The rooms measured three metres by one and a half and were 'unworthy of a civilized nation'.[37] In these hovels the most frightful abodes of all were the tiny, irregularly shaped lairs boxed in beneath the flights of stairs. In all respects the *fondaci* were synonymous with the final depths of human misery, and were referred to by contemporaries in Dantean terms as 'the pits of hell'.[38] The Swedish doctor Axel Munthe, who visited a number of these pits as a volunteer during the 1884 epidemic, described them as 'the most ghastly human habitations on the face of the earth'.[39]

The London *Times* published a description of a representative *fondaco* that went a considerable way to justifying Munthe's hyperbole. The article urged:

Imagine the doorway of a cave where on entering you must descend. Not a ray of light penetrates into it except by the one aperture you have passed through; and there, between four black battered walls and upon a layer of filth mixed with putrid straw, two, three, and four families vegetate together. The best side of the cave, namely that through which humidity filtrates the least, is occupied by a rack and manger to which animals of various kinds are tied; a horse it may be or an ass, a calf, or a pig. On the opposite, a heap of boards and rags represents the beds. In one corner is the fireplace and the household utensils lie about the floor. This atrocious scene is animated by a swarm of half-naked dishevelled women; of children entirely naked rolling about in the dirt, and of men stretched on the ground in the sleep of idiocy. Such is a Neapolitan *Fondacho* [*sic*]. Multiply it by thousands. Remember that a hundred thousand beings at least have no other shelter; that they only live on fruit and vegetables, on snails and onions; without even changing their rags once in a year; without water except such as flows in a dense impure rivulet winding through those lanes.[40]

Fondaci were justly notorious. In 1884 they housed a population that was estimated to number between 30,000 and 90,000 inhabitants.[41] The wide margin of error allowed by City Hall in compiling its estimate is itself a measure of the prevailing neglect. But the full horror of the Lower City was the condition of the apartments located at ground level and known as *bassi*. The *bassi* were hardly more salubrious than the more infamous *fondaci*. Here, sleeping on straw mattresses on mud floors, two families normally shared one room of an average size of seventy to eighty cubic metres.[42] A population as large as the city of Bologna lived in such accommodation. The *bassi* housed the overwhelming majority of the Neapolitan poor in a social condition that, in the words of the American Consul, 'defies belief'.[43] 'The word "home",' he continued, 'as understood in the US and Germany and England is unknown here ... With the Neapolitan working man and woman life is a perpetual struggle for existence.'[44]

The residents of the *bassi* in the Largo S. Erasmo ai Granili in the *sezione* Mercato described themselves as 'forced to live on the actual inside of a sewer'. 'The houses', they explained,

> lack a proper sewer main. There is only a simple cesspit that acts as the receptacle for the filth from the various soil-pipes about. When the pit itself is full, it overflows, flooding the courtyard, and it becomes necessary to wade through that disgusting slime in order to enter one's home, and all through the stubborn neglect of the landlord. The putrid exhalations are the cause of many fevers.
>
> And what can one say of the water? The well is surrounded by soil-pipes that leak and make the water revolting and full of insects – to the point that it becomes impossible to use even for the washing of clothes.[45]

In addition to the *bassi* and *fondaci*, which provided permanent abodes, there was the problem of the large transient population of the city. This broad swathe of humanity was predominantly male, impoverished and illiterate. It included the elderly, emigrants awaiting departure, bricklayers, street pedlars, vagrants and new arrivals seeking employment – people who could not name the Prime Minister of their country and who were uncertain of their age and of the identity of their father.

Most numerous in their midst were the quasi-nomadic builders who lived in villages and small towns in the Neapolitan hinterland where the cost of living was lower. They returned to their homes on Saturday, but stayed in Naples during the week.[46] The chronic super-abundance of labour in the city drove their wages down and crippled the development of labour organizations and strikes.

The unhappy result was that a thirteen-hour workday – the norm in the trade – was barely sufficient to provide a subsistence living for a man and his family. A Neapolitan bricklayer, rough carpenter, house painter or stone mason could expect to spend three-quarters of his income on food alone – despite a diet consisting of bread, macaroni, bean soup, fruit and vegetables.[47] Wages were abysmally low in relation to the cost of living in a major metropolitan centre. Expressed in 1884 US dollars, the daily pay for unskilled, heavy manual labour in the building trades ranged in 1884 from $0.29 to $0.39. A day of labour hewing stone or painting walls from sunrise to sunset was insufficient to purchase a kilo of meat, which cost from $0.44 to $0.50. Ten days were required to meet the monthly rent of $3 or more for a single room in the most squalid Neapolitan tenement.[48]

Such earnings, in any event, were notional because of the permanent insecurity of employment in the construction trade. If inclement weather, a shortage of materials, saints' day observances or the financial embarrassment of a contractor stopped work, the labourers were dismissed instantly and without compensation for the hours lost. On average, a bricklayer or mason worked only 270 days a year. Wages, moreover, were commonly paid in arrears. To meet current expenses, therefore, the worker was dependent on obtaining credit at exorbitant rates. The engineer Alfredo Minozzi explained,

> The woodworm gnawing at the workers' budget is usury, which reaches incredible rates of interest. For instance, a labourer seeking a loan of ten lire to purchase flour does not receive the money in cash. What he gets instead is an advance of so many kilos of flour at a cost above the market value, and with the obligation to repay the creditor one lira a week for each of the following fifteen weeks – that is, 50% interest in three months, and with no deductions.[49]

Thus driven by low pay, debt, uncertain prospects, and the aspiration to return with savings to their villages, the builders sought temporary accommodation on the cheap in Naples. They found it in the *locande* in the vicinity of the harbour in the borough of Porto, in streets like the via del Lavinaio. Here they paid from 2 to 4 lire a night for a mattress in a room that they shared with assorted other 'bohemians of labour' who lived rough in the former capital.[50]

The institutions where they resided played an important and unhappy part in the medical and social history of Naples. The *locande* were located in buildings indistinguishable from the surrounding tenements except that the landlords had transformed the flats into workers' dormitories where impecunious men slept nine or ten to a room. In these dreary and unregulated barracks all the worst sanitary features of the Lower City were reproduced – overcrowding, vermin, lack of light and ventilation, the absence of water and lavatories. The medical consequences of the Neapolitan *locande* fit a more general European pattern. Already in 1855 the London physician and epidemiologist John Snow observed of the first cholera pandemic in Britain that unregulated 'common lodging-houses, in which several families were crowded into a single room' played a strategic role in the introduction and spread of the disease in urban centres throughout the kingdom.[51] In a recent study of the same epidemic, Michael Durey confirms this observation by pointing to the heavy mortality from cholera among the 'wandering tribes' of vagrants, huxters, showmen and wayfarers, who were the principal denizens of these squalid institutions.[52] In Britain, an Act of Parliament successfully regulated the sanitary conditions in boarding-houses after the first epidemic of cholera, and prevented their playing the same role in later outbreaks.[53]

In Naples, however, *laissez-faire* continued until the twentieth century in the matter of the *locande*, despite their notorious insalubrity. These sordid hostels were already known, for instance, for their major role in the spread of typhoid.[54] The particular contribution of the boarding-houses to the history of cholera was that they provided an ideal means for the disease to gain entry to the city. In the epidemics both of 1884 and of 1910–11, cholera arrived in Naples with emigrants who slept in the lodging-houses of Porto until their departure. Once admitted with the travellers to the hospitable environment of the lodging-houses, cholera claimed its first victims among the builders who shared the emigrants' rooms. The disease then journeyed with their slops and their dejecta to the unprotected water-tanks and wells of the neighbourhood on the way to becoming a widespread epidemic. In his account of the devastation of 1884, Vincenzo Pagano paid particular attention to the *locande*. In time of epidemics, he argued,

> The borough of Porto is the first to suffer because it is more exposed than any other neighbourhood in the city to imported diseases as a result of its traffic with the sea. In this borough are located countless boarding-houses which are the gathering places by night of the most unhappy people of the lowest social classes.[55]

The mechanisms involved in the establishment first of a localized neighbourhood outbreak and then of a general city-wide epidemic are best understood in terms of a common nineteenth-century distinction between two levels of Asiatic cholera – 'sporadic' and 'epidemic'.[56] What the distinction highlighted was not the presence of two separate diseases, but the same disease propagated in two different manners. 'Epidemic' cholera was a violent and seemingly arbitrary explosion of unrelated cases throughout a city, and it depended upon the general contamination of the municipal water supply. Once the vibrio had reached the river, reservoirs and wells of a city, it struck victims on a grand scale throughout the urban area, claiming lives that had no relationship with one another.

Water-borne epidemics were so devastating that they obscured the presence of slower, more limited means of transmission. The disease commonly spread, however, along chains of person-to-person communication. An outburst of this sort was known to contemporaries as 'sporadic' cholera because it manifested itself in clusters of victims concentrated in restricted areas – a neighbourhood, a particular street, even a single dwelling-house. A 'sporadic' outbreak could exist alongside a more general epidemic, unnoticed in the midst of the larger disaster. It could also unfold as a limited flare-up of cases separated entirely in time and space from a broader and more violent spread of disease. In 1884 and 1910, the appearance of 'sporadic' cholera in the borough of Porto marked the prologue to catastrophe.

'Sporadic' cholera thrived on the overcrowded conditions that were so widespread in Lower Naples. When a single room served at once as sick-room, kitchen, living-room and bedroom for seven to ten people, there were multiple opportunities for the disease to spread from the first victim to those who shared his accommodation. John Snow, who first unravelled the complex aetiology of cholera, explained in reference to London that,

> The bed linen nearly always becomes wetted by the cholera evacuations, and as these are devoid of the usual colour and odour, the hands of persons waiting on the patient become soiled without their knowing it; and unless these persons are scrupulously cleanly in their habits, and wash their hands before taking food, they must accidentally swallow some of the excretion, and leave some on the food they handle or prepare, which has to be eaten by the rest of the family, who, amongst the working classes, often have to take their meals in the sick room: hence the thousands of instances in which, amongst this class of the population, a case of cholera in one member of the family is followed by other cases[57]

The sick-room frequently served as a store-room for the provisions of a family or the wares of a street vendor, and in such cases it was difficult to ensure that the copious, clear evacuations of the patient never reached the produce. Buckets used to fetch water, wash utensils and store goods were also imperilled, especially since they could serve multiple other functions involved in attendance upon the sick. The dangers were compounded by the absence of light, which rendered the contaminating 'rice-water stools' virtually invisible. In such circumstances, first the *locande* and then the surrounding *bassi* and *fondaci* of the Lower City experienced long chains of person-to-person infection that struck down handfuls of victims until a more general explosion occurred when the bacilli reached the municipal supplies of water.

SANITATION

The condition of the streets themselves was a significant additional factor in undermining health. As cholera approached in 1884, the Old City was in imminent danger of choking on its own refuse. In this metropolis without plumbing the walls of the buildings functioned as public urinals and the streets served as cesspools. Some of the accumulating filth was also of animal origin. Many of the ground-floor entrances on every lane opened onto stables for the horses and donkeys of carters and coachmen, and onto sheds for the cows that provided 'filth, stench and poor milk'.[58] More widely scattered throughout the buildings in every neighbourhood were smaller animals on whom people depended for their livelihood – sheep, goats, dogs, and poultry. In the slums of Naples the distinction between urban and rural was blurred. Traditional rural occupations persisted in the centre of the greatest Italian city. Numerous goatherds, shepherds and drovers plied their trades, and their citified beasts added both their dung and their carcasses to the general filth.

Various crafts also generated noxious byproducts that propagated disease. Butchers and fishmongers emptied their slops into gullies that already stank. The *caionzari* and *sevaioli*, the makers of catgut and tallow – two important Neapolitan products – disposed of great quantities of offal and animal fat from the slaughter-houses. Their notoriously filthy workshops were the source of 'mephitic effluvia' and 'putrid drippings' that poured into the streets.[59] The owners of vegetable stalls and the street fryers of pizza all left their mark. Ragpickers, employed in one of the busiest trades of the Lower City, recycled vast heaps of used clothing that proved lethal in time of cholera.

The laundry business caused special concern to public health officials. Prosperous residents of the Upper City entrusted their clothes to washerwomen from neighbouring communes. They descended upon the metropolis in large numbers on fixed days of the week, removed the dirty linen to the countryside for cleaning, and then returned it the following week. Here was a certain means of conveying disease to the surrounding countryside. Even the cleansing practices of the poor gave rise to serious dangers. Residents of the Lower City normally did their own laundry. Since, however, there were no laundering facilities in private homes, and since the municipality provided no public wash-houses, the normal practice was to do the washing at wells located in courtyards and in the city streets. All too often linen from the sick-room, sometimes pilfered by residents who sought to profit from the misfortunes of their neighbours, found its way among the rest. The women who performed this work were themselves at risk, and the slops they generated carried deadly germs to drains, cisterns and wells.[60]

Seriously unhealthy to the residents were the small brass foundries that occupied ground-floor premises in many streets of the Lower City. There were fifty such foundries in the *sezione* Pendino alone in the summer of 1884.[61] Lacking chimneys for the escape of the fumes they emitted, they filled the narrow, airless lanes with pungent fumes that corroded the lungs of the tenants above and forced them to close their shutters even in the heat of the summer. A particularly hazardous by-product of the casting of zinc – a constituent element of brass – is arsenic that, according to the municipal sanitary officials, found its way into the streets in copious amounts. The angry residents of the Vico Strettola agli Orefici, a densely populated street with several foundries, protested that there was not a family in the neighbourhood without at least one member who was ill from the occupational diseases of the brass-founders.[62] But most disturbing from the standpoint of infectious disease was the discovery that the master founders reduced their costs of production by engaging in a highly illegal trade in recycled zinc coffins from the municipal cemetery.[63]

For a city with such severely polluted public spaces, an efficient municipal cleansing service was a vital means of self-defence against germs. Unfortunately, the Neapolitan Department of Sanitation was unequal to the task of disposing of the vast quantities of waste that fouled the streets and squares afresh every day.

Since few streets except the main thoroughfares were paved or boasted drains, the main responsibility for the removal of waste fell to patrolling dustmen and their carts. Regrettably, they found the teeming, narrow alleys of the lower boroughs impossible to negotiate, with the result that the most densely populated lanes, where the risks were greatest, were never visited or swept.

Even the roadways accessible to the street-sweepers derived only a limited benefit from the service. The irony of the Department of Sanitation, as municipal councillors frequently protested, was that it never contemplated cleansing as its objective. Dustmen were employed for the modest purpose of preventing the accumulating refuse of the city from rising to the upper storeys and paralysing every activity.

Four hundred Neapolitan dustmen began their day with the so-called 'general sweep'. This early-morning activity was in reality not a sweep at all, and it accomplished nothing that its promising title suggested. It was a rough sorting operation intended to clear the streets of obstruction. From the general accumulation of rubbish, the 'sweepers' separated the largest and most visible items, which they gathered into piles for disposal later in the day. The problem of omnipresent excrement of human and animal origin was not addressed. Sewage was left where it lay or, in the few streets so equipped, consigned to the drains. Only the piazzas and paved boulevards such as the Via Toledo and the Via del Duomo, were periodically washed. Water only aggravated the condition of the back lanes and alleys, where it spread a putrid slime. Most of the streets of Naples, therefore, were cleared, not cleaned.[64]

A further deficiency in the sweeping service was that it confined itself to the streets themselves. Municipal dustmen did not undertake the removal of domestic waste or the emptying of the 4,000 cesspits located in tenement courtyards.[65] These chores on which the health of the city depended were left to private initiative. Only the prosperous few who could afford commercial cesspool dumpers and removal men benefited. The rest of the population turned to the streets as the only alternative. There they generated a problem of such proportions that it overwhelmed the 'general sweepers', who devoted themselves to the manageable issue of litter.[66]

The disposal of the mounds of refuse heaped by the 'sweep' created additional problems. Disposal was a separate service that was leased to private contractors. In the afternoon, when the sweep was completed, the dilapidated tip-carts of the contractors appeared, drawn by ageing donkeys. Each conveyance was accompanied by a young boy, whose labour cost little. The boy's job was to gather up the rubbish in a bin and to hurl it into the cart. Because his height was seldom equal to the task, the emptying of every bin-load produced a shower of stinking debris that cascaded over the sides. Furthermore, since the cart was uncovered and was carelessly filled, a portion of the load was lost overboard as the tip-cart made its awkward progress through the streets. This problem was compounded by the fact that there were no dumps within the city limits. Every cart, therefore, travelled to the distant municipal tip near the Maddalena Bridge on the eastern extremity of town. A portion of the work achieved by the sweepers in the morning was thus undone in the afternoon.[67]

The unsanitary condition of the streets was of particular importance in a city with the overwhelming density of population that afflicted Naples. The houses were so cramped, so unpleasant and so lacking in facilities that the people of the Lower City led their lives out of doors. Food was prepared, sold and eaten in the streets. Children played, adults practised their trades, and people socialized – all in the midst of an evil putrefaction. That all of the activities of life were pursued in so poisoned an environment brought danger.

Furthermore, the disposal of waste provided a hazardous link between the streets and cesspits of the city and the market gardens of the adjacent province. Much of the produce consumed in Naples was cultivated in the delta of the Sebeto river to the east of the city in such communes as Barra, Portici, Ponticelli, San Pietro a Patierno and San Giovanni a Teduccio. The private dustmen who emptied the pits added to their income by selling their noxious product as fertilizer to the peasants known as *padulani* who supplied the city with vegetables. In addition, the manure available in the streets was so abundant that peasants from the Neapolitan hinterland made periodic forays with their carts to collect precious cargoes for their fields. The green vegetables that fed the city were grown in untreated human and animal faeces. This practice of 'sewage farming' enabled microbes originating in the city to reach the farthest boundaries of the province and then to return to town in wagons loaded with tomatoes and heads of lettuce. Furthermore, the fields to the east of Naples were crisscrossed with waterways that served the multiple purposes of irrigating the land, disposing of waste and washing clothes. En route to town, the peasants frequently dipped their green vegetables in these polluted streams to keep them fresh for market. By these various means the vibrio was able to complete a round-trip journey from mouth to privy and back.[68]

WATER

To live in such conditions was to risk disease. But since cholera is most widely spread by contaminated water, particular attention must be paid to the water supply and sewage systems of the city. Drinking water for the 500,000 residents of the city came from several sources. Again, there was a major distinction between the Upper and Lower Cities. The Neapolitan nobility and the bourgeoisie drank rainwater collected and stored in private and well-maintained water-tanks. The Lower City relied on a variety of less trustworthy sources. The most important were the Bolla and Carmignano aqueducts, and the 4,500 wells dug in the calcareous tufa beneath the streets and still in use in 1884.[69] These supplies were universally acknowledged to be inadequate as the volume of water supplied to the city had not expanded in 250 years despite the expansion of the population and the diversification of its demands for water. The average supply of water for all purposes was 45,000 cubic metres a day, as it had been since the completion of the Carmignano aqueduct in 1627.[70]

More important than the deficient quantity of water, however, was the fact that all three supplies were severely polluted.[71] The water provided by the Bolla and Carmignano aqueducts was lethally corrupted even before it reached the city. The more extreme case was that of the Carmignano. Every stage of its lengthy journey of 43 kilometers from the springs near Montesarchio was marked by fresh contamination. From its source the water flowed in a covered conduit as far as Maddaloni. Thereafter it traversed the countryside of Campania in an open canal, passed through the town of Acerra, and then flowed again through the fields to the gates of Naples. There – too late – the water was channelled into an enclosed conduit that distributed it to the city. Having reached the main suburban ring road called the Foria, the aqueduct divided into two branches. One flowed along the city walls to power the municipal mills; the other branch supplied conduits running beneath the city streets that filled the 2,000 cisterns of the Lower City operating in 1884.[72] By lowering buckets into the tanks, which were usually sited in courtyards, the inhabitants obtained the water they needed for drinking and for all domestic purposes.

At every point from source to storage-tank the Carmignano waters were exposed to the risk of contamination. Leaves, insects and debris were blown into the open canal. Peasants illegally retted hemp in the stream, laundered their garments, and disposed of their household waste and the carcasses of farm animals. Horses quenched their thirst in the flow, while mud and manure used to fertilize the fields drained into the aqueduct after every rain or seeped through the porous stone sides. Particularly after a storm, the water arriving at the city gates was brown and thick with sludge. The watermen who regulated the supply interrupted the flow for long periods, allowing the sediment to settle before they released the stream into the Lower City. The problems afflicting the Bolla on its course to Naples were similar, but the quality of the water was better, if only because the distance it traversed across the plains of the region – five miles – was so much shorter.

Having arrived beneath the streets of Naples, the Carmignano and Bolla waters rapidly experienced further deterioration. The aqueducts and the sewer mains ran in parallel adjacent lines underground. Since both were made of porous limestone, their contents slowly intermingled as liquid from each seeped into the soil and through the walls of the other. The high level of reciprocal exchange between aqueduct and sewer was demonstrated in the summer of 1884 when the city took desperate measures to improve its sanitation. Carbolic acid was poured into the sewers to disinfect them and sulphur bonfires were lit in the streets to purify the air. Distressed residents promptly complained of the taste of sulphur and acid in their drinking water.[73]

Thus laden with bacteria, the water poured into the water tanks beneath the tenement courtyards. Unfortunately, the process of contamination continued unabated. Since the storage cisterns were also built of local limestone, surface-water continually seeped into them. In the many buildings where cesspits were sited adjacent to the tank, the bacterial exchange was immediate and overwhelming. Even in dwellings where cesspits were more distantly located, dangers abounded. Tenants were not always accurate when emptying their slops; and the pits, rarely emptied, frequently overflowed. Such polluted surface-water percolated downward and into the supply.

Finally, the water tanks suffered from the same neglect as the buildings. Most were never cleansed or repaired, so that their sides were cracked, broken and coated in layers of accumulated filth. Since the underground trenches that supplied the tanks flowed from tenement to tenement, everyone was at the mercy of his neighbours upstream. The use of buckets had a direct medical consequence. Rarely washed, they lowered their microbial bounty into the cisterns as easily as they raised water out of them. For these reasons, the storage tanks had an evil reputation. Those who dwelt on the ground floor normally turned to public fountains for their drinking water, reserving the supply in the tanks for other domestic purposes. The residents of the upper floors, for whom it was easier to lower buckets than to carry pails up the stairs, made the greatest use of the tanks and fell victim most frequently to diarrhoeal diseases.[74]

Despite such misadventures, those residents of Lower Naples who drank Carmignano and Bolla water were thought fortunate. The third major source of drinking water within the city walls was the network of underground wells that yielded a supply that was slimy, foul-tasting and sometimes deadly. The wells, usually located like storage tanks in building courtyards, experienced all of the risks that followed automatically from their location, their limestone construction, and their total neglect. The ageing masonry was cracked and chinked so that surface-water, infallibly finding the shortest path, seeped through the sides without passing through the natural filtration process of slowly percolating through the soil. All too frequently users avoided the labour of transporting the water needed for domestic purposes. Instead they used it directly *in situ*, washing linen, performing ablutions, rinsing chamber-pots. The slops then rapidly rejoined the supply, whose abundant cargo of bacteria was ready to be drawn again. A further hazard was the universal use of buckets rather than pumps to draw the water – a practice that contaminated the wells just as it did the water tanks.

In addition, however, well-water originated in the worst sources in the city. The wells were supplied by a series of five sluggish underground streams that flowed to their basin beneath the city and into the sea. These streams were the final repositories of all the waste that saturated the soil of the most densely populated city in Europe – a city of constantly seeping sewage pipes, leaking cesspits, and putrefying waste emptied onto unpaved streets that were never swept. In the course of an epidemic, bacteria from the human gut were rapidly recycled through the intermediary of the wells. Those who drank from them dominated the mortality rolls, especially in the heat of summer when thirst drove them to lower their buckets again and again.

An extensive report on the condition of the wells in the borough of Pendino during the 1884 epidemic was provided by the Medical Officer of Health for the *sezione*, Federico Sirignano. Sirignano and his colleagues visually inspected all of the wells of the borough. Although they made no bacteriological analysis of the water-content, their findings were a vivid reminder of the conditions that destroyed the health of Neapolitans. Sirignano was obliged to order the closure of over 300 wells in the borough as a result of their construction and the visible contamination of the water they contained. As he explained,

> By means of careful investigations carried out in all the dwellings of the borough of Pendino ... , we had the occasion to observe a large number of wells that do not conform in any respect to the necessities of hygiene.
>
> Most often located ... adjacent to domestic latrines, from which they are sometimes separated only by thin partitions, the wells directly absorbed the effluvia of faecal materials, and there was no shortage of instances in which the privies and wells were in direct mutual communication. On that basis it is easy to appreciate that, when drawn, the water from these wells was cloudy, disgusting to taste, and reeking with a nauseating smell of ammonia. Such water was evil not only because of filthy seepage but also on account of the fact that solid materials were to be found floating suspended within it.'[75]

Naples provided a classic illustration of the warning made by Robert Koch – that the recourse to tank-wells is the most hazardous and 'irrational' method of procuring underground water.[76]

SEWERS

The defects of the sewer system completed the sanitary havoc created by the water supply. All leading sanitary authorities regarded the 180 kilometres of pipes that formed the Neapolitan sewer network as dangerously obsolete. They had not been constructed originally on the basis of a coherent plan or a unity of sanitary criteria. Instead, they had been laid piecemeal as the city expanded. Never renewed, the system had fallen by 1884 into a state of terminal disrepair. The purpose for which the system had been constructed detracted from its effectiveness. The function of the Neapolitan sewers was drainage rather than the removal of domestic waste. For this reason, water-closets were a rarity, with the result that the populace was compelled to have recourse instead to cesspits, to the courtyards and to the streets. As the American Consul observed, a feature of Neapolitan life in 1884 was that 'there are no plumbers as a class in Naples, there being no such system of water pipes or water supply as exists in the United States'.[77]

Indeed, as there were only thirty-nine main collector sewers in the commune, most streets enjoyed no provision of any sort. By the 1880s, in any case, the antique network was approaching a state of paralysis. In the densely populated quarters to the east of the Via Roma, where the system was most extensive, many of the sewers were over 250 years old. These aged conduit-pipes were broken; they were porous and of insufficient diameter; they numbered countless blockages in their course; and the linkages were no longer firmly sealed. No provision was made for their ventilation, and traps were almost unknown. This was the reason for the endless seepage that poisoned the drinking water and for the unbearable stench for which the Lower City was justly famous. The soil itself was a black compost where human manure had percolated for centuries.

The problem of leaching was compounded by improper maintenance, which allowed an ever-thickening layer of sludge to clog the mains. The pipes, in any event, were too narrow and too brittle for proper repair and cleansing. The difficulty was made more acute by the insufficient gradient of the conduits that crossed the Neapolitan plain. Confounded by the topography of streets that ran only a few feet above sea level, the architects of the original networks had laid their conduits perilously close to the horizontal. This original defect was compounded in 1740 by the construction of the Via Marina, the raised coastal road that skirted the harbour. This project further reduced the inadequate slope of the collector pipes. The results were a chronically sluggish flow that lingered in the mains; a proclivity to obstructions that produced stagnant pools throughout the network; and a tendency for the sewers to regurgitate their contents through the drains after the least rise in the level of the sea.

Worst of all, the system disgorged its entire load of raw, untreated waste directly into the Bay. All fifty-four of the outfalls of the system were located on the shore within the city limits. The result was unfortunate for the appearance of the Neapolitan beaches, which were streaked by the passage of reeking, black, slow-moving streams. More serious were the consequences for public health. Bathing in the turbid waters of the Bay, even in direct proximity to the sewer outfalls, was a popular recreation. This practice was a direct means of spreading infection. Still more alarming to sanitarians were the consequences for the diet of the population. Shellfish – mussels, oysters and crabs – were abundant and inexpensive. They therefore formed a staple item in the diet of the city. After feeding on human excrement, however, they were dangerously contaminated and formed an ideal vehicle for the transmission of cholera, especially since a common preference was to eat them raw.[78] Furthermore, in a city where water was in permanently short supply and salt bore the burden of taxation imposed by a state monopoly, sea water from the Bay was widely used in the making of bread.[79] Thus conceived to meet the needs of an early modern city and improperly maintained thereafter, the sewers contributed liberally to the long Neapolitan history of epidemics.

POVERTY

Aberrant housing, impure water, an antique sewer system and deficient sanitation – these were four of the high-risk factors that exposed the people of Naples to the danger of epidemic disease. There were other important considerations, of which the most important was poverty. Cholera thrives on poverty because the poor, through malnutrition and intestinal disorders, are predisposed to contracting the disease. A major cause of the ravages of 1884, therefore, was the economy of the Lower City.

The dominant feature of the economy, as of every facet of Neapolitan life, was the enormous disproportion between the size of the population and the limited resources available. By the time of the 1884 catastrophe, Naples had become the symbol of the intractable 'Southern Question' in Italian history. The former capital of an impoverished kingdom, modern Naples was neither modernizing nor developing. Under the old regime the city had existed largely on the stunted basis of royal favour. The capital enjoyed a position of monopoly as the obligatory entrepôt for the commerce of the whole Mezzogiorno. The exported produce of southern agriculture and pastoralism – wheat, wine, olive oil, wool, cheese – passed through Naples on the way to northern Italy, France and England in exchange for the finished products of the industry of northern Europe, such as clothing, and the luxury products of the colonial trade – sugar, spices, tobacco.

A problem of this pattern of development was that the economy of the city was geared to marketing rather than production, to services and the retail trades rather than to industry. Furthermore, a large proportion of the wealth generated in foreign trade failed to stimulate the local economy because so many of the merchants were foreigners who exported their profits instead of investing in the local economy. In addition, as an exporter of raw materials and importer of industrial goods, Naples faced the long-term problem that the terms of trade were unfavourable to its own wealth and economic well-being. Too little capital was generated for re-investment and the modernization of the productive structures of the city. The privileged role conferred on Naples in relation to the rest of the Mezzogiorno also meant that the Neapolitan economy was artificially based – dependent, that is, on the continued position of the city as the capital of the kingdom. Naples thus became an emporium with archaic social and economic structures not unlike those of a contemporary Third World capital. At the time of unification the city lacked an adequate productive base to support its enormous population.

Despite the absence of industry or of stable prospects for employment, the population of the city had swollen as early as the seventeenth century to make Naples one of the great European capitals. The poverty of southern Italian agriculture yielded a continuous stream of immigrants, and every poor harvest or fall in the price of wheat quickened the flow. Despite its frail economic base, the city remained an unfailing magnet for the destitute. In an effort to prevent subversion and riot in time of hardship, the Bourbon Crown had equipped the city with enormous stocks of grain to supply the population in time of dearth and to control price levels. It also had a large-scale network of charitable associations for the elderly, the indigent and the chronically ill that had no parallel anywhere in the provinces. Most importantly, the city generated a vast demand for the services of the unskilled and the illiterate – domestic servants, porters, huxsters, builders and pedlars. It was the misfortune of Neapolitans that supply constantly outstripped demand.

Count Giusso, a leading financial expert, Mayor and Director of the Banco di

Napoli, presented a clear description of the economic cul-de-sac in which the city found itself.[80] In his budget report for 1881 he reasoned:

> Although Naples is the largest city in Italy, its productive capacity bears no direct relation to the number of its inhabitants ... Naples is a centre for consumption rather than for production. This is the principal reason for the misery of its populace, and for the slow, almost insensible, increase of that misery over time ... If we want the city to prosper, we must discover and promote ways of putting it to work.[81]

Before unification, as after, the great majority of Neapolitans lived in poverty, squalor, and ill health. There was a privileged minority of merchants, nobles, industrialists, functionaries and members of the liberal professions. They lived in the Upper City or in such isolated pockets of gentility as the Via Toledo in the Lower. For the mass of the working population, conditions were stark. This point was carefully noted in 1884 by the American Consul, who compiled a report on 'wages and conditions of labor in Naples' for the benefit of the Department of State and its attempt to provide an exhaustive comparative survey of the conditions of labour throughout Europe.[82] As the Secretary of State explained in his introductory letter to Congress, the purpose of the investigation was to support American employers by providing them with comprehensive information on the employment practices of their competitors abroad and on the habits, political sentiments and wages of the men and women they might wish to recruit. Reliable information on the relations of capital and labour in Europe was also the necessary basis for public debate and official policymaking on the labour question in the United States.[83] The consular service, the Secretary suggested, provided the most extensive network available for gathering and collating the necessary data. This survey and especially the local response of Frank Haughwout, the American Consul at Naples, are important sources on the living conditions prevailing at the time of the cholera epidemic. Haughwout concluded that,

> the rate of wages in all branches of labor in Naples is very low. To this fact is due much of the misery, poverty and degradation of the working classes ... Among them there is a total absence of ambition and desire of bettering their condition and, further, the amount of wages they receive is not in proportion to the work done by them.[84]

'It is said', he elaborated, 'that the Neapolitan workman ... generally dies in the same station of life as that in which he began work. His earnings are not sufficient for more than the actual wants of the day on which they are received and no provision can be made by him for old age and sickness.'[85]

According to the Department of State, average Italian wages were the most meagre in Europe, and Neapolitan wages were the lowest among major Italian cities. The most fortunate Neapolitan wage earners were the limited numbers of male industrial workers – dockers, engineers, metallurgical workers, and labourers for the railroads and trams. Competition in a radically overcrowded labour

Table 1.6. *Average industrial salaries and wages in Naples, 1884*

Occupation	Wage (US dollars)
Director	$48.25 per month
Chief miller	$77.20 per month
Office clerk	$25 per month
Night watchman	$17.30 per month
Shipping clerk	$11.58 per month
Ship carpenter	$0.77 per day
Workman	$0.48 per day

market depressed their wages. The result was that they earned a fraction of the pay of their colleagues in identical jobs in Milan, Turin, or Genoa. The earnings of the average worker, according to the American Consul, were not sufficient to allow the annual purchase of a change of clothing and his garments were always acquired second-hand.[86] Calculated in American dollars ($1 was equal to 1.93 lire), the average wages in Neapolitan factories, mills and shipyards in 1884 were those listed in Table 1.6.[87] The typical daily industrial wage of less than $0.50 compares with the prices for necessities of life in the city given in Table 1.7.[88]

In Neapolitan conditions, therefore, the average unskilled worker employed for the standard ten- to twelve-hour day earned no more than the cost of four kilos of macaroni, and four days' work would be required for the purchase of a pair of shoes at the market rate of $2.00 a pair. But factory operatives were few in number in backward Naples, and they occupied a position of relative privilege. Mill hands, ship carpenters and stevedores enjoyed the benefit of steady employment and the approximation of a living wage.

In the backward urban economy the industrial working class could be considered the local aristocracy of labour – provided that one considers only adult males. By contrast, the average daily wage for women in the city was only $0.30. Many earned as little as $0.10; and the American Consul was unable to locate any who earned more than $0.40. The largest single concentration of women consisted of the 2,400 cigar-makers, some as young as fourteen years of age, employed in the state-owned tobacco plant. The cigar-makers earned only $0.20 to $0.32 a day,[89] they were supervised by an all-male corps of foremen and directors, and they suffered especially harsh conditions. In the terse comment of the consular report, 'No means are taken for the safety of the employees in such cases.'[90] The tobacco workers were the only female factory operatives in Naples, partly because of the prevailing job segregation in the city and partly because the textile industry, which was the principal international employer of female industrial workers in western Europe at the time, did not exist within the walls of the city. In its report on female labour in Naples, the American Consulate listed the following occupations in addition to the tobacco trade:

Table 1.7. *Prevailing prices in Naples, 1884*

Item	Price (US dollars)
Meat	$0.44 to $0.50 per kilo
Macaroni	$0.10 to $0.12 per kilo
Fish	$0.15 per kilo
Bread	$0.07 to $0.09 per kilo
Tomatoes	$0.20 per kilo (winter), $0.02 per kilo (summer)
Potatoes	$0.02 per kilo
Fruit	$0.04 to $0.10 per kilo
Wine	$0.07 to $0.15 per litre
Cauliflower	$0.02 per head
Peas	$0.06 per kilo
Rent	$3 per room in a *basso* per month

teachers, agricultural workers, coral workers, sewing women, workers in the construction of buildings, fruit vendors and hucksters, telegraph officers, money changers, water sellers and carriers, household servants and nurses ... The proportion of numbers which is to be assigned to each class cannot possibly be given. There is nothing to which one can look for such information.[91]

In the building trade, women did not perform the same tasks as men. They were employed exclusively for the heavy labour of carrying stone and timber.

For both men and women, factory labour was the exception. Far more numerous were the tens of thousands of craftsmen in a multitude of tiny workshops located throughout the Lower City. Some of the trades had flourished in earlier centuries, such as the glass, pottery, silk, leather, carpet, wool and goldsmith crafts. By the nineteenth century, however, the undercapitalized workshops of the city were caught in a downward spiral of decline. Small shops were unable to modernize their methods of production; they had no access to credit facilities; and their livelihood was threatened by the competition of machinery and the influx of unskilled and inexpensive labour. Despite long hours, the traditional crafts barely yielded a subsistence for those who practised them. Their members shared a common hardship with the artisans who catered to the daily needs of the population – bakers, butchers, cobblers, seamstresses, blacksmiths, cabmen and joiners – and with those numerous factotums of the city, the domestic servants and porters. At the bottom of the pay-scale for men, daily wages for tailors reached $0.29, for tanners $0.39, for hatters $0.40, for horse-shoers $0.39, and for gardeners $0.29. No figures are available for servants.[92]

The disadvantages of Italian and especially Neapolitan craftsmen in comparison with their counterparts elsewhere were noted by the Department of State. Comparative figures for selected general trades demonstrate the low general level of remuneration of Italian tradesmen. Since, according to the American findings,

Table 1.8. *Male wages in selected trades in Europe, 1884*
(expressed in 1884 US dollars)

Trades	Countries				
	Germany	France	England	Belgium	Italy
Bricklayers	$0.70	$0.96	$1.26	$0.76	$0.70
Masons	$0.78	$0.89	$1.28	$0.87	$0.60
Blacksmiths	$0.67	$0.97	$1.23	$0.90	$0.60
Tailors	$0.57	$0.84	$1.23	$0.93	$0.67
Bookbinders	$0.70	$0.86	$1.13	$0.89	$0.63
Coopers	$0.66	$0.93	$1.25	$0.86	$0.43
Printers	–	$1.10	$1.20	$0.99	$0.77

there were no significant differences in prices among the nations of the West, it is possible to compare the norms prevailing elsewhere directly with the earnings of Neapolitans, as in Table 1.8.[93]

A special and wretched case was that of the 10,000 fishermen and their families who lived in the neighbourhood of S. Lucia, one of the most unhealthy slums in Naples.[94] The men of S. Lucia were small-scale, short-distance seamen with antiquated equipment and 3,000 tiny boats. In good times they could hope to earn 180 lire a year. They were poor because they were far too numerous for the polluted Bay, which had been overfished for generations by means of illegal nets with a narrow mesh. The unregulated fishing industry of the Bay, and the men engaged in it were in steady decline as every boat further depleted the stock and undermined the livelihood of its rivals. The fishermen were also squeezed in the marketplace, where they faced the competition of long-distance importers and where they sold their catch, not directly to the public, but rather to merchants who in turn distributed the produce to the city's fishmongers. The middlemen profited from an overcrowded industry to drive prices down. The fishermen of S. Lucia also suffered from being in daily contact with waters contaminated by untreated sewage. Particularly when they included shellfish in their own diet, they were exposed to immediate danger. In 1884 S. Lucia was among the earliest and most tragically visited quarters of the city.

Descending further in the social scale, one encounters the myriad Neapolitans who earned their living directly in the streets. It was characteristic of the ailing local economy that tens of thousands of people subsisted by peddling their wares amidst the filth of the city lanes and alleys. It was these impoverished entrepreneurs who gave Naples its feverish activity as a great emporium. These men and women were not workers, but 'ragged-trousered capitalists' who filled a bewildering variety of roles that baffled all efforts at quantification. A local authority termed them 'micro-industrialists'.[95] The elite of the streets were the newspaper vendors who practised only one trade year-round and enjoyed a stable remuneration. The other huxters were 'gypsy merchants', authentic nomads of the marketplace who moved from activity to activity as opportunity dictated. There were sellers of vegetables, chestnuts and shoe laces; purveyors of pizzas, mussels and recycled clothes; vendors of mineral water, corn cobs and candy. Some of the men completed their activity by acting as messenger-boys, distributors of commercial leaflets or private dustmen who emptied cesspits or removed domestic waste for a few centesimi a week. Others acted as professional mourners paid to follow the hearses bearing the bodies of substantial citizens to the cemetery at Poggioreale. By their presence, hired paupers swelled the attendance, allowing the genteel classes to confirm their popularity and their sense of power.[96] Certain occupations not listed by the United States consular authorities involved only women, who contributed to the family budget by taking in washing, repairing wicker chairs and selling matches.

The most monstrous feature of the city, however, was that its social structure genuinely approximated the shape of a pyramid. Broadening remorselessly from top to bottom, it rested on the most abject and numerous stratum of all – the unemployed. Precise quantification of the unemployed in the city is impossible. Census figures are of little value because census-takers were unable to reach or define a population that was constantly in the process of re-inventing itself, that was often semi-nomadic, that lived in tenements where officials never entered, and that could neither read nor understand the bureaucratic language of Italian officialdom. There are, however, suggestive estimates by local experts such as the socialist councillor Leone, who represented the Lower City and was a careful student of its social problems. In 1902 he informed the city council that of the Neapolitan population of half a million people 200,000 (40 per cent) were permanently unemployed. To convey the full magnitude of the problem, Leone noted for comparison that London, with a population of 5,000,000 had only 100,000 unemployed.[97] Nowhere else in western Europe was there such a concentration of the totally destitute, of people who woke in the morning not knowing when they would next eat, or where they would sleep. Here were the recruits for the Neapolitan armies of beggars, prostitutes and criminals, and here were ready candidates for the cholera isolation wards. A disproportionate share of economic hardship was borne by women. In 1884 the city reported that three-quarters of the women of the Lower City lacked any occupation – a rate that was approximately double that of men.[98]

A city already desperately poor in the first half of the century experienced a steady economic and social decline in the second. A major cause for the continuous expansion of misery after 1861 was unification itself, which destroyed the greatest resource the city possessed – its status as a royal capital. With the overthrow of the Bourbons, the port and the arsenal languished; the luxury trades withered; and the rich veins of royal patronage and military spending were exhausted. According to the municipal authorities, Naples lost 24,000,000 lire a year in public spending.[99] The completion of the great Adriatic trunk railway line redirected the exports of Apulia and the Abruzzi away from Naples direct to the North and beyond the Alps. At the same time the free-trade policy of Liberal Italy cost Naples its privileged position in the commerce of the South and exposed its producers to competition from the economically advanced North.

With the completion of unity in 1871, many wealthy property-owners abandoned Naples for the new capital in Rome. A massive flight of capital accompanied this northward migration.[100] Nor did the middle classes who remained effectively defend the interests of the former capital. With their traditional training in law and medicine, they advanced no strategy of economic development and they avoided risk by investing their funds in urban property, money-lending and land. The productive economy of the ex-capital city was starved of capital and credit. Hardship in Naples was thus created by an enormous surplus population that swamped the city's urban infrastructures and opportunities for employment, but it was greatly exacerbated by the free-trade priorities of the ruling classes of the North and by the lack of vision of the local elites. [101]

A further major factor was the tax regime of United Italy, which imposed on its citizens the highest burden in Europe. Comparing the taxes of the old regime with those of the new, the city council calculated that the aggregate tax contribution assessed against the inhabitants of Naples rose from 7,000,000 lire a year to 20,000,000 – without counting the additional levies of local government.[102] With regard to local government, the strategy of the parliament in Rome was to minimize the burdens of the exchequer by devolving on the *comune* the responsibility of providing for education, health and welfare and by stipulating that these essential services be financed locally.

In communes where the local economy was strong, such a policy produced no ill effects. Naples, however, was the poorest of the major cities in the kingdom, and it lacked the wealth to fund the services needed to protect the vital interests of its population. The regressive tax regime of the kingdom widened the gulf in social provision between wealthy and depressed municipalities, between North and South. Neapolitans, because they inhabited the poorest commune in Italy, were caught in an ever tightening poverty trap. The disadvantages facing the Palazzo San Giacomo can be clearly understood by a consideration of the municipal budget.

The backbone of local government finance was the hated consumption levy known as the *dazio consumo*. The *dazio* was a tax collected on all the prime necessities of life. Under its provisions, Naples became a 'closed' city with barriers at every point of entry. At the barriers the compulsory excise was collected on all articles brought into the city to be sold retail. This customs duty was borne disproportionately by the poor, and its effects were calamitous. The first consequence of the *dazio consumo* was radically to increase the cost of living, placing many foodstuffs beyond the reach of large swathes of the Neapolitan population. Under the tax system imposed by the Piedmontese, the local government of Naples lived, in the expression of one of its aldermen, by thrusting its hands into the pockets of the poor.[103] During the years 1870–5, for instance, the population was assessed for sums varying from 9.9 to 11.7 million lire annually through the consumption levy alone.[104]

A second result was no less disastrous. The local administration was crippled by being made financially dependent on the contributions of the destitute. Because the yield of the customs duties was necessarily inelastic, the city had no opportunity to finance major initiatives to confront its severe and growing social problems through programmes of urban renewal, sanitation and poor relief. Naples instead found itself forever on the verge of bankruptcy. A succession of mayors and aldermen responsible for finance in the decades after 1861 described the financial plight of the city as 'ailing' and 'abnormal', and blamed the *dazio* for the malaise. The largest item of expenditure, at 38.5 per cent of the 1876 budget, was the servicing of the municipal debt.[105] The history of Liberal Naples could be written, argued Alderman Pizzuti in 1873, 'in terms of the unending struggle against limited resources, unlimited needs, and the anxious expectation of a balanced budget'.[106] The *dazio* was also inefficient as a source of revenue because it was exorbitantly expensive to collect, requiring the deployment of teams of armed municipal guards at every barrier. Collection of the consumption levy in 1876 absorbed 4.8 per cent of the city budget – as compared, for example, with the 4.1 per cent allocated for education.[107] Understandably, the consumption levy was detested by the populace and inflamed social tensions.

The executive committee of the Neapolitan town council also suffered from a failure of will. At the turn of the century a commission of enquiry led by the Ligurian technocrat Giuseppe Saredo was appointed by parliament to examine the conditions of local government in the city. Saredo accepted that the city had been placed in an impossible position by Italian tax legislation, but he also reported that the officials in Palazzo San Giacomo compounded the difficulty instead of attempting to alleviate it. It had become the practice of the aldermen to attend to the interests of their electors rather than to the more pressing needs of the populace. Rather than attempting to compensate for the glaring inequality of the consumption levy by introducing proportionality in the other secondary taxes that fell within its jurisdiction, the Neapolitan municipal council aggravated the unequal burden falling upon the poor by reproducing the regressive principles of the *dazio consumo* in all of its levies. The council consistently gave tax relief to the wealthy by relying on indirect rather than direct taxes.[108] No attempt was ever made to institute a progressive tax reform.

Poverty bred poverty in a tragic downward spiral. No more important example in the life of nineteenth-century Naples can be found than the movement of rent. Rent was the major item in the family budgets of the poor, and any increase directly caused the populace to skimp on food. In the hundred years ending with the First World War, rents in the city moved steadily and dramatically upward. Part of the explanation was simply the effect of supply and demand on the crowded Neapolitan plain where empty sites for construction had long ago disappeared.

Rent increases far outstripped the sluggish population growth of the city.

Table 1.9. *Naples: average rent per room (1806 = 100)*

1830	150
1850	225
1860	315
1885	504

Rents in Naples were said to be 'rising every day'[109] while the population experienced no parallel growth in prosperity. By the end of the century rent had increased fivefold while the inhabitants of the city had grown poorer. Ironically, moreover, the highest rents per square metre were for the most dismal rooms in the slums. Because these rooms cost the least in absolute terms, the demand for them was greatest. Unhappily, the demand for slum accommodation grew with increasing poverty, thus giving further twists to the rent spiral affecting those least able to pay. If the rent of an average room in the city of Naples is set at an index of 100 in 1806, the expense of the same room took the upward direction in the course of the century shown in Table 1.9.[110] It is easy to comprehend, then, that rent accounted for 40 to 60 per cent of family expenditure.[111] In this way rent directly set narrow parameters for health and longevity by depleting the funds available for food, clothing and heat.

The pricing of food – a critical factor in the health of the Lower City – obeyed different principles. The high cost of produce reflected the predations of organized crime. Naples possessed in the Camorra one of the most powerful criminal associations in modern European history. Like the Sicilian Mafia, the Camorra clothed itself in populist rhetoric, proclaiming itself the champion of the poor and the defender of the South. It veiled the reality of the unpitying oppression that it meted out. The Camorra adopted mysterious jargon and rites that mimicked those of a secret society; it flaunted a pseudo-chivalric code of 'honour' among its members; and it created a mythology of distributive justice in which it claimed the role of urban Robin Hood.[112]

In reality, however, the Camorra was itself a symptom of the social pathology of modern Naples, and it added immeasurably to the burdens of the poor. Captain Carlo Fabbroni of the *carabinieri*, who was charged with repressing the Camorra in the Neapolitan hinterland, expressed the matter with clarity in 1911. He rejected the chivalric 'window-dressing' of the organization as a charade designed to 'inflame the minds of the young and the ignorant'. 'The Camorra today', he argued, 'is an association for the purpose of making money and nothing else, for making money at any cost by milking the weak in the most dishonest possible manner.'[113] A vital example is the contribution of the Camorra to the ruinous cost of living that destroyed the health of the population. The means was monopoly pricing imposed by violence.

With its stronghold in the Lower City, the Camorra is best understood as a means of market rationalization. The destitute furnished the mass of members of the Neapolitan underworld,[114] and in a society dominated by mass unemployment and poverty, there was a constant threat of an oversupply of recruits to the life of crime. The criminal trade, like virtually every other craft in the city, was in danger of being swamped. The Camorra restored order and profitability by rigidly and violently restricting entry to the profession. What was not to be tolerated was freelance criminality. For criminal purposes the city was divided into fourteen families or 'societies', one to each neighbourhood where the organization had an effective presence. In some cases the territory claimed by a 'society' corresponded to one of the administrative boroughs of the city as in Mercato and Pendino, but more frequently the territory was smaller, with a preponderance of 'societies' in the Lower City.[115] Within its territory a Camorra 'society' was not a kinship network, but a monopoly that enforced its claim to a percentage of all illegal activity. The Camorra ruled without competition in its chosen domains of prostitution, illegal gambling, 'protection', money-lending and theft. The Camorra was a guild by other means: it protected the standard of living of its members by a rigid policy of exclusion guaranteed by the threat of violence. In a city famous for criminal activity, the striking feature of illegality, according to the police, was that almost every illegal deed had the sanction of the Camorra.[116]

Through the monopoly of criminality in a neighbourhood and the willingness of its members to resort to violent means, the Camorra achieved a domination over large areas of the economic and political life of the city. An important premise for the establishment of its power was the weakness of authority under both the old regime and the new. In their final years before the national revolution, the Bourbons made use of the services of *camorristi* to enforce, if not law, then at least a kind of order. As the inspector in command of the police in the borough of Montecalvario explained in 1875, 'Under the old regime of the Bourbons, the Camorra was an underworld society in the service of crime and the authorities ... who not only tolerated but also protected it.'[117] After the change of regime, the new Liberal administration in the city confronted a turbulent interregnum. To secure control, it colluded with organized crime. Liborio Romano, who presided over the change of regime in the city, made use of the Camorra as an auxiliary police force.[118] Thus the Camorra thrived as never before during the Risorgimento because authority was weak and for a time it was the only organized force in Naples.[119] In every sphere its influence was also favoured by the small-scale operations, the weakness, and the lack of organization of its victims. Large-scale industry, major landowners, an organized working class and consumers integrated into a highly developed civil society would have been less susceptible to its predations. But the isolated, demoralized and impoverished members of the Neapolitan *plebe* were ideal for victimization. As Marc Monnier wrote,

> Individuals were scattered, and this population of isolated people could offer no collective resistance to the oppression of powerful and violent minorities. The only ones to possess an organization, they dominated and triumphed with impunity.[120]

In this fragmented civil society the Camorra established a well-organized protection racket at the expense of defenceless small retailers, who passed a share of the cost onto consumers in the form of higher prices. By intimidation, blackmail, and favouritism it 'made' the elections of councillors and deputies. The Camorra also gained powerful friends by eliminating their rivals for contracts for the performance of municipal services. In this manner the 'low Camorra' of the streets increased its influence by gaining access to the collusion of the powerful. The shadowy 'high Camorra' of polite society was created. In this way the political process in the city failed to represent the interests of the voters of the Neapolitan plain. The effect of the 'Society' on both the politics and the health of the city could be seen whenever handsome contracts to perform such essential services as waste removal or management of the slaughter-house were awarded with little expectation of performance or no concern for the protection of the public interest. More directly important for medical history was the monopoly by the Camorra of the wholesale trade of every product that entered the city.

A well-documented case is that of the meat trade, which was considered at length by the Saredo report.[121] The Neapolitan slaughter-house, located in the suburb of Poggioreale and managed by a contractor, was, Saredo observed, 'the running sore and shame of Naples'.[122] Here the Camorra reigned supreme. Health regulations were ignored, so that the premises were rarely washed; the meat of superannuated farm animals who had perished of disease masqueraded as beef or lamb; taxes were never paid to the city; and peasants, shepherds and drovers who delivered their animals were obliged to pay protection money, to hire unnecessary labourers supplied by the management of the abattoir and to accept fraudulent weights without demur. The meat sold for distribution to the consumer was often of mysterious origin, of suspect freshness and of highly inflated price – to the detriment of the health and the budget of the population.

The meat trade, however, is only one illustration of the situation prevailing within the produce markets. In 1874 Alderman Luigi Simeoni reported to the city council the results of an extensive official investigation into the high cost of foodstuffs. A major cause of the high prices and poor quality of fruit, flour and vegetables in the Neapolitan markets, the study revealed, was the influence of organized crime.[123] The cost of produce in Naples, Simeoni explained, was 'intolerable' and higher than in other urban centres in the peninsula. The claim that the Risorgimento had established free trade throughout the kingdom was a fiction.[124] Instead, Naples was permanently affected by artificially inflated prices. In Neapolitan markets, consumers were the victims of every sort of abuse. At the same time peasants and market gardeners were forced to sell their goods solely to the Central Market and 'to accept whatever prices the Camorra imposes'.[125]

In 1875 the officers commanding the police in the twelve boroughs of the city were asked to file reports on organized crime within their jurisdictions. Their replies indicated the extent to which markets were controlled by *camorristi*. The professions most commonly exercised by the underworld were those with a strategic role in the circulation and distribution of goods – dockers, porters, hawkers, cabmen, butchers, tavern keepers – people 'who set sales prices', in the words of one police inspector.[126] The organization had a marked commercial vocation.[127] Confirming that the conditions denounced by the Simeoni Committee in 1874, the police enquiry in 1875, and the Saredo Report of 1901 were permanent features in the 'City of the Sirens', Dr Giuseppe Semmola revealed in 1909 that identical conditions still prevailed in the distribution of every variety of foodstuff. The Neapolitan populace was the victim of the 'abnormal, illegal and immoral conditions' imposed by the Camorra.[128]

Poverty in Naples, then, was the result of a series of mutually reinforcing factors – overpopulation, the change of regime in 1861, the absence of industry, high rents, low wages, a high burden of indirect taxation, high food prices imposed by organized crime and neglect or collusion by the municipal authorities. The effects on the health of the population and its vulnerability to epidemic cholera were direct. Already in the first half of the century the Neapolitan physician Salvatore De Renzi noted that the population of the Lower City was extensively affected by malnutrition. The signs he reported as typical of the inhabitants of the four boroughs of the Old City were: pallor; excessive body weight; a pervasive listlessness and lack of energy that he termed, in accordance with contemporary medical fashion, a 'lymphatic constitution'; cachexia; chronic constipation; hemorrhoids; and, among women, chlorotic anaemia and amenorrhea.[129]

In the decades after unification, both poverty and malnutrition increased substantially. Two clear indications of poverty – homelessness and begging – point clearly to this conclusion. In the decades after unification mendicants became an important preoccupation of the city council. In 1874, for example, the councillors were alarmed by the ever-growing numbers of beggars on the streets of the former capital. City Hall was concerned because beggars were a disagreeable nuisance to worthy citizens and tourists, because there were many occasions when homeless paupers died on the streets, and because vagrants constituted a charge on the municipal budget. Councillor Castellano explained that their numbers had 'increased to extraordinary proportions'.[130] Similarly aroused, Mayor Nicola Amore in 1883 returned to the theme. Amore declared himself disgusted by the 'swelling numbers of the poor who circulate not only in the back streets of the city but even along the main thoroughfares where ... the children go so far as to stop carriages until they are given money.' Such people, he argued, were a public scandal that ought to be repressed because so many of them were unworthy, able-bodied paupers who should be repressed in the name of morals, order and hygiene.[131]

If a swelling problem of vagrancy suggests poverty, there is also direct evidence that the family budgets of the mass of the population of the city came under stark pressure following 1861. As the population of the city grew, its consumption of foodstuffs, which already suggested pervasive malnutrition, declined both per capita and even absolutely for the city as a whole. Despite an increased population, Naples consumed less food in 1884 than it had before 1861.[132] The food that it ate, moreover, was substantially poorer in quality.

On the eve of the 1884 epidemic, the diet of the Neapolitan *plebe* was almost exclusively vegetarian. During the winter months it consisted of macaroni, adulterated bread, and pizza flavoured with green peppers and beans. As a result of this regimen, the winter and spring were seasons of constipation and hemorrhoids. In the summer and early autumn instead, the poor of Naples devoured prodigious quantities of fruit. In the interest of economy, they purchased spoiled or unripe figs, plums, apricots, cherries, pears, apples and grapes. The disagreeable effects of this summer diet were indigestion, gastric disturbance and diarrhoea. In October there were drinking excesses associated with the popular festivities known as the *ottobrate* when the first stocks of cheap new wine became available after the grape-harvest.

The relationship of such a regimen to the outbreak of cholera was direct. Malnutrition, through mechanisms not yet fully understood, lessens the resistance of the organism to infection. A sound diet is the first rampart in the body's system of defence. More immediately, however, the excessive consumption of under- and over-ripe fruit and new wine directly predisposed the digestive tract to cholera. A widely accepted tenet of nineteenth-century epidemiology was that cholera outbreaks, both in the individual and in the general population, were preceded by a phase of 'premonitory diarrhoea'.[133] The concept of 'premonitory diarrhoea' is now largely discredited as it is well established that Asiatic cholera can attack both the individual and a society without warning. There is no period of grace in which the vigilant can take effective preventive measures either individually or collectively. The idea of 'premonitory diarrhoea' in a different sense, however, had a sound historical and epidemiological foundation. Cholera was often preceded – and to some degree facilitated – by otherwise unrelated diarrhoeal illnesses resulting from improper diet.

The history of the 1884 epidemic in Naples confirms this point. Cholera struck when the summer heat drove the people to drink more frequently from suspect wells and storage tanks, producing widespread outbursts of gastro-enteritis. There was then a recrudescence in the autumn coincident with the popular celebrations and binges of October. October wine predisposed the digestive system to attack by neutralizing the acidity of the stomach.

The suspect diet that put the Lower City at risk was aggravated by a rebellious aspect of human nature. The poor of the city did not plan their family budgets in a rational manner, practising strict economy on inadequate income and maximizing their expenditure on food. Instead they reacted to poverty by dreaming of a miraculous escape and entrusting their fate to fortune. The wretched inhabitants of the Old City voluntarily submitted to what was, in effect, yet another heavy tribute that resulted in further skimping and privation. The national lottery was one of the great resources of the exchequer, generating a revenue by the 1880s of nearly 80 million lire. Despite its poverty, Naples bore an overwhelming share of this disguised taxation, contributing 21 million lire to the national total of 80 million.[134] The weekly draw on Saturday afternoon became the passion of the Lower City, where it was fuelled by popular superstitions that attributed magic powers to certain numbers. People already indebted and suffering from malnutrition squandered their resources by purchasing tickets in the hope of solving every problem with a single lucky tern.

In her novel *Il paese di Cuccagna*, Matilde Serao placed the lottery at the centre of her Dickensian portrayal of Neapolitan life in the 1880s. Her protagonists, all of whom inhabited the Lower City, were drawn remorselessly to self-destruction and to the ruin of their families by their incurable addiction to gambling. To place their weekly bets, they skimped on food and heat, pawned their last possessions, and fell into the devouring power of clairvoyants who claimed the magic gift of predicting winning numbers.[135] Serao stressed that her fictional account was a faithful depiction of the destructive power of the most insidious of Neapolitan misfortunes. If every third shop in the Lower City were a lottery office, she argued, they would all be full on Friday evening and Saturday morning as the betting deadline approached.[136] Poverty, illness and death inexorably followed.

Marcellin Pellet, the French Consul, confirmed Serao's observation. He noted during his sojourn in the city that

> In Naples the passion for the lottery reaches a frenzy. It has become an epidemic disease. Everyone plays in the hope of winning either the necessities or the luxuries of life. The most impoverished workers, scullery-boys, cabmen, cooks, matchstick vendors, and beggars all go without food in order to make their weekly bets ... But it is among the poor that the disease is most widespread and most devastating. Everyone, without exception, plays in some quarters of the Old City ... The lottery, therefore, is the scourge, the tapeworm, of the Neapolitan people.[137]

One need only add that Pellet considered only the official state lottery. Alongside it illegal numbers games were sponsored by the Camorra, which accepted small bets from those who could not afford tickets in the state lottery. In this underground lottery – the *gioco piccolo* – further fabulous sums that the poor could ill afford served only to strengthen the most vicious source of their tribulations.[138]

PUBLIC AUTHORITY AND PUBLIC HEALTH

Placed so severely at risk by the conditions in the former capital, the Neapolitan population urgently required sanitary vigilance as the threat of epidemic cholera approached. It was the misfortune of the city that no sentinels had been posted. The explanation for the neglect from which the city suffered so violently in 1884 involves the politics of both the national and the municipal governments.

At the national level, the Risorgimento embodied an 'administrative revolution' by which the modern state was created with resources and power far beyond the scope of the backward dynasties of the old regime. With its assistance, a transformation in public health was imaginable, and Neapolitans began to elaborate schemes for the sanitary renaissance of their city. Unfortunately for Naples, the Liberal regime faced more pressing problems in the first decades of unification than disease and sanitation. The parliament at Montecitorio was concerned with such preoccupations as the counter-revolutionary rebellion in the South known as 'Brigandage'; the ambition to complete national unity by capturing Rome; the establishment of the legitimacy of the new national institutions and laws; the balancing of a budget gravely compromised by the expense of the wars of unification; the progress of the economy; and the resolution of the thorny question of relations with the Church.

In these circumstances, the new regime gave priority to the essential instruments of power – the army and the economy. Since Italy was still a poor, preponderantly agricultural nation, the means remaining to confront the other serious problems of the nation were severely limited. Public health suffered because it was low in the order of national priorities.

It was not only a matter of scarce resources, however. Liberal Italy was a conservative regime in which the discontents of the poor received little attention unless they posed a threat to public order. Unification had been accomplished through the conquest of the whole of the peninsula by its most independent and commercially advanced part – the northern kingdom of Piedmont. Fearing popular initiative as subversive and potentially uncontrollable, the Piedmontese leaders had taken care to achieve their objective by diplomatic and military means in which the masses played no part. Antonio Gramsci described this process as a 'passive revolution' because the mass of Italians was thereby eliminated from the political process and from the life of the nation. As a result, the new state lacked a broad legitimacy, and the immense gulf between the 'real Italy' of the Italian population and the 'legal Italy' of the official institutions became a commonplace of Italian political thought.[139]

Nowhere in the nation were the consequences more evident than in the South. The Piedmontese were poorly informed about conditions in the Mezzogiorno, and their approach to southern problems was calculated to confirm the relative disadvantages of Italy's poorest regions. The northern conviction was that the South possessed great natural resources which were prevented from bearing fruit by the illiberal institutions of the old regime. It was necessary only to replace these structures with progressive Piedmontese models to free the economy of the South from its shackles. Thereafter a policy of *laissez-faire* rather than remedial action was considered appropriate. Since the voice of ordinary southerners found no expression in a parliament where a narrow suffrage and a property qualification restricted election to wealthy notables, the result in matters affecting public health was neglect.

At the national level, the Italian parliament created no Ministry of Health. Instead, it relegated the problem to a department within the Ministry of the Interior directed by a layman with no medical qualifications. This Department of Public Health throughout the period leading to the epidemic of 1884, functioned as little more than a postal address. With a skeletal staff and a minimal budget, it took no major initiatives and made little effort even to enforce existing legislation in the field. Thus, although the law stipulated that every commune appoint a public health doctor or *medico condotto* to attend to the needs of the poor, still by 1878 over 2,000 communes had failed to make appointments to the position, and these offending municipalities were concentrated in the South, where the need was greatest. Similarly, the Department ignored sanitation in penal institutions and at the workplace, and it allowed considerations of economy to prevail in the administration of the hospital service. The Department commissioned few studies of the health needs of the nation and undertook no planning to confront the possible contingency of epidemic disease. When cholera nevertheless appeared in each of the first three decades after 1861, the state responded with hurried and inadequate improvisation.[140] As the disease approached again in 1884, the Royal Hygiene Society protested that, in what was ostensibly a modern state, the administration of public health was crippled by rickets.[141]

Unhappily for Neapolitans, there were no countervailing forces at work on the local level. On the contrary, the same processes that fostered sanitary neglect in Rome were reproduced in microcosm in the chambers of the Palazzo San Giacomo. One factor was financial. National fiscal policy provided the constraints within which local decisions were taken. State policy devolved the responsibility for education, health care and sanitation upon local government, which had to finance these services from its own resources. In impoverished Naples, the inevitable result of such a strategy was that City Hall had no resources to meet the urgent needs of the population.

In any event, the composition of the municipal council ensured that the needs of the unemployed, the homeless and the under-nourished who formed such a large proportion of the population were not prioritized. In Naples the result of unification was to produce what, paraphrasing Gramsci, might be described as a 'revolution without a revolution', that is, a political transformation accompanied by a minimum of social and economic consequences and an absence of popular involvement. The Liberals who assumed the governance of the city after the overthrow of the Bourbons had no radical ambitions for change, and they were content to make their peace with the established local elites. Protected by the bulwark of the property-based male franchise, these elites dominated local affairs as the grand electors of the city.

The councillors were not, of course, unanimous in their views. On the contrary, the council was divided by 1884 into three major political factions. The first was the Historical Right organized by the local 'Constitutional Association'. The Right represented continuity with the original political aspirations of moderate Piedmontese Liberalism. Mayor Nicola Amore, who faced the emergency posed by the return of Asiatic cholera, was the leader of the Right. The second faction was the Historical Left represented by the Neapolitan 'Association of Progress'. The Left was the loyal opposition that advocated more audacious reforms and greater attention to the needs of the city. Finally, there was the Catholic faction of notables termed 'clerico-moderates' who fought elections under the banner of the 'Association for the Interest of the Economy'. They were unhappy with the Risorgimento and the resulting secularization of political life, but they urged that Catholics make their peace with the new order.

For the purposes of municipal governance, the presence of three large political factions complicated the task of implementing a coherent line of policy because there was no stable majority among the councillors. In the decade prior to 1884 mayors from the three competing currents succeeded one another as local authority lurched from crisis to crisis.

What was common to all of the eighty Neapolitan city councillors was the narrowness of their social and class origins. Chosen by thousands of propertied electors in a great metropolis, the councillors were unrepresentative of the general population. According to the electoral law of 1882, the franchise was restricted to males over the age of twenty-one years of age who satisfied the requirement of literacy by means of a certificate of primary education and who met one of the following property qualifications:[142]

taxpayers: a contribution of 19.8 lire a year in direct taxes
tenant farmers: annual rent payments of 500 lire
sharecroppers: holdings assessed for 80 lire in annual taxes
householders: annual rent payments of 150 lire

Nationally, this law entitled 7 per cent of the population to vote. In the the twelve boroughs of Naples the resulting electorate was restricted as Table 1.10 demonstrates.[143] Elected on the basis of such a franchise, the men who assembled in the chambers of the Palazzo San Giacomo were bankers, merchants, industrialists, aristocrats and professionals who possessed a university education and conducted their business in the foreign language of Italian rather than Neapolitan dialect. They were separated by a social abyss from the city at large.

Political corruption increased the distance between governors and governed. At the turn of the century the famous lawsuit of the Neapolitan deputy and Camorra boss Alberto Casale against the local newspaper, *La Propaganda*, revealed a systematic falsification of the electoral will of the population. Beginning with the precedent created in the 1870s by the Liberal Deputy Rocco De Zerbi, powerful figures in the local administration comprehensively perverted the electoral process, eliminating opponents from the registers of eligible voters; bribing undecided citizens with contracts, employment and cash; and hiring members of the criminal underworld to disrupt the campaigns of the opposition. On polling day in *sezioni* like Vicaria it was unsafe for the supporters of rival political factions to walk the streets. Elections conducted in such a fashion undermined the legitimacy of those in office.[144]

Only by recalling this rarefied social composition of the city government, and the illegal means that maintained it, is it possible to explain the sanitary conditions in which the inhabitants of the *bassi* continued to live. Ironically, all

Sanitary anxieties

Table 1.10. *Eligible voters in Naples for the*
municipal elections of 1875

Sezione	Voters
S. Giuseppe	1,900
Montecalvario	2,567
Avvocata	2,437
Stella	2,437
S. Carlo all'Arena	1,465
Vicaria	2,780
S. Lorenzo	1,555
Mercato	1,286
Pendino	1,089
Porto	1,587
S. Ferdinando	2,808
Chiaia	1,619
Total	23,135

three of the factions represented in the city council acknowledged the severe problems of the city, and each proposed reforms. The city commissioned studies of the great issues of housing, sanitation, water supply and sewerage. In the decade leading to 1884, the leader of the Left (the Duke of San Donato); a Catholic (Count Girolamo Giusso); and the dominant figure of the Right (Nicola Amore) served successive terms as Mayor, and each launched his mayoralty with the promise of ambitious programmes of urban renewal. The difficulty was that public health, although an officially recognized necessity, was always a consideration that followed far behind the need to balance the municipal budget and behind competing projects that enhanced prestige, patronage and the loyalty of the grand electors.

The achievements in practice since unification in the domain of public health were minimal, even nil. Eminent professors of medicine prepared extensive reports and recommendations, but 'those reports lie gathering dust ... unread, unopened'. Professor Ciro Marziale, in disgust, sent a copy of his proposals for the city to London, where he was honoured for his efforts and awarded the Order of the Bath.[145]

While the city drank contaminated water and scattered its waste in the streets, the councillors embellished the seafront of Chiaia with the handsome promenade of the Via Caracciolo for the benefit of the aristocracy; they provided illumination for the elegant commercial boulevardes of the Via Toledo and the Via Chiaia; and they voted subsidies of 300,000 lire a year for the opera season at the San Carlo Theatre.[146] The executive committee (*giunta*) awarded handsome terms to its contractors; granted licences to its friends; employed inflated numbers of clients who knew how to vote on election day; attended to the *per diem* and travel expenses of its members; granted lucrative subsidies and pensions; and drew up electoral lists.

Only the immediate threat of an epidemic produced a sudden flurry of activity. Councillor Gennaro Barbarisi described the *modus operandi* of the Town Hall as it confronted the first cholera epidemic to strike Naples after unification. At the earliest news of suspect cases in 1865, he reported,

> As usual in the case of cholera and all epidemic diseases, we begin by denying their existence, then we move to a time of doubt. We only accept the reality of their presence when it is too late to take preventive action.[147]

As soon as the emergency was over, Naples returned at once to its 'original neglect'.[148]

The major epidemic of 1865–7 and the smaller outbreak of 1873 both left the city no better organized than they found it. In 1884 Naples remained unimproved, and it still lacked a plan of self-defence. The correspondent of the *Corriere della sera* took the measure of the stagnation that prevailed in all sanitary matters on the basis of his own personal experience. Having lived through the disaster of the 1860s, he remembered the promises that were made to demolish the *fondaci*, improve the insalubrious quarters, build low-cost housing, modernize the sewer network, and supply the city with pure water. 'Now', he wrote in distress,

> twenty years have passed, and another cholera epidemic has arrived. I find that the aristocratic upper quarters of the city have been renewed, but the low-lying quarters where the people live have deteriorated further. The diet remains inadequate, the wine is still adulterated, and the water is both insufficient and more contaminated than ever.[149]

The Saredo enquiry exposed the inveterate practice of neglect that affected matters of public welfare. In 1900 Saredo reported that Naples was the city with the most urgent health needs in the kingdom. Nevertheless, the Town Hall spent less than 1 per cent of its budget on sanitation and hygiene, or less than 0.40 lire per inhabitant. More than twice the amount, both per capita and as a proportion of total municipal expenditure, was spent in Milan and Turin, where the needs were far less urgent.[150] Among all major Italian cities, Saredo concluded that, 'Naples more than any other is burdened by debt, and spends the least per resident on education, health and public works.'[151]

Saredo's views in this respect echoed the conclusions already reached by the mayors of the city. Reviewing the accomplishments of the municipality since unification, Mayor San Donato informed his colleagues in 1876 that the legitimate expectations of the citizens had all been disappointed. 'In the past sixteen years', he reported,

> Naples has accomplished nothing resembling the transformations that have taken place successfully in other Italian cities, such as Milan and Florence. Our programmes have remained in the realm of ideas, or else they have been aborted or left miserably unfinished. Naples is in a state of both absolute and relative neglect. This is true even though the city has made many heavy sacrifices.[152]

Naples, San Donato concluded, lived in a state of 'deadly inertia', surviving by a succession of short-term expedients.[153]

Thus the origins of the municipal regime in the 'passive revolution' of the Risorgimento had serious consequences for health. But there was an additional result that affected the relations between Town Hall and the populace when the *giunta* attempted to undertake emergency measures in a time of medical crisis. The remoteness of the authorities from the population made this unpopular local regime fragile and therefore vulnerable during an emergency. This consequence became evident during the epidemic of 1884, when its brittle authority floundered and the Mayor and his aldermen risked losing control of events.

The city council had only a limited legitimacy among the people the respectable classes termed the *popolino* – the 'humble folk'. Expressed in Gramscian terms, the municipal government lacked hegemony in the Lower City because the institutions of civil society through which power is transformed into 'consent' were rudimentary. The mass of illiterate and impoverished citizens were beyond the reach of schools, newspapers, political campaigns, and conscription.

Furthermore, the distinction between benign *laissez-faire* and culpable neglect is a fine one, and there were factors at work that caused the inhabitants of Naples to view their governors as responsible for their hardships. One factor was the growing burden of regressive indirect taxes collected by the municipality, the most onerous and deeply unpopular of which was the consumption levy already considered. A further cause of distrust was the fact that another of the direct causes of impoverishment – the spiralling cost of rent – could be attributed to the Town Hall. Many councillors acted in their private capacity as urban landlords – to such an extent that in the new century the socialist paper of the city was to term them 'our landlord-councillors'. In addition, the benevolent associations (*opere pie*) and the Bank of Naples over which City Hall exercised control also owned extensive urban properties. The municipal councillors on their boards of directors did not, however, intervene to impose rent control. Indeed, the city government was consistently solicitous of the prerogatives of private property. As the Head of the Municipal Department of Engineering, Giulio Melisurgo, explained, one of the reasons for the unhealthy condition of housing in Naples was that the city had never enacted a building code imposing minimum standards on landlords.[154]

Finally, there was a religious division between the people of Naples and their governors. Unification had taken place against the opposition of the Church. The Risorgimento entailed the creation of a secular regime at odds with the Vatican. Pope Pius IX declared himself a prisoner in the Vatican, and ordered that Catholics should play no part in the political life of the state. In Naples, where the Church had enjoyed a position of privilege and power under the absolutist order, the clergy opposed both the national state and the Liberal Town Hall. The result was a distance from the population among whom the Church exercised a large measure of influence.

Naturally, the religious issue requires qualifications and distinctions. Popular religion among the poor and illiterate is better described as pagan superstition than the official theology of Rome. Furthermore, the lower clergy were often of humble social origins and nourished their own grievances against the rigid and hierarchical authority of the bishops. Parish priests often had a more audacious political vision than their social and ecclesiastical superiors, and there were many who favoured an accommodation with the local authorities. There was even among the Catholic laity a current of clerico-moderates who contested municipal elections, sat in the city council and shared in the responsibilities of aldermanic office. Nevertheless, the dilemma for the occupants of the Palazzo San Giacomo was that the Church possessed a more continuous and visible presence in the Lower City than the municipal officials, and the teachings it imparted weakened the authority of office-holders who swore loyalty to King Victor Emmanuel.

Commenting broadly on the attitude of the population towards the municipal authorities, Raffaele Parisi commented,

> The dominant factor is distrust. After twenty-four years distrust is now bursting out among the people because the ruling classes ... have done nothing for their moral and material betterment. When we walk through the sunken and filthy streets of Mercato, Porto and Pendino, we find them just as they were in 1860.[155]

In articles in the press he reiterated that everywhere he encountered 'a lack of confidence, or rather a total suspicion of all authority, of all public officials, high and low'.[156] Parisi knew the Lower City well because he served throughout the epidemic in 1884 as the Deputy Director of the volunteer service in the anti-cholera campaign. His views were echoed by the prefecture, which used terms such as 'weariness' and 'scepticism' to describe political life in the former capital.[157]

Thus when the city council sought at last to take vigorous measures to combat the epidemic, there was no time to overcome the legacy of neglect and distrust. When notices went up throughout the Lower City in September 1884 proclaiming that the municipal officials were interested, almost for the first time, in the health of the people, the response was scepticism. It further transpired that the measures the city intended to take were violent and draconian. The city proposed to send armed municipal guards and unknown health officials into the homes of the poor to carry away their critically ill relatives and to destroy their personal effects. Under the pressure of such a threat, the simmering suspicion of authority turned into terror and a desperate resistance.

DOCTORS AND HOSPITALS

Such distrust extended specifically to physicians in the city, despite major advances in the position of the Italian medical profession since unification. As the *Lancet* recognized, the Liberal regime provided a favourable environment for advances in the standing of medical practitioners. After 1861 state encouragement of education, the identification by the national movement of progress with science, the constitutional guarantees of freedom of association and the lifting of censorship enabled the liberal professions to flourish.[158] Commenting in 1876, the journal observed that, 'Medicine, as a science and as an art, is advancing in Italy, her professional journals are improving in quality as well as augmenting in numbers, and a more practical spirit presides over her medical congresses.'[159] Furthermore, political unity promoted professional unity. After 1861 the Italian Medical Association, founded in Piedmont in 1850, established its presence throughout the peninsula, and it was followed in 1874 by the National Association of Medical Ethics.[160]

Naples in particular enjoyed a prestigious position as one of the foremost medical centres in the nation. With the only school of medicine in the South of Italy, the University of Naples possessed one of the largest and most prestigious medical faculties on the Continent. It enrolled 2,000 students in 1884 and boasted a distinguished professoriate, which included such luminaries of the international scientific community as the psychiatrist Giuseppe Buonomo, the clinicians Errico De Renzi and Mariano Semmola, the hygienist Marino Turchi and the bacteriologist Arnaldo Cantani.[161] Neapolitan physicians published seven of the sixty-eight medical journals in Italy, including the *Rivista clinica e terapeutica*; staffed eight hospitals; and organized a range of societies capped by the prestigious Royal Neapolitan Academy of Medicine and Surgery. Such was the fame of the elite of local practitioners that throughout the Mezzogiorno, aristocrats and the wealthy middle classes with serious medical complaints, as well as poor people with access to patronage, aspired to a consultation with a Neapolitan professor of medicine. It was emblematic that, at the time of his final illness in 1883, Don Fabrizio, Prince of Salina and protagonist of Giuseppe Tomasi di Lampedusa's novel *Il gattopardo*, travelled from Palermo to Naples for the opinion of Professor Mariano Semmola.[162]

A major irony was that the presence of a centre of medical excellence was of little relevance to the health of most Neapolitans. One reason was that the medical profession of the province of Naples, consisting of 1,195 physicians in 1886, was divided into two vastly unequal components. The overwhelming majority of these doctors were involved in private practice and had little professional contact with the impoverished inhabitants of the Lower City. Outpatient care for the general population was provided through the services of a mere 154 public health doctors (*medici condotti*) for the whole of the province.[163] In 1900 the city itself, permanently short of funds, employed only eighteen public health doctors, plus seven more for the four 'villages' in the immediate hinterland. Even if the average *medico condotto* had been highly qualified, motivated and devoted to his[164] duties, there were too few practitioners to provide even a skeletal service for so large and unhealthy a population. If only for reason of numbers, the public health doctor was inevitably a remote figure rarely seen in the alleys of the Lower City and seldom present in the medical dramas of everyday life.

The assumption of a conscientious and dedicated service, however, is unrealistic and makes it impossible to comprehend the antipathy of the people towards the municipal doctors that was so prominent a feature of the tumults of 1884. In practice, the *medici condotti* employed by local government were newly qualified junior doctors hired on the strength of the qualification that their employment, which was a legal obligation of local government under Italian law, would weigh as little as possible on the city budget. *Medici condotti* in Liberal Italy were poorly remunerated, demoralized by the impossible task they confronted, and denied authority either within the profession or in the larger community. Their standing in the eyes of the public was compromised further by the conditions of their appointment and tenure. In Neapolitan circumstances, the *condotte mediche*, like all municipal offices, were filled on the basis of favouritism, nepotism and clientage. As the Saredo enquiry revealed at the turn of the century, the municipal service 'left much to be desired'.[165] Many Neapolitan public health doctors, far from dedicating themselves to the public welfare, were pluralists who 'were distracted from attending scrupulously to the needs of the poor'.[166] Some maintained more lucrative private practices; others held hospital and teaching appointments, sometimes requiring their presence on a daily basis outside the city; and many lived far from their offices and were unavailable when emergencies occurred.[167] In any case, the poor were deterred from seeking their assistance by the fact that, although a consultation was free, the commune made no provision for the cost of medicines and any prescribed dietary regimens. In general, Saredo concluded, the inhabitants of Lower Naples had recourse to a doctor 'only in the most serious emergencies', and many residents not only had never been examined by a physician but did not even know that public health doctors existed.[168] Inevitably, the *medici condotti* inspired little confidence among the people. Eminent professors like Cantani and Semmola had enormous prestige, but the mantle of their authority did not envelop the young men who held municipal appointments. They were virtual strangers in the community.

The scarcity and inadequate quality of the attention provided free to the public were major sources of the hostility that confronted municipal doctors when they sought to intervene energetically in the Lower City during the emergency of 1884. Aspects of private practice compounded the problem. A glaring contradiction was that, while the public service was starved of personnel, the private sector suffered from glut. Under the existing distribution of income and demand for medical services, there was an oversupply of physicians, with over 1,000 physicians already competing for scarce clients and the medical faculty awarding hundreds of additional degrees every year in a city in which there was no market for their skills. The profession was divided, therefore, between an elite of society physicians and professors of medicine on the one hand and a medical surplus army that 'lived from hand to mouth' in educated poverty. So great was the problem that the profession was seriously concerned about a crisis of recruitment in which it was failing to attract into the profession the most able and ambitious young men. There were serious implications as well for morale and for the standing of practitioners in the public eye.

The quality of hospital care further complicated the crisis and undermined public health. There were eight civilian hospitals in the city, all originally established under the aegis of Catholic benevolent associations known as *opere pie*.[169] With the political revolution of 1861, the hospitals became hybrid institutions. They gained access to municipal finance, and in exchange they became publicly accountable for their performance and representatives of the city council became members of their boards of governors. The wards of these institutions were important points of contact between private physicians and the poor because hospital appointments formed part of the private sector. This contact was not likely, however, to have served the interests of the city or to have improved the relations between doctors and patients.

On the contrary, the hospitals of Naples contributed heavily to poisoning the atmosphere between the medical profession and the people. One reason was the confessional legacy. There were glaring contradictions between the terms of the medieval benefactions that had founded the hospitals and the changing medical requirements of a modern metropolis. A major example is that the *opere pie* had been instituted to give as much attention to the spiritual well-being of their patients as to their physical needs. A major portion of the income from their endowments, therefore, was allocated to devotional rather than curative purposes. In 1886, for instance, the combined *opere pie* of Naples province spent 4,341,655 lire on charitable purposes, of which 2,229,874 were allocated for hospital treatment and care, 231,911 for medicines, and 1,001,471 for religious devotions.[170] Similarly, physicians, employed for purely secular objectives, often found themselves in conflict with the sisters of charity. These nuns acted as nurses on the wards, but formed part of a very different disciplinary structure, lacked formal medical training and saw their task in religious rather than scientific terms.

Furthermore, the stipulations of long-deceased benefactors rather than the emerging medical needs of the population and the evolving boundaries of medical specialisms dictated the parameters of the service provided by individual infirmaries. An obvious example was the Pilgrims' Hospital, which was founded to care not for Neapolitans but for pilgrims from afar who were suddenly stricken ill or injured in accidents while visiting the reliquaries and holy shrines of the city. For similar testamentary reasons, the Loreto met the needs only of the male residents of the great Neapolitan poorhouse, the Albergo dei Poveri, even turning away seriously ill patients who collapsed at its doorway; the Hospital of Santa Maria della Vita served as the counterpart of the Loreto for the female paupers residing in the poorhouse; and the Hospital for Incurables treated only a narrowly circumscribed range of chronic illnesses. The Pace and the S. Eligio hospitals attended to the acute illnesses of Neapolitans, the former treating men and the latter women. Moreover, in a century which began with the celebration of the Paris Clinic as the incarnation of modern, scientific medicine, Naples possessed only the Gesù e Maria as a place of instruction and a source of clinical knowledge. By 1884 the Gesù e Maria was a dilapidated relic – crumbling, overcrowded and unhygienic. Finally, and most troubling of all in a city repeatedly devastated by epidemic disease, Naples possessed no institution at all to cope with the sudden emergencies created by infectious and epidemic diseases. The city council found itself in the untenable position of expecting a return of the cholera while having no facility that could accommodate and isolate the victims.

Thus religious obligations and the original terms of benefactions seriously distorted the structure of hospital provision in the city and drained resources from purely medical requirements. Most crippling of all, however, was a severe long-term financial crisis, which prevented the hospitals of the city from providing even the semblance of a service that was adequate by contemporary standards for one of the largest and most needy cities in Europe. The income from the endowments of the *opere pie* and the allocations of a city council in financial disarray were woefully inadequate to meet the medical needs of half a million inhabitants. For this reason there was in the closing decades of the nineteenth century a consensus among contemporary commentators that Naples faced a severe hospital crisis. The hospitals in the city lacked a sufficient supply of beds and facilities; the buildings were inadequately maintained; the staff was neither sufficiently numerous nor fully trained; and the morale of the physicians was low. Inevitably, standards of care were affected, and this fact surrounded the institutions with an evil reputation. When cholera returned, Neapolitans were terrified at the thought of being forcibly hospitalized.

PART II

The public epidemic of 1884

2

From Provence to the Bay of Naples

Before reaching Naples in the summer of 1884, cholera had long been expected. The endemic home of the disease was in the Ganges–Brahmaputra Delta in West Bengal. Until the nineteenth century, the *Vibrio cholerae* had proven too perishable to survive the journey from the sub-continent to western Europe. In the new century, however, the steamship and the railroad transformed the length of voyages. At the same time the growing economic and military presence of the British in India multiplied the contacts between East and West. The medical consequence was that cholera for the first time acquired the means of spreading far beyond its original Asiatic habitat.

Six times between 1830 and the First World War cholera spread from Bengal to the West along two great microbial highways. To the north it followed the trade routes to the Punjab, Afghanistan and Persia. Having crossed the Caspian Sea, the germ passed into Europe at Astrakhan and Orenburg, and then journeyed up the Volga to Moscow and the heart of the continent. Alternatively, cholera travelled to the south – overland to Bombay and Madras, then by sea to Ceylon and Jedda. It then accompanied the pilgrims to Mecca, and dispersed with them to Egypt and the Mediterranean seaports.

The renewed menace to Naples began in 1881, when the bacterium began its fifth and penultimate voyage to Europe. In 1883 it reached Egypt with Muslim pilgrims and with Indian troops serving in the British army of occupation. The frightful carnage in Egypt, where 60,000 people perished in the course of a few months,[1] raised the alarm throughout the Mediterranean. Carefully following the progress of the epidemic, the Italian authorities grew apprehensive, but were reassured as cholera seemed to reach no further west than Alexandria. From Naples the American consul reported in late June that the Egyptian disaster had caused 'great alarm' and that, as a precaution, the state had re-activated the quarantine station on the neighbouring island of Nisida, where all vessels bound for Naples from Egyptian ports were directed.[2] In July 1883, unknown to Italian officials, there was in fact a brief but undisclosed flare-up at Marseilles. This outburst was confined to seven cases and two fatalities that were all kept secret

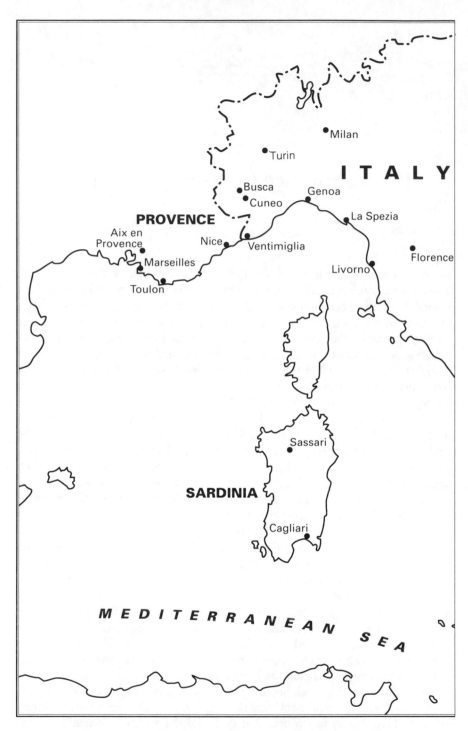

Map 2.1 Italy and Provence

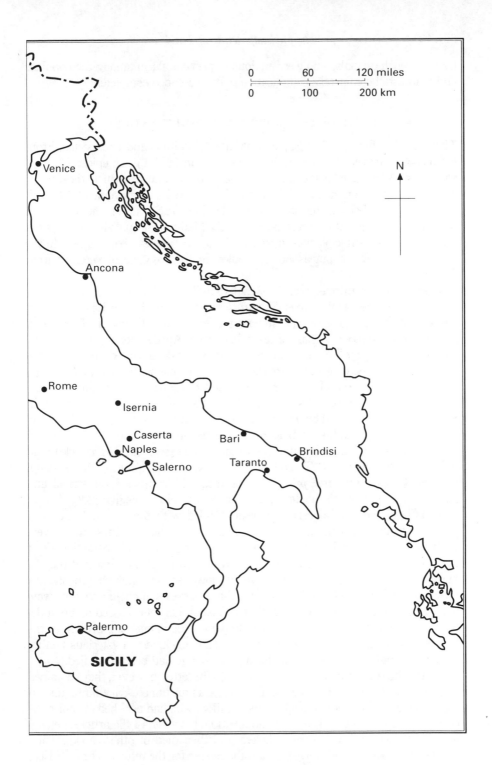

0   60   120 miles

0   100   200 km

N

Venice

Ancona

Rome

Isernia

Caserta

Bari

Naples

Brindisi

Salerno

Taranto

Palermo

SICILY

by the French officials, who were anxious to prevent alarm among the populace and to forestall commercial complications.[3] Italy escaped completely.

KNAPSACKS, GERMS AND IMMIGRANTS

The road that finally led to Naples was more circuitous and unexpected. From India cholera travelled east as well as west, and in 1884 a great epidemic swept south-east Asia, then in the throes of the colonial war by which the French established their domination of the future Indo-China. The movement of French troops and ships between the naval base at Toulon and Saigon via the Suez Canal provided the vibrio with a direct passage to the Mediterranean. With good reason the fifth cholera pandemic was known in Europe as the 'eastern plague'.[4] In the late spring of 1884 it put ashore at Toulon in the baggage of veterans from Tonkin.

There were unconfirmed reports of cholera at Toulon by local doctors as early as April when the naval steamer *Shamrock* arrived from the Far East. It carried suspect baggage and a marine suffering from severe diarrhoea. There was, however, no evidence of a chain of cases linking the April sufferer to the full-scale outburst in late June.[5] A more probable and better documented vehicle for the transmission of the cholera to Provence was the transport vessel *Sarthe*, which returned to Toulon on 3 June after delivering provisions and ammunition to the French forces in Tonkin. Its return, after a passage of forty-five days from Saigon, had been delayed by an outbreak of cholera among the crew. The vessel was placed in quarantine at Saigon, disinfected and scrubbed. Its cargo was unloaded and fumigated. The naval authorities then gave the *Sarthe* a clean bill of health and ordered it to Toulon. Since no cases occurred during the crossing, the vessel was given 'free *pratique*' – or medical clearance – on arrival and allowed to dock. Only the medical officer on board voiced misgivings.[6]

In its hold the *Sarthe* carried knapsacks filled with the personal effects of sailors and marines who had perished in the Far East, and these items were auctioned for the benefit of the fleet. French naval regulations forbade the sale of the clothing and linen of men who had died of cholera, stipulating that they be burned in Tonkin. There was controversy, however, over how rigorously this provision was enforced, and it is possible that the goods of cholera victims were among those sold to the crew of the fleet in Toulon harbour. Folded damp in the hold of a ship, such items were widely known to be dangerous, even after the six-week crossing from Tonkin. There were rumours that a mysterious fatality among the engine-room personnel during the voyage had been concealed.[7]

Even if the regulations had been enforced to the letter, however, they contained two important and fatal loopholes. The first was an unnecessary ambiguity. It was mandatory that the personal effects of sailors who had perished of cholera be consigned to the flames. There was no mention, however, of the articles belonging to men who recovered from cholera and then died of other causes. Their articles were packed and stowed aboard the *Sarthe* for the return to France. Here was a careless oversight. The second loophole reflected instead the still imperfect understanding of the aetiology of cholera. Mild cases were not recognized as Asiatic cholera, and the dangers posed by asymptomatic carriers were still unknown. Thus the unhappy transport arrived with live cholera bacilli aboard.[8]

The results were soon apparent. During the second week in June the knapsacks from the *Sarthe* were emptied and their contents sold in the Toulon barracks and aboard vessels anchored in the harbour. On 14 June the first case appeared when a sailor aboard the *Montebello* was stricken, followed the next day by a fellow member of the ship's-company. Other cases then broke out on the *Jupiter* and the *Alexandre*. It is impossible retrospectively to establish the responsibility of the *Sarthe* – or any other vessel – with absolute certainty. The fact that the first victims of the epidemic were sailors and marines, however, clearly established the connection between the epidemic and French military action in the Far East. The populace immediately made the link, and there were widespread demonstrations against the government of Jules Ferry and its policy of colonial expansion. Frank Mason, the American Consul, informed Washington that, 'The epidemic that now prevails at Marseilles and Toulon is Asiatic cholera, imported, beyond all reasonable doubt, from Saigon, China, by the French transport *Sarthe* to the port of Toulon.'[9]

The sufferers were removed to the Naval Hospital ashore for treatment, and their illness was kept secret by both municipal officials and the national government in the hope that the disease might be contained as effectively as the Marseilles outburst the year before.[10] Matters became more serious, however, on 21 June when the first civilian was stricken – a student at the lycée who had no contact with the fleet. The disease had gained a wider circulation. On 23 June there were ten cholera deaths in the city – three in the Naval Hospital and seven among the civilian population. The news was made public that cholera was at large in the city.[11] By 26 June thirty-two people were being treated in the cholera wards in Toulon and at the St Mandrier Hospital in the neighbouring town of La Seyne.

Toulon was vulnerable to epidemic disease. This great naval base was in a severe state of sanitary neglect that prompted *The Times* to describe it as a 'sink of putrefaction'.[12] The city possessed no sewerage or drainage system. The inhabitants emptied their chamber-pots in the streets, where the gutters poured into a single open canal that crossed the city in an evil-smelling flow. The canal in turn discharged the collected waste of 60,000 people into the shallow, tideless port. There, compounding the problem, a great breakwater prevented even the slightest rill from entering and clearing the harbour. The port was in constant danger of being silted up, and it remained navigable only by means of an annual dredging that released such overwhelming and foul exhalations that local doctors regarded the clearing measures as a danger to health.

The slums of the Old City provided additional opportunities for infectious diseases to flourish. Here poorly paid workers from the arsenal and their families lived in crowded and unventilated tenements that were dark, squalid and damp.

Most lethal of all was the water supply, which originated beneath the city streets in wells that were badly maintained and subject to constant contamination. Here even in normal years rates of mortality were frighteningly high.[13]

The sombre medical news in Toulon directly menaced its neighbour to the west – Marseilles, the third largest city in France.[14] The authorities, therefore, took immediate measures to combat the danger. All arrivals by sea from Toulon were subject to quarantine; the former imperial Pharo castle was requisitioned as a hospital for epidemic diseases; the railway station was placed under surveillance; the streets were washed and sprinkled with carbolic acid as a disinfectant; the sewers were flushed; and all dredging operations in the port were halted to prevent miasmatic effusions. The Mayor and the town council at Marseilles called unsuccessfully for still more rigorous measures. They appealed to the military to establish a *cordon sanitaire* to seal Toulon hermetically from the outside world. The Deputy Mayor also proposed official censure of the naval authorities for their negligence in handling the *Sarthe* and her cargo.

Unfortunately, it was too late for both censure and prevention. The nine days of secrecy between the first case on 14 June and the official acknowledgement of cholera on the twenty-third had allowed the disease to spread. On 25 June a marine who had recently arrived in Marseilles from Toulon before the quarantine was instituted was stricken, together with a labourer resident in the city.[15] By the 28th the press proclaimed that cholera had broken out in both of the great seaports of Provence.[16]

This announcement caused consternation not only in France but also throughout the Italian peninsula. The French epidemic became the leading item of news in the press. Events in Provence also gave rise to debate in the Chamber, and they formed the staple of conversation. The municipal council of Naples discussed the outbreak and heard a statement from Mayor Nicola Amore on 25 June – the day following the announcement in Toulon.[17] One reason for such concern was geographical: Provence was perilously close to the frontiers of Piedmont. Furthermore, there was constant traffic between the ports of the two nations. More importantly, in time of epidemic the medical fortunes of southern France and Italy were linked by the massive immigration of Italians into Provence. In the early 1880s approximately 50,000 Italians crossed the French border every year in search of work.[18] The census of 1881 revealed that there were 240,733 Italians in France. The largest concentrations were in the departments of Bouches du Rhone and the Var, where there were 66,663 and 21,363 Italians respectively. Through them a cholera epidemic in France –and especially Provence – directly threatened Italy.

Nearly half the Italians in France were ex-peasants from the hills of Piedmont, who were joined by smaller contingents from Lombardy, Venetia, Tuscany and Emilia, and a trickle of emigrants from the Mezzogiorno, including some Neapolitans. Most were former small proprietors and leaseholders who had been driven off the land in Italy and attracted to France by the prospect of employment. Economic hardship drove tens of thousands of northern Italian peasants over the border to France. With the completion of a single world market, small producers growing wheat on dwarf plots with antiquated methods were unable to compete with the modern farms of the American mid-west or the black soil regions of the Russian Empire. As the price for wheat in Italian markets fell, peasants faced mounting debts and arrears. They also suffered from rising population, which placed growing strains on scarce resources; from the regressive Italian tax system; and from the enclosure of common land, which entailed the abolition of traditional rights of pasturage, gleaning, and gathering wood. A poor harvest or the death of a farm animal was frequently sufficient to transform a peasant into a migrant worker.

The causes of the exodus to France were documented by the Mayors of Cuneo province in Piedmont, the province that contributed the largest number of emigrants to the flow. They completed a questionnaire for the Ministry of Agriculture, Industry and Commerce in 1885 explaining the factors that led to emigration. In nearly all cases the explanation was poverty, which was vividly demonstrated by the fact that the departing peasants normally took with them only the money required to reach their destinations in France.[19] The Mayor of Busca, a commune that contributed disproportionately to the trans-Alpine migration, described the forces behind the movement as 'high taxes, failed harvests, especially of beans, and the low prices of produce'. [20] In the same vein, the Mayor at Cocconato mentioned 'bad agricultural years and the excessive sub-division of property'.[21] Generalizing with regard to the province of Alessandria, the Prefect wrote that, 'The difficult circumstances of the lower classes explain the phenomenon of emigration ... It is most common in the poorest communes of the province, where the aridity of the soil and the conditions of industry leave many people without resources.'[22]

In France the Italian immigrants supplied the large demand for low-paid, unskilled outdoor labour.[23] The Piedmontese lived in Provence as nomads, moving from job to job as navvies, dockers, miners, farm workers, domestic servants, street sweepers, waiters, and builders.[24] At Marseilles, at Toulon, and in the surrounding departments the Italians were a despised minority holding the lowest-paid, dead-end jobs. They occupied the worst slums, ate the most unwholesome diets and suffered the highest rates of illiteracy, disease and death. They were detested by the French middle classes for their poverty and by the workers as competitors who drove wages down. The Italian Consul at Marseilles noted in the spring of 1884 'an ever-growing antipathy towards our people, whom the French workers regard as formidable rivals'.[25] Although the overwhelming majority of the Italians were from the North, the French contemptuously termed them 'the Neapolitans' and not infrequently met them with violence. A genuine anti-Italian xenophobia developed, culminating in 1893 in the murderous witchhunt at Aigues-Mortes in the department of the Gard, where eight Italians were killed and fifty wounded.[26]

This barely tolerated Italian population was particularly susceptible to epidemic cholera. Indeed, the reason for the intense interest of Italians in the events of southern France was the fact that their compatriots were most at risk from epidemic disease. Marseilles and Toulon, where the cholera struck earliest and hardest, contained the largest concentrations of Italian workers – 60,000 at Marseilles and 10,000 at Toulon. It was they who endured the worst social and hygienic conditions in two seaports universally recognized as highly insalubrious. Having begun in the French fleet at Toulon, the disease moved rapidly beyond its original maritime niche. In July cholera ravaged the slums of the inner city where the Piedmontese construction workers lodged. They were employed in the public-works programme of improving the fortifications of the city and modernizing the arsenal. In July 1884 they fell ill in alarming numbers. The course of events at Marseilles was similar. There the first victims were native-born seamen, but the disease soon spread to the Italian quarters, where it raged with unequalled ferocity.

The official statistics of mortality at Marseilles in 1884 clearly demonstrate the unhappy fate of the Italians. The city numbered 340,000 inhabitants, of whom 60,000 (17.6 per cent) were of Italian origin. Between the onset of the epidemic in June and its end in October, 1,781 residents perished of cholera. Of the victims, 464 (26 per cent) were Italian immigrants. Thus for every thousand inhabitants, 4.34 Frenchmen died, but 7.82 Italians.[27] But these figures understate both the total mortality in the seaport and the unequal tribute of death paid by the immigrant population. The published rates of death make no allowance for the policy of repatriation adopted by the French and the Italian authorities. The immigrants were considered dangerously infectious by their hosts and perilously vulnerable by their own consular officials. The governments both in Paris and in Rome, therefore, took vigorous measures to hasten their departure. As a result, tens of thousands of Italian citizens left Provence in the early weeks of the epidemic. Therefore, the real rate of death among the severely depleted population that remained was undoubtedly higher than calculations based on residence would reveal. Furthermore, the French figures take no account of deaths that occurred among the medical refugees after their departure. And, finally, it was common knowledge that some cholera deaths were concealed while others were registered under false diagnoses by officials whose interest was to minimize the crisis in public health. The *New York Times*, wisely avoiding the temptation to quantify, noted simply that, 'A very large proportion of the victims at Marseilles and Toulon were Italians. Even in those sinks of contagion the Italians were dirtier than their native neighbors and they suffered more.'[28]

THE EMERGENCE OF TERROR

From the standpoint of the events about to unfold in Naples, the trials of Piedmontese bricklayers in Provence were of considerable significance. A marked feature of the Neapolitan tragedy was the extent to which cholera created not only a medical but also a social emergency. The basis of the social crisis was a pervasive panic among the populace. The news of the first deaths in Toulon,

The Times reported, caused a 'great scare' in Naples.[29] On 24 June – the day after the epidemic was officially confirmed in France – the Neapolitan daily *Piccolo* declared that Neapolitans had been 'seized by a great fear' and that 'in the city nothing else is spoken of'.[30] Stoking the very fear it described, the paper announced the following day that 'Cholera, then, is at our gates in the most threatening possible form, implacable in attack and as sudden as lightning.'[31] Naples, it concluded, was already doomed.

This cholera phobia grew daily and immeasurably increased the sufferings caused by the disease, giving rise to various acute forms of collective hysteria – headlong flight, riot, religious revivalism, the abandonment of the ill and the murder of doctors. It is important, therefore, to explain the panic. Part of the explanation is provided by such factors as the severity of cholera itself; the almost equal violence of the remedies applied by physicians; the memory of the carnage experienced in the epidemics of previous decades; the severe disruption of the economy that the epidemic left in its wake; and the misguided preventive measures undertaken by the state. It would be wrong, however, to explain the alarm that gripped Naples in the late summer and autumn of 1884 solely on the basis of developments within the boundaries of the city itself. The cholera epidemic arrived from France with a rich prior history and mythology of its own. This recent past was well known to Neapolitans because of the terrifying accounts by veterans of the French outbreak of their experiences in Provence and of the violent welcome they received on reaching Italian soil. These accounts were retailed directly by returning emigrants, thousands of whom were compelled to make an extended stay in the Bay of Naples. These first-hand reports were supplemented by the press, by wall posters throughout the city, and by multi-headed rumour. The terror that spread through Naples had a foundation in the odyssey of Italians fleeing southern France.

In Provence a distinguishing feature of the 1884 epidemic was the alarm that it aroused. A major reason was the official policy of encouraging the populace to take flight. On the day after the public acknowledgement of Asiatic cholera in Toulon and Marseilles, wall posters appeared inciting the inhabitants to save themselves by escaping. The basis of this advice was the medical theory of 'localism' or 'miasmatism' then dominant in the French medical profession and internationally best associated with the Bavarian hygienist Max von Pettenkofer. The localists' view that cholera was an atmospheric poison was neither new nor universally accepted by European cholera experts. For the previous half century, since the first European cholera epidemic in the 1830s, an important debate in the international medical community with regard to cholera, yellow fever and plague was the opposition of 'contagionists' and 'anticontagionists'. Recent research, especially by Margaret Pelling, has established that the terms of this debate were complex; that the lines of division were fluid and shifting; and that there was room for a wide spectrum of intermediate positions. The profession was not neatly split into two clearly demarcated and warring camps. There were, however, two contrasting poles of opinion that produced heated exchanges.[32]

Contagionists tended to argue that the three great epidemic diseases of the century were spread from person to person in the manner of smallpox and syphilis. For the anticontagionists, instead, cholera was not communicable but, like malaria in the medical literature of the period, resulted from a general contamination of the environment that struck down those most susceptible. 'Localism' was a specific variant of the anticontagionist position.

The most rigorous version of 'localist' theory was Pettenkofer's 'ground-water' philosophy. Pettenkofer assumed the existence of a choleraic germ responsible for the disease. The germ did not, however, cause the disease directly by being transmitted from person to person. Its effect was mediated by a process of fermentation in porous, humid and alluvial subsoil rich in decaying organic matter. Under appropriate local conditions of topography, climate and pollution, the germ could thrive, emitting poisonous effluvia into the atmosphere that affected individuals who were predisposed by their constitution, diet or temperament. Based on painstaking topographical studies of major centres afflicted by cholera and on extensive epidemiological studies of previous pandemics, Pettenkofer's analysis provided a highly plausible explanation of many of the great 'cholera mysteries' that so puzzled the nineteenth-century medical profession. Pettenkofer conveniently explained why physicians and nurses attending cholera patients were rarely attacked themselves, why cholera showed a marked predilection for certain seasons of the year, why cholera did not persist permanently in the localities it attacked, and why the disease repeatedly devastated certain cities, such as Marseilles, while avoiding others of comparable size and commensurate urban problems, such as Lyons. Pettenkofer's theory was elegant, and it took into account the various 'germ theories' that became increasingly fashionable among cholera researchers from Filippo Pacini in the 1850s to Robert Koch in 1883. The great difference that set Pettenkofer apart from the 'contagionist' germ theorists was his insistence that 'germs' caused cholera, not directly, but indirectly through their poisoning of the atmosphere under certain specific local conditions of climate, soil and season.[33] More complex in his position than earlier 'anticontagionists', Pettenkofer preferred to call his view 'contagio- miasmatic'[34] or 'ecto-genous'.

In previous epidemics 'localism' had never received the rigorous and sophisticated formulation given to it in Pettenkofer's 'ground-water' doctrines; nor had the theory held such sway among the French officials responsible for public health. In 1884 the mayors of Provence, the naval command at Toulon, and the ministry in Paris adopted the localist position that choleraic germs, having fermented in the polluted subsoil and harbours of Toulon and Marseilles, had poisoned the atmosphere. The major thrust of the 'localist' position was extensive sanitary reform as a long-term measure of prophylaxis. Pettenkofer's position logically implied the clean-up of the environment. In the midst of a cholera epidemic, however, the view that the air is fatally poisoned leads to the immediate recommendation of flight. Pettenkofer himself argued that one means of escaping cholera was to flee the locality. The 'rapid evacuation' of centres of infection, he argued, was always a 'salutary measure'.[35] 'Those who lived in decimated areas could be removed and lodged in barracks or tents during the season.'[36]

Flight, of course, was no novelty in the history of epidemic disease as Boccaccio, Chaucer and Defoe remind us. Escape, however, was a course of action normally undertaken by a wealthy elite with means to finance the journey. A distinctive aspect of the events in Provence in 1884 was the attempt by the Toulon authorities to evacuate the entire population. Indeed, Mayor Dutastata, the most committed of all the advocates of flight, attempted to transform the traditional social bases of the exodus from a major epidemic. Toulon, the first European city to face the return of Asiatic cholera, actively promoted the departure of the indigent. Calculating that the poor were most at risk, Dutasta and his colleagues attempted to disperse them as a measure of public health.

On 24 June 1884 the local government at Toulon covered the city walls with posters calling on the people to abandon the town at once. The administration also gave particular thought to the most disadvantaged sector of the population – the immigrants from Italy. The Mayor, accompanied by the Deputy Prefect, the police commissioner and the Italian consul, visited the immigrant quarters in the Rue Navarin and advised Italian nationals to depart immediately.[37] Evacuation was the mainstay of policy. Echoing this officially sanctioned strategy, the local press urged departure. On the second acknowledged day of the epidemic *Le Petit Var* advised that, 'Many of our fellow residents have already left Toulon for the countryside or the interior of the Department. They have behaved wisely. The sooner we leave the city, the sooner we shall overcome the evil influences presently at work among us.'[38]

Policy successfully reinforced popular alarm. By 25 June – two days after the first announcement of the outbreak and a week after the first suspicious cases had spread alarm among the populace – 25,000 people had fled Toulon.[39] The station was jammed with desperate travellers. Unseemly scenes took place, and there were fist-fights for tickets. To finance their departure, the poor pawned their last possessions. Such was the run on their funds that the pawnbrokers were compelled to suspend operations and to borrow the needed capital.[40] Savings banks too were emptied of their deposits.

The roads were soon crowded with the carts of the poor loaded with all their belongings. In its hasty instructions to depart, the commune had given little thought to possible destinations. The countryside of the Var was soon filled with indigent workers bivouacking under trees and desperately looking for wild vegetables and fruit to assuage their hunger. Their state was one of 'abject and pitiful poverty'.[41] Despite their own fear and the encouragement of both the Toulon authorities and the Italian Consulate, however, large numbers of the poorest and most stricken sector of the populace – the 'Neapolitans' – felt trapped and unable to flee. Crowds of these penniless immigrants gathered outside the Consulate demanding free and immediate passage to Italy.[42] The municipality intervened on their behalf, providing 500 tents for their immediate use and calling upon the Italian state to implement their rapid repatriation. The government of Agostino Depretis responded to the emergency. Free rail tickets to the frontier were issued, and steamships were chartered to furnish passage. By 4 July *The Times* reported that Toulon had become a ghost town, deserted by 40,000 of its 60,000 civilian inhabitants, plus the 10,000 sailors and marines[43] of the port, who were moved to camps in the mountains.[44]

Mayor Dutasta was harshly criticized for creating a panic by the intemperate tone of his advice and by what *The Times* termed his 'ridiculous official placards'.[45] Many doctors, however, argued that fear itself was the best preventive measure of all because it so effectively promoted flight. The leading cities of Provence – Marseilles, Nîmes, Arles and Aix – all witnessed similar headlong flight. Only the proportions involved were different, because most of the communes of Provence adopted a policy of *laissez-faire* instead of actively stimulating a general evacuation. Marseilles illustrates the difference. By the middle of July 100,000 people had departed from the great Mediterranean port. This was a substantial exodus by any standard, but it affected less than 30 per cent of the population as opposed to the 65 to 75 per cent who fled Toulon.[46]

The atmosphere in Provence as it was experienced by tens of thousands of fleeing Italians is best described as social hysteria. The great cities were rapidly depopulated while within them belated sanitary measures were adopted that spread gloom and a sense of crisis. The streets were sprinkled with carbolic acid in an attempt to 'drown' the choleraic germs; tar and sulphur bonfires were lit at every corner to purify the air; public gatherings of every kind were forbidden; railroad passengers and their baggage were fumigated; and the sewers were flushed. The urban landscape was suddenly transformed beyond recognition by fire, pungent smoke, the unfamiliar smell of acid and the near-desertion of the streets. In this threatening environment all economic activity halted as factories and shops closed. Provisions became nearly impossible to find, and those who remained anxiously watched for the first premonitory symptoms, convinced that they were inhaling poison with every breath.

The Cholera Committee of the Academy of Medicine noted in disgust the 'excessive emotion' of the people – an emotion that 'dishonours our manhood'.[47] Signs of hysteria were everywhere. When a sailor aboard the steamer *Mistral* fell ill en route from Marseilles to Toulon, the captain and crew abandoned ship and took flight in the woods ashore.[48] Magistrates, municipal councillors, and health officials deserted their posts and escaped for their lives, including the grave-diggers of Toulon and the laundresses of the cholera hospital. The undertakers and the washerwomen were replaced by convicts who were pardoned in return for their hazardous service.[49] The atmosphere was made still more tense by an outbreak of cholera-inspired crime. In the half-abandoned cities of Provence burglars raided homes and looters plundered shops.

There was even a wave of cholera-suicides. Among the victims was the editor of the newspaper *Le Petit Var* and owner of a bathing establishment who faced financial ruin as a result of the calamity.[50] A young ship captain named Belot, suddenly afflicted with diarrhoea, thought that by destroying himself he could save his wife and children.[51] A stricken labourer leapt from a third-storey window to avoid being taken to hospital.[52] Five shopkeepers took their lives in the first week of July when trade collapsed and their livelihood vanished.[53] Rumour added to the anxiety by inflating the number of those who had killed themselves. It was widely reported, for instance, that the captain of the *Sarthe*, horrified at having unwittingly unleashed the epidemic, had taken his life.[54] 'The populace', wrote the *Corriere della sera*, 'is alarmed beyond the power of words to express.'[55] *The Times* noted that they were 'beside themselves' with fear.[56]

In this highly charged atmosphere superstition transformed natural events into dismal portents of doom. In the last days of June the weather turned stiflingly hot and Toulon was invaded by swarms of mosquitoes, just as in the great catastrophe of 1865 when 1,000 *toulonnais* had perished.[57] A frightened population interpreted the occurrence as an evil omen presaging calamity.

The theology of cholera generated further dismay when the clergy fulminated that the disease was the wrath of God. The biblical interpretation of death and disease is categorical: they are the 'wages of sin' visited upon mankind for disobedience to the Lord. Life and longevity, by contrast, are rewards for observing divine law and the commandments.[58] Mortality became Adam's fate as a result of his original transgression in the Garden. The only ambiguity was whether the cause of divine punishment was the Fall of Man in a general sense, or the specific evil of particular communities and individuals.[59] When individuals alone were stricken, the evidence in the Bible is divided. On the one side stands the example of King Herod. When he was smitten by the Angel of God and eaten by worms, there was no doubt that his own sin had brought about his fate.[60] On the other hand, in the case of a man who was blind from birth, Jesus taught his disciples that 'Neither hath this man sinned, nor his parents.'[61]

In the collective calamities of epidemic diseases, however, the emphasis of Holy Scripture is unambiguous. Pestilence is unmistakably divine retribution unleashed by the moral shortcomings of the sufferers. There is only one view, for example, of leprosy. Miriam,[62] Gehazi[63] and Uzziah[64] were stricken and their skin turned 'white as snow' for rebellion, greed and overweening pride. Even more dramatically, plague was specially reserved for foul crimes and irreverence. Thus the Angel of the Lord smote the Philistines for stealing the Ark of God. The Lord 'threw them into distress and plagued them with tumours, and their territory swarmed with rats. There was death and destruction all through the city.'[65] Similarly the Egyptians were condemned to pestilence for the Pharaoh's crimes of abducting Sarah and of hardening his heart against the Israelites and refusing to let them go. Epidemic disease was invariably a sign of sin.

Cholera, of course, was a new disease never mentioned in the Old Testament or the New. There was a broad consensus among churchmen, however, that the biblical view of leprosy and plague was applicable to cholera as well. In accordance with this interpretation, some priests on both sides of the Alps castigated the sufferers. The Bishop of Fréjus and Toulon issued a pastoral letter describing the cholera as 'the chastisement of Heaven' for a straying people, a well earned reproof for a flock that had left the way of the Lord.[66] The Cardinal Archbishop of Paris blamed the people for their hostility to religion and urged repentance.[67] The disease did not have natural causes, but originated in 'the spirit of revolt' against the Divine Will and in 'atheistic negations'. His advice, therefore, was not to resort to public health, but to imitate the example of Hezekiah, who fell ill with a carbuncle, but prayed, repented and was delivered.[68] Still more explicitly, the Archbishop of Marseilles and the clerical party interpreted the epidemic as the punishment that Frenchmen had brought on themselves by their materialism, their republicanism, and their votes for Radicals. Summarizing the conduct of the French clergy, the *New York Times* reported,

> The better part of the priests are doing their job nobly, but a few ignorant bigots among them have made themselves responsible for much of the mischief by seizing the opportunity to preach the doctrine that the plague is the result of the spread of radicalism.[69]

Thus the people fled, some of them with the fear in their hearts that they were being pursued by God.

On reaching Italian soil, the refugees often found that, there too, religion could add to the terrors of the homeward journey. In Italy as in France, the epidemic was regarded by the Church as a divine punishment. An illustration of the views the fugitives from Provence encountered after crossing the frontier is the work of Giuseppe Ferrigno, Dean and Professor of Theology at the seminary of Palermo.[70] For Ferrigno, the disease attacked Italy because, despite being a city of God, it had begun 'to listen to the bewitching sirens of the land of Egypt' and 'to plunge its greedy lips into the putrid fountains of Babylon'. The sin of the people was to heed the corrupting, secular doctrine of the Enlightenment. In its name Italians had rebelled in the Risorgimento, had turned against the Church, and had adopted Liberalism as their faith. Angered by the Italians' crime, the Lord scourged them with cholera. A year of Divine Judgment, argued Ferrigno, had come to Zion.[71] 'Haughty city,' he wrote to his countrymen, 'save yourself, if you can, from the thunderbolts of the Lord!'[72]

Ferrigno seemed almost to rejoice at the punishment of the Almighty. His glee was exceptional. The substance of his position, however, was sanctioned by the highest authorities in the Catholic Church in Italy. The archdioceses most violently stricken during the course of the epidemic that arrived from Toulon were Naples and Palermo. In both cities the cardinal archbishops circulated pastoral letters devoted to the cholera that were published with approval in the papal daily *Osservatore romano*. Their views strictly followed the Old Testament. Guglielmo Sanfelice, Archbishop of Naples, called on priests 'to persuade the faithful to placate the wrath of God so that He may call a halt to the scourge; to observe more carefully the Divine Law and the laws of the Church; to practise penitence and deeds of charity; and to avoid dissolute behaviour'.[73] Still more emphatically, Archbishop Celesia of Palermo reminded the faithful that it was a

Christian duty to recognize cholera as 'one of the scourges that God uses to punish the sins of men and the transgression of His law, and to recall them for their own good to contrition and repentance'.[74]

The Jesuits elaborated on the causes that had led the Lord to strike down the Italians and the French. According to their journal *Civiltà cattolica*, the epidemic served a salutary and timely purpose. God chastised His people for the familiar catalogue of moral failings – blasphemy, secularism, materialism, indifference to the teachings of the Church. In a bitter reversal of the famous charge by the Liberal Massimo D'Azeglio that violence and repression had been the fruits of papal rule before the Risorgimento, the Jesuit review argued that the misery caused by the return of cholera was the moral outcome of a generation of Liberal misgovernment.[75]

The original note sounded by the Jesuits was the notion that the deaths of tens of thousands of people also served a positive function. Asiatic cholera was a great educator, a *maestro*. Half a century of unavailing attempts by scientists and statesmen to control, prevent and cure the new plague demonstrated the weakness of human reason. In 1884 the people learned at last to jeer at mayors, prefects, cabinet ministers and doctors who were all powerless to help them. Cholera, therefore, was a much needed reminder of the infinite power of the Lord and of the need for faith in Revealed Truth. It demonstrated the impotence of science and exposed it to ridicule. As the nation faced the threat of painful and sudden death, only the Church had the means to provide solace, counsel and the hope of relief. The loss of so many lives was the modest price men paid for the salvation of their immortal souls.[76]

Furthermore, the disease could remind Christians of the errors of infidels. This theme ran through *Civiltà cattolica* from its first articles on cholera in 1865 – the first epidemic year since the founding of the monthly journal in 1850 – through 1911, the last major outbreak in Italy. In 1865 *Civiltà cattolica* reminded its readers that Europe was stricken as a result of the Muslim pilgrimage to Mecca, where 'peoples from every pagan sect' gathered together in 'nauseating filth'.[77] Moreover, as its first measure of public health at Rome, which was still under papal administration, the Holy See ordered a campaign to cleanse the Jewish Ghetto.[78] In 1910 the journal regarded gypsies as the source of the scourge.[79]

The Christian view of cholera as divine punishment for sin increased the hardship of the return journey of the refugees from Provence. More was involved, however, than biblical exegesis. Some clergymen even tempered the rigour of the doctrine of sin. For Archbishops Sanfelice and Celesia, for example, any direct condemnation of the victims of disease for their sins was tempered by the obligation of Christian charity towards them and by the recognition that the ways of God were always mysterious. Among the laity, however, there was a pervasive form of popular religion and superstition that contradicted all obligations of charity. This view was that sufferers were suspect and dangerous, both medically and morally. Such an interpretation was taken up with ardour by opponents of the Republic in France and of the Liberal state in Italy. In both countries the clerical right fanned the flames of Catholic prejudice to stir up opposition to regimes they hated. The correspondent of the *New York Times* observed that, 'The clerical party in France and Italy naturally, and doubtless honestly, takes the ground that the cholera is a scourge set upon the people because of the irreligion of their rulers.'[80]

The fact that the returning travellers were poor – 'third-class passengers' in the euphemism of the press – heightened suspicion by adding a dose of class prejudice, which combined in many places with a xenophobic view of outsiders. In newly and imperfectly united Italy, a 'foreigner' was frequently the resident of a different region or province. The result was a potent mixture of fear and moral outrage that led communities throughout the Italian peninsula to turn the returning emigrants away, greeting them with hostile demonstrations and armed vigilante groups. The first boatload of refugees from stricken France was met with such a demonstration in Naples. In Calabria terrified peasants opened fire on arriving railroad carriages and tore up the tracks, and villagers in Sicily attacked boats as they docked.[81] Everywhere the press described an atmosphere of 'panic', 'anarchy' and 'untold bad feeling'.[82]

If officials and priests, then, contributed to the panic, the medical profession played an important and highly visible part. The stakes involved in the medical diagnosis of the outbreak at Toulon had enormous political implications that thrust the luminaries of the French and European medical community into the limelight. The French Government was reluctant to admit the possibility that cholera had been imported from Tonkin for three important political reasons. The first was that the peregrinations of the *Sarthe* raised doubts about the competence of the French navy and the adequacy of French sanitary regulations. A second reason for extreme reluctance to accept a diagnosis of Asiatic cholera was that it threatened the economy of the nation, disrupting trade and the tourist industry. The third reason for reticence, however, was the most sensitive of all: to admit that cholera had been brought from Tonkin was to discredit the colonial mission of France in the Far East. The very first rumours of cholera in Provence brought trouble for the government and even the regime. Graffiti began to cover the walls of Toulon denouncing the ministry of Jules Ferry and calling for him to be lynched for a war that brought only epidemic disease to France. Scrawled across the city were such slogans as 'Death to Ferry!' 'Lynch Ferry!' and 'Tonkin has ruined France.'[83] The press began to castigate the policy of colonial expansion for exposing the French to disease, while the political Right and the clerical party began to see in public health a weapon to assail the Republic.

It was not only in the interest of science, therefore, that the government turned to the Academy of Medicine, appointing two of the most distinguished experts on its Hygiene Committee to conduct an official enquiry into the health conditions of Provence. Dr. Brouardel, the chairman of the Committee, and Dr. Proust arrived in Provence on 24 June with a heavy burden of political and medical responsibility. Their conclusion, announced in a series of despatches to Paris in the following week, brought temporary comfort to the navy and the state. The disease that had broken out in the South of France, they argued, was not Asiatic cholera at all, but benign 'cholera nostras' – simple diarrhoea – that was due to local causes and was not infectious. The *Sarthe*, the navy and the war for the future Indo-China were absolved of all responsibility.[84] Speaking for the government, the Minister of Trade, Hérisson, announced in the Chamber of Deputies on 27 June that the suspect cases in Toulon were not epidemic 'Indian cholera' but 'local cholera'.[85] This soothing conclusion was supported by the Inspector-General of the Sanitary Service, Dr Fauvel. In Fauvel's opinion, the disease was only 'sporadic' rather than 'Asiatic' cholera – a much milder and non-epidemic illness endemic to hot Mediterranean seaports in summer. As Fauvel revealingly stated at the opening of his speech to the Academy on 1 July, 'If it were only a question of scientific interest, I would not insist with such energy on my point of view. But unfortunately the reticence of my colleagues has damaging consequences for my country.'[86]

The difficulty with this reassuring and painless diagnosis was that it conflicted with reality. Every day that passed heightened public awareness that Provence was in the throes of an epidemic of Asiatic cholera and that local doctors, the naval command, the municipalities of the region, and foreign governments were taking measures in accordance with this fact. Brouardel reluctantly and publicly changed his opinion of the illness afflicting the South. In so doing, however, he merely added to the confusion. By 1 July he adopted the untenable position that the epidemic was indeed Asiatic cholera, but only a mild form that need not cause alarm. Meanwhile Fauvel and other members of the Academy loudly maintained their original position – that only cholera nostras was involved. In opposition, Louis Pasteur contended that the course of previous epidemics at Toulon demonstrated that the current outbreak was clearly Asiatic cholera. Fauvel's argument, he continued, was 'void and irrelevant to present circumstances'.[87] The effect of this sterile controversy was to discredit doctors in the eyes of the public. Eminent members of the Academy of Medicine were publicly divided in a heated and acrimonious debate that perplexed and mystified the nation. In August the Academy expressed grave concern at the impression the debate had made on public opinion.[88]

Confusing matters further, the German Government sent Robert Koch to Provence to report on the outbreak. During the Egyptian epidemic of the year before, Koch had discovered and named the micro-organism responsible for cholera; and he subsequently demonstrated its presence in the stools of cholera patients in Calcutta. The outbreak in Toulon gave him the opportunity to confirm his theory in a European context. During his stay in the South of France, however, Koch created an international incident when he held a public interview at the end of the first week of July. He declared that the disease had, beyond all reasonable doubt, been transmitted from the Far East; he castigated his French colleagues for their incompetence; he denounced the measures undertaken by the local authorities in Provence as useless or positively harmful; and he ventured the terrifying opinion that the epidemic in progress would rapidly sweep the whole of the continent.[89] In reply, the doctors from Marseilles reported that they regarded Koch's view that the *Vibrio cholerae* was the causative agent of the disease as merely one of many still unproved hypotheses; and Koch's great rival, Louis Pasteur, defended the sanitary measures undertaken by French local governments. This bitter and highly public division further undermined the authority of physicians. Furthermore, Koch's dire forecast and the enormous publicity given to it produced a general consternation. According to the *New York Times*, Koch's prediction raised the alarm to new heights and unleashed a 'vast exodus' from the region.[90]

But relations between French doctors and the victims of cholera, among whom there were such disproportionate numbers of Italians, were strained beyond a simple 'crisis of authority'. This aspect of the events of Provence is important because it provides part of the explanation for a pronounced trait of the later Neapolitan epidemic – the mortal antagonism of the people towards the doctors of the city. An aversion so profound that it sometimes led to assault and murder was stoked anew by the quality of the early contact between indigent Italian patients and the physicians of Marseilles and Toulon. Many aspects of this contact seemed almost designed to kindle suspicion and hatred. The best documented illustration is that of the cholera wards at the Pharo Hospital at Marseilles, the storm centre of the epidemic in Provence. A young English doctor, Paul Bassano, was employed there during the outbreak. He reported his observations to the *New York Times*, which corroborated them by sending its own correspondent to visit the Pharo. Both the English physician and the American journalist were shocked by what they witnessed, particularly during the early weeks. Conditions improved later, but for an understanding of events in Naples the first weeks were decisive.

A characteristic of the Marseilles hospital was the class warfare that was waged on its cholera wards. There the patients, overwhelmingly drawn from the poorest economic strata, were separated from the doctors by a yawning social chasm. According to the *New York Times* correspondent, the physicians at the Pharo regarded these victims as a formless mass of illiterates, paupers and immigrants whose individuality and personal fates were of no interest or concern. Constantly smoking cigars that were thought to purify the air and create a protective screen between the sufferers and themselves, the French doctors on the ward discussed cases 'as lightly as a shoemaker would tell you when you could have your boots.'[91]

Such disdain was corrosive of trust, which was further destroyed by the sinister reputation that the cholera ward acquired as a place of painful and deadly medical experimentation rather than cure. The poor of the city preferred to die at home rather than be treated at the Pharo. Undoubtedly a large part of the reputation surrounding the hospital was simply due to the hasty improvisation from which the institution suffered at the outset of the emergency when it lacked staff, medicines, and 'needful appliances'.[92] Fear itself complicated the task of the physicians because patients avoided the hospital until the most advanced stages of the disease and arrived already dying. The systems of cholera management practised at the Pharo were unexceptionable. They included the treatment widely recognized as best practice by the standards of the day – the administration of opiates (laudanum orally and morphine by subcutaneous injection) to relieve the spasms and diarrhoea that were two of the most distressing symptoms of cholera. The Pharo was also among the many medical centres that attempted in the course of this pandemic to replace lost bodily fluids by subcutaneous injections of saline solutions. Where the French hospital departed from accepted practice and generated anxiety among its patients was in experimenting with two systems of therapy that were its own innovation in the medical history of the fifth cholera pandemic – electric shock and the inhalation of pure oxygen. Electric treatment – a clear example of 'heroic medicine' administered to patients already in a state of total prostration and acute shock – was particularly mysterious and gave rise to daemonic reports by convalescents and survivors.[93]

More important, however, than the therapeutic principles of the Pharo was the exceptionally high mortality from which it suffered. In this respect the Marseilles hospital provided material for the already active imagination of a frightened population. In the early weeks of the epidemic, large numbers of cholera patients were admitted to the Pharo, but almost none returned as the hospital experienced a fatality rate of 95 per cent among its patients. Only later in July did this terrifying percentage fall to 65 per cent, which was still somewhat higher than contemporaries believed to be the result even in cases that received no medical attention.[94] Here was a statistical foundation for what the press reported as the 'almost incredible' hostility between the working-class population of Marseilles and the medical profession – a hostility that made it unsafe for a doctor to walk the streets of the city. Indeed, several physicians were assaulted when they ventured abroad, and carts bringing patients to the hospital were mobbed.[95]

The position of Italians in Provence was especially dramatic. The Italians were an unwelcome minority with a history of violent and exploitative relations with the French. They had also been urged by their host nation and by their own consular officials to depart forthwith. Now their relatives, friends and acquaintances began to disappear in frightening numbers behind the gates of the Pharo, and the few convalescents to emerge brought with them brutal and, no doubt, exaggerated reports. It was an easy step for overwrought minds to suspect that the distant physicians of the Marseilles cholera ward were involved in a diabolical plot to rid Provence of a surplus population of unwanted foreigners by mass murder. The seeds for such a conclusion had already been sewn by rumour. Wide currency was given in France to reports that medical men in Berlin had greeted the cholera as a useful form of genetic hygiene. It swept away the weak and the poor – those members of the population who were least fitted for the Darwinian struggle for existence. With the aid of epidemic cholera, their suspect and unwanted heredity could be eliminated, thereby improving the race and ameliorating the social question. This view bred a generalized antipathy towards physicians and all officials thought to share the Prussian eugenic position.[96] Working people speculated that French doctors were in league with the government in seeking to further the good work of the disease. The result was a rampant poisoning hysteria that ran ahead of the epidemic and prepared bitter social conflicts when it arrived.

Finally, the anxiety of the returning Italians had a material basis. Cholera confronted them with economic ruin. From the end of June they were suddenly made unemployed, and repatriated to a country whose poverty they had fled. The return journey was long and arduous as a result of Italian sanitary regulations, and during the trip the fugitives were forced to deplete their savings and to endure the confiscation of their personal effects. What awaited them in Italy was also uncertain and foreboding. If cholera broke out in Italy as well, the lesson of their experience in Provence, where all economic activity had ceased, was far from reassuring. The Italian economy, in any event, was undergoing the difficult process of adjustment to the world that had been created by modern means of transport. Suddenly confronted with the competition of more advanced industrial and agricultural powers, Italy faced a crisis of falling prices, reduced exports and structural adjustments. There were particularly acute tensions in 1884 because of poor harvests due to unseasonable rains and the vine disease of peronospera.[97] For the thousands arriving from Provence, there was little prospect of rapid employment. All too representative was the example of the Neapolitan worker Salvatore Nappa, who first lost his job as a labourer at Marseilles and then forfeited both his belongings and his savings at the frontier quarantine station. In the middle of the summer he found himself destitute in his native city, poorer and less likely to find work than when he first left.[98]

PEST-HOUSES AND SANITARY CORDONS

With the departure of tens of thousands of Italians from France, many of them exporting the vibrio as they fled, the further course of the epidemic was determined by Italian public health policy. The government of Agostino Depretis in this respect made medical history. It made a desperate attempt – the last on the national level in European history – to protect the nation by employing the arsenal of defensive measures developed in the seventeenth century as means of combatting bubonic plague – quarantine, lazarettos and sanitary cordons. These measures had made an important contribution to the elimination of the plague from Europe, and the hope lingered that they would prove effective against cholera as well.[99]

Against plague the first steps towards the establishment of a comprehensive system of preventive health measures were taken as early as the fourteenth century during the Black Death. Beginning in the city-states of Italy, authorities across Europe began to enact detailed and systematic 'plague regulations' to prevent and combat the disease. The specifics varied from place to place, but there were certain common strategies underlying the first attempts at public health in time of plague. Accepting the premise that plague was contagious, communities sought to insulate themselves from infection by forcibly banning the entry of travellers and goods from suspect areas and by isolating patients, burning their personal effects and sealing their houses. Most frequently when the authorities took action, they also banned public assemblies; ordered the removal of waste and the cleansing of streets; purified the air by burning sulphur in public squares; regulated the burial of the dead; and recruited personnel to enforce the emergency decrees and maintain order.

Despite this widespread evidence of improvisation and ingenuity by beleaguered officials and terrified communities, and despite occasional local successes, the attempt to contain the Black Death was largely unavailing. Ironically, the fact that the complex aetiology of plague was not understood was not the primary reason for this failure. On the contrary, the existing theory of contagion proved adequate in the seventeenth and eighteenth centuries to permit the eradication of the disease from western Europe – even though the complex interactions of microbes, rodents, fleas and people in causing plague were not fully explained until the twentieth century. The explanation for the failure of the anti-plague measures of the late Middle Ages is more administrative than conceptual. The varied and uncoordinated initiatives of decentralized authorities were unequal to the challenge of bubonic plague. The turning point occurred when the disease returned to the West in the seventeenth and eighteenth centuries. Then the prophylactic ideas inspired by contagionist medical theory were rigourously applied on a regional or national level and backed by the power of the early modern state.

An influential model of success in the defence against plague was the Venetian Republic in the seventeenth century. Venice was motivated by the permanent vulnerability that resulted from its extensive commerce with the Levant. The Venetian idea was that it was possible to insulate the great Adriatic port from any further invasions of plague from the sea. Their defensive measures rested on the inaccurate theory that the disease was a contagion that spread from the bodies of infected patients into the atmosphere. To seal the city off from the deadly contagion, the authorities constructed an enormous pest-house or lazaretto on an outlying island. All ships arriving from the eastern Mediterranean, where plague was endemic, were directed there for quarantine. A vessel from a suspect port was impounded, scrubbed and fumigated; the crew and passengers were disembarked and isolated; and the cargo, together with the personal effects of all those on board, was unloaded, turned in the sun and fumigated. Only at the expiration of forty days of quarantine were the goods, ship and travellers released from detention and allowed to enter the city. The reasoning was that isolation should be sufficiently long for any pestilential vapours from the bodies of the people, the bales of goods or the hull of the ship to be harmlessly dissipated. Behind its defensive ramparts, the Republic would be saved from infection.

Simple in principle, the establishment of maritime quarantine required a series of preconditions. The lazaretto was in effect a fortress where thousands of passengers and crew had to be policed, provisioned and isolated from all contacts with the city. Beyond its walls, it required a strong naval presence to compel unwilling and possibly terrified captains to anchor within its waters, and to prevent all attempts at escape or evasion. Within its precincts, the lazaretto functioned on the basis of detailed and complex regulations ensuring that thousands of passengers in different stages of their quarantine would be isolated not only from outside contacts but also from each other; and that the whole of each ship's cargo would undergo elaborate rituals of purification. The system worked most effectively when it was buttressed by regular intelligence on the health of the Levant provided by consuls stationed in all of the great plague centres of the East. Thus the procedures of effective maritime quarantine presupposed both a long experience of the disease, and the prior establishment of the bureaucratic, naval and administrative power of the emerging modern state.

Although the Venetian system of quarantine worked effectively in practice, the medical theory underlying it was seriously flawed. There were no pestilential miasmas that could be dissipated by prolonged exposure to the air; bubonic plague was not spread by simple contagion; and many of the rituals of purification were to no effect. But the imposition of lengthy and militarily enforced isolation upon all vessels arriving from the East was highly successful. The traditional length of quarantine – forty days – had no empirical foundation. The period of detention was suggested instead by Hippocratic doctrine and by the biblical travails of Christ in the wilderness. Since forty days substantially exceeded the incubation period of the plague, however, quarantine effectively guaranteed that any people or goods released were medically harmless. Quarantine was long enough to ensure the death both of the infected fleas needed to transmit the disease and of *Yersinia pestis*, the plague bacillus itself. Furthermore, the elaborate rituals of the lazaretto prevented the ship- borne black rat, that great bearer of fleas, from disembarking. Thus an inaccurate theory produced workable administrative procedures for dealing with the spread of bubonic plague by sea. The Venetian lazaretto demonstrated in practice that it could protect the city from disaster.

Within a generation the other major Mediterranean ports of western Europe engaged in the eastern trade also equipped themselves with lazarettos – Naples, Genoa, Valencia, Marseilles, Palermo, Corfu. By the end of the seventeenth century the menace to Europe from the sea had been sharply diminished. Plague continued to be imported, but it was contained with only two major failures. In 1720 bubonic plague spread from the lazaretto to the city of Marseilles, where it laid waste to the city, killing 60,000 of the 100,000 inhabitants. And in 1743 a ship from the East was allowed to anchor at Messina, which had no lazaretto, instead of being diverted first to Naples for the required forty days. The result was the last great outburst of sea- borne plague in western Europe.

But if maritime quarantine insulated the West from infection by sea, there remained the menace of overland trade arriving from Turkey through the

Balkans. Here the decisive intervention was that of the Hapsburg Monarchy, which in the eighteenth century divided East and West by means of a *cordon sanitaire*, a great swathe of soldiers stretching across the Balkan peninsula. The Austrian cordon was 10 to 20 miles wide and 1,200 miles long. It consisted of a permanent line of soldiers and sentry posts stationed to prevent anyone from passing, and with orders to shoot on sight any person attempting an illegal passage until he or she had undergone quarantine. One of the great armies of Europe thus assumed the task of isolating western Europe by land, just as the maritime lazarettos isolated it by sea.

Other nations also deployed their troops to surround and isolate local outbreaks of plague when they appeared. This strategy was successfully adopted in France, for instance, when the authorities confined the great Marseilles plague of 1720–2 within the borders of Provence and a portion of neighbouring Languedoc. Troops with orders to shoot on sight blockaded the roads, patrolled the coast, and halted river traffic. They also enclosed the territory within a great plaguewall hundreds of kilometers long protected by a moat, ramparts and periodic sentry-posts, and extended by the natural barriers of the Rhone, the Durance and the Verdon Rivers. At the same time naval vessels prevented ships from leaving the infected ports of Marseilles and Toulon. On land, the first line of defence was reinforced by secondary cordons manned by patrols recruited by individual communities to preserve their immunity. The measures of the civil authorities in southern France were reinforced by the threat of excommunication pronounced by the Church against anyone who attempted evasion. The rest of the nation was thus effectively isolated by military and religious blockade from all intercourse with the affected provinces. The isolation of Marseilles was not lifted for four years. Half the population of Marseilles perished, but France and the rest of Europe were saved.[100]

Finally, as the Ottoman Empire collapsed in the first half of the nineteenth century, the newly independent states of the Balkans imitated the Hapsburg success on their own territories. By 1850 bubonic plague, the immemorial scourge, was eliminated from the whole of Europe. The proportion of the victory that was due to the measures of quarantine, sanitary cordons and lazarettos rather than other factors is unknowable. The final conquest of the plague perhaps owed much to such imponderables as sanitary and dietary improvements, possible changes in the ecology of fleas and the replacement of the sociable, flea-bearing black rat by the retiring brown. The important point in understanding the response of European states to cholera is that the administrative procedures devised at Venice by sea and by Vienna on land were highly visible and were given full credit by governments and doctors. They also provided at least a measure of hope when a new and mysterious pestilence appeared from the East.

Thus when Asiatic cholera first invaded Europe in 1830, there was a strong temptation to resurrect the defences that had proved effective as a shield against the plague. The policy of combatting cholera by quarantines, lazarettos and sanitary cordons was carried out by the Romanov, Hohenzollern and Hapsburg autocracies during the first European encounter with the new threat.[101] The problem was that Asiatic cholera was not bubonic plague. The two diseases are transmitted in entirely dissimilar manners – one by flea-bite and the other by the ingestion of contaminated food and water – and measures effective against plague proved powerless to halt the advance of cholera.

After carefully studying the great experiment in central and eastern Europe at defeating cholera with anti-plague defences, Britain in 1831 drew the conclusion that they were useless. As the epidemic advanced across the continent, the Central Board of Health in London considered sanitary cordons and the employment of 'expurgators' to convey the victims to pest-house quarantine under military supervision. The vision of the Board was of a 'hedge of soldiery' outside afflicted towns and within 'a horde of expurgators descending on the house with carts and conveyances'.[102] The failure of such policies in the east, however, led the authorities to abandon the scheme, which was never revived in England. The British medical profession denounced the deployment of military force against cholera as 'folly' that failed to achieve its purpose while raising the spectre of riot and civil war.[103] Russia, Austria and Prussia also rapidly dismantled their coercive sanitary regime as ineffective.

The French government drew the same lesson. As the epidemic advanced towards its borders, the Academy of Medicine sent two of its most respected members – Auguste Gerardin and Paul Gaimard – to the Russian Empire to study the disease and the effectiveness of the various measures adopted to combat it. Their first visit to the Estonian capital at Revel persuaded them of the futility of militarily enforced isolation. Revel had been protected with the utmost rigour by a ring of soldiers, but it fell victim to a terrible outbreak that the cordon seriously aggravated. The residents, imprisoned within the city,

> isolate themselves with a zeal that seems to become the one fixed idea of their existence. All communication with the outside world is abruptly halted, so that in the space of a few days the city is seized with a general terror, forced to live on its own resources and compelled to make immense sacrifices to meet the pressing needs of its population. Thus the city traps within its perimeter all the factors needed for the active propagation of the epidemic it seeks to combat.[104]

The experience of Revel was repeated in city after city in the Russian Empire. Similarly, the Prussians attempted to defend themselves by means of a double line of 60,000 men along their eastern frontier. The cordon was maintained with the utmost rigour and at enormous cost, but with no demonstrable effect on the progress of the epidemic. The chief result of the sanitary zeal of the Prussian state was to spread terror among the people. The French investigators could only conclude in the strongest possible terms that cordons and quarantines were not only useless but positively dangerous.[105]

In the half century between the practical demonstration during the first pandemic of the failure of land-based quarantine as a defence against Asiatic cholera and the outbreak of the epidemic in Provence, the international medical community exhaustively debated the issue and explained the reasons. The experience of the first pandemic was regarded as conclusive, and this evidence was supplemented by the failure of quarantines in Malta in 1865 [106] and in Egypt in 1883. The Egyptian experience was the most recent. There the cholera spread throughout the country 'notwithstanding cordons maintained with a degree of severity and cruelty almost unexampled'.[107] By 1884 there was little unanimity among doctors with regard to most aspects of cholera. But on this question, more than on any other affecting the disease, there was a substantial measure of consensus among the leading authorities. Miasmatists and proponents of the *Vibrio cholerae*, Pettenkofer and Koch, Pasteur and Virchow, the French Academy of Medicine and the British Medical Association, the most eminent cholera authorities in Italy and the leading medical journals – all were united in condemning any public health policy that relied upon land-based quarantines, lazarettos and sanitary cordons.[108]

Sanitary cordons, it was widely agreed, were useless in halting the advance of cholera for a variety of reasons. There was a division of opinion as to whether cholera was water-borne or air-borne, and whether it was a disease caused by a micro-organism or a poisoning of the atmosphere arising from soil contaminated with decaying organic matter. Whether one accepted the germ theory of Koch, the 'contagio-miasmatism' of Pettenkofer, an intermediate 'contingent contagionism', or one of the other less widely shared views, however, there was general agreement that the disease could not be contained by military means. Koch's vibrio could elude sanitary cordons by flowing past them in water-ways, and Pettenkofer's effluvia were no more amenable to soldiery. Furthermore, it was accepted by nearly all investigators that there was a fatal difference in timing between the pace of the disease and the ability of the state to deploy troops. All too commonly the army sealed off a locality from which the disease had already moved on. Indeed, the fear of being trapped behind a line of soldiers virtually ensured concealment and flight at the first rumours of sickness within a community. Therefore, the attempt to enforce isolation had the ironic effect of both rapidly disseminating cholera more widely and creating a long delay before officials were first informed of suspect cases.

In the dawning age of scientific medicine, sound public health policies depended on accurate and prompt information. The threat of military force was instead the best way to sever the lines of communication between the populace and the authorities. Worse still, to move large numbers of soldiers, largely drawn from high-risk social groups, from locality to locality in unsanitary conditions was itself an excellent means of spreading an epidemic. A large part of the history of cholera was the story of the movement of young men in uniform. Similarly, to assemble large numbers of indigent and often unhealthy people in hastily improvised lazarettos, as the advocates of the policy of force proposed, was to expose the surrounding locality to serious risk. The lazaretto employed in the defence against plague had successfully reduced this danger by conscientious fumigation. But as Koch himself explained in his visit to cholera-stricken Marseilles, fumigation was useless as a prophylactic against cholera because the danger now travelled in the guts of the victims and not, like the flea, on their clothes.

Furthermore, the enemies of sanitary cordons argued, the idea that cholera could be combatted by deploying troops was dangerous because it created a fatal illusion. The best means of defence against cholera involved long-term and costly improvements in housing, diet, sewerage and water supply. To think that soldiers hastily deployed when the disease had already broken out could contain an epidemic of Asiatic cholera was to undermine the whole cause of sanitary reform. In Europe, by the 1880s the temptation to resort to cordons was strong only in relatively poor countries which had grossly neglected their cities. Cordons and lazarettos had become the poor man's self-defence.

Finally, there was an argument based on the weighing of costs and benefits. Sanitary cordons were blunt instruments of violence. Their deployment imposed upon communities already facing a terrible disease the additional burden of economic disruption and the terror of being indefinitely confined among the dead and dying. Cordons also encouraged waves of lawlessness and vigilante terror in communities not yet reached by the epidemic. Instructed by the state that the way to salvation was through the use of force, citizens in countries adopting the policy of military anti-cholera campaigns made savage attempts to isolate themselves from the danger arriving from without. The experience of sanitary cordons in the first pandemic taught the lesson that the military response caused greater social dislocation and hardship than the disease.

In 1874 the emerging consensus on the issue of land-based quarantine was registered by the Third International Sanitary Conference that met in July at Vienna. The nineteen nations represented at the conference passed a resolution condemning coercive anti-cholera measures – with the assent of the Italian delegation.[109] The eminent Neapolitan pathologist E. De Renzi, who was soon to direct the medical campaign against the epidemic in the borough of Mercato, reflected the orthodox position within the profession when he declared that land-based quarantines were 'a barbaric system, unworthy of the modern era, and utterly ineffective'.[110]

It was hardly surprising, therefore, that most European nations reacted to the threat from Provence by rejecting the rigours of military measures of self-defence. Britain, France, Germany, Switzerland, Austria-Hungary and Belgium immediately condemned the idea of sanitary cordons. More surprising was the contrary decision of Spain and Italy. The Italian decision in the matter of cordons, pest-houses and quarantine is of particular interest because, as the Neapolitan medical profession noted, 'never before had there been recourse to such a vast and rigorously devised system of measures of repression and containment'.[111] The strategy of coercive self-defence was applied to the letter. For that very reason, Italy became a vivid illustration of the uselessness of the anti-plague defences when deployed against the very different disease of Asiatic cholera. Despite being the country in western Europe to rely most zealously on sanitary cordons in 1884, Italy became the nation most ravaged by the disease. Against the advice of the best contemporary medical opinion, Agostino Depretis and the Secretary-General of the Interior, Giovanni Battista Morana, wagered on the analogy between cholera and plague as they revived the anti-plague protective system in the great emergency of the summer of 1884. Realizing that Italy lacked the defences recommended by the international medical profession, the Italian state belatedly resorted to measures that could be hastily improvised and that could at least re-assure the population that the government was responding vigorously to the crisis. In the haste of the emergency, Depretis and Morana dispensed with the advice of the medical advisory committee appointed to counsel the government on measures of public health – the Superior Health Committee (*Consiglio Superiore di Sanità*).[112] The Committee was not consulted in part because the policy to be pursued was at variance with the growing consensus of the medical profession.

Unfortunately, the desperate gamble of Depretis and Morana confirmed the warnings of the physicians in every respect. Cholera evaded the army and the pest-houses and raged unchecked throughout the nation. According to official estimates, cholera killed 50,000 Italians between 1884 and 1887. Particularly sobering to officials was the comparison between 1884 and 1865, when cholera invaded Liberal Italy for the first time. In 1865 the state opted to reject coercive measures, employing neither cordons nor pest-houses. It was not clear, however, that liberal means of prevention had served the nation less well than the attempt to repel the disease with military force. In 1884 cholera spread more extensively and more rapidly than in 1865, invading 858 communes as opposed to 348. Furthermore, the number of fatalities was almost identical in both years – approximately 12,000 deaths from cholera.[113] Although its contribution to the protection of the nation, therefore, was dubious, the military strategy was expensive, costing the treasury 1,781,560 lire.[114] In addition, as medical authorities had long suggested, the coercive experiment fuelled hysteria and social tensions. Morana himself concluded that experience demonstrated the 'practical uselessness of this rigorous procedure'.[115] In 1885 the Italian attempt to contain cholera by anti-plague means was abandoned.[116] Having witnessed the Italian debacle, the International Sanitary Conference meeting at Rome in 1885 reaffirmed the futility of *cordons sanitaires* in the fight against cholera.[117]

The medical profession had warned that reliance on cordons and land-based quarantines was the alternative to sanitary reform practised by nations guilty of gross neglect. Italian policy in 1884 was illustrative of the truth of this indictment. The decision of Depretis and Morana to resort to coercion was not the result of a considered sanitary strategy but a desperate measure based on the awareness of the extreme vulnerability of the nation. With Asiatic cholera rampant in Provence and multitudes of emigrants returning in terror, the threat to the health of the nation was direct and immediate. Confronted with this emergency, Italy was unprepared and defenceless. There had been no sanitary movement; there was no adequate public health infrastructure of cholera hospitals, public health officials and stocks of necessary supplies; there were few communes with pure water or facilities for the removal of waste; and there was no tradition of trust between the medical and state authorities on the one hand and the public on the other. Despite the long Italian experience of epidemic cholera and the awareness of the manner in which unsanitary conditions predisposed the nation to attack, Italy was as unprepared in 1884 as it had been a generation before when confronted with disaster in 1865 and 1866.

In this climate of sanitary neglect, the decision to resuscitate the anti-plague measures of coercive prophylaxis was a desperate gamble. Knowing that there was little hope of containing cholera once it crossed the frontier, the authorities turned to the most reliable instruments of the kingdom – the army and the police – to seal the borders and insulate the nation from disease. Such a decision was also politically expedient. As soon as the outbreak at Toulon was confirmed on 23 June, there was great pressure in Italy for the state to act vigorously. On 24, 27 and 28 June deputies in the Chamber questioned the government on its plans to defend the nation and demanded action. In the days that followed, the press helped to ignite a national cholera-hysteria, and communities throughout the peninsula began to undertake violent measures to isolate themselves from the threatening contagion. According to the medical student from Montepellier, Alexandrine Tkatcheff, who volunteered her services in Naples, the cordons responded above all to a psychological need. They provided reassurance as communities menaced by an invisible invader sheltered behind a protecting wall of rifles and bayonets.[118] In pursuing this strategy, the Italian Government placed itself at odds with the medical profession, but it gained the support of the general population. The American Deputy Consul-General, Charles Wood wrote of Depretis that, 'The Government has seldom been more strongly supported by the people than it is now in the precautionary measures it has taken against the epidemic.'[119]

Hasty improvisation characterized Italian policy. The decision to resort to quarantine, lazarettos and cordons was taken almost immediately after the announcement of the outbreak in Provence. Throughout the epidemic that followed, however, the details of the instructions emanating from Rome changed continually, revealing considerable hesitation and uncertainty. The length of quarantine, the status of Sicily and Sardinia that could be considered as special cases because of their geographical isolation; the feasibility of attempting militarily to encircle great metropolitan centres such as Naples as well as smaller towns; the recommended techniques for fumigation and disinfection – all of these issues were continually debated and the decisions taken were just as often revised. The first instructions, issued on 28 June, ordered a period of three days of quarantine, which was extended to five on 7 July and to seven days on the twenty-second.[120] In his official report on the epidemic, Morana acknowledged that he had entertained doubts from the start about the wisdom of the policy on which the ministry had embarked. But the public and their representatives in parliament demanded dramatic measures.[121] Paradoxically, a bold and resolute military policy was enforced with vacillation and inconsistency, generating suspicion, fear and an ever-growing sense that the state had lost control of events. It was all too apparent that Morana was fully aware of the strenuous medical objections to his policy. 'Anarchy' was the term that recurred in the press in reference to Italian public health.

Patterned after the measures that were thought to have rid Europe of the plague, Morana's strategy had both land-based and maritime components. By land, Italy attempted militarily to seal its border with France. The tens of thousands of fugitives from Provence arriving by road and rail were stopped at the frontier and interned for observation and seven days of quarantine in hastily equipped lazarettos, the most important of which were the great pest-houses of Pian di Latte near Ventimiglia, and Bardonecchia. At Pian di Latte 16,050 returning Italian emigrants were quarantined between the end of June and the end of the year, and at Bardonecchia 8,856.[122] The principal quarantine facility – the lazaretto at Pian di Latte – consisted of sixty hectares of olive groves and vineyards in the delta of the Latte River rising above the main railway line just inside Italian territory. Armed with the right of eminent domain, the state requisitioned the whole of the area, including the seven villas located on it, and encircled the perimeter with sentry-posts and armed sentinels. First- and second-class passengers enjoyed the relative comfort of the villas; women travelling third class occupied temporary wooden sheds; and third-class males slept on the ground in army tents.[123]

Smaller lazarettos, sometimes no more than a cluster of tents, were organized at thirty other border crossings and Alpine passes, including Clavières, Piccolo S. Bernardo, S. Dalmazzo, Crissolo, Piattamola and Quarcino. This network of pest-houses, anchored by the facilities at Pian di Latte and Bardonecchia, and buttressed by a cordon of troops guarding the frontier to prevent evasion, constituted the forward line of defence. Only after the sanitary authorities issued travellers with a *patente nette*, or clean bill of health, were they allowed to proceed. As French physicians who inspected the Italian quarantine installations noted, it was no small triumph of organization that the great lazarettos at Pian di Latte and Bardonecchia successfully interned thousands of indigent refugees, some of whom succumbed to infection during their detention, without experiencing a major disaster on the premises. The patients were effectively isolated from their fellow internees and a major outbreak was forestalled. Neither Bardonecchia nor Pian di Latte became a necropolis.

To safeguard the nation and reassure public opinion, the ministry also ordered rituals of purification. Upon their release from quarantine, all passengers and their effects were either fumigated with sulphur and chlorine or disinfected with carbolic acid, corrosive sublimate, or bichloride of mercury. Like quarantine itself, fumigation and disinfection were held in low regard by the medical profession. They were ineffective because the vibrio travelled securely in the intestines beyond the reach of the fumigators. The only certain medical effects were to irritate the lungs, to impregnate the clothing with a strong odour denoting cleanliness, and to burn the skin. There were also, however, secondary political effects. Fumigation and disinfection calmed public anxiety and created the impression that the state was responding vigorously to the crisis. The elaborate ritual performed at the border was duly repeated on municipal authority at railway stations throughout the peninsula.[124]

The sealing of the border with France perhaps delayed the spread of cholera to Italy. Precision on this point is impossible because so many cases were never reported, or were inaccurately diagnosed. The first Italian officially to fall ill of cholera on Italian soil, however, was a worker who arrived at Ventimiglia from Toulon on 26 June. He was successfully detained at Pian di Latte and isolated.[125] The cordon and quarantine had met the first challenge, and the inevitable was briefly delayed. To have expected the cordon permanently to prevent cholera from entering Italy – or even to provide a lengthy reprieve – was unrealistic on several grounds. The line of sanitary defence was permeable because of medical uncertainty regarding the incubation period of cholera. As a result, some travellers from France were released from observation prematurely, only to be stricken in their native towns and villages. At Saluzzo in Cuneo province a veteran of the Ventimiglia facility sickened on 27 June and died the following day. Similarly, on 18 July at Lucinasco in Porto Maurizio province a cholera death occurred in the person of a woman returning from Provence who had just been released from detention at Pian di Latte.[126]

More important than accidental failures of detection, however, was intentional evasion. The Piedmontese fugitives knew the hills and mountains of the region, and they were motivated by desperate fear to escape detection. As every medical authority anticipated, they employed a thousand ruses to evade the sanitary regime that had been established along the border. Large numbers of terrified refugees crossed the border at night via unguarded hills, mountains and woods. And they carried the cholera with them. At La Spezia, the official report on the outbreak of cholera in the city noted that a serious danger had been posed by 'the return of many workers to the city and its hinterland, many of whom had crossed the frontier clandestinely without undergoing quarantine at Pian di Latte'.[127]

The failure of the system slowly became evident as isolated cases of infection were reported in villages scattered across Piedmont, Liguria and Tuscany. Because the water supply of a major centre had not yet been contaminated, there was no sudden, explosive outburst at first. The disease spread slowly in tiny clusters based on person-to-person contact. By the end of July, over seventy people had died of cholera in eight provinces (Turin, Alessandria, Massa, La Spezia, Livorno, Genoa, Porto Maurizio and Savona).[128] In August the infection seemed to have escaped all control, spreading almost daily to a new province. By the end of the month deaths from cholera had been registered in twenty-one provinces.[129] In addition, the first violent epidemic outburst occurred in the second half of August in the village of Busca, which had played such a prominent role in the migration of Piedmontese to France. Of the 9,000 inhabitants of Busca,

152 died of cholera.[130] The cordon along the French border was becoming increasingly irrelevant to the health of Italians. As *Le Temps* observed, by mid-August Italy reached the absurd position of having more cases of cholera on its own side of the cordon than on the French.[131] On 12 September Depretis finally recalled the troops.

But the strategy of land-based quarantine involved more than a single cordon of soldiers along the French border. It also implied the deployment of defensive lines in the rear in case the frontiers were breached. When foci of infection appeared on Italian soil, the army and police were charged with enveloping them in secondary cordons intended to isolate affected communities from the rest of the nation. In July alone troops surrounded seventeen communes as the Department of Public Health attempted to prevent the disease from spreading further.[132]

This procedure of imprisoning entire populations within the boundaries of the commune where they resided reproduced at home the experience at the border: cholera advanced relentlessly, ignoring the presence of the military. The Italian experiment in 1884 demonstrated yet again the inability of land-based quarantines to contain Asiatic cholera. Blunt and unwieldy, a sanitary cordon is unequal to the task of combatting an epidemic when timely information and a rapid response are required. The cordons deployed on Morana's orders were counterproductive, hastening the propagation of disease rather than arresting it. The inhabitants of centres where infection broke out were terrified by the prospect of being besieged by the army and confined within reach of the disease. Since the cordon isolated a locality economically as well as medically, it served in effect as a total blockade. The population was therefore threatened not only with illness but also with economic collapse, hunger and financial ruin. Not surprisingly, when cases first broke out, the reaction of friends, family and neighbours was to conceal the illnesses from the authorities and to make good their own escape. There was a fatal difference in time between the ability of the vibrio to move forward and the capacity of the state to respond by despatching troops. The normal pattern was for the army to isolate communities from which the cholera had already spread.

In addition, the troops themselves helped the disease in its progress. Living in improvised encampments with poor sanitary conditions, Italian soldiers and policemen paid a heavy tribute to the disease. In 1884, Asiatic cholera became the fourth leading cause of death among the 212,000 Italian infantrymen, claiming the lives of 192 enlisted men.[133] Just as in warfare, their junior officers died in even greater proportions, as twenty-three lieutenants succumbed. At the same time fifty-eight policemen died of cholera (see Appendix, Table A.1). In this situation, there was no answer to the question of who was to cordon the cordons. As the military lines were re-deployed and their members rotated, the men carried the infection with them as they moved.

If land-based quarantines and sanitary cordons were powerless to stop the disease, they did produce important side effects. They led to a breakdown of public order and to a rapid escalation of the cholera-terror. By embarking on the strategy of military prophylaxis, the Italian state inevitably fulfilled a dramatic but unintended educational role with regard to the attitude of the Italian people towards epidemic disease. The state in effect informed the populace that strangers were responsible for cholera, that all outsiders were suspect, and that every community could best save itself by employing violent means to turn them away. Under the influence of this lesson, towns and villages where the disease had not yet penetrated began to clamour for military protection, especially in localities that had a history of epidemic cholera and therefore felt exposed and vulnerable. Since the army lacked the troops to secure every locality against unwanted outsiders, communities began illegally to organize their own armed self-defence, often at the initiative of the municipal authorities. The summer of 1884 was a time when the lives of 'foreigners' were at risk in many regions. Numerous returning emigrants unintentionally arrived in Naples after being forcibly repulsed at every other station along the line.[134]

The conviction that foreigners were dangerous shaded imperceptibly into the suspicion that they were malevolent and filled with criminal intent. In this way a great poisoning hysteria swept the nation and especially the South, where previous experiences of cholera revived fearful memories, where illiteracy and superstition were most pervasive, and where confidence in the Italian state was weakest. Calabria and Sicily were the storm-centres of the poisoning frenzy and of the improvised sanitary cordons composed of villagers and townsmen armed with hunting rifles. Of Calabria, far from the front lines of the anti-cholera campaign, Morana reported:

> Here more than anywhere else there was a deeply rooted opinion that cholera was spread by design. Every traveller was looked upon as a poisoner. Every commune wished hermetically to seal its borders and to cut itself off from the rest of the nation. Bands of vigilantes went on patrol, ready to open fire on any unknown person who ventured near.[135]

Railway lines and harbours became the focal points for public outrage. At Reggio Calabria, at Cosenza and at towns and villages throughout the region – Pizzo, S. Biase, Dasa, Nicotera, Filadelfia, Policastro, Longobucco – crowds laid siege to stations, tore up lines, and opened fire on passing trains. Armed men kept anxious watch over ports and fishing villages, and fired on boats that attempted to dock or moor. Frightened citizens also gathered in front of town halls calling for immediate action, and riots began when their demands went unheeded.

Indeed, the example of rigour set by the state implied that no vigilance was excessive. The most important and widely publicized case was the martyrdom of La Spezia,[136] the first important city to experience a major outbreak and to be cordoned off for the duration. La Spezia was the Italian Toulon – a great naval base and arsenal with a population of 31,565 people.[137] The city had grown feverishly as a result of the naval expansion launched by Depretis. In the decade before 1884 the population of the city had doubled, overwhelming the existing supply of accommodation and the local sanitary facilities. La Spezia, like Toulon, rapidly acquired a reputation for sanitary neglect.

La Spezia, therefore, provided an environment where cholera could thrive, and the population anxiously followed events after the disease appeared in Provence. The first reported case was that of the cobbler Domenico Gianazzi. He died on 22 July following three days of celebrations and riotous drinking to mark the return of a relative from Toulon who had successfully eluded the border guards and escaped quarantine. As this first case remained an isolated event, no dramatic measures were taken to isolate the city. In the following month down to 22 August there were two further deaths from cholera, both of which were thought to have been successfully isolated. Later investigations revealed, however, that there had been a continuous trickle of suspiciously rapid deaths diagnosed as enteritis or meningitis, and that numerous fugitives had arrived secretly from Provence. The disease reached La Spezia and spread further without the knowledge of the state. When the presence of cholera in the city was officially proclaimed, there was widespread mirth that the doctors and sanitary officials were the last to know what everyone else had already heard.

By 22 August, however, cholera had contaminated the water supply of the city. Instead of isolated and unreported cases, there occurred a major epidemic that could no longer be concealed. A cordon encircled the commune and remained in position for forty-five days. Unfortunately for the nation, there was an interval of a day between the sudden outbreak on 22 August and the arrival of the soldiers to take up their positions. During this interval there was a great exodus of 10,000 people who gathered up their essential possessions and fled the city. The reaction of those who remained was described by Dr. Francesco Pierotti, who wrote the official municipal account of the epidemic:

> Only those who lived through those dreadful days can understand the impact of that senseless sanitary measure on the morale of the entire population. There was an inexpressible anguish and a feeling of dismay that invaded the minds of even the calmest and most courageous inhabitants as they realized that they had been caged in like so many rabid dogs – and to no useful purpose.[138]

The sufferings of La Spezia became an object-lesson and a warning to the nation. The authorities of the city protested repeatedly to the government, demanding that the cordon be revoked as its only effect was to add the calamity of hunger to the havoc of disease. In an account of the travails of the city, Stefano Oldoini explained:

> The sanitary blockade, in an industrial centre like La Spezia, which was accustomed to importing its provisions from outside on a daily basis, entailed two disastrous consequences – famine and the cessation of all productive activity. Thus many families were suddenly placed in the position of being unable to procure the means of subsistence, especially as prices rose precipitously. No one will ever be able form an adequate conception of the sufferings of the citizens of La Spezia

during those long forty-five days of blockade, trapped amidst fear, hunger, and the devastation of the disease.'[139]

By mid-September there were two days of violent tumults in the city as the desperate inhabitants rioted and attempted to break through the military lines by force.[140] With the example of La Spezia in their minds, Italians sought by every available means to avoid a similar fate. In such circumstances, fear itself proved capable of creating nearly as much disruption as the disease, and the quelling of disorder was itself a means of spreading cholera.[141]

Easily bypassing the sanitary barriers erected by the state, refugees from France and the exotic disease they imported advanced unimpeded towards Naples. By the middle of July there was an outbreak in the town of Isernia in Campobasso province just across the regional border. This outbreak followed the return of 200 labourers from Provence, and the extensive commerce between Isernia and the ex-capital of the South posed a major danger.[142] In an all too frequent pattern, however, the first cases of cholera at Isernia were concealed from the authorities. The state learned of the disease only after many of the veterans of Provence and their local contacts had moved on. One of them was the carter Antonio De Vita, who arrived in Naples on 11 August.

One theory of the origin of the Neapolitan outbreak – a theory which included the Mayor among its proponents – was that the disease entered the city with De Vita, who was seized with cramps and diarrhoea in the streets of the *sezione* Mercato on 21 August. He was conveyed to the local charity hospital of Loreto, where he perished three days later.[143] An alternative speculation also pointed in the direction of Isernia. According to this view, cholera reached Naples not with the unfortunate De Vita but with troops stationed at Isernia who were redeployed at Naples. The basis for this opinion was that there were in fact soldiers and policemen who had fallen suspiciously ill on their return to Naples after tours of duty in the province of Campobasso.[144]

If Isernia was indeed the source of Neapolitan misfortunes, it demonstrated a severe shortcoming of military strategies of public health – the inability of the authorities to respond to crises with a speed equal to that of the disease. The city council at Palazzo San Giacomo requested that a sanitary cordon be deployed to isolate Isernia, only to be informed that the national authorities regarded the cases that had occurred in the province of Campobasso as too isolated and scattered to merit the measure. Nicola Amore, on his own authority, therefore ordered the municipal guard to stop everyone seeking to enter the city for examination and questioning. Passengers arriving by rail were ordered to alight at Casalnuovo and people journeying by road were intercepted at the customs barriers. Any traveller regarded as suspect by reason of either health or place of origin was to be detained for observation on one of three quarantine vessels stationed in the harbour.[145]

As with the cordons ordered by the state, so too this local measure of self-protection was badly timed. It was probably also misdirected. In the atmosphere of distrust and concealment that marked the Italian epidemic, it is impossible to know with certainty when the cholera first entered the city. The land route via Isernia is plausible, but it overlooks the fact that there were persistent rumours of mysterious illnesses in the city from at least the beginning of August – well before the arrival of De Vita and the soldiers released from duty in the sanitary cordons to the north of Campania. Giuseppe Somma was the first doctor in Naples to return a diagnosis of cholera when he attributed the death of the child Antonio Sera in the borough of Porto on 17 July to the disease imported from Provence. Somma recalled, however, that many of his colleagues greeted his suggestion with horror, 'almost as if I had committed a crime!'[146]

In the absence of laboratory confirmation, it is possible that Somma's disquieting report was premature, that it was itself an indication of the anxiety gripping the southern metropolis. Whatever the nature of Antonio Sera's affliction, however, there is strong evidence that cholera was present in the city by early August. For this reason, the dominant conviction soon emerged among informed observers that the long-expected disease finally arrived not by land but by sea – as a direct result of the quarantine measures taken under Morana's direction.

One measure was particularly suspect. Immediately after the adoption of the military strategy of self-defence along the French border, it became apparent that land-based lazarettos were unable to cope with the flood of refugees seeking repatriation. The state therefore re-activated three maritime pest-houses originally built for the containment of plague at the ports of Venice, La Spezia and Naples. The lazarettos were located, respectively, on the off-shore islands of Poveglia, Varignano and Nisida.

The Poveglia pest-house was re-opened as a contingency measure in the event that the disease appeared unexpectedly in the Balkans or the Hapsburg domains, and it never functioned in practice during the epidemic. The lazarettos at Varignano and Nisida, however, played a major part in Italian public health policy. Their function was to receive the overflow that could not be accommodated at Pian di Latte and Bardonecchia. Elderly tramp steamers such as the *Città di Napoli*, the *Malabar*, and the *Città di Genova* were chartered to bring third-class travellers from Ventimiglia, or else to ferry them directly from Toulon and Marseilles. From the arrival of the first ship at Varignano on 27 June until the de-commissioning of the facilities at the end of the year, 7,597 people underwent fifteen days of quarantine at Varignano in the Bay of La Spezia and some 3,000 more at Nisida in the Bay of Naples.[147] Passengers and crew were landed on the islands until the facilities were overcrowded, and then the excess passengers were accommodated on the decks of the ships themselves, which were anchored in the harbours of the lazarettos and isolated by the Italian navy.

From the outset the Varignano and Nisida lazarettos aroused bitter opposition. A large measure of the controversy reflected the geography of the facilities. The islands were located in the immediate vicinity of major cities, both of which were known to be highly unsanitary and both of which had repeatedly experienced devastating epidemics of infectious diseases. Nisida, for instance, was the nearest of the islands in the Bay of Naples. It was literally within hailing distance of the fashionable Coroglio beach, which was only five miles from the centre of the city. To critics, it seemed unwise, even perverse, to transport thousands of travellers, some of whom would inevitably prove to be carriers of cholera, to islands so close to great population centres that were universally recognized as highly vulnerable to the disease. Already during the cholera scare of 1883 when the Nisida facility had been briefly activated to quarantine Egyptian ships, B.D. Duncan, the American Consul in Naples, expressed concern. The Nisida quarantine station, he wrote, 'is so near the city that were the malady to break out there it is considered that it would be almost certain to spread'.[148]

The populations of both La Spezia and Naples were incensed at the decision from the day it was announced, and the local authorities protested to Depretis and Morana. The first ship to dock at Nisida was the *Sampiero* from Marseilles, which anchored on 11 July with 125 passengers aboard. At Naples thousands of demonstrators, led by two of the deputies from the city – Rocco De Zerbi and Pasquale Billi – marched first to Nisida and then to the town hall at Palazzo San Giacomo to demand that the order to intern refugees from Provence in the Bay of Naples be rescinded.[149] The march itself demonstrated the proximity of the lazaretto to the heart of the city. Looking back in December on a decision that had tragic consequences, Depretis admitted in parliament that:

> The Government recognizes all the problems posed by the use of the lazarettos of Nisida and Varignano. The nearness of Nisida to such a great population centre as the city of Naples, we must not deceive ourselves, is a permanent danger.... The location is one that fully justifies the apprehensions of the Neapolitan people.
>
> I do not hesitate, however, to announce that the intention of the Government is to dismantle the lazaretto at Nisida and to provide for maritime quarantine in another manner, constructing a pest-house on another site that does not present the same difficulties.
>
> I must say the same about the lazaretto at Varignano. It possessed many attractions because of its site, its size and the security of the anchorage it provided in the vast Gulf of La Spezia. But since La Spezia became our chief naval arsenal, since thousands of workers were concentrated there, and since the population of the city and its sanitary conditions have demonstrated the perils of choosing it as a location, the Government also plans to abandon the lazaretto at Varignano, and to make other provisions.[150]

While admitting in principle the peril that the quarantine stations at Varignano and Nisida had posed to the ports in their vicinity, Depretis resolutely denied that in practice the epidemic in either city began as a result of the system he had devised. The Prime Minister exculpated himself and the Italian navy, which administered the three maritime lazarettos. Other health authorities took a far less sanguine view. Unfortunately, there is no adequate study of Nisida and its bacterial relationship with Naples – only a bland report by F. Fiorani, the Chief Medical Officer of the Italian navy, who defended the officials stationed at

Nisida and asserted that Italian sailors had performed their duties to the letter.[151] Like Prime Minister Depretis, Fiorani accepted that the lazarettos of Varignano and Nisida were located in hazardous positions, but he denied that the risks had led to any practical consequences.[152] His anodyne conclusions were more reassuring to naval pride than they are convincing to the dispassionate observer. Even on narrow technical grounds, Fiorani's optimism seems excessive. The period of quarantine at Nisida was fifteen days, whereas the incubation period for cholera, according to his own observation, often exceeded eighteen. Furthermore, Fiorani doubted the efficacy of the disinfectant procedures then in use. It follows from his own argument that Nisida probably released people and effects that were still highly infectious.

More careful official investigations at Varignano than Fiorani's apologetic defence revealed serious failures that provided numerous and repeated opportunities for infection to spread to La Spezia.[153] The implications for its sister facility in the Bay of Naples are obvious. At Varignano, the reports explained, naval regulations stipulated the total isolation of the pest-house from the city. All of the personal effects of cholera patients within the island hospital were to be burned, and all intercourse with the shore was severely forbidden. In reality, however, the municipal Health Officer of La Spezia concluded, the supposedly impenetrable barrier interposed between the lazaretto and the seaport was porous. Dr Pierotti explained that,

> Everyone understands that, however vigilant the authorities were, it was virtually impossible to avoid contacts and commerce between those undergoing quarantine and the city, both through the necessity of provisioning the island and through the greed of those who sought to profit through a commerce in clothing and other items with infected people. There were those who gave no thought to the danger to which they exposed themselves and others.[154]

James Fletcher, the American consul at Genoa, elaborated:

> The report is ... , that after their days of quarantine had expired, those refugees were allowed to take their mattresses and other bedding ashore with them. After landing they disposed of the infected stuff to the highest bidder. Such being the case, it is easy to account for the sudden outbreak of the cholera at Spezia. Another reason is also given, to wit, that many fugitives escaped ashore during the night, and took their infected clothing with them, the quarantine regulations being rather loose at the time, owing to the small guard stationed along the harbor. There is little doubt but these reasons are correct.[155]

Here was a substantial danger, and it was no accident that the first officially recognized cholera victims in La Spezia were laundresses. Officially, the washer-women in the vicinity of the harbour laundered the uniforms of sailors in the navy and merchant marine. In addition, however, they were strategically placed to supplement their income by engaging in the illegal recycling of bed-linen and garments from Varignano. All too often they were unaware of the hazard they incurred. On 12 August the washerwoman Carolina Tarantola fell ill and died, but only after informing her attending physician that she had purchased forbidden second-hand clothing from Varignano.

Another danger that beset Varignano and Nisida no less than land-based Pian di Latte and Bardonecchia was the risk of discharging passengers and crew before the incubation period for cholera had run its course. Once released, some fell ill, creating a serious danger. At La Spezia this threat was realized on 2 August. On that day the ship *Città di Genova*, which had transported 'third-class passengers' from Marseilles and Toulon, discharged its crew from observation and allowed them to disembark. On the following day the ship's cannon summoned the men back aboard because one of them had taken violently ill while ashore. At the same time, there were unconfirmed rumours that a steady trickle of passengers had secured their release from the lazaretto by bribing the guards. Even simple carelessness carried serious risks. A mattress used by a patient at Varignano was thrown into the Bay as a rapid means of disposal. Unhappily, it floated, and was retrieved by a fisherman from the nearby village of Riomaggiore. The fisherman and his family were soon stricken with the disease.[156]

For all of these reasons, Pierotti's conclusion with regard to the role of Varignano in the epidemic at La Spezia was categorical: the lazaretto in the Bay was the direct source of the infection that scourged the city.[157] A similar conclusion seems warranted for the much greater tragedy that, soon after La Spezia, overtook Naples. At the very least, the coercive measures of self-defence adopted by the Italian authorities had signally failed to protect the nation. From the end of June scattered cases began to occur in provinces throughout the north and centre of Italy, reaching as far south by August as Isernia. Then during the month of August there occurred in rapid succession three violent epidemic eruptions, each more devastating than the last – the Piedmontese village of Busca with 150 deaths, La Spezia with 610 and finally Naples with many thousands.[158] On 17 August – several days before the attack that struck down the carter from Isernia – Dr Somma made his second alarming diagnosis, and this time other authorities confirmed the presence of cholera in the *sezione* of Porto.[159] On the same day the Naples cemetery recorded the first burial of a cholera victim, who had died the day before.[160] The epidemic was beginning in earnest.

Neighbouring Nisida was a probable source of infection. The volume alone of people, baggage and boats arriving from infected France to be quarantined so close to the city border raises suspicion, as Depretis acknowledged. Between the time of its opening on 24 June and its closure on 22 December, Nisida processed 47 steamships, 402 sailing vessels, 5,417 crew members and 3,627 passengers.[161] The traffic, in the view of the authorities, at once reached 'vast proportions'.[162]

Particularly hazardous for the health of Neapolitans were the early weeks after the lazaretto in the Bay of Naples first became operational. In that period the facility was in a state of administrative confusion and disarray. As the anxious reports from the captain responsible for order on the island indiciated, the institution that had been conceived as the front line of the Italian defence against cholera was in fact in no condition to receive the mass influx of indigent passengers for whom it was responsible. The Italian navy assumed responsibility for isolating Nisida by sea, and the army established a sanitary cordon on the Coroglio beach that faced it by land.[163] On the island itself, however, the task of preserving order and enforcing sanitary regulations was entrusted to untrained, uneducated and undisciplined casual labour. The guards were civilian workers 'recruited from the lowest social classes'.[164] They were issued with uniforms and entrusted with the well-being of the nation – some of them against the express protest of the Director of the lazaretto, A. Di Martino.[165] These men commanded no authority, and the regime that they devised rapidly led to bitter protest, tension and unrest. Here was a consequence of an administrative practice dating from the founding of the Nisida facility in the seventeenth century. The lazaretto was regarded by the authorities not as a type of hospital requiring qualified personnel, but as a semi-penal institution where it was appropriate for discipline to be entrusted to men hired as prison guards.[166]

The main issue causing disturbances at Nisida was that the guards entered into an agreement with the suppliers of provisions to the island to defraud the detainees of their money and possessions. For their daily ration of soup, bread, wine and meat – items deemed to present no threat of gastro-intestinal disturbance – the passengers from France were charged the 'exorbitant' rate of two lire a day.[167] If they had no money, they were compelled to exchange their clothing and personal effects for food. Here, commented one official, was 'unbridled greed'.[168] The issue was more than one of justice. The suppliers and guards had found a means of defeating the whole purpose of quarantine. The garments, linen and blankets of people suspected of infection were illegally smuggled ashore, laundered and sold in a manner all too reminiscent of La Spezia. One is entitled to speculate that such enterprising guards and purveyors of food may also have been open to bribes to transport passengers ashore before the expiration of their term of detention. The *Osservatore romano* reported just such a case. After parting with a fistful of money, a passenger from France was secretly landed ashore after only a few hours of quarantine.[169]

Further speculation about the role of Nisida in bringing the epidemic to Naples is tempting because veterans of the Nisida lazaretto, like all impoverished transients passing through the city of Naples, would have found temporary accommodation in the *locande* in the neighbourhood of the docks pending their departure to their homes. And as the Royal Italian Society of Hygiene noted in its deliberations, it was in the *locande* of the sezione Porto that disquieting reports of diarrhoeal diseases began to circulate during the month of July.[170] Although Dr Somma was the only physician to advance a diagnosis of cholera, these early reports are intriguing. It is also significant that, from the first week of August, the Neapolitan daily newspaper *Roma* recorded a series of 'false alarms' – mysterious deaths officially recorded as 'apoplexy', 'fulminant apoplexy', and 'infantile cholera'.[171] Finally, on 24 August, *Roma* announced the first corroborated case of cholera in the city – in the person of the bricklayer Nicola Ciliento, who was taken ill in a *locanda* in the Via Porto.[172]

The theory that Nisida was the likely source of the epidemic is further corroborated by the locality and timing of the eruption that followed. The sezione Porto was the centre of the Neapolitan cholera epidemic. There it graduated from a 'sporadic' outbreak of individual cases such as would occur through person-to-person contact to become a violent epidemic throughout the whole of the Lower City at the end of August and beginning of September. Such an interval would be the time required for the vibrio to move from the labourers' barracks, where it was confined to clusters of single victims, to contaminate the wells and the waters of the harbour in order to produce a general catastrophe. The repeated passage of former emigrants on their release from Nisida would also provide a possible source of multiple contamination, which would escalate into a major epidemic more surely than a single carrier from Isernia or elsewhere. The Nisida hypothesis implicates not a single person but a constant flow of people as the origin of the sufferings of 1884. Here was the most likely pathway by which cholera travelled from Provence to reach a city that was much at risk.[173] Edward Shakespeare, the United States Commissioner charged by President Cleveland with investigating the epidemic, concluded that at both La Spezia and Naples cholera arrived by sea in the company of returning emigrants – despite, or perhaps because of, the lazarettos intended to protect the nation.[174]

3

Death in Naples, 1884

Having reached the *sezione* of Porto, cholera first spread as a slow succession of isolated cases. During the twenty-four hours from midnight on Monday 1 September, however, the disease suddenly erupted as a full-scale epidemic. On that day 122 people were stricken and 82 died.[1] Ironically, after the alarms of August, the emergency found Naples unprepared. During the final week of August a wave of panic had swept the city following the first official bills of mortality and seven acknowledged cholera-deaths. The churches filled, votive candles were lit, and the populace prayed to placate the wrath of God. On Saturday the 30th there was the reassuring news that there were no new cases. This report was greeted as a divine sign that the city had been spared. Sunday, 31 August, therefore, witnessed an orgy of excess as Neapolitans celebrated their deliverance with riotous drinking, a binge of eating and noisy processions in the streets.[2]

Superstition increased the certainty that disaster had been averted by the will of God. On Friday there was a demonstration at a primary school in the Lower City.[3] During the preceding days rumours concerning the still-mysterious disease and unaccustomed measures to disinfect the school premises had given rise to wicked suspicions in the minds of anxious mothers. They gathered in an angry crowd outside the school to remove their children from authorities they suspected of malevolent intentions. The fact that the municipal health inspectors arrived in force, accompanied by a detachment of armed guards, heightened the atmosphere of distrust. The tumultuous confrontation that ensued ended only after the large-scale deployment of police and *carabinieri*. These events at the school created a stir throughout the city centre.

For many inhabitants, the demonstration seemed a portentous omen. As a result, the weekly lottery was besieged by people wishing to place the numbers 52, 61, and 94 – numbers that were deemed to represent significant statistics in the events at the school (fifty-two screaming mothers, sixty-one infant children, and ninety-four policemen). When these very numbers were drawn as the winning tern on Saturday, the belief that the city had experienced a miracle became a settled conviction. The inclination to rejoice was fuelled by the sum of two million lire paid to the many holders of the lucky combination. The Sunday celebration, the press reported, was 'a day of general intemperance'.[4]

After the premature festivities, the people were unprepared for the terrifying notices that appeared on Monday and Tuesday. Unhappily, the weekend revelry contributed to the sudden upsurge in mortality during the following week by increasing the vulnerability of the population to gastro-intestinal disease. The immoderate consumption of wine, especially the chemically adulterated product so widely consumed in Naples, undermines the major line of bodily defence against cholera – the acidity of the digestive juices. In addition, the over-ripe and inexpensive figs, prickly pears and melons that were so copiously eaten induced diarrhoea and indigestion. These disturbances radically reduce the time of digestion and therefore the period that the cholera bacterium spends in the hostile environment of the stomach. The Sunday festivities produced an acute manifestation of a phenomenon first noted by Robert Koch. In cholera epidemics, he observed, the highest numbers of cases normally occurred on Mondays and Tuesdays – 'thus on days preceded by excessive eating and drinking'.[5] In Naples, the ill-timed joy of deliverance helped to bring on the day of reckoning.

The city governors were no better prepared than the people they administered. The municipal plan for defence against Asiatic cholera was devised by two members of the executive committee (*giunta*) of the city council – Nicola Amore, the mayor, and Teodosio De Bonis, a Professor of Medicine at the University and the alderman responsible for the municipal Department of Health. Initially, Amore and De Bonis chose to shelter under the protective umbrella of the *cordons sanitaires* of the state. The only early initiative of the city was to station its own guards at the customs gates and the railroad station as the last bulwark against infection. When the vibrio evaded all detection and appeared in the Lower City, the administration found itself without a coherent strategy.

Since the first decade of Italian unification, a succession of medical and hygienic experts had identified the major risks to public health and proposed far-reaching solutions – sewers, a protected supply of water, the rehousing of the poor, the sealing of the wells, rigorous inspection of markets. As social conditions deteriorated under the Liberal regime, three of the most able and far-sighted Mayors – the Duke of Sandonato, Count Girolamo Giusso and Amore himself – made sanitary reform a central focus of their political platforms. Nicola Amore emerged as the dominant figure in the city council in September 1883, and he was elected Mayor the following May. Placing resanification at the heart of his political vision for the city, he proclaimed that his ambition was to become 'the Mayor of the sewers'.

The problem was that the chronic shortage of funds prevented the administration from acting on the recommendations of its own experts. The ambitious structural reforms of San Donato, Giusso and Amore were impossible to realize without major new sources of capital. In the absence of such fundamental renewal of the sanitary infrastructure of the city, no short-term local plan to defend the city from cholera had any realistic chance of success. With the outbreak of the disease at Toulon, the Amore administration faced a peculiarly unhappy dilemma. Having commissioned extensive analyses of the sanitary problems of the city, the Mayor and the aldermen fully understood the vulnerability of the city to a return of the epidemic from the Ganges. If the national defences failed to keep the comma bacillus at bay, emergency measures at the local level offered little ground for optimism.

As early as 25 June, the day after the confirmation that cholera had broken out in Toulon, De Bonis assessed the threat to Naples in a meeting of the city council.[6] Naples, he explained, already possessed a high rate of death by infectious disease and 'today we do little to follow the feverish activity of all the major cities of the civilized world in the field of public health'.[7] Although he sought at the time to assuage anxiety by denying that the city was in imminent peril, he later admitted that 'we were deeply worried, conscious as we were of the unfortunate hygienic circumstances of our city'.[8] Indeed, the dangers to the health of the city that he enumerated were so overwhelming that they constituted almost an invitation to fatalism – contaminated drinking water, a polluted subsoil, overcrowding, the lack of a sewerage system. Thwarted in its commitment to full-scale urban renewal, the Amore administration in the summer of 1884 lapsed into resigned near-passivity.

As events unfolded in Provence and in the North of Italy, the reaction of a despairing Town Hall passed through three phases.[9] The common feature of all three was that the disease far outpaced the tardy response of a demoralized municipality. From the day that news of the outbreak at Toulon reached Italy on 25 June until 18 July the administration opted for inaction. During this period the Town Hall chose to rely on the rigorous preventive measures undertaken by the state, thereby demonstrating a fundamental weakness of the reliance on *cordon sanitaires*: they relieved local officials of a clear sense of obligation.

Unhappily, by the middle of July the disease had successfully crossed the border and numerous cases were occurring in the North. On 18 July, therefore, Nicola Amore initiated a new phase in the health policy of the city by requesting that his executive committee be granted emergency powers to take whatever measures it deemed appropriate to face the gathering crisis. Although armed with such extensive powers, Amore failed during the five weeks after 18 July to undertake a more energetic course of action. Instead, the *giunta* limited itself to establishing the structures needed to introduce draconian measures if necessary. The Mayor convened the Municipal Sanitary Committee to coordinate the anti-cholera campaign and seconded one of its members to supervise the initiatives of the individual *sezioni*. Each *sezione* in turn appointed a Borough Sanitary Committee whose purpose was to inspect the borough in order to identify the major sanitary perils that needed to be confronted. The boroughs also hired additional doctors as emergency public health officers. Pendino, for example, which in normal times employed three *medici condotti* for its population of 34, 895, increased its complement to thirteen.[10] Thus organized, the responsible authorities engaged in learned discussions of the latest discoveries of Robert Koch and of the relative merits of various chemical disinfectants.

Having prepared to prepare, the city waited, and vital time was lost. Frank Haughwout, the American Consul, was of the opinion that municipal policy between 2 August and 23 August was particularly negligent. It seemed as though officials chose to reassure themselves more than to defend the city. Thus when the first suspect case occurred on 2 August, followed by others with identical clinical symptoms and fatal outcomes, the city issued no health bulletins and responded in an altogether 'desultory way'. Officials declared that the suspect cases were only 'sporadic' rather than 'epidemic' cholera, and that it was too late in the season for the disease to spread. Timing and especially the imminent onset of the powerful southerly wind or *scirocco* would protect the city from further danger.[11]

Vincenzo Muro, a physician who served as a volunteer throughout the epidemic, castigated City Hall as 'indolent' and 'remiss'. The sanitary campaign in Naples was a 'sad spectacle'. Of the practical results of the summer of self-defence, Muro recalled:

> If some day our descendants were to read that, when they learned that the arrival of cholera in Naples was imminent, the city fathers did not equip even one hospital to even a minimal standard of care, then they would shake their heads and regard such a report as vicious libel . . .
>
> *On 7 September 1884, when cholera was laying waste to the city, when the victims of the epidemic were numbered in the hundreds, the Conocchia Hospital – the only one available – did not even possess beds to accommodate the sufferers!!*[12]

A substantive policy of preventive health – the final phase in the evolution of local policy – took effect only when the onslaught of epidemic cholera had already begun. When cholera attacked the borough of Porto in the final week of August, the Town Hall at Palazzo San Giacomo finally undertook an active campaign to combat the danger. The theoretical basis of the Neapolitan anti-cholera defence was the 'miasmo-contagionist' theory of Max von Pettenkofer, which provided the dominant understanding of the disease within the Neapolitan medical profession. De Bonis positively proclaimed himself a disciple of the Munich hygienist.

In time of cholera, the logic of Pettenkofer's analysis was that the essence of a sound defensive strategy was twofold – to kill or isolate the invading germs before they found a niche in which to ferment in the Neapolitan subsoil, and at the same time to cleanse the environment in order that the vibrio would find the habitat of the metropolis inhospitable. The implication for policy was a widespread attempt at disinfection, purification and isolation.

The first means adopted by the Municipal Sanitary Committee was to remove cholera patients from their homes and to isolate them at the Conocchia Hospital for Infectious Diseases, which was re-opened for the purpose. When the borough authorities in any part of the city were informed of a suspect case, they were instructed to dispatch two teams of health officials to the spot. The first team consisted of a doctor accompanied by an escort of municipal guards and a cart. Their purpose was to confirm that the illness was suspicious, and to convey the sufferer to the Conocchia. The second team was a disinfection squad. Its mission was to fumigate the premises; to burn the victim's clothing, mattress and bed-linen; and to disinfect the building with antibacterial acid solutions. If the patient was already dead, or died during the journey to the hospital, there were strict regulations concerning the burial arrangements for the corpse. The cadaver was immediately to be transported by municipal hearse to the specially designated Cholera Cemetery at Poggioreale, and buried within twenty-four hours in a mass grave steeped in corrosive sublimate. By these procedures the health officials sought to ensure that germs from the bodies of cholera victims did not gain access to the contaminated subsoil of the city, where they would ferment and emit pestiferous exhalations.

At the same time that De Bonis attempted to isolate the cholera germ, he launched a large-scale effort to disinfect both the likely niches where it could ferment and the conduits that led to them. For this reason he ordered the whitewashing of the *fondaci*, which had been identified as major risks to health and which had been ravaged by the disease in previous epidemics. He then gave instructions that the street-sweeping service be intensified. Health officials also began to empty cesspits, to close wells that were visibly contaminated, and to wash the sewer mains with sulphur, carbolic acid and aluminium chloride. Since Pettenkofer reasoned that the air as well as the earth could be poisoned, the city also initiated a campaign to cleanse the atmosphere itself by lighting sulphur bonfires at every street corner or public square. These bonfires were one of the aspects of the epidemic that most impressed contemporaries. The acrid sulphur fumes caused the population to choke and gag, and they even induced death among those suffering from respiratory afflictions.[13] Alexandrine Tkatcheff, the volunteer from Montpellier, recalled,

> I shall never forget, and the Neapolitans still less, the famous sulphur bonfires. In ordinary times fresh air is in short supply in the Lower City; with the arrival of cholera, it became impossible to breathe even on the highest points of Upper Naples. As soon as evening fell, sulphur was burned everywhere – in all the streets, lanes and passages, in the middle of the public squares.
>
> How I hated those sulphur fumes! ... The sulphuric acid cauterized your nose and your throat, burned your eyes, and desiccated your lungs.[14]

But the fires were thought to preserve the city twice over. The heat and fumes purified the air, and the ashes left on the ground helped to disinfect the soil.

Miasmo-contagionism had additional repercussions for municipal policy. The theory directed attention to filth and to noxious odours. Under its influence, Town Hall ordered that certain industries notorious for their effect on the environment be removed from the centre of the city. This prohibition particularly affected horse butchers, the rag trade and the catgut industry. Localist theory further underlined the importance of 'predisposing factors' in explaining who contracted the disease. Among these factors overcrowded living conditions and poor diet were of particular importance. De Bonis and his colleagues accordingly attempted to address the most infamous instances of overcrowding in the city. They arranged temporary accommodation for homeless people and for the residents of certain *fondaci*, *locande*, prisons and public insane asylums. They also sought to provide the inhabitants of the Lower City with the means to follow what contemporary medical fashion regarded as a diet unlikely to produce gastro-intestinal disturbances – a diet based on wholesome bread, soup and meat. To achieve this end, Town Hall opened soup kitchens that by mid-September served approximately 18,000 rations a day, and it issued a city ordinance regulating the price of meat within the city. Inspectors also descended in large numbers on the city markets, where they paid particular attention to the stalls of fishmongers and fruit vendors, and where they confiscated adulterated wine.

Finally, the city posted notices and distributed pamphlets advising the people of individual measures of prevention that they could take to protect themselves and their families. These suggestions for private self-defence illustrate most of all the social gulf between the councillors and the city they administered. The advice was sensible in theory, but it was impossible for the inhabitants of the *sezioni* of Porto and Mercato to follow. The Municipal Sanitary Committee recommended that the people drink pure water, preferably boiled and uncontaminated by faecal matter; that they live in clean and well-ventilated rooms; that they eat a well-regulated diet consisting above all of meat and animal products; that they avoid public lavatories; and that they dismiss all strong emotions. Ideally, it was best not to think about the disease because anxiety lowers the resistance of the body.[15] Such 'popular instructions', moreover, were published in Italian rather than Neapolitan dialect.

As Amore and his councillors well knew, and as the Jesuits observed with malicious satisfaction, the desperate measures taken in September were far too late to forestall disaster. The vibrio had already reached the Neapolitan water supply, and the disease erupted with explosive force throughout the Lower City. The most violent epidemic since 1837 had begun.

THE ONSET OF THE EPIDEMIC

Cholera profoundly affected every aspect of life in Naples. By the end of the epidemic when the last cholera victim, Rosa Romano, was interred on 15 November, the municipal cemetery had recorded 7,143 deaths from the disease[16] and the administration a total of 14,233 cases.[17] Despite a duration of only two and a half months, cholera became the leading cause of death in the city for the entire year of 1884, and it provided Naples with the highest rate of death among all the major cities in the nation – 447.6 fatalities for every 10,000 inhabitants.[18]

Table 3.1. *Causes of Death in Naples in 1884*

Cause	Deaths per 10,000 inhabitants
Smallpox	0.1
Measles	7.3
Scarlet fever	0.9
Diphtheria	3.9
Croup	1.9
Typhoid fever	6.4
Asiatic cholera	139.3
Malaria	0.9
Puerperal fever	0.2
Syphilis	2.5
Other infections	5.6
Tuberculosis	28.6
Pleuritis, bronchitis and pneumonia	83.1
Enteritis and diarrhoea	20.4
Accidents	3.7
Suicide	0.4
Other causes	141.3
Total	446.5

Expressed in terms of victims per 10,000 residents and in accordance with contemporary medical diagnostic fashion, the leading causes of death in Naples in the year were listed by the Department of Statistics as shown in Table 3.1.[19]

In the view of many informed observers, however, these official figures seriously underestimated the real mortality from Asiatic cholera because of widespread concealment and underreporting. The American Consul, Frank G. Haughwout, informed the Department of State that the official statistics relating to cholera in the city were mendacious and not to be relied upon. He reported that the actual number of deaths even before the end of September exceeded 9,000.[20] Similarly, on 27 September, when municipal sources listed 10,000 cases since the onset of the epidemic, *The Times* asserted that a more honest estimate would be 18,000 to 20,000.[21] Many of the deaths officially recorded as due to 'other causes' were perhaps disguised cholera. Even if one accepts the Neapolitan bills of mortality uncritically, however, the death of thousands of people and the illness of many thousands more in the space of ten weeks was a major cataclysm.

The tremendous impact of the disaster on the imagination of the population is better understood by recalling the radically uneven distribution of the deaths during the seventy-seven days when cholera ravaged the city. From scattered individual cases in August, the officially acknowledged mortality suddenly climbed without warning to 80 deaths on the first of September, over 100 on the sixth, and 200 on the seventh. The disease reached a furious climax when 500 people died on 10 September and as many more on 11 September.[22] The impression made on the city is even more comprehensible if one accepts the view of the American Consul, who testified that the real number of deaths on those two terrible days was 2,800. Such was the horror that the administration concealed the reality from the public by distributing the corpses more evenly over the surrounding days and inventing more reassuring numbers.[23]

The decline of the disease from its peak was less precipitate. The daily bulletins recorded 445 deaths on the twelfth, 303 on the fifteenth, 152 on the twenty-second, 85 on the twenty-fifth, and 33 on 4 October. When only 8 deaths were recorded on 7 October, there were widespread hopes that the visitation was over. There was a recrudescence on 10 and 11 October, however, when 62 and 70 deaths were registered. Mortality declined to single digits again only on 27 October. Thereafter isolated cases broke out until the final death on 14 November.

The graphic representation of the cholera deaths in the city did not take the form of a smooth, even arc. Instead, the line plotted by the September deaths rose upward almost vertically and then fell away from the apex in a more gentle gradient to form the hypotenuse of a nearly perfect right-angled triangle. Such a dramatically uneven distribution of mortality maximized the consternation caused by the epidemic. The people who experienced the sudden explosion of cases lacked the retrospective assurance that the disaster would prove self-limiting. The immediate impression was that all of Naples was dying. The comparison made by the physician Eugenio Fazio was that of a 'raging forest-fire, terrifying and uncontrolled'. This great outburst 'did not follow the normal course of ordinary epidemics with their gradual and regular expansion'.[24] Stunned by the sudden and unexpected news of the outbreak on 1 September, the whole of the city was paralyzed with fear by the fifth.[25] The lasting impact of the epidemic of 1884 on the consciousness of the people was heavily influenced by the unprecedented intensity of the deadly days of September. The total mortality of 1837 exceeded that of 1884. In 1837, however, the epidemic lasted six months, whereas in 1884 the deaths occurred in a period of two and a half and the vast majority in the single month of September.[26]

Just as the impact of the cholera was heightened by its uneven distribution over time, a further factor magnifying its influence was its radically unequal geographic spread. The epidemic was overwhelmingly concentrated in the four *sezioni* of Porto, Pendino, Mercato and Vicaria. The figures provided by E. De Renzi, one of the most eminent Neapolitan physicians, establish this point with dramatic clarity. Although De Renzi's statistics seriously understate the total mortality from cholera, his primary concern was to indicate the severe inequalities among the twelve *sezioni* of the city. In that respect his conclusions are suggestive and unimpeachable (see Table 3.2[27]). The shock of the disease was enhanced by the striking concentration of the deaths in the four most populous boroughs of the city. According to many witnesses, the 1884 epidemic was the most terrifying that the city ever endured. The Deputy from Udine Giovanni

Table 3.2. *Cholera in the* sezioni *of Naples, 1884*

Sezione	Population	Deaths	Deaths per 1,000 inhabitants
Pendino*	34,895	871	24.96
Mercato*	55,538	1714	30.86
S. Lorenzo	22,302	122	5.47
Vicaria*	63,736	1031	16.17
S. Carlo all'Arena	28,401	171	6.02
Stella	40,693	179	4.40
Avvocata	39,428	120	3.04
Montecalvario	44,733	183	4.09
Chiaia	36,611	162	4.42
S. Ferdinando	36,985	139	3.75
Porto*	38,487	874	22.70
S. Giuseppe	19,333	185	9.56

Billia, who was present in Naples in September, announced in parliament that, 'The cholera epidemic of 1884 was greater than all others that have afflicted us, not because of the number of victims it claimed, but because of the indescribable panic that took possession of the people.'[28]

Just as in Provence in June and July, the reaction of those with means was to take flight. The first week of September produced a general exodus. 150,000 citizens deserted the city – virtually the whole of the middle classes and the aristocracy.[29] Occasionally, too, public officials deserted their posts and joined the flood of fugitives. The most prominent municipal officer to decamp was Errico Guida, the Deputy Mayor responsible for the administration of Vicaria, the largest borough in the city.[30] Dr Eugenio Fazio recalled the atmosphere:

> I shall not forget the panic that seized the population in the early days of the epidemic ... There were people who had hardly glimpsed the first official notice when they fell into a state of nervous hysteria. Restless and agitated, they knew that they could not endure this test of their courage. Without delaying a moment, without settling their business affairs or tending to family concerns, they rushed as if possessed for the safety of distant, humble villages.[31]

The prevailing doctrine of miasmo-contagionism reinforced the frenzy to depart. If the disease lurked in the subsoil and poisoned the air of the city, as localists contended, then flight was a rational measure of prophylaxis. Indeed, physicians with a clientele sufficiently wealthy to afford the journey advised their patients to escape. In the affluent borough of S. Carlo all'Arena, for instance, Dr G. Ciaramelli, a member of the Municipal Sanitary Committee, subscribed to Pettenkofer's theory. On that basis he reasoned that,

> Removing oneself from the localities where the epidemic is raging most furiously is a preventive measure of capital importance.
> I advised my patients and my friends to take this course of action ... At the very

least one must presume that those who leave a centre of infection will develop cholera in a milder form because they will no longer be surrounded by a poisonous environment.[32]

Ironically, Naples emptied itself of the residents least at risk – the people whom the physician Eugenio Fazio termed the 'civilized element' of the city.[33] The railroad stations and the roads leaving the city experienced pandemonium as genteel throngs attempted to escape for their lives. They scattered in all directions – to nearby Salerno, to more distant Foggia, to the villages of Calabria, to Rome, and to Florence. Twenty-five thousand prosperous Neapolitans decamped to Rome alone, where they occupied buildings still under construction on the famous seven hills. Anxious people with fewer funds sought refuge in the Upper City of Naples itself – on the Vomero and Posillipo hills, where rooms were rapidly made available at fantastic rents. Only the poor – Fazio's *popolaglia* or 'rabble' – remained behind. As the American Consul noted,

> Those who were left in the city of Naples were the poorer classes, the tradespeople, those in the employ of the various departments of Government service, the employees of private business houses, soldiers and marines, and those entirely dependent for their support upon their daily work.[34]

Such a massive emigration was possible because the state made no attempt to seal off its greatest city with a *cordon sanitaire*. The purpose of the coercive sanitary apparatus was to protect the great population centres of the nation. Now that the epidemic was raging in Naples, the regime of coercion had lost its *raison d'être*. Furthermore, completely to isolate the largest city in the kingdom with its impossible surrounding terrain would have required the deployment of nearly the entire Italian army. The danger to public order was incalculable. In September, therefore, the nation tacitly adopted a new policy of sanitary liberalism in Campania.

Having established the numbers of victims, the rates of death, the population of the city, and the extent of the exodus, one can then express the experience of the city in statistical terms that better capture the impact of the disease on those who lived through it. At the outset of the epidemic there were 461,962 inhabitants in the city, or 97,966 families averaging 4.7 members each.[35] Since approximately 150,000 people fled at the outset of the cholera, 310,000 people remained, or 65,800 families. On the assumption that the conservative figures of roughly 7,000 deaths and 14,000 cases are correct, and on the basis of the fiction that the disease was evenly spread throughout the city, then there was a case of cholera in every fifth family in Naples and a death in every ninth in the space of only eight weeks. But, since the risk of disease and death was much higher in the Lower City, and since the real figures for victims of cholera were probably substantially higher than the official estimates, the experience of the inhabitants of the Old City was even gloomier.

Abandoned and fearfully stricken, Naples in September 1884 lost all sign of animation. With the employing classes safely abroad, all economic activity ceased. The port was idle; shops, cafés and restaurants were closed; and the boarding-houses stood empty. The streets were nearly deserted, and the only sound was that of carpenters hammering together the wooden coffins of the poor. The few passers-by held handkerchiefs containing aromatic herbs and camphor to their noses to ward off lethal exhalations. These pedestrians scurried to their destinations, fearful that friends and family had fallen victim to the disease during their absence. As one observer wrote,

> Hardly anyone walked the streets. Those who did were few in number, and they wore an expression of misery. They moved slowly and painfully, fearful for their own lives, and uncertain of the survival of their loved ones. Returning home, they could easily find them ill in bed, or taken to the hospital, or transported to the cemetery.[36]

In a similar spirit, the Vatican newspaper observed,

> The people are silent, disconsolate and tearful. The *signori* take no notice because they are far away from Naples or in the countryside. The foreigners have all fled, and the hotels are empty. The streets are deserted, the shops are empty ... and not a living soul spends a farthing.[37]

The aspect of streets in the Lower City was particularly lugubrious. Omnibuses functioning as municipal hearses stood draped in black in all the principal squares. Too wide to pass through the narrow *vichi*, they served as collecting points where the daily cadavers of a neighbourhood were gathered. In place of these overly wide vehicles, stretcher-bearers were dispatched down the lanes, preceded by town criers calling for the houses to yield up their dead. At frequent intervals these mournful visitors passed priests and their assistants bearing the viaticum to administer extreme unction. The local custom of closing the courtyard entrance of buildings where a death had occurred in sign of mourning dramatically revealed the press of funereal business. There were many streets where every building was closed. The Via della Duchessa, which experienced thirty deaths in a single hour on 10 September, was such a street.

So unrelenting was the demand for both stretcher-bearers and priests that they were unequal to the task, and bodies remained uncollected and unanointed for days at a time. In some streets newspaper correspondents observed that there was not a soul left who was not either ill or dying.[38] In the *sezione* Mercato 'deplorable scenes' ensued. Here the streets were filled with the wailing of men and women whose spouses had died in agony without attendance, and who found themselves alone with bodies that were beginning to decompose. The neighbours, fearing contagion, were in a state of panic and agitation.[39] A different problem sometimes arose. When a sufferer died, all too commonly no one remained to identify the corpse. As the epidemic reached its height, the city was unable to bury its dead. The atmosphere, commented the *New York Times*, was reminiscent of the plague, and the public morale was 'worse than it is possible to describe'.[40]

Superstition added a further element to the atmosphere of the nearly empty

streets. A traditional observance in the Lower City was the cult of saints –
especially the Madonna, Saint Anne and Saint Gennaro, the patron saint of
Naples. These saints fulfilled the functions of the ancient household gods and
they had been worshipped for centuries at outdoor shrines erected in countless
niches carved out in the walls of buildings. At the time of unification, the Liberal
administration, at odds with the Church, had removed the shrines, plastered over
the niches and whitewashed the images.

When the wrath of God smote the city in September, the people revived the
immemorial tradition. They hurriedly re-opened the niches and restored the
shrines, where they gathered in fervent prayer and prostrated themselves on the
ground, hoping by self-mortification to win intercession and forgiveness. These
gatherings bore witness to a religious delirium that swept the city along with the
cholera. Rumour and credulity sometimes brought devotion to a fever-pitch. An
example was the report that at the church of San Gennaro the Madonna had
stepped down from the altar to bless the congregation. Hundreds of people
rushed to the church, forced the troops in attendance to open the bolted door, and
fell upon their knees before the icon 'praying, weeping, beating their breasts and
invoking her aid'.[41]

Less dramatically, the people thronged the churches where there were relics of
saints whose aid could be invoked, such as the church of Saint Brigid and the
church of the Most Holy Virgin of the Shelter. Here crowds gathered day and
night in prayer and hopeful vigil. The most frequented shrine of all was the tiny
church of Saint Frances in the Vico Giardinetto a Toledo, where unending lines of
people filed past the effigy of the saint to touch the garments and objects
associated with her life. These were thought to possess a magical power to ward
off the disease.[42] Divination was also much in vogue. On 15 September, an
overcast day after heavy rains, a stir of emotion swept the city. A great flock of
birds was said to have descended through the clouds, and the event was
interpreted as a sign of divine grace proclaiming the salvation of the people.

A more menacing development was the formation of impromptu processions
of penitents carrying sacred images, chanting psalms and demanding financial
contributions of anyone they encountered in their progress from shrine to shrine.
These latter-day flagellants, who occasionally numbered as many as a thousand,
spread fear wherever they passed. The contributions they sought – ostensibly for
the purchase of candles and the support of the orphans of cholera victims – were
compulsory, and people who refused were set upon and beaten. Condemned by
both Church and State, which together banned public assemblies during the
epidemic, the processions attracted the desperate, who used them as a means of
extorting money in this time of economic collapse and universal unemployment.[43]

In addition to the streets themselves, there were other localities in the Old City
that contributed to the prevailing atmosphere of despair and menace. The city
halls of the boroughs of Porto, Pendino, Mercato and Vicaria, where by law
deaths from cholera had to be reported, were such places.[44] Here the registry
offices were overwhelmed by the volume of business they suddenly confronted.

Recently bereaved relatives gathered at the borough premises in queues that stretched far into the streets. The extent of the emergency was starkly displayed in long columns of human misery. In the lengthy delays that ensued there was ample time for the exchange of alarming news and exaggerated rumour. Citizens on gloomy errands regularly witnessed distressing scenes of grief. Not uncommonly there were moments of panic when people who had arrived in a state of health were suddenly attacked by cholera where they stood and collapsed in agony. Unhappily, many Neapolitans experienced more than one loss and returned to the borough offices again and again. The reports they took back to their neighbours and their families could only heighten the tension. Reporting on conditions he witnessed at the offices of the borough of Mercato, the most devastated in Naples, Vincenzo Pagano wrote,

> It would be impossible to describe the distress that reigned in the municipal offices of that *sezione*. It was the sorriest spectacle imaginable. People who went to the offices to report the death of a relative were attacked by cholera there on the premises, so that very, very often employees witnessed the offices flooded with vomit, and they were compelled to assist the sufferers.
>
> The street passing in front of the town hall of the borough was frequently choked with stretchers, hearses, and conveyances for the doctors of the city, or the White Cross, or the Green Cross. There was a great coming and going, and the anguish of the public was overwhelming as people sought help, subsidies, rations, accommodation, linen. People even left the bodies of dead children on the steps to be transported to the cemetery.[45]

Even more alarming were the long vigils at the gates of the four cholera hospitals – the Conocchia, the Maddalena, the Piedigrotta and the Vittoria. Since these unfamiliar infectious disease hospitals were surrounded by high fences and cordons of municipal guards to ensure their isolation, they were forbidding – even sinister – in appearance. As crowds of friends and relatives waited at the gates for news of critically ill patients, the sights they witnessed were calculated to instil alarm. As the epidemic gained in force, there were continuous arrivals of stretchers and cholera-carts and ominously frequent departures of hearses bound for the cemetery. Since the fatality rate at all four hospitals was desperately high, the news from the attendants who brought periodic reports from inside was predominantly tragic. Statistics for the Conocchia, Maddalena and Piedigrotta hospitals during the epidemic vividly illustrate this aspect of the epidemic (see Table 3.3[46]).

To wait outside the hospital gates was to gain the vivid impression that all of the poor were being destroyed. At the Maddalena, which opened on 7 September as the largest of the cholera hospitals, the fearful climax of the epidemic was unmistakable. In the twenty-four hours from 9 September to 10 September there were 200 deaths on its wards and an unending succession of departures to the cemetery. The terse comment of the Naples correspondent of the papal newspaper *Osservatore romano* was, 'Frightful'.[47]

This impression was strengthened by occasional moments of horror. One such

Table 3.3. *Success of treatment in the Neapolitan cholera hospitals, 1884*

Hospital	Admissions	Discharges	No. deaths	% deaths
Conocchia	714	279	435	60.9
Maddalena	1,053	397	656	62.3
Piedigrotta	92	49	43	46.7

instance occurred at the Conocchia Hospital, where a delirious cholera patient hurled himself from a window to his death on the pavement below.[48] The tension mounted further when reports of conditions inside leaked out. The hospitals were ill-equipped for the catastrophe they faced. The Conocchia, the first of the four installations to open, possessed only 150 beds when the epidemic first exploded. To cope with the surge of patients, the institution accommodated desperately ill men and women in the corridors, on the floors, on the stairs. It ran short of supplies and equipment of all descriptions. The standard of care was also erratic as a result of the impossible burden of work that was borne by doctors and attendants. Despite the best efforts of the medical staff, therefore, the Conocchia and its sister facilities were soon surrounded by fear and rumours of malevolence.[49]

As at the Pharo, a considerable portion of the dread surrounding the Neapolitan cholera hospitals was unmerited. The high rates of mortality suffered by their patients were due in large measure to factors other than the prevailing standards of care and systems of management. In Naples, hospitals were places of last resort where the poor were taken in desperation at advanced stages of the disease. Cholera wards in other European cities achieved similar results for the same reasons. The point here is not to indict the hospitals but to explain the popular perception that they were death-houses.

SYMPTOMS

In this tense and gloomy climate, the medical drama taking place inside the hospital gates added immeasurably to the fear. It would be misleading to treat epidemic diseases as so many interchangeable causes of death. On the contrary, the particular symptoms of each specific disease set an indelible stamp on the social responses it evokes. Thus the distinctive pathology of cholera produced reactions that set it apart from other infectious diseases. Asiatic cholera above all was highly conducive to widespread terror.

The horror this disease aroused was not simply a result of the number of dead it left in its wake. Nowhere did cholera unleash a demographic catastrophe comparable with the Black Death in Europe, or smallpox and measles among native Americans. In terms of sheer mortality, cholera did not compare with the great contemporary killer disease of tuberculosis, which caused over fifty thousand deaths a year in Italy. Tuberculosis, however, was familiar, omnipresent and slow. It reaped its great harvest silently, almost imperceptibly.

Consumption, moreover, was a disease of the lungs, where it established a respectable infection that wasted away the flesh in harmony with bourgeois notions of propriety and Christian theology. Tuberculosis was even ennobling. It affected monarchs, inspired operas and helped to form the slender modern European ideal of feminine beauty. Thomas Mann, that contemporary chronicler of genteel perceptions of disease, charted every medical particular of the sanatorium.[50]

Even syphilis had its devotees and admirers. Syphilis was agonizing, disfiguring and potentially lethal, but at least it struck all levels of the social pyramid without distinction. Its dissolute connotations, furthermore, enabled it to provoke mirth and levity regarding the 'clap'. Alternatively, some transformed the disease into an emblem of iconoclasm, sexual conquest and bold rejection of hypocritical conventions. Flaubert and Baudelaire treated their illness with bravado. The syphilitic could even become the hero of the picaresque novel.

Cholera instead enjoyed no positive associations. It was a vile disease of the gut irredeemably linked with filth and poverty. This malady seldom affected the nobility and the literati of Europe; nor could it be contracted in defiance of social conventions. It is impossible to imagine a choleraic heroine of the opera pouring forth her insides upon the stage or the romantic protagonist of a novel celebrating his diarrhoea as a proof of daring. For Thomas Mann, whose *Death in Venice* deals with the final pandemic to afflict Europe, cholera served as a symbol of the final 'bestial degradation' of the writer Gustave von Aschenbach.[51] It is revealing that Mann spared his subject the indignity of detailing his symptoms. Aschenbach made medical history by becoming the only cholera victim ever to die peacefully asleep in a deck-chair. Tellingly, in his novel *Mastro-Don Gesualdo* even the naturalist Giovanni Verga dealt with the disease in Sicily in apocalyptic terms as a social cataclysm that spread terror, disruption and death.[52] The fate of individual sufferers was lost against the larger epic canvas. Verga too avoided medical particulars. Cholera was too disgusting.

This plague from the Ganges was all the more terrifying because there was no cure. When the disease attacked Europe in 1884, it was inevitable that the majority of cases would terminate in death. Cholera was a mysterious and foreign killer that struck with fearful rapidity and despatched its victims in transports of pain for which there was no reliable means of palliation. It was a fulminant disease that ran its course in hours or days at most. The sudden mortality of cholera was 'more like the desolation of warfare than the progress of disease.'[53] A robust and healthy traveller could begin a journey by train, be overcome and die before reaching his destination. The intervening hours were a trauma not only for the victim, but also for those who witnessed his or her torment.[54]

After being ingested, the *Vibrio cholerae* first encountered the hazards of the acidic process of digestion. In robustly healthy subjects, the invading parasites were unlikely to survive. Various circumstances, however, could transform the odds. If the number of bacteria swallowed was sufficiently large, if indigestion speeded the passage through the stomach, or if the resistance of the subject was compromised by illness, then the vibrio could reach the safety of the small intestine. The warm alkaline environment of the bowels provided the ideal conditions for the germs to flourish and to multiply with great rapidity, especially in the ileum. In time the flagellum or tail that furnished the vibrio with its motility enabled substantial numbers to propel themselves through the mucous lining and to attach themselves to the intestinal wall. The centre of infection had been established.

Curiously, the immune system of the body was normally capable of destroying the attacking micro-organism. In one sense, the infection was self-limiting. The misfortune for the victim in severe cases was that the body's triumph over the microbial invasion normally occurred too late. Illness resulted not from the presence of the germ and its activity in life, but rather from its death. The destruction of the bacterial cell released the poison it contained – one of the most powerful toxins in nature. This enterotoxin caused the classic symptoms of the disease. Its effect was to reverse the normal action of the intestinal wall. In health, the intestine is porous in only one direction, allowing nutrients to be absorbed from the digestive tract into the blood stream but blocking any reverse flow from the circulatory system into the gut. Under the influence of the choleraic entero-toxin, the intestinal wall became porous in both directions, allowing the liquid portion of the blood to drain backward into the bowels. When this reversal of natural functioning began, the sudden onset of illness occurred, marked by a massive and unstoppable purging. The matter expelled, however, was not excrement but blood fluid – the famous 'rice-water stools' of cholera. In conjunction with the purging, there was normally an equally violent vomiting in which 'the fluid vomited poured out from the mouth like water from the spout of a well'.[55]

The severity of the attack varied widely, depending on such imponderables as the number of bacteria ingested, the length and acidity of the digestive process, and the general health of the victim. The mildest cases were asymptomatic, and the heedless carriers were a danger only to others. Their infection was demonstrable only by the bacteriological examination of their faeces. At the opposite extreme, the onset was so violent that the victim died instantly before there was time even for symptoms to appear. Here was the origin of the dreaded 'dropping cases' that first spread consternation across Europe in the 1830s as people suddenly collapsed and died without warning in the streets.[56] This was *cholera sicca* – dry cholera.[57] Between the two poles, every gradation was possible, but it was estimated in Naples in 1884 that for every three people who became ill from the vibrio, one developed the full clinical tableau of classic Asiatic cholera or *cholera gravis*.[58]

In such severe cases, the result of the disease was the equivalent of rapidly haemorrhaging to death. The sufferer's blood fluid gushed forth at the lethal rate of up to one litre per hour. With the rapid loss of even two-thirds of its fluid constituents, the blood thickened to a dark tar that refused to circulate, depriving the tissues of oxygen and the body of heat. Body temperature fell to 95 or 96 degrees Fahrenheit. Reduced to this 'algid state', the patient was rapidly transformed beyond recognition. The still-living body was 'cadaverized', assuming in half a day the cold touch and hideous aspect of an aged, shrunken corpse after a prolonged wasting illness. Within hours the livid face withered into a deathmask with cavernous eyes that were dry, lifeless, and surrounded with great dark circles. As the tear ducts no longer secreted, the whites were irritated and bloodshot beneath lids that were permanently half-opened. The skin was wrinkled, the cheeks were hollow, and the teeth protruded from receding blue lips that no longer closed. The tongue grew dry and thick, resembling the leather soles of a new pair of shoes, and the breath blew cold. As the blood pressure fell, the pulse weakened dangerously and the lack of circulation caused every system to collapse, while death approached from acute shock. There followed in kaleidoscopic succession nausea with vomiting that was frequently as copious as the diarrhoea, dizziness, unrelenting hiccoughs, chills, tormenting thirst, asphyxia, cramp and searing abdominal pain. The ordeal was all the more agonizing because the intellect remained unimpaired to the end.

Two of the symptoms were particularly distressing to onlookers as well as unbearable for the patients – the cramps and asphyxia. The contraction of muscles starved of oxygen and salts by the circulatory collapse was sometimes so violent that a muscle or tendon was torn. Not infrequently the cramps themselves became the cause of death. In such cases there were such severe spasms of the laryngeal muscles that swallowing and breathing became impossible. A clear description of these cramps and their effect on those who observed them is that of the nineteenth-century cholera expert A J Wall, who wrote:

In extreme cases, nearly the whole of the muscular system is affected – the calves, the thighs, the arms, the forearms, the muscles of the abdomen and back, the intercostal muscles, and those of the neck. The patient writhes in agony, and can scarcely be confined to his bed, his shrieks from this cause being very distressing to those around him.[59]

Continuing with regard to the gathering threat of suffocation, Wall added:

The patient usually complains of feeling cold – a great aggravation of his sufferings – ... and to crown all his tortures a distressing dyspnoea that threatens to suffocate him supervenes. He raises himself as well as he can to aid his respiration, and restlessly throws himself from side to side, crying out frequently on account of the cramp or for more air ... .[60]

In a short time the respirations, which had only been 20 or 40 a minute, will rise to 30 to 35. The chest movements are also greatly exaggerated, and the nostrils dilate widely at each inspiration. But with all this extra movement there is an intense feeling of dyspnoea and impending suffocation; and it will be noticed that, as the dyspnoea increases, the colour of the skin becomes perceptibly darker.[61]

If the patient nevertheless survived the first day of his or her affliction, a second stage of the disease began – the phase of 'reaction' or 'choleraic typhoid' in the current medical terminology.[62] After the high drama of the algid or 'collapse' phase, the period of reaction was relatively uneventful. The clinical signs of acute cholera subsided, or were even reversed. Temperature returned to the body and often led to fever. The evacuations, dyspnoea and cramps abated. The pulse and blood pressure gathered strength, and colour returned to the skin. There was a strong superficial appearance of improvement.

Throughout the hours of the collapse stage, the aspiration of the physician was to enable the patient to survive into the period of reaction. The prognosis, however, did not improve significantly because the second phase of cholera was no less deadly than the first. In the state of extreme prostration to which the victim had been reduced, recovery was less probable than the onset of an array of complications that cholera brought in its wake. In his or her weakness the patient was all too likely to succumb to pneumonia, uraemia, meningitis, or gangrene of the nose, the extremities, or the male sexual organs. So severe was the exhaustion that the patient often lapsed into coma. The most common complication of all, however, was uraemia, which accounted for nearly a quarter of the entire mortality from cholera. Choleraic uraemia resulted from the mechanical obstruction of circulation through the kidneys as a result of low blood pressure. The consequences were total renal failure, the suppression of urination, general toxaemia and death.

This haunting spectacle spread terror all the more rapidly in Naples because the whole drama so often took place as a public spectacle. One reason was inherent in the disease itself – the frequency with which unsuspecting citizens were attacked without warning in public places. In the queues at the city halls of the *sezioni*, in the ever-crowded churches, in the streets and in the courtyards of buildings people suddenly fell to the ground in all too evident torment. Such incidents formed an integral part of every epidemic of Asiatic cholera. Two aggravating circumstances, however, were more peculiarly Neapolitan. The first was the length of time that, all too often, victims were compelled to lie where they fell. Passers-by and neighbours were too frightened to lend assistance, and the overwhelmed municipal services were slow in responding to calls for assistance, particularly in the desperate days in mid-September when the mortality rose to its peak. The other circumstance was that large numbers of Neapolitans, in their dread of authority, resorted to concealment. As a result, the violent ordeal of the cholera sufferer very often ran its course in the home among terrified relatives and friends.

A further feature of Asiatic cholera that distinguished it from other epidemic diseases and added immensely to the havoc it created was the age profile of its victims. Cholera disproportionately struck down adults in the prime of life. This aspect of cholera made the disease seem peculiarly unnatural and foreign to the experience of the people. All of the familiar, infectious diseases endemic to Naples – smallpox, measles, gastro-enteritis, typhoid, tuberculosis – primarily affected either infants and children or the elderly. Furthermore, the predilection of cholera for young and middle-aged adults, who were the financial mainstays of families, maximized the economic and social misery it caused. The 'abnormal' incidence of cholera by age was part of the accepted wisdom of nineteenth-century Europe. In every pandemic observers commented in horror upon the overrepresentation of breadwinners among those struck down by the disease. Historians subsequently have repeated their views. Roderick McGrew, the authority on cholera in Russia, noted that this aspect of the disease 'was a basic fact of cholera's epidemiology which subsequent experience confirmed again and again'.[63] More recently but in the same vein, Patrice Bourdelais and Jean-Yves Raulot observed with regard to the French experience of cholera that, 'The curve of the graph of cholera mortality climbs steadily upward from the age of fifteen.' There is no variable, they concluded, as sharply marked as that of age in determining risk from the disease.[64]

Neapolitans in 1884 viewed the disease in the same manner. An important and influential example is that of Dr E. De Renzi, who directed the health service in the borough of Mercato, where the decimation of the disease was greatest. De Renzi was struck by the predominance of young and middle-aged adults among the victims of the epidemic, and he produced statistics to illustrate his perception. His figures understate the real mortality in the *sezione*, but the point they establish is his view of the relative proportions of the various age groups. De Renzi's table is replicated as Table 3.4.[65] The most striking feature of this table is the tally of just seventy-six children under the age of five among the 1,704 people who died. In 'normal' years the population of infants was decimated by gastro-intestinal diseases to such an extent that they dominated the mortality lists. For De Renzi, therefore, cholera was particularly unnatural and threatening. As a further consequence, the progress of this disease was marked by the sudden destitution of orphans, widows and elderly dependents.

By modern accounting standards, De Renzi's figures are inconclusive because they take no account of the proportion of the various age cohorts among the overall population. They are important as they stand, however, as an expression of attitudes. It was not necessary, in De Renzi's view, to prove the relative immunity of children to cholera because his intention was merely to repeat a universally accepted commonplace about the disease. And, whether true or not, this contemporary 'common sense' regarding cholera is a vital part of the explanation of the terror that it aroused. Adults in nineteenth-century Europe felt a particular dread of cholera in part because they believed that it specifically targeted them and that it threatened to leave their dependents without provision.

It is important to stress this point about nineteenth-century beliefs because of a recent polemical point made by Richard Evans, the historian of the cholera epidemic at Hamburg in 1892.[66] With regard to the mortality of children, Evans charges that the historiography of cholera needs to be thoroughly revised. Historians of cholera, in his view, have been seriously misled by accepting the opinion of commentators at the time such as De Renzi, who relied on statistics that are 'worthless' and need to be discarded. When the age profile of the general

Table 3.4. *Age at death of cholera victims in
the* sezione *Mercato in 1884*

Age	Deaths
0–5	76
6–10	217
11–20	328
21–40	584
41–60	322
over 60	177
Total	1704

population is taken into account, and when due allowance is made for diagnostic uncertainty and for the frequently mistaken attribution of the death of children to the familiar diseases of gastro-enteritis and *cholera nostras* rather than Asiatic cholera, Evans argues that an entirely different picture emerges. In Hamburg, the unexpected 'truth' was that cholera was no different from other infectious diseases: in per capita terms, it claimed its victims disproportionately among the most vulnerable age groups in the population – young children and the elderly. The same point, he asserts, is valid elsewhere, and the unchallenged opinion of nineteenth-century Europeans with regard to the mortality of children from cholera should be overturned. In his words, 'Drastic though such a conclusion may seem, therefore, it seems that all statistics on the age structure of victims in the cholera epidemics of the 1830s must be dismissed as worthless.'[67]

Apart from the issue of whether the experience of a single year in one city is a valid basis for wholesale retrospective re-diagnosis, Evans misses a major point. Even if false, the contemporary 'common sense' regarding cholera is itself an important fact that needs to be understood if one hopes to explain the reactions of the population to the disease. Cholera was experienced with terror because of what people *believed* its consequences would be. In that sense, De Renzi's statistics are accurate even if they are 'wrong': they embody the reality of *mentalités* – of attitudes towards the disease.

There is a further point, however, that needs to be made. At least in Naples, the best available evidence suggests that the accepted opinion of contemporaries regarding the incidence of cholera by age was medically and statistically accurate. The Department of Statistics systematically measured the rate of death from cholera for various age cohorts of the population, and produced the figures in Table 3.5.[68] In Italy in 1884, as contemporaries recognized, cholera was different from other infectious diseases in that it did not decimate the population of children. In this sense, it was not a 'normal' disease, and was therefore greeted with particular fear.

The unexpectedly low mortality of small children corresponds with what is

Table 3.5. *Rates of death from cholera by age group: Italy, 1884*

Age cohort	Deaths per 10,000 inhabitants of the age group	
	Males	Females
Birth to 1 year of age	8.2	8.9
2 to 5 years of age	14.0	14.7
6 to 10 years of age	12.1	11.2
11 to 15 years of age	7.8	7.1
16 to 20 years of age	7.2	7.2
21 to 40 years of age	12.1	11.8
41 to 60 years of age	13.7	12.9
61 to 80 years of age	20.5	20.5
Over 80	39.6	37.8
Average of all ages	12.6	12.3

known about childhood immunity and behaviour. Infants, for example, were protected from the contaminated water supply of the city by breastfeeding, a variable that Evans does not take into due consideration. He stresses the fact that Hamburg was anomalous in terms of the ever-increasing abandonment of 'natural feeding' after the introduction of the rubber teat at mid-century.[69] Evans does not, however, relate this factor to the high local incidence of cholera among small children in 1873 and 1892. Recent epidemiological investigations carried out in the twentieth century during the course of the seventh pandemic in Asia, Africa and Latin America have underlined the significance of breastfeeding in providing children with a substantial immunity to the disease. Researchers have established that lactating mothers pass protective antibodies against cholera and other enteropathogens to their infants.[70] A study of cholera in Bangladesh, for example, notes that,

> Children from two to nine years of age are hospitalized for cholera five times more often than are infants and children of breast-feeding age, suggesting that components in breast milk may provide some protection against severe disease.[71]

Breast-fed babies therefore possessed a significant immunity to the disease. The evidence from Bangladesh suggested the conclusion that,

> Interestingly, infants less than 1 year old rarely contract cholera ... We suggest that the relatively low incidence of cholera in infants in these studies and in areas where cholera is endemic is due to parentally transmitted serum IgG vibriocidal.[72]

Behavioural patterns reinforced the protection conferred by antibodies. Young children in Naples had a low degree of exposure to many of the most important potential sources of contamination. They were unlikely to eat large quantities of shellfish, to swim in the harbour, to wash the linen of sufferers or to indulge in alcohol and the October celebrations. For such epidemiological reasons, the conclusions of contemporaries seem plausible.

In addition to the fear generated by what Neapolitans considered the unnatural age distribution of death from cholera, post-mortem observations spread further alarm. Even after death the pathology of cholera created terror. In life, the cholera sufferer mimicked death; in death, the victim imitated life. A feature of the disease was an eerie post-mortem muscular twitching that caused the limbs to contract and shake. In an age of diagnostic uncertainty and distrust of authority, the result was a widespread suspicion that cholera was not a disease but a crime. In a paper to the Westminster Medical Society in 1849, the London practitioner Dr W.F. Barlow had warned of the contractions that frequently occurred after death. 'These movements', he noted,

> occurred after dissolution, and lasted for a very considerable time. The muscles of the arms, chest, and legs, and, in one of these examples, those of the face, were observed to be affected, some muscles being much more influenced than others. Some of the movements in respect of form were not unlike those of volition.
>
> Attention was directed to the terror which they had caused to ignorant persons and persons not ignorant; they had given rise to unfounded notions of persons being buried whilst yet alive. They had been seen by friends, to their extreme amazement, as they were watching the bodies of their deceased relatives; and it was necessary, with the view of preventing groundless alarm and false conclusions, that all persons who might come in contact with the corpses of those who had perished from cholera should be informed that it was by no means extraordinary for such actions to be witnessed after death in this disease.[73]

As a result, the municipal hearses that moved slowly through the narrow streets of Naples sometimes seemed disturbingly alive with movement. The air teemed with rumours of macabre deeds and malevolent plots.[74]

Municipal funerary regulations reinforced apprehension. The bodies of those who died of cholera were to be confiscated by the commune, transported without accompaniment by public conveyances to the newly commissioned Cholera Cemetery, and buried within twenty-four hours in mass graves steeped in corrosive sublimate. The bodies of victims from the Lower City were thus removed from the care of friends and relatives and conveyed for burial in urgent haste. They were trundled in heaving cholera vans beyond the city limits to Poggioreale and laid in paupers' plots pending final exhumation and disposal in unmarked ossuaries. By decree, only municipal guards and cemetery employees were allowed in attendance.

These provisions were deeply resented because they removed the means of expressing grief. They denied survivors the opportunity of taking their leave, and they prevented relatives and friends from bearing witness and affirming their solidarity. The Mayor's funeral edict clashed headlong with the traditions of the community and the rituals of the Church. In addition, the city ordinance aroused a real and reasonable fear of premature burial. Since contemporary scientific criteria for distinguishing life and death were highly uncertain, the immemorial customs of the wake and the funeral procession were more than signs of respect for the dead. They were also guarantees against untimely inhumation. Such caution, eminent physicians warned, was urgently necessary in cases of cholera because of the remarkable similarity between death and the symptoms of the disease. Filippo Pacini, the anatomist who isolated the *Vibrio cholerae* in relative obscurity three decades before the famous intervention of Robert Koch, had long warned against the danger of seeming death. In every cholera epidemic, he argued, numerous patients were buried alive. In 1884 Arnaldo Cantani, the most celebrated living Italian authority on the disease, repeated Pacini's warning. Of all diseases, he suggested, cholera was the one most likely to result in premature burial.[75]

The Cholera Cemetery, isolated, forbidden and unfamiliar, was the source of such persistent alarm that the city ordered the establishment of an observation shed where the bodies of victims were placed in open coffins on arrival. Here municipal guards were stationed to reassure the populace by keeping a twenty-four hour vigil, watching for signs of life in lieu of absent relatives.[76] Even then, Pacini's disciples argued, there was still cause for anxiety because the only medically certain sign of death was the onset of putrefaction, which required a minimum of thirty-six hours.[77] This fear of premature burial became a generalized terror throughout the city when news circulated of an authenticated case of what everyone dreaded. The Vatican correspondent wrote:

> The Municipal [Sanitary] Committee visited the Cholera Cemetery and discovered the case of a poor unfortunate who had been buried alive. The foot of the coffin where the man lay was found kicked out, exposing two stockinged feet. Everyone is most alarmed, reasoning that what could happen to one could also happen to many.[78]

TREATMENT

It is important to stress that each particular epidemic disease is unique in its symptomatology and therefore in the social responses it evokes. Asiatic cholera is radically different from other epidemic diseases both in its psychological resonance and in the social history that it leaves in its wake. Furthermore, each pandemic that swept Europe between 1830 and 1911 was distinctive in terms of the treatments that the medical profession employed to combat it. As a result, each epidemic was experienced differently by those who lived through it and consequently must be studied in its own specific therapeutic context.

What took place in 1884 behind the gates at the Conocchia, on the wards at the Maddalena, at the bedside in the borough of Mercato? What weapons did physicians deploy in their battle with this deadly tropical disease for which there was no remedy? What ends did they have in view? Where were the divisions within the profession with respect to alternative curative strategies? The answers to these questions are important for understanding the Neapolitan epidemic that arrived from Provence, the fear of doctors it created, and the desperate responses of the city at large. The lines of division within the debate over therapy were paralleled by marked differences in the reactions of Neapolitans to illness and the promise or threat of care. Treatment was central to the course of events.

In the half-century since the first cholera pandemic struck the West in the 1830s, a sea-change had occurred in therapeutic fashions, as John Harley Warner has explained in a recent work.[79] It is important not to misunderstand this transformation by viewing it in terms of any simple idea of progress from ignorance to knowledge, from blind empiricism to science. The physicians who first attempted to treat the victims of Asiatic cholera in the era of the Bourbon King Ferdinand II were no less 'scientific' than their successors in the reign of Umberto I of the House of Savoy. What occurred is better conceived as a shift in the understanding of science itself, as a swing from one pole to the other in a debate as old as medical thought.

From Hippocrates and Galen physicians had inherited a divided legacy in regard to the vexed issue of the source of medical knowledge. On the one side of this epistemological divide was the view that knowledge originated in direct empirical observation and experience at the patient's bedside; on the other side was the aspiration to base knowledge on theory and deduction from first principles within a rationalistic system. In the nineteenth century this bipolarity took the form of a clear opposition. On the one side stood the empiricism of the Paris Clinic, which dominated progressive medical thinking at the time of the first cholera visitation. On the other side was the rationalism of the German laboratory, which captured the imagination of practitioners confronting cholera in the aftermath of the microbiological breakthroughs of Robert Koch. The first pole dominated medical fashion in the first half of the century; the second was in the ascendant at the time of the Neapolitan misfortunes of 1884. They were separated by a mid-century generation of doubt when doctors had largely lost faith in Paris without yet hearing the hopeful news from Berlin.

European physicians initially responded to the ravages of cholera by having recourse to the traditional procedures in the armamentarium used to restore the patient to his or her natural state. Doctors were not certain whether cholera was one disease or several, whether it was contagious, whether it was a new malady imported from without or an extreme form of the familiar *cholera nostras* or 'European cholera' – summer diarrhoea. The dominant belief, however, was that, like other diseases, cholera resulted from a morbid inflammation, an over-excitation of the system. The cause of this excitation was deemed to be a poisoning of the nervous system by malignant miasmas. The ganglionic and sympathetic nerves were seen as the primary seats of the disease, and the collapse of other bodily systems – digestive, respiratory and circulatory – were thought to be secondary effects occasioned by the intoxicated ganglia.[80] Only the supposition that the nervous system was afflicted, it was argued, would account for the general systemic nature of the cholera attack, which affected every bodily function.[81]

Physicians holding this nervous explanation of the aetiology of the disease regarded the dramatic symptoms of cholera, especially the diarrhoea and vomiting, as attempts by the body to rid itself of the infectious matter. 'Nature,' commented Dr J. Johnson of the Westminster Medical Society in London, 'appears to make violent, but too often unsuccessful, efforts to restore the broken balance of the circulation and to re-establish the secretions by sickness and purging.'[82] Accordingly, the indication for treatment, was to assist the body in its natural defence of evacuating the morbid material. Doctors therefore sought to enhance the evacuations at both ends of the digestive tract. Furthermore, since the symptoms were so overwhelming, medical intervention had to be correspondingly heroic. Until the second half of the century, the reigning dogma among practitioners confronted with devastating tropical diseases was that 'a severe disease requires a severe remedy'. As late as 1869 a doctor could still report in the *Lancet* that, 'The prevailing idea seems to be that the acute diseases of India are so rapid in their course that gentle measures cannot be of any service, and violent remedial treatment is therefore imperatively called for.'[83]

Traditional depletive therapies were essentially symptomatic. They included bloodletting by venesection, dry cupping and leeches to draw off poison and to relieve congestion by easing the flow of circulation. Considerable ingenuity and perseverance were sometimes required. Since the quantity of blood in the veins was inadequate and they were frequently difficult to locate, practitioners had recourse to major vessels, including the jugular, and to repeated attempts.[84] Dr H. Bell, a prominent English physician who treated patients during the first cholera pandemic explained:

> In no case in which it has been possible to persevere in blood-letting, until the blood flows freely from the veins, and its colour is recovered, and the oppressed chest is relieved, will the patient die from the attack of the disease...
>
> The blood ought to be allowed to flow, until the natural current in the veins has been restored... If opening one vein be not sufficient, let others be tried; and, until the disease yields, the practitioner must persevere in his endeavours to accomplish this great object.[85]

A second front in the battle to save the patient's life was the digestive tract itself, which was assaulted with the most powerful weapons available. Physicians inundated the intestines with violent cathartics – calomel, colocynth, croton oil and castor oil. They also plied the patient with emetics such as ipecacuanha, which was extensively tried in Naples during the first pandemic in 1836 and 1837;[86] tartar emetic; mustard; zinc; and even salt water. 'Full vomiting' and violent retching were deemed to have the highly beneficial side-effects of driving blood into the capillaries and stimulating the circulation.[87] Bloodletting, therefore, was especially productive during vomiting spasms.

There followed the 'sweating treatment' in which sudorifics were administered, and the patient was then submerged in hot water, wrapped in flannels, and piled high with blankets. Dr Mitchell of London described the technique:

> I then lay the naked body on the sheet, and having covered the abdomen with a bag of hot sand or salt, as hot as can be agreeably borne by the patient, and also having placed hot bags of sand or salt to the soles of the feet, I wrap the body closely in the

sheet, confining the hands and arms to the sides, within the sheet. I then roll the body tightly in the first, then the second, third, and fourth blanket, over which I place as much other warm clothing as I can collect, or else a light feather bed. This soon produces great perspiration; in some cases, in half an hour, in others, in a longer period, which I allow to be kept up from one to two, and even three hours ... My hopes of success depend on producing an active perspiration ...[88]

Ingenious practitioners even devised a mechanical steam cage – the 'hot-air bath' in which they encased their patients, hoping to assist them in discharging the toxin through their pores.[89] On some occasions blisters were raised with boiling water or cauterization with the intention of bringing the blood to the surface.

The therapeutics of depletion possessed an extraordinary persistence even in the face of repeated failure. One reason was the legacy of religion. The concept of elimination as a mode of treatment was based on a quasi-theological notion of the diseased patient as a person possessed by an evil force. In 1869 the English physician Francis Anstie observed that certain therapeutic ideas 'were ante-cedent to the birth of scientific physiology'. In explanation, he argued that those notions were, "the direct result of those old theoretical ways of regarding vitality which looked upon disease as an invading demon, which fastened itself with savage grasp upon some portion of the body for which it had a malignant liking'.[90]

Anstie referred specifically to the practise of counter-irritation, but what he said was equally applicable to depletion. The point was that the nineteenth-century physician still engaged in a secularized rite of exorcism. Cathartics, venesection, emetics and sudorifics were the instruments employed to cast out 'morbific demons' and restore the sufferer to health. Strategies for treatment reflected what William Gull in 1872 called 'the old theological notion ... that an evil spirit entered the sick man'.[91] Depletion therapy was powerfully rooted in a still religious cosmology.

Depletion also owed its hold on the medical imagination to tradition and professional identity. Venesection was, quite simply, what physicians did. The lancet was the symbol of their art, and it lent its name as the title of some of the most prestigious journals in the profession. Bloodletting was the mark of the regular physician, separating him from empirics and linking him to an unbroken therapeutic tradition stretching back to Hippocrates. It conferred legitimacy, and doctors were reluctant to acknowledge their disillusionment.[92]

After extensive trials as the dominant therapy throughout the West in both the first and second pandemics, eliminant therapy fell into disfavour. By mid-century it was almost universally abandoned in the management of cholera patients. Depletion hastened death by enhancing the fatal loss of bodily fluid and by increasing the prostration of the sufferer. It was widely reported in the medical press that patients subjected to its rigours experienced considerably higher rates of death than those whose diseases were allowed to run their natural course. In 1855, for example, the *Lancet* conducted a comparative statistical survey of the rates of death of patients under the various competing therapeutic systems – the alterative (i.e., by means of calomel), the stimulant, the astringent, and the eliminant. Its most striking and forceful conclusion was that,

> The Eliminative method, whether carried out by exciting to vomiting or purging, by giving castor oil or tartar emetic, is injurious in the premonitory diarrhoea, and the most fatal of all methods in actual cholera.[93]

Depletive therapies were said to result in a death rate approaching 80 per cent. By the 1860s leading physicians could announce the demise of elimination in the treatment of cholera patients,[94] and in 1870 the *Lancet* editorialized that purgatives 'cannot eliminate morbid poisons' and were unavailing against Asiatic cholera.[95]

Although depletion was the strategy of choice for European practitioners in their first encounters with Asiatic cholera, the crisis created by the mass devastation of the disease and the all too evident inability of physicians to contain it encouraged desperate alternative initiatives of the most varied kind and a lively professional debate about the relative merits of different approaches. On the analogy of the first 'miracle' drugs – mercury in the treatment of syphilis and quinine in the care of malaria – physicians often sought the specific or 'grand remedy' for cholera. Through much of the century there was an enduring vogue in mercury and especially its derivative, calomel.[96] The fashion persisted despite the objections of eminent critics who noted that the absorptive powers of the patient in the algid stage of cholera virtually cease. As a result, small doses of calomel had no effect while large doses accumulated, unabsorbed, in the gut until the onset of the reaction stage, when a sudden rush of mercury into the system occurred, unleashing the complications of ptyalism. Trusting in serendipity – described by one authority as 'wild haphazard experiment'[97] – doctors dosed their patients with quinine as well or randomly deployed the most potent medications in the materia medica – arsenic, strychnine, prussic acid,[98] and phosphorus.[99] In Italy in the 1860s there was a great vogue for ammonio-citrate of iron.[100]

Many doctors supported such courses of treatment with the theory of counter-irritation, a concept that verged dangerously close to the medical heresy of homeopathy. According to the counter-irritant doctrine, poisons that produce symptoms resembling those of a particular disease can be administered to stimulate the resistance of the body to the malady itself. Alternatively, a lesion induced by the physician – through cauterization or scarification, for instance – would mobilize the healing powers of the body against the disease as well as the more recent wound. To create an 'artificial disease' or 'remedial injury' by medical means was to assist the sufferer in his or her struggle with the natural disease. Arguing the case for arsenic, surgeon S. Dickson explained his stance in these terms:

> Of all the various modes of treatment resorted to in nervous disease, is not counter-irritation the most generally efficacious? Zinc, arsenic, and copper, are called tonics; may they not rather be termed irritants, seeing that when they

produce cures in ague, epilepsy, gout, palsy etc., they do so only by establishing an analogous disease? They act, in a word, by counter-irritation.... The poison of arsenic, and of certain snakes, produces a train of symptoms analogous to cholera. The natives of India treat the bite of the cobra de capello successfully with arsenic. Ought not this to be an inducement to give it a fair trial in cholera?[101]

Other healers sought not to enhance the symptoms manifested spontaneously by the disease as their depletion-minded colleagues advocated but rather to suppress them as dangerous rather than life-supporting. For this purpose they turned to sedatives and antiphlogistics, especially the opiates – laudanum and morphine.[102] The opiates, which were administered extensively during all six of the pandemics that afflicted Europe, were thought to sedate the poisoned and overexcited nervous system, to ease the cramps, and to slow the diarrhoea. At the same time it was common to make use of astringents such as copper sulphate, iron, acetate of lead and chalk as antidiarrhoeics. To halt the vomiting, they employed the drastic anti-emetic hydrocyanic acid. During the early decades of the century, the antiphlogistic or 'physiological' treatment, made famous by François Broussais in Paris, also implied bloodletting to lower the general inflammation.[103]

Alternatively, some physicians attempted a diametrically opposed procedure, hoping not to sedate but to stimulate. Their gamble was that the administration of tonics would help to revive the flagging animal energy of their patients. This restorative strategy involved camphor, alcoholic beverages, ether, ammonia, capsicum, musk and even opium – the same drug employed by the advocates of sedation but now adopted with a contrary purpose. An additional medication employed by the champions of stimulation was strychnine, the poison favoured also by counter-irritant and homeopathic theories. Now it was seized upon as 'the most powerful cerebro-spinal stimulant known', and the one hope of restoring a nervous system slipping inexorably into general paralysis.[104]

Devising a wholly different approach, some imaginative doctors attributed the cause of death in cholera to the severe chemical alterations that it produced in the composition of the blood. Beginning during the 1830s with Jaehnichen in Russia, François Magendie in France, and William O'Shaughnessy and Thomas Latta in Britain, a current of physicians attempted to thin the blood, replace its lost fluid content and oxygenate it. For this purpose, they experimented with subcutaneous and intravenous injections of saline and other solutions;[105] and with the copious oral administration of liquids 'resembling as near as possible the serum, with albumen, muriate and carbonate of soda'.[106] This line of experimentation led ultimately in 1909 to the development by Leonard Rogers of successful rehydration therapy – the foundation of modern cholera therapeutics. It also led in the early pandemics to a variety of therapeutic cul-de-sacs, when doctors injected substances that proved rapidly lethal, such as warm milk,[107] and attempted transfusions of the healthy blood of animals and random human volunteers.[108] Only saline solutions provided sufficiently rewarding results to encourage persistence.

Unfortunately, in the nineteenth century, physicians injected so-called isotonic saline solutions – solutions equivalent in salt content to that of blood itself. The idea was to replace like with like. Only in the new century was it discovered that the body retains only hypertonic solutions – solutions much richer in salt than natural body fluid. For that reason, the injected liquid only poured forth again, producing striking but fleeting improvements in the patient's condition. Another problem was that, in an era still innocent of the germ theory of disease, there was no understanding that the solution injected had to be sterile, with the result that the patients frequently succumbed, if not to cholera, then to septicaemia. The temporary results of this procedure were so dramatic, however, that the path of rehydration was followed with ever-changing refinements from the first pandemic of Asiatic cholera to the last. The spectacular effects that could be achieved, if only briefly, were described by the *Lancet* in a case treated in England during the first British experience with the disease:

> In one case, nearly 7 lbs. were at once thrown in to the median basilic vein, and in nine hours 15 lbs. were infused. But in this very case – a desperate example of the last stage of a protracted attack of cholera, after excessive purging and vomiting had drained the body almost dry – when the pulse had been imperceptible for hours, the skin livid, and the voice lost, *the patient completely recovered!* While the injection was performing, the pulse rose, the heat returned, the lividity disappeared, the countenance became florid and beaming, in short the patient underwent a change more like the workings of a miraculous and supernatural agent, than the effect of the interposition of medical science.[109]

It was unfortunate that, as usual, the remission was fleeting, and that the patient subsequently died.[110]

Finally, there was every manner of idiosyncratic experimentation. On the theory that cholera was a nervous disorder, doctors in many countries attempted to treat what they hypothesized was an electrical malfunction of the system with galvanism.[111] Physicians also persisted in prescribing inhalations, most frequently of oxygen, but also of chloroform and ether in the later epidemics of the century.[112] There were even attempts to treat cholera by mechanical interventions such as the 'corking-up method', which was an effort to halt the lethal evacuations by plugging the bowel with wax[113] or by a more elaborate roller and plug.[114] At Berlin in 1849 the cholera-hospital employed the 'cold-water system' designed to restore animation. Patients were stripped, placed in an empty tub, and then repeatedly drenched with buckets of iced water intended to arouse their declining animation.[115] And in the 1860s sufferers were girded in the 'cholera belt', a flannel bandage wrapped tightly around the abdomen to sustain warmth and to bind the system against collapse.[116]

It would be instructive to trace the history of therapeutic endeavours in their specific relations to individual outbreaks of cholera and the responses they evoked among the population. Unfortunately, such an approach is not characteristic of the literature on European cholera to date. Historians have dealt all too briefly with therapeutics, have neglected comparisons between different epidemics, and have often failed to relate the practice of physicians at the bedside to the reactions of the population at large. The discussion that follows is intended as a partial counterweight to this imbalance and as a point of eventual international comparison between the Neapolitan case and other experiences. As the doctors at the Pharo Hospital in Marseilles discovered, certain forms of treatment were perceived by patients as needlessly painful, as forms of human vivisection or even as simple murder. Therapy in this manner played an important part in surrounding certain medical facilities or even at times the whole medical profession with suspicion, fear and resistance.

Furthermore, as doctors and medical journals lamented, the very lack of agreement within the profession with regard to treatment undermined the confidence of the public and made patients unwilling to submit to certain heroic medical procedures. In the pages of the Neapolitan journal *Rivista clinica e terapeutica*, the local physician T. Senise, reflecting in 1885 on the events of the preceding year, argued that the disorders that beset the city were in large measure a product of the lack of confidence in the medical profession. By publicly confessing their ignorance and loudly proclaiming their disagreements, Neapolitan physicians lost their claim to authority in the eyes of the populace. It was incumbent upon the profession to maintain an official posture of unity and self-confidence. In any case, he observed sardonically, medicine was no more impotent when confronted with cholera than it was with other diseases.[117]

From the standpoint of the experience of Naples in 1884, the chief point to be made is that none of the initiatives taken in the course of half a century of experience with cholera had yielded positive results. All had failed so comprehensively that some scientists argued that a cholera victim had better odds of survival if he avoided medical attention entirely. The results of this history of disappointment were twofold. The first result was that at least certain negative advances had been made in the sense that various blatantly ineffective treatments were discarded. There are no records, for instance, that any Neapolitan physician in 1884 opened the veins of cholera victims, exhibited strychnine or prussic acid, administered blood transfusions, or experimented with purgatives and emetics.

There was a second and more far-reaching consequence. In the decades after mid-century there emerged a powerful current that Warner terms 'therapeutic gloom'[118] within the international medical profession. Despondent doctors, who formed a dominant element in Naples, rejected all received therapeutic approaches as useless, or worse. In addition, they reached the radical conclusion that doctors facing cholera should eschew the very attempt to cure. Instead of 'treating' sufferers, the despondent school argued that physicians should avoid harming the patients entrusted to their care. The doctor could not assume the task of combatting cholera because he possessed no understanding of what the disease was or where it was located. Therapeutics, therefore, should be minimal, consisting of the attempt to fortify the stricken body so that it would be able to fight cholera alone.

Such an approach was not new. In the course of each epidemic there were physicians who were deeply affected by their impotence and who concluded that all of the remedies in vogue had only one consequence – to torture helplessly exhausted patients in the departing hours of their lives. After witnessing three years of fruitless therapeutic experimentation, large numbers of doctors by 1833, for example, had reached the judgment that they preferred to do nothing and to trust instead to the healing power of nature – the *vis medicatrix naturae*. In Paris, the *Lancet* remarked, this attitude was shared by the majority of practitioners. Despairing after persistent failure, they 'seem content with allowing nature "to work out her own salvation", if she will, without any interference on their part'.[119] What was new in the second half of the century was that this spontaneous attitude of therapeutic minimalism was elaborated into a conscious methodology.

In Naples in 1884 the most influential advocate of this strategy, which he termed the 'physiological treatment of cholera', was the eminent Professor of Medicine Mariano Semmola, the editor of one of the major medical journals published in the city, *La Medicina contemporanea*. His views were widely shared, particularly by the older and more senior physicians who had experience of previous outbreaks and of innumerable disappointments with therapies once recommended as highly efficacious. More Parisian than the Parisians, these doctors endorsed the most far-reaching possible rejection of medical rationalism, of systematic theory, and of heroic therapeutic interventionism.

On the other side of the debate were the proponents of a new rationalism and of therapeutic optimism, led by Arnaldo Cantani, the foremost Italian authority on cholera and a Professor at the University who directed operations in the municipal cholera hospitals. Cantani and his followers enthusiastically embraced the new model of German science, looking to the laboratory bench and basic science as the sources of medical knowledge and of the answers to the epistemological doubts of their colleagues. They heralded the discovery of the *Vibrio cholerae* by Robert Koch as the key to unlocking the riddle of therapeutics. Koch had isolated what they termed the 'cholera virus' – the specific cause of the disease. Furthermore, by cultivating the vibrio in a variety of laboratory mediums, the Berlin microbiologist had revealed its properties and the peculiarities of its life-cycle. Especially important for Cantani was the demonstration of the preference of the bacillus for alkaline conditions and of its vulnerability to acidity. Extrapolating from the test tube to the clinic, Cantani postulated that since he now knew which organism caused cholera, where to find it in the gut and how to kill it with acid, then he was in a position to cure its victims.

In their rush of therapeutic optimism, the Neapolitan rationalists were more Germanic than the Germans. By September 1884, when Cantani began to experiment on patients, German laboratory science had not announced the cure for a single disease. Indeed, a considerable leap of faith was required to sustain the belief that to know the specific cause of cholera was also to know its specific cure. Koch's discovery was barely a year old, and his vibrio was far from universally accepted by the profession as the pathogen responsible for the disease.

For technical reasons, scientists attempting to confirm the Berlin doctor's claims by identifying the cholera germ in the gut of deceased patients, in stool samples and in contaminated water supplies often failed to make positive determinations. The reason was that the gelatine-cultivation method that Koch first developed was not sufficiently reliable, especially when used by investigators who lacked a long experience of microscopy. Bacteria other than the *Vibrio cholerae* were commonly found in the human intestine and in contaminated water. In gelatine, these other germs proved hardier than the cholera germ. They reproduced more luxuriantly than the comma bacillus, overgrowing it and preventing its characteristic colonies from being observable. Furthermore, the isolation of the *Vibrio cholerae* in suspect water posed complicated technical problems. Even the most lethally polluted stream or well was not equably contaminated throughout and it was always possible to draw samples in which no cholera bacteria were present, just as in a lake filled with fish it is easy to draw buckets of water that are fish-free. It required nearly a decade of refinement and the development of the alternative technologies of agar-and peptone-cultivation before Koch could announce methods of isolating the germ that were sufficiently infallible to convince sceptics.[120]

Furthermore, by the outbreak of cholera in Naples, Koch had not fully persuaded the medical profession because his initial attempts to offer proof that he had found the specific cause of cholera omitted a necessary step in logic. By skillful microscopy and good fortune, Koch was able to demonstrate that wherever there was cholera the investigator could always find the *Vibrio cholerae*. This, however, was only circumstantial evidence. Koch was unable to provide the missing causal link – to prove, that is, that the vibrio not only accompanied cholera but actually caused it. Indeed, the evidence seemed to point the other way because attempts to induce cholera experimentally failed. Guinea-pigs, mice and monkeys remained obstinately healthy after being fed massive doses of the germ. In addition, several eminent scientists critical of Koch performed auto-experiments, swallowing cholera-cocktails without ill effect. An important example was Edward Emanuel Klein, the great English authority on cholera and opponent of Koch's conclusions. He dosed himself with the vibrio in the midst of the Naples outbreak.[121] Klein also replicated Koch's methods and reported that his conclusions were unsound.[122]

Here, then, was a vital flaw that was made all the more damaging because Koch himself, in a previous incarnation, had vehemently insisted on rigour in the matter of causation. Indeed, the famous 'Koch's Postulates' that he had elaborated before turning to cholera insisted that an organism thought to cause a disease must be shown to induce the disease experimentally in animals before it can be accepted as the cause. In time, Koch would provide the necessary demonstration by developing the technique of injecting cholera germs artificially into the peritoneal cavity of animals rather than administering them orally. And in 1892–93 painstaking research into the aetiology of the cholera outbreak at Hamburg and Altona provided irrefutable epidemiological proof of the role of the vibrio in the transmission of the disease.[123] In 1884, however, it still required as much faith as logic to accept Koch's claims.

Finally and most importantly, Cantani's therapeutic conclusions were foreign to Koch's own thinking. The Neapolitan doctor's speculations were not rewarded by an endorsement from the master in Berlin. The implications of Koch's discoveries for the eradication of Asiatic cholera were enormous. They provided physicians with a reliable means of diagnosing the disease and of taking effective measures of public health to prevent outbreaks. What Robert Koch did not offer, however, was a system of cure.

At stake in the debate between the partisans of Semmola and those of Cantani was more than a stance on the abstract issue of medical epistemology. The implications for both physicians and patients were far-reaching. For physicians, the questions touched the core of their identity and their ethics as practitioners. To follow Semmola meant to take a stand on the bedrock of medicine as an art guiding the physician as he does battle with disease on the field of the patient's body. In this contest the sole criterion for victory was the restoration of health to the individual sufferer and the only guide to practice was accumulated experience at the bedside. To embrace Cantani's reasoning, by contrast, was to declare that medicine was not an art but a science in which universal principles discovered in the laboratory were the only authoritative guides to practice and that success could be measured by the advance of knowledge even if the individual patient was lost. Indeed, Cantani's approach implied both human experimentation and animal vivisection. For G. Manfredonia, an attending physician at the Hospital for Incurables, to accept Cantani meant to reject the past traditions of Italian medical practise and to opt instead for an alien 'Germanic analysis' that had seduced the 'medical youth' of the nation.[124]

For the cholera victim, the consequences were also starkly contrasting. For Semmola, the theoretical dictates of the rationalist system-makers were to be rejected absolutely as dangerous in principle and lethal in practice.[125] For the despondent practitioner, who accepted that there was no specific cure for the disease, there were only two stances that could be defended at the bedside. The first was a traditional symptomatic approach, which dictated that the physician take moderate action to oppose each symptom as it arose, using the well-tried weapons of the armamentarium whose effects were known, antagonistic to the disease and predictable. An experienced practitioner adopting this approach would suppress intestinal inflammation with astringents; general prostration with stimulants; algidism with alcohol and artificial external heat; and paralysis of the heart with sulphuric ether. 'This kind of treatment,' Semmola argued in a typical suggestion of his minimalist approach,

> when it is managed within certain limits, and when one does not demand too much from it, is productive of favourable results, with this fundamental condition, that one must not use agents which shall produce profound and unknown disturbances, and that the actions of the agents used shall be evanescent.[126]

Manfredonia and Giuseppe Amalfi were representative of therapeutic minimalism in the treatment of cholera. They believed that practitioners had for too long vainly chased the chimera of the specific cure. This search had failed entirely, doing incalculable harm to patients in the process. It was time instead, they reasoned, to return to the one agent – opium – whose use was vindicated by long experience. Opium did no actual harm if administered in small doses and it demonstrably alleviated the most painful symptoms of the disease. Manfredonia and Amalfi, therefore, drastically simplified their curative interventions, reducing them to the exhibition of a single medication in small doses.[127]

Although Semmola applauded such modest symptomaticians as at least harmless, he advocated instead the second of his two 'reasonable' therapeutic stances. This was his own method of 'physiological treatment', which was still more self-effacing. Semmola worried that to suppress symptoms was to create two pernicious side-effects. The first was that the symptomatic strategy inevitably involved the administration of poisonous substances whose negative consequences would be fully apparent only as the patient convalesced. The second, and still more important, defect was that chemicals powerful enough to suppress the symptoms of a disease as violent as cholera would also 'paralyze the spontaneous resources of the system' that were essential to recovery. Furthermore, Semmola believed that not too much importance should be attached to symptoms, especially in Asiatic cholera. The essence of the disease was the poisoning of the nervous system, which could affect any bodily function. The specific symptoms that resulted in each individual patient were merely the impact of the affected nerves on the inherited weaknesses of the particular victim. A sufferer with a weak stomach, for instance, would be most affected in the digestive system and one with a weak heart in his circulation.

Semmola, therefore, rejected an approach that prioritized symptoms. There remained only the physiological approach. 'I call physiological treatment', he explained, 'that which, without disturbing the system with powerful medicinal actions, proposes only to increase by all means the resistance of the vital economy against the successive invasions of the choleraic poison.'[128] The essence of the therapy was its avoidance of heroic and invasive methods. Semmola relied on the precept that he treats best who treats least. The first requirement of this treatment was 'absolute and rigorous repose' of the whole body and especially of the organs attacked. Since the digestive tract was the organ most directly and universally affected by Asiatic cholera, the indication for the patient was complete and total fasting. No substance of any kind was to be swallowed. Even a few drops of consommé, he suggested, acted like a mitrailleuse placed in the hands of a deadly and powerful enemy.

Since fever and bodily heat are the natural modes of resistance to infection, a second aspect of physiological care was to apply external heat, preferably in the form of a warm bath administered at the first sign of diarrhoea. In the fully developed algid state a bath would require too great an exertion and, as experience suggested, produced no more effect than the attempt to heat marble. Adopted at the earliest moment, however, the warm bath tonicized the system. By stimulating the peripheral nerves, it had a reflex effect on the circulation. Heat also favoured perspiration, which eliminated the choleraic poison. Alternatively, reasoning that fever was the natural defence of the body against disease, some followers of Semmola sought to raise the body temperature internally by chemical means. An example was G. Ciaramelli, whom we have encountered recommending flight from the borough of S. Carlo all'Arena. He injected his patients with what he considered a fever-inducing 10 per cent solution of iron citrate.[129]

A final component of Mariano Semmola's approach was the exhibition of small doses of laudanum. Unlike the symptom-suppressors, Semmola did not aspire to end the diarrhoea with opiates, and he insisted that the quantities given should be far smaller than those required for that ambitious purpose. He aimed only at fortifying the nervous system, slightly deadening its hyper-sensitivity so that it would be placed in the most advantageous condition to withstand the cholera poison – provided, of course, that not too much was expected. Nothing more could be usefully done in the algid stage of Asiatic cholera.

Arnaldo Cantani advocated a radical alternative in the management of cholera patients – an alternative that was imitated elsewhere throughout the fifth pandemic both in Italy and elsewhere.[130] A follower of the latest developments in Berlin, he agreed with Semmola in rejecting traditional symptomatic approaches to the treatment of the disease. Cantani's reasons, however, were wholly at odds with Semmola's position. Cantani concluded that, instead of growing more modest in their therapeutics, physicians should become more resolutely interventionist. He argued that practitioners should take advantage of recent developments in microbiology to go far beyond the mere suppression of cholera symptoms. Cantani advocated instead an all-out assault intended to seek out the invading microbe and destroy it. His programme of 'rational therapy' was avowedly experimental and based on theory derived from the laboratory rather than clinical experience. His ambition was to take advantage of the discovery that the vibrio is susceptible to acid. For that purpose, he instituted a treatment involving two phases.

The first phase was an attempt to restore sufficient strength to the patient's body to enable it to benefit from the subsequent victory over the microparasite. With that end in view, the new rationalism had recourse to saline injections, which were known to provide at least a fleeting improvement in the condition of the sufferer by counteracting the inspissation of the blood. Regarding intravenous solutions as highly dangerous procedures that placed too sudden a strain on the heart, Cantani called instead for more gradually absorbed subcutaneous injections. Since this method was more readily tolerated by the patient, up to three litres could be injected at a time, and the procedure could be repeated as long as purging persisted. Known as hypodermoclysis, the method involved simultaneous injections into the abdomen on both sides of the body. To reduce the acidity of the blood, which he regarded as a contributory cause of death, Cantani added sodium chloride or carbonate of soda to the injected solution.[131]

After the course of saline injections had improved the general condition of the patient, Cantani then launched the more innovative second phase of his therapy. This was the frontal attack on the cholera germ and it involved a procedure that he termed 'enteroclysis' and that he had first developed in the treatment of dysentery. It consisted of the irrigation of the ileum with warm carbolic acid, which had demonstrated its potency as a disinfectant and which had achieved international prominence in the 1860s when Joseph Lister had made use of it to pioneer antiseptic surgery. Since Koch had now demonstrated that the *Vibrio cholerae* thrives in an alkaline environment and perishes in acid, Cantani intended, as he wrote, 'to render the intestinal contents acidic for a time'.[132] The flushing of the bowels would also assist the body in ridding itself of the toxic cholera-matter while the astringency of the fluid would slow the purging.

The bacillicidal acidic solution that Cantani employed consisted of a concentration of 1 gram of phenol crystals in 2 litres of a mixture of distilled water and alcohol. (Alternatively, some of Cantani's followers employed 15 grams of tannic acid to 2 litres of water.[133]) The serum was heated to a temperature of 38 to 40 degrees Centigrade to help raise the algid body temperature and then forced by means of a powerful enema into the ileum, where the cholera germ nestled. The enema was so designed that the force of the flow would overcome the resistance of the ileocolonic valve that separated the large intestine from the small. The force of the flow was imparted by gravity. The carbolic acid solution was allowed to descend from an altitude of 3 metres from a raised container down a tube and into the rectum.[134]

Carbolic acid, of course, is highly corrosive and toxic. Cantani argued, however, that the intestine in the algid state is incapable of absorption so that the danger of toxicity to the system would be minimal. Indeed, he reasoned that the failure of absorption caused by the disease would allow irrigations to be attempted at levels of acidity that would prove lethal in a healthy subject but that were necessary to effect the desired disinfection. Furthermore, Cantani called for experimentation with still higher acidity and trials of a wide variety of disinfectants for purposes of comparison—boric acid, thymol, iodine, salicylic acid, tannic acid, potassium permanganate, sulphuric acid. He expressed his therapeutic intention as follows:

> Enteroclysis brings the disinfecting liquid into direct contact with a wide intestinal surface. By this means alone, and by no other, can one hope seriously to disinfect the intestine. In all cases it is certainly possible in this way to disinfect the entire colon as well as the caecum, and in the many cases in which the rising water succeeds in opening Bahun's valve, it is possible to disinfect the small intestine as well. Thus the disinfectant, although tolerated by the patient, comes into direct contact with the cholera germs and either kills them or at least paralyzes them and renders them less harmful.[135]

The alcohol in his solution would also, he hypothesized, produce a 'useful topical effect.'[136]

All the while that the procedures of enteroclysis and hypodermoclysis were being carried out, Cantani continued to treat symptoms energetically. He gave instructions for the injection of ether as a stimulant, the exhibition of laudanum and cognac, massages for the relief of cramps, hot baths and hot compresses. In some cases the inhalation of oxygen was also indicated.

In reply to Cantani's suggestions, Semmola responded in a vitriolic manner, charging the rationalists and the advocates of intestinal irrigation with 'scientific charlatanism'. He charged that, 'The specific remedy, in cholera, or the quinine of cholera, so to speak, has not yet been discovered, and I am constrained to believe that it will never be discovered by rational means, that is to say, by means of the laboratory.'[137] The resort to theory denoted a 'deplorable pathological and clinical confusion'. Indeed, although he respected Koch and believed that his ideas would prove fruitful, Semmola argued that, for the sake of cholera patients, he almost wished that Koch's discoveries had never been published, such was the suffering and unnecessary death caused by intemperate followers like Cantani.

An extensive critique of Cantani's procedures appeared in Semmola's journal, *La Medicina contemporanea*, written by the editor, Gaetano Rummo.[138] Like Semmola, Rummo argued that Robert Koch's discoveries had led to a better understanding of cholera, but not to an improvement in the treatment of victims. Hypodermoclysis first attracted his fire. The procedure, he argued, presented a series of unresolved technical problems. There was a significant risk of embolism through the injection of air; it was impossible to administer fluid rapidly enough to compensate for loss by purging; and the technique required constant vigilance throughout by experienced physicians, who were already overburdened in the midst of an epidemic. In addition, a matter of principle arose because the only evidence in favour of hypodermoclysis was that put forward by ardent partisans.

With respect to enteroclysis, Rummo's conclusions were more comprehensively negative. He presented three major grounds for rejecting Cantani's intestinal irrigation. Cantani's argument held no validity in the first place, Rummo argued, because it was based on the assumption that it was possible for an enema to impart sufficient force to the flow of acidic fluid to open the valve between the small intestine and the large. Only in this manner could the phenol reach the germs it was intended to kill. In practice, however, the fluid seldom, if ever, rose beyond the colon. Secondly, in Rummo's view, the whole idea of killing the cholera germs with acid was absurd. What killed the patient was not the germ but the poison that it released. Therefore a more reasonable suggestion would be to introduce an antidote to the poison rather than a germ-killing acid. (Indeed, in the aftermath of the epidemic Cantani began to conduct experiments on dogs, searching for an antidote to the cholera poison that could be introduced by enteroclysis.)[139] Finally, by its very nature, the procedure placed the life of the patient in a crossfire between the cholera poison on one side and, on the other side, the poisonous acid introduced as an enema. If the patient failed to die of cholera, then he would be killed by the acid. The clinic, Rummo argued, invalidated abstract theories borrowed from the laboratory.

The opposition between the curative strategies of Semmola and Cantani was institutionalized in early September 1884. The municipal anti-cholera campaign endorsed the rationalist therapeutics of enteroclysis. Teodosio De Bonis was an avid supporter of Cantani's approach who had devised a portable enteroclysis kit that doctors could take with them to patients' homes, and he participated in clinical trials of the procedure at the Conocchia. De Bonis also secured the appointment of a fellow admirer of German science, the famous psychiatrist Buonomo, as Director of the hospital service and of Cantani as a consulting physician at the Conocchia.[140] Young devotees such as Orazio Caro[141] and Alfonso Montefusco, who at a later stage in their careers were to direct the municipal anti-cholera campaign of 1910–11, were hired as residents. As a matter of policy, therefore, the Conocchia, the Maddalena, the Piedigrotta and the Vittoria became centres of experimentation in a hopeful burst of enthusiasm to discover the cure for cholera through the application of Koch's laboratory discoveries to clinical practice.

Here was a factor that contributed to the anxiety of relatives who waited outside the gates, to the reluctance of patients to be hospitalized, and to the violent resistance to municipal doctors. Enteroclysis was a drastic, experimental and painful procedure. It was also lethal: it was not by coincidence that the Neapolitan cholera hospitals had uncomfortably high death-rates well in excess of the 50 per cent that contemporaries expected in untreated cases.[142] At the Conocchia, the young Montefusco noted that 75 per cent of the patients treated by hypodermoclysis died. So devastating was the procedure that Buonomo gave instructions that trials involving it be halted.[143] The results of enteroclysis were hardly more encouraging. The consequences, Montefusco reported cryptically, 'did not correspond to our expectations'.[144]

E. De Renzi, who directed the municipal medical campaign in the strategic *sezione* of Mercato, accepted the logic of Cantani's position. He nevertheless made observations on its practical results that were less than reassuring. He carried out clinical trials of a slightly modified version of 'physiological treatment', using injections of caffeine, quinine, ether and ammonia as stimulants to increase vitality and restore the pulse. De Renzi followed these with hypodermoclysis and enteroclysis practised with iodine as the intestinal disinfectant. He remained convinced of the correctness of the approach, but he admitted that the trial of iodine ended in death and that hypodermoclysis,

> which gave rise to such hopes, has only dashed them. My own personal experience, and that of my colleagues, has been negative. Personal vanity and other motives may surround the procedure with a false aura of success, but the dispassionate examination of clinical facts has, in my view, definitively condemned hypodermoclysis as a remedy for cholera.[145]

Apart from acidic irrigation, the Conocchia was the theatre for two speculative procedures introduced by traditionalists who were not persuaded by Cantani's attempts to find and kill the vibrio but who sought a more aggressive approach to therapeutics than Semmola's minimalism. One strategy they adopted was a revival of galvanism; the other was the administration of strychnine.

Three objectives underlay the electrical treatments. The first was based on the widely held theory that cholera was an electrical malfunction of a central nervous system, poisoned by the cholera toxin. To jolt the system into normal functioning, the physicians applied electrodes to the abdomen of the sufferer or lowered him into an 'electric bath'. Alternatively, electricity was employed as a means to revive a failing circulation. Finally, electrical treatment was believed to produce quantities of ozone that was deemed to be a powerful disinfectant. To witness the electric ordeal was alarming to fellow-sufferers and convalescents. Similar experiments had led to ill feeling in Provence.[146]

The second experimental idea – the resort to strychine – was also based on the concept of cholera as an intoxication of the nerves. Strychnine, once used as a counter-irritant, had been restored to a favoured place in the armamentarium by late nineteenth-century practitioners as a means of stimulating the spinal cords of the victims of paralysis. Reasoning that cholera itself was a violent form of palsy, municipal doctors employed the drug on sufferers and claimed 'splendid successes'.[147] Therapy thus affected popular responses to the epidemic. The Conocchia cholera ward, where physicians administered ratsbane, was one of the plausible sources of the poisoning hysteria.

The opposition of the population to municipal doctors and the phobia of poisoning that swept the Lower City were frequently denounced by the press and the authorities as based on ignorance, superstition and hysteria. It is worth noting, however, that the popular reaction had a basis in experience and that the idea of poisoning, exaggerated by frenzy and desperation, had a small kernel of truth. Cholera victims did not want to be the subjects of tormenting experiments that visibly concluded most often in failure. And they were all the more resolute in their position because, even in the medical profession in Naples, the municipal approach to treatment was the subject of fierce debate. The irrigation of the intestines with acid, the use of electrodes and the administration of strychnine were drastic therapies that were not legitimated by a consensus of medical opinion. Indeed, by the end of the first week in September, the people were offered an alternative. Alongside the official anti-cholera effort, a volunteer organization was founded. It was called the White Cross, and its Medical Director was Mariano Semmola.

The populace at large could not, of course, have understood the niceties of the debate between the followers of Semmola and the partisans of Cantani. It could not have known in detail of the procedures that were adopted on the cholera wards nor of the rationale for the therapies followed by doctors at bedsides in the Lower City. On the other hand, as Georges Lefebvre demonstrated in his classic study of the 'Great Fear' that swept the French countryside in the summer of 1789, rumour is a swift, inventive and powerful social force.[148] Like a raging brush fire, it requires only scattered fuel to sweep all before it. Naples in 1884 provided ample fuel for the flames. One element was simply the contrast between the openness of the White Cross doctors, who attended to sufferers in their own homes, and the secrecy of the four closed and forbidding hospitals manned by the municipal physicians directed by Cantani and De Bonis. The contrast between the two approaches was itself a factor that stoked the rumours surrounding the hospitals and created a dread of what was occurring on their wards. In a time of crisis, mystery bred suspicion. In so tense an atmosphere, occasional remarks by the enthusiastic and often untrained White Cross volunteeers casting doubts on the rival procedures followed by the city would have provided combustible material. Furthermore, some few distorted and distressing pieces of information inevitably filtered through the hospital gates. Discharged survivors, priests, and off-duty orderlies, attendants and nurses periodically brought tales of painful and suspicious experiments to a waiting city. Reaching a wide audience through such channels, enteroclysis, however misunderstood, played a part in sharpening social conflict.

RESISTANCE AND REVOLT

In early September the growing fear was transformed into urgent panic. Cholera brought normal life to a halt and replaced it with a constant effort to escape sudden and painful death. It also threatened the survivors with economic ruin by creating universal unemployment and by destroying the financial mainstays of families already stricken with poverty and grief. The resulting anguish manifested itself somatically in medical symptoms that were widespread among a people trapped by poverty in a dying city. Eugenio Fazio diagnosed the malady as 'nervous erethism' and chronicled its physical signs. Unendurable tension, he recorded, produced an abundant array of disorders – palpitations of the heart, a pronounced loss of appetite, nausea, indigestion, intestinal rumblings, a sense of oppression, psychic and bodily inertia and nervous tremors. Men became sexually impotent, and women experienced severe menstrual irregularities. Fazio also noted that hysteria, normally regarded as a psychological complaint of women, now afflicted both sexes equally and in its most pronounced forms.[149]

In addition to the physical and psychic disorders that affected individuals, the panic also manifested itself in a collective outburst of mass pathology. During September 1884 a great phobia of poisoning gripped the city of Naples. Fearing that the municipal officials were engaged in a diabolical plot to eliminate surplus population, the people reasoned that cholera was literal class warfare. The health officials, doctors and municipal guards who suddenly appeared in the back lanes of Old Naples were the agents of a deadly conspiracy. Their mission was to kill off the poor, and their weapon was poison.

Such a response, of course, is unintelligible except in the context of the long-term and deeply rooted suspicion of the people towards authority. With this long background of distrust, the popular imagination in 1884 found evidence everywhere for the malevolence of officials. Contemporary medical discourse was an important consideration. The contagio-miasmatic theory which dominated official and professional discussion interpreted cholera as a poison released into the environment by bacteria that had found suitable telluric conditions in which to ferment. In the opinion of many, the symptomatology of the disease reinforced this view of the aetiology of the disease. The symptoms of cholera, that is, were consistent with a general systemic poisoning. In its clinical features, cholera bore more resemblance to arsenical poisoning than to the course of any other known disease.

The impoverished and frequently illiterate inhabitants of the Neapolitan *bassi*, *fondaci* and *locande* did not read learned medical journals, attend meetings of the Neapolitan Academy of Medicine, or participate in conferences at the University. There were, however, numerous conduits through which some of the tenets of official medical doctrine were transmitted to the populace at large, forming what became the prevailing common sense with regard to cholera. As the disease approached the city, the authorities had attempted to prepare the population for the sanitary measures they intended to take if need arose. An integral part of this preparation was the circulation throughout the Lower City of wall posters, notices and pamphlets stating the official view of the disease in terms accessible to laymen. In addition, there were residents who read the newspapers, or had contact with public health officials, or attended the demonstrations against the Nisida lazaretto.

Still more unmistakable was the decoding by the people of the actions of Town Hall. The lighting of bonfires, the cleansing of sewers, the whitewashing of buildings, the sudden attention paid to wells and the flight of the wealthy were deeds rich in meaning. A medical lesson was implicit in the new fashion to tie an aromatic handkerchief around the neck before venturing abroad. The message conveyed, however, was often radically different from the one intended. It was unfortunate for officials that the idea of poison passed into popular consciousness, and that the people formed their own opinion in the vital matter of who was poisoning whom.

The state had already informed the nation that human agency was the cause of the epidemic. Lazarettos, quarantines and sanitary cordons were premised on the notion that people spread cholera. These health measures all implied that some individuals were dangerous and in need of confinement. The Catholic Church reinforced the lesson imparted by the state. The doctrine that epidemic diseases were the wages of sin concentrated attention on the dark deeds of men and women. It may even have been psychologically reassuring to invoke a wicked but comprehensible explanation for disaster. Far more unsettling was the idea that catastrophe had no meaning, that it resulted from the movement of microscopic creatures. Even the medical profession was divided over the plausibility of the germ theory. Popular culture instead resolutely personified cholera: the contemporary nicknames for the disease were 'the gypsy' and 'the wandering Jew'. The people were on the lookout for culprits.

The experience of the population with the disease itself was also educational. Like the doctors, laymen were struck by the dramatic symptoms exhibited by the victims. They were impressed, too, with the extraordinary age and class profiles of the sufferers. The cholera seemed uncannily to demonstrate a strategic purpose. It all too clearly targeted adults in the Lower City – the mainstays of the community and the very people who were of the age to bear children. If the *signori* intended in one cruel stroke to destroy the poor and to solve the problem of overpopulation, they could not have chosen their victims with greater accuracy.

Furthermore, unaccustomed as they were to attentions from their governors, the people of the city were able to observe a simple correlation. In normal years, the municipality practised *laissez-faire* in matters of public health, and there was no cholera. Suddenly, in the late summer of 1884 the authorities switched to a very different strategy of assiduous interventionism. Without warning, officials who did not visit the back lanes of Mercato and Pendino from one year to the next arrived in force and multiplied their attentions. They fumigated, inspected, disinfected, whitewashed, swept, medicated and interned. Concurrently with this frenzy of activity, the epidemic erupted in full force. The more intensively the officials interfered, the more savagely the cholera raged. To worried and suspicious minds, there seemed to be good reason to see here a relationship of cause and effect.[150] Moreover, it was only natural to note that the employees of the city drew lucrative salaries while the outbreak lasted. They might logically be thought to have an interest more in the perpetuation of the cholera than in its termination. The volunteer Alexandrine Tkatcheff explained that, 'The crowd did not understand why death struck them and not the rich. They believed that the doctors were paid to spread the cholera and kill off the ill ... because the people were too numerous.'[151]

Most important of all, however, in establishing a widespread conviction of poisoning in Naples was the sinister appearance of official health policies. The visits by municipal medical and disinfection teams had the appearance of a police manhunt or a military operation. As Nicola Amore admitted, the teams made the serious mistake of making a great show of force when they began their operations at the start of the month. To encourage compliance, they arrived at tenements with their weapons drawn, and they behaved towards distraught residents like an army of occupation in enemy territory. People who had no previous contact with the medical profession were suddenly ordered, sometimes at night, to surrender critically ill relatives to undergo compulsory treatment alone at a distant hospital that was rumoured to be a death-house rather than a curative establishment. They were also compelled by force to relinquish precious clothing and bedding to be destroyed by fire and to allow strangers to enter their homes to fumigate and disinfect. All too commonly the gravediggers who were sent to bear bodies to the cemetery drank heavily to stiffen their courage. They then arrived intoxicated, foul-mouthed and belligerent in the homes of people terrified or in mourning.[152] The *Osservatore romano* commented,

> The conduct of the authorities contributes mightily to the terror of the citizenry. As soon as a person is found to suffer the least disorder of the stomach, his home is invaded by municipal guards, police and doctors. ... In short, while it is possible to admire their energy, everyone condemns their behaviour. The guards and doctors act with such lack of concern and with such highhandedness that Mayor Amore

himself has felt compelled to send instructions in the matter to all twelve Deputy mayors of the city.[153]

The local paper *Roma* appealed to the responsible authorities to order their subordinates 'not to descend to acts of violence without cause'.[154] It seemed implausible to residents that the city was acting for their benefit.

Municipal actions were also suspect because they violated established gender roles. As the Bureau of Statistics noted, it was more acceptable in Italian popular medical culture for men to be hospitalized than for women. In 1886, for example, men were far more likely to be admitted to hospital, recording 193,135 admissions in the whole of the kingdom as opposed to 117,200 admissions for women.[155] Regarding the hospital, where all physicians and governors were men, as the antithesis of the role of the family in times of illness and as a negation of their traditional skills in folk medicine, women resisted seeking medical care and hospitalization until their diseases were far more advanced and desperate. For this reason, once admitted to hospital wards, women stayed far longer for treatment. In 1886, the 3,793 female hospital patients in Naples province stayed for an average of forty-nine days, as opposed to the average of twenty-nine for their 6,084 male counterparts.[156] For the same reason, women were significantly more likely than male patients to die before being discharged, recording a rate of 13.7 deaths per hundred discharges in all of Italy, in comparison with 11.1 for men.[157] These two facts reinforced women's perception of the hospital as an alien and threatening institution. It is readily comprehensible, therefore, that the entry of uninvited male doctors into their homes issuing orders for their forcible removal to distant cholera wards was a source of particular alarm to the female population of the Lower City. Understandably, women played a leading part in popular resistance to the municipal anti-cholera campaign.

Finally, the convictions of the population regarding the malevolence of their governors need to be seen in the context of the remarkable care with which the epidemic of 1884 seemed to choose its victims. Official statistics eloquently confirm the impression of contemporaries that the disease struck overwhelmingly at the most impoverished social classes. Unfortunately, as there are no comprehensive figures indicating the social composition of the victims of cholera in the city of Naples, it is necessary to make use of aggregate national statistics.

In Italy as a whole, the Department of Statistics (*Direzione Generale di Statistica*) recorded 14,299 deaths from cholera in 64 communes between the first death at Saluzzo on 19 June 1884 and the last at Gaeta on 17 December.[158] For our interest in Naples, the regional and provincial breakdown of the 14,299 deaths is important, as Table A2 in the Appendix demonstrates. Among the sixteen regions of Italy, five (Apulia, Calabria, Basilicata, Sicily and Sardinia) were either totally untouched by cholera or experienced fewer than six deaths from the disease. At the other extreme, Campania stood apart as the region most overwhelmingly afflicted with 8,424 cholera deaths. In Campania itself, moreover, the province of Naples accounted for 7,994 of all recorded cholera deaths, and the city itself for 7,123. Virtually half of those who died of cholera in all of Italy, therefore, were Neapolitans. Since the epidemic of 1884 was so preponderantly a Neapolitan disaster, national figures regarding the social composition of the victims inevitably shed considerable light on the local course of the disease.

The usefulness of the national statistics is further enhanced by the accident of the manner in which the figures were compiled. The Neapolitan authorities were unusually diligent in recording the vital statistics of those who were buried. According to the Department, deaths in Naples were 'comprehensively reported'.[159] Elsewhere, such information was not provided for 6,971 of the victims.[160] Because of the variable manner in which local authorities recorded mortality statistics, therefore, national figures published by the Department of Statistics concerning the age, sex and occupation of those who died of cholera in 1884 were overwhelmingly based on Neapolitan data. When these tables are used as sources of information on Naples alone, however, allowance must be made for a certain margin of error due (1) to the 'contamination' of the Neapolitan statistics concerning 7,123 people with a small proportion of 205 non-Neapolitans and (2) to the fact that, although Neapolitan officials diligently registered the age, sex and occupation of all officially reported cases, not all of the cases or deaths that occurred in the city were reported.

According to the Department of Statistics, cholera in 1884 became the fifth leading cause of death in Italy, accounting for 5.8 per cent of all deaths occurring during the year, even though it was primarily confined to a single city. Dividing the male population over 15 years of age into fifty-nine occupational groups, the Department then provided the absolute numbers of deaths from Asiatic cholera for each group and measured the proportion of cholera deaths in relation to the total deaths from all causes for the members of each occupation. It then compared the rate of mortality from cholera for each group with the national 'average' of 5.8 per cent. The results demonstrated that certain occupations and classes were heavily overrepresented among the 3,403 male victims of the disease aged 15 or over for whom information was provided. The most afflicted social groups were those endangered either because of their impoverishment or because of specific risks associated with their profession. In terms of the measurement by proportion, brass founders, who exercised their trade in the midst of the most notorious slums in Naples and who dealt in illegally recycled coffins, paid the highest toll of all with 29.6 per cent of the deaths among them being attributed to cholera. Other employments with mortality rates from cholera far in excess of the average were ragpickers (21.5 per cent), hawkers and huxters (20.7 per cent), policemen (17.5 per cent), unskilled labourers (17.0 per cent), hairdressers (16.2 per cent), kilnmen (14.7 per cent), charcoal burners (12.5 per cent) and messengers (11.7 per cent).[161] (Poverty, however, should be conceived as a necessary condition for a high rate of death from cholera, but not a sufficient cause. Some of the poorest professions in the nation, such as the beggars, porters and bakers escaped relatively lightly. With regard to the apparent good fortune of beggars, however, one suspects that a certain number of mendicants were concealed among the 403 men listed as 'other professions or profession unknown'.)

Absolute numbers formed the second means of measurement of the incidence of the disease by occupational category. The results, although somewhat different, confirmed the stark impression of the link between disease and poverty. Of the fifty-nine occupations listed, six contributed more than 100 victims: manual labourers (285), soldiers (182), clerks (162), carpenters (156), day labourers (126), and shopkeepers (110).[162] Complete figures are provided in Appendix A.

The available statistics for the incidence of cholera among women shed less light on the relationship between the disease on the one hand and class status or occupational group on the other. Women contracted cholera and died in almost identical proportions as men, and the Department of Statistics recorded the profession of 3,234 women over 15 years of age who died of cholera. The Department made less effort, however, at precision with regard to the occupation of women victims, dividing the female population into nineteen categories rather than fifty-nine as it did with regard to males. Furthermore, as a result of the prevailing sexual division of labour in the Neapolitan economy, approximately two-thirds (2,131) of the women who died from the epidemic were listed in the official tables as homeworkers (*'attendenti alle cure domestiche'*), a category that provides little insight into relative social and economic standing. The second largest category, with 357 deaths, was that of 'profession unknown'. It is difficult, therefore, to draw meaningful conclusions in regard to occupation and class on the basis of the statistics regarding women.[163]

At the apex of the male social pyramid, the professional and privileged classes were poorly represented among the cholera dead in terms of both proportion and number. Landlords, priests, lawyers and doctors, for instance, made minimal contributions to the bills of mortality in 1884: only 1.5 per cent, 3.0 per cent, 4.9 per cent and 5.2 per cent respectively of their members who died succumbed to Asiatic cholera. Among women, the grouping listed as 'wealthy' also enjoyed a figure of just 2.5 per cent. The general lack of affliction among such privileged members of society confirmed the populace in its view of the epidemic as a malevolent plot. Because of their involvement with sufferers, doctors seemed especially suspect: only thirteen physicians died as a result of the epidemic of 1884. It appeared sinister that the profession that was most extensively exposed to the disease remained mysteriously almost immune. Wherever doctors appeared in the Lower City, large numbers of people around them perished, but the medical men themselves seldom if ever succumbed.

That physicians, priests and municipal officials lived in the midst of cholera but rarely contracted it is not, in retrospect, mysterious. These visitors to the tenements of the Lower City did not eat meals or drink water during the course of their rounds, and they did not sleep in the *bassi* or *fondaci* to which they were called. They also took no part in the excesses of the popular festivals, and a well-regulated diet added to their immunity. The fact that professional men and women worked in the severely decimated back streets of Old Naples did not mean that they shared the risk factors that undermined the health of full-time residents.

Furthermore, educated members of the middle classes benefited from the profoundly unequal distribution of information concerning measures of individual self-defence against cholera and of the means to apply those measures in practice. Here was a respect in which the final pandemics of cholera accentuated class disparities. In the early visitations of the disease the mechanisms by which cholera was transmitted were entirely unknown. It was virtually impossible, therefore, for anyone to take effective individual precautions against infection, except by having recourse to the ancient expedient of taking flight. After half a century of experience with cholera, however, by the 1880s advances in the understanding of the aetiology of the disease enabled physicians to identify many of the factors that most strongly exposed individuals to risk and to offer practical advice on improving the odds against infection.

The work of epidemiologists and sanitarians such as Snow, Pettenkofer and Koch had resulted in a series of prophylactic procedures that individuals could follow to protect themselves. These measures were widely disseminated by public health pamphlets, wall posters, articles in the press and the counsel of medical personnel. Educated men and women were aware of the utility of boiling water; practising scrupulous personal hygiene; avoiding fruit, vegetables, seafood and alcohol; and of submitting themselves to disinfection after visits to cholera sick-rooms. The memoirs of doctors involved in the anti-cholera campaign record the vigilance that they exercised to avoid contamination. They were not, of course, totally immune: even Mariano Semmola, one of the most eminent authorities on Asiatic cholera at the University and a leading figure in the battle against the epidemic, was taken seriously ill in the course of his duties. But the odds had been enormously lengthened.

For the inhabitants of the slums, however, illiteracy, poverty and the distrust of authority made such advice inaccessible, or rendered it impossible to follow and difficult to accept. In Neapolitan conditions, the advance of knowledge served in 1884 to deepen the inequality of death among the social classes of the city. The people of Naples drew their own conclusions about the reasons for such striking disparities; they grew resentful and suspicious; and they rebelled against every aspect of the municipal strategy of collective self-defence. The press reported that the Lower City seethed with 'class hatred'[164] and officials complained unhappily of the 'indescribable resistance opposed by the lower classes [*popolo minuto*] to the measures that were intended for their salvation'.[165]

One aspect of this resistance was ritualized public defiance. The municipality had posted notices giving dietary advice, recommending above all the avoidance of un- or over-ripe fruit. It then attempted to enforce this suggestion by a rigorous inspection of market stalls, where officials ordered the confiscation and destruction of suspect produce. Superstition here clashed headlong with public policy. The people believed that to acknowledge danger was to make it more likely. To reassure themselves by a gesture of bravado, they responded by holding a series of public alimentary demonstrations. Crowds gathered in the squares in front of the Palazzo San Giacomo and the town halls of the *sezioni*. There they set basketloads of figs, prickly pears and melons on the ground. Members of the public, sometimes led by vendors eager to reassure their customers, proceeded to consume the forbidden fruit in enormous quantity. The crowd applauded, placed wagers on which binger would eat the most, and shouted mocking invectives at the authorities inside the adjacent offices.[166]

A similar defiance greeted other aspects of the intended municipal campaign to combat the epidemic. When workers arrived in the Lower City to light sulphur bonfires to purify the air, crowds often gathered, uncomprehending of the purpose of the flames. For the residents, the fires were unpopular because of their unpleasant effects. They produced pungent fumes and drove whole armies of sewer rats into the streets. The citizens prevented the workers from carrying out their assignment or put out the flames as soon as they had been kindled.[167]

The population regularly ignored the Mayor's decrees banning public assemblies of all descriptions. Penitents wearing crowns of thorns, carrying crosses and images of saints, and attracting hundreds of followers refused to disband. Openly flaunting their disobedience, the processions grew more rather than less numerous as September advanced. Undeterred, they continued to make their rounds of devotion and extortion. In mid-September, too, Neapolitans celebrated the traditional festival of Piedigrotta without regard to Nicola Amore's ban or his prophylactic advice. The festival was observed in the normal manner as a pagan ritual marked by excesses of fruit, uncooked vegetables and wine.[168]

The requirement that every case of gastro-intestinal disorder be reported to the authorities met with a more sullen opposition. An epidemic of concealment accompanied the epidemic of disease. Throughout Naples families refused to report illnesses, shielding the victims of cholera from medical attention and protecting their property from destruction. When physicians nevertheless appeared unasked, dying men and women refused to take their prescriptions or barricaded themselves in their hovels. People preferred to die unattended where they lay rather than be delivered into the hands of the city.[169] On numerous occasions neighbours and friends gathered around. Hoping to unmask a scoundrel, they forced the unlucky doctors to dose themselves with their own medications.

Dr Gallinari, a public health officer in the *sezione* Porto, suffered this tribulation as he made his way through the streets to attend a patient. A passer-by suddenly collapsed in front of him, exhibiting all the signs of Asiatic cholera. As he knelt to assist the man, a throng of suspicious inhabitants assembled. Unsure of Gallinari's intentions, they compelled him to open his phials of laudanum and alkermes and to consume their contents.[170]

Often the arrival of doctors and their escorts was the flashpoint for violent confrontation. It was dangerous in late August and September 1884 for municipal health teams to appear in the Lower City. Everywhere hostile crowds gathered, hurling insults and accusing them of murder. Frequently they were stoned, pushed down stairs or beaten. Similar receptions were accorded to stretcher-bearers who arrived, unbidden, in the midst of mourning to take possession of the body.[171] The newspapers were filled with reports of 'tumults', 'mutinies' and 'rebellions'. The accounts written by physicians apply to the people such epithets as 'beasts', 'mob', 'idiot plebeians' and 'inhuman rabble'.[172] Nicola Amore wrote in consternation that, 'As soon as the lower classes see doctors and guards, they hurl missiles at them. The people surround them and rain upon them blows of blind fury. Many, many guards and numerous doctors have been hit and injured.'[173]

The meaning of these occurrences was made apparent in the *sezione* Mercato. There the municipal doctor Antonio Rubino learned to his cost how perilous an official visit could become. On 26 August, in the company of policemen, Rubino was sent to examine a stricken child in the Borgo Loreto, one of the most insalubrious slums of the city. There he was met by an excited assembly of residents, armed in anticipation with sticks and cobble-stones. On seeing the doctor and his guards, they shouted 'After them! After them! They've come to kill us!', and gave vent to their fury.

Shaken but unhurt, Rubino was rescued by the fortunate arrival of twenty-five *carabinieri*, summoned by a passing street-sweeper. By then the crowd numbered several hundred, and the arrival of the troops inflamed the situation. The assault on the doctor now escalated into a violent affray as Rubino's assailants began to stone the military police. A street battle ensued, and the troops gained control only by drawing their weapons and opening fire.[174]

Nor was Rubino the only doctor who had to be rescued by the army. A physician called to treat a woman suffering from a chronic complaint found her symptoms suspect and announced his intention to summon the stretcher-bearers. Alarmed by the doctor's diagnosis, the residents of the building seized the offending medic and hurled him into the courtyard. There they pelted him with stones and rotten fruit. When he sought to escape, they gave chase. Terrified, he found refuge in a neighbouring barber shop and ventured forth only after a detachment of *carabinieri* arrived and put his tormentors to flight with unsheathed sabres.[175]

There were also scenes of vengeance. An example was the attempted homicide perpetrated by a certain Cervinara, a grocer in the Lower City. His young son had fallen ill of cholera in the last week of August, and had been taken to the Conocchia Hospital. There he died. Grief-stricken and convinced of foul play, Cervinara and his brothers armed themselves and forced their way through the hospitals gates and onto the wards, intent on killing the attending physician. Only the presence of the chaplain prevented bloodshed. He calmed the frenzied visitors until orderlies came to his aid, disarmed the men and took them into custody.[176]

The arrival of the distraught Cervinara was not the only violent incident to occur on the wards of the Conocchia. On 27 August a further conflict took place when the hospital was invaded by three men from the city – Luigi Giannattasio, Ernesto Lancellotti and Guglielmo Ferraro. They had a relative in common who had been stricken by the disease and taken to the Conocchia by force for isolation and treatment. Distraught and fearful for the well-being of their kinsman, they invaded the hospital determined to liberate the patient. When the Conocchia porters attempted to evict them, a fracas ensued. Summoned to restore order, the police arrested the trio and enforced a sardonic sequel. Deeming that the three intruders by their presence on the wards had been exposed to contagion, the *questore* (Chief of Police) ordered that they in turn be fumigated, disinfected and quarantined at Nisida.[177] The liberators were themselves incarcerated.

On several occasions as the epidemic reached the height of its fury, the tensions of the city unleashed full-scale insurrections. Two such occasions occurred with the opening of the new cholera hospitals of the Piedigrotta and the Maddalena to supplement the severely overburdened Concocchia. These new institutions were fearfully unwelcome in the neighbourhoods where they were sited. Cholera hospitals were the most dreaded feature of the municipal plan to save the city. They were regarded by the people as places of horror – charnel houses from which no one ever returned. Cholera hospitals, furthermore, were considered a lethal danger not only to their patients but also to everyone in their vicinity. To a city now schooled in the perils of miasmas, it seemed perverse or even diabolically malevolent to concentrate large numbers of contagious people exuding fatal exhalations in densely populated neighbourhoods.

The first explosion of protest occurred on Tuesday, 9 September when the city announced the opening of a second hospital for infectious diseases. The site of the city's second cholera hospital was the former military hospital of Piedigrotta, now hastily transformed to accommodate civilian cholera patients. To reach the Piedigrotta, the cholera vans and stretcher-bearers would have to cross the *sezione* Chiaia, which had been largely spared by the epidemic. To many who lived in the borough, the passage of ill patients through their streets was tantamount to a collective sentence to death. When the first stretchers appeared, they were met by a crowd of terrified residents. When the porters attempted to proceed, they were attacked and forced to retreat, dropping their charges in the street as they ran off in headlong flight.

Exulting in this sudden triumph, the crowd grew larger and more purposeful. Fearing the arrival of authorities intent on enforcing the will of the City Hall, the people hastily erected barricades and gathered paving stones, sticks and missiles of every description. Some residents also equipped themselves with firearms. When the municipal guard arrived in force in the late morning, a pitched battle ensued in which the city police sustained many injuries and finally withdrew. In the afternoon, the cavalry arrived and attempted to force a passage. They too were driven off. Calm was restored only when parish priests intervened as mediators, bearing the message that the city had capitulated and would avoid the streets of Chiaia as a means of reaching the Piedigrotta.[178]

An almost identical scene took place at the opposite end of the city – in the east near the Maddalena Bridge over the Sebeto River that marked the municipal boundary. There in the second week of September the army cleared its barracks. The municipality transformed them into the third and largest of the cholera hospitals. On 14 September, the first attempt to transport patients to the new facility developed into a violent revolt as the inhabitants released their fury at the expense of the first unlucky porters to attempt a passage through the streets of the borough of Vicaria. From the upper storeys the residents hurled benches, tables, mattresses and stones, critically injuring two porters and seriously wounding several others. They then blocked the streets in open rebellion.[179]

The fear of painful death also caused violent tumults in two of the city's eight prisons – the Carmine and the San Francesco, each of which held approximately a thousand men in detention. There tensions had mounted with the first approach of cholera in August. Part of the protest that followed was based on the long-term conditions that prevailed in these facilities. Conducting an investigation into the disorders that had broken out the previous summer, the local newspaper *Roma* concluded in 1885 that the prisoners' protest was founded on the 'intolerable state' of the municipal jails. The city prisons were sordid, unhygienic establishments with an unhappy history of disease. They were described as damp, airless and overcrowded, 'fit only to destroy the health of robust inmates and to worsen the condition of those already unwell'.[180] During previous cholera epidemics, they had been savagely decimated. Acknowledging the dangerous overcrowding and the pervasive filth of the jails and attempting to prevent the recurrence of earlier calamities, the city instituted a harsh new regime in the prisons.

The purpose was to save life, but the effect was to create terror. The prison governors suddenly ordered a change of diet, banning the ever-suspect fruit and vegetables to which the inmates were accustomed and putting them instead on a diet of rice, meat, broth and water acidulated with vinegar to destroy dangerous microbes. They then declared that the prisons were to be sealed from all contact with the outside world. Transfers of offenders within the penal system and court appearances were deferred. Post was banned, all visits were cancelled for an indefinite period and cholera wards were established in every institution. The prisoners were suspicious of the motives of the new regime; the cholera wards were mysterious in function; and the isolation magnified fear, severing all contact between the men and their friends and families.[181] It was also unnerving that the warders and guards were granted hazard pay for the duration of the emergency.[182]

When the epidemic exploded in the city and the first scattered cases broke out within the prisons, the convicts developed the certainty that they had been shut inside to die. At both the Carmine and the San Francesco the fear exploded into a mutiny. The prisoners attacked the warders, clambered onto the roofs, and attempted to force the gates, shouting 'Help! We don't want to die! Let us out!' The fate of the convicts provoked an answering protest in the streets outside, where crowds gathered in sympathy, denouncing the authorities and demanding the release of the men inside. The prison governors lost control, and order was restored only when the army was sent in.[183]

So pervasive and determined was the opposition of people throughout Lower Naples to the sanitary campaign of the city that by the second week in September it had rendered much of the municipal plan nugatory. Every initiative under-taken by the authorities provoked a violent backlash. In the domain of public health, Naples was approaching a state of near-anarchy. *The Times* correspon-dent announced that the city was afflicted with something far worse than the epidemic – a state of 'medieval ignorance and superstition'.[184] Realizing that he was rapidly losing control of events and that the cholera was sweeping all before it, the Mayor of secular Italy's largest city took in the first week of September the unprecedented step of appealing for help to the Cardinal Archbishop.

EPILOGUE: EPIDEMICS AND POISONERS

The poisoning frenzy that raged in the Old City in 1884 was not, of course, a novelty in the European experience of epidemic diseases. The history of both bubonic plague and Asiatic cholera was marked by bouts of collective fury directed at scapegoats held responsible for diabolical crimes. In both the four-teenth century and the seventeenth, the ravages of pestilence were made more frightful by murderous waves of xenophobia and antisemitism. Frenzied mobs, convinced that the disaster was the work of demonic criminals, conducted witchhunts at the expense of foreigners, religious minorities and such marginal members of society as lepers and pilgrims.[185] In Italian history the most famous episode of this poisoning mania – its notoriety ensured by the attention it received from the *philosophe* Cesare Beccaria and the novelist Alessandro Manzoni – was the so-called *colonna infame* (the 'column of infamy') of the 1630 epidemic of plague in Milan. This sinister incident involved the torture and execution of hapless foreigners suspected of being *untori* – spreaders and smearers of the poison responsible for the catastrophe that had overtaken the city.[186]

After plague had been banished from most of Europe in the eighteenth century, the arrival of cholera as the most dreaded disease of the modern era generated renewed outbursts of collective pathology directed once more at the suspected agents of a monstrous conspiracy. As at Naples in 1884, cholera epidemics gave rise in many nations to serious social tensions, leading to riots, mass flight and assaults on doctors and officials. Contemporaries who experi-enced the cholera pandemics after 1830 immediately drew parallels between the tumults that followed in the wake of the two great epidemic maladies of modern times. Manzoni, who wrote the history of plague and experienced the first cholera pandemic, called attention to the similarity of the social response to the two diseases. Describing the conviction of the Milanese population that foreign agents were at large daubing the city walls with poison to spread the plague, Manzoni noted in 1842 that, 'Anyone who contemplates this deeply rooted superstition, this mad fear of an imaginary crime, inevitably recalls the similar events that took place in various parts of Europe, just a few years ago, in the time of cholera.'[187] In the same vein contemporary physicians, journalists and politicians described the events unleashed by the cholera phobia as 'plague scenes' and 'medieval fear'. In the midst of the first epidemic to visit the British Isles, the physician James Johnson speculated that, 'The cholera-phobia will frighten to death a far greater number of Britons than the monster itself will ever destroy by his actual presence.'[188]

The poisoning hysteria of the first cholera pandemic in the 1830s, when the disease inexorably swept all before it, was the most tumultuous and the most nearly reminiscent of the plague. Among European nations the extreme case was Russia, where the consequences of the epidemic were apocalyptic. In Russia not only did the disease cause a terrifying mortality but the regime also magnified the terror by a violent and coercive strategy of public health. The Romanovs reproduced some of the social consequences that accompanied the plague by reviving the anti-plague public health policies of early modern political authorities. Furthermore, the war waged by the regime to suppress the uprising in Poland gave credence to the widespread Russian belief that the foreigners in their midst were Polish agents sent to kill them off en masse by poison. The results were outlined by Roderick McGrew, who observed that,

> The poison hysteria was actually an effort to rationalize the darkling fears which the cholera's recurrence produced, and since poison was an instrument used by human agents for special ends, the hysteria focused on particular scapegoats. The most popular villains were Polish agents and foreigners in general, though both physicians and government officials were also included. By mid-summer a mass phobia had set in which affected the educated and the illiterate alike. The former were able to rationalize their stories by reference to public problems and private greed, but for the masses a spirit of evil had entered the land, and no one was immune. The poison scare played a part in the Petersburg cholera revolt, in the risings in the Novogorod military colonies, in the riots which occurred in Staraia Russia, but it also appeared away from these centers of unrest.[189]

On a far smaller canvas, the Sicilian domains of the Bourbon crown presented a comparable spectacle. There too the state adopted military measures of public health, and a brutal history of violent repression by the Neapolitan rulers of the island made it plausible for the population to imagine that the disease was instead a genocidal final settling of scores. Indeed, Professor E. Albanesi, the foremost Sicilian authority on cholera and the President of the Sanitary Council of Palermo during the outbreak of 1885, explained the Sicilian poisoning psychosis as the popular response to the violent military campaign of General Declaretto, who used the cholera epidemic of 1837 as a pretext to institute a 'government of military terror in Sicily, which lasted without interruption until 1848'.[190] The Bourbon general, Albanesi concluded, 'seized this opportunity to persecute and torture some of our greatest patriots, and to snatch from Sicily every trace of freedom. This is why the people believe in poisons, which they fancy the Bourbons scattered in order to render the island miserable, and to deprive it of every former privilege.'[191] In this climate, Sicily during the cholera invasions of the 1830s and the 1840s experienced the violent confrontations and all-pervading panic described by Giuseppe Verga in his novel *Mastro-don Gesualdo*.

Even in Britain and France, where the fear of the disease was not exacerbated by warfare and military measures, the deadly first pandemic produced poisoning manias and violence. In Britain the epidemic coincided unhappily with a wave of public suspicion of doctors unleashed by revelations of widespread body stealing by 'resurrection men' who supplied the anatomy theatres of professors of medicine. In such a context, rumours abounded that cholera was a conspiracy to increase the supply of human cadavers by murder. Only a flashpoint was needed to produce scattered deeds of violence of the kind described by Michael Durey, R.J. Morris and Norman Longmate.[192] Between February and November 1832, Durey estimates, some thirty riots took place, 'varying considerably in intensity, from what contemporaries called "petty tumults", in which small groups of people hurled stones and assaulted doctors, to large-scale riots involving hundreds'.[193]

Similarly, in France the disease was widely 'denounced as a criminal enterprise conducted by the authorities or by the privileged classes'.[194] In Paris – 'the scene of such melancholy events as will form one of the most gloomy pages in the history of pestilential disease'[195] –there were two days of rioting in April 1832 by the ragpickers of the city against the genteel classes, whom they regarded as assassins. Foreigners were thrown into the Seine, and there were numerous demonstrations against hospitals and attacks on doctors.[196]

But even in the light of so many disturbances across the whole of Europe, the direct parallels that have been made between plague and cholera in terms of the social response they evoke are based on literary licence – a point that must be stressed in order to understand the historical particularity of the events of 1884. The level of violence against scapegoats accused of spreading cholera never approached the frenzy of the pogroms and witchhunts of the early modern world. Asiatic cholera produced less extreme popular reactions than plague because of three interrelated categories of factors – the very different nature of the disease itself, the changes that had occurred in the societies that experienced the malady, and the very different sanitary policies adopted by the modern state.

The first factor – the differing natures of the two diseases – is the most obvious and perhaps the most crucial. Cholera never produced a social pathology commensurate with that of bubonic plague because it never exhibited a comparably devastating and indiscriminate mortality, and it never continued to claim its victims for so protracted a period of time. With vastly reduced mortality and duration, cholera epidemics also gave rise to more limited explosions of social paranoia. Not only, however, was cholera different as a disease from plague, but also the societies it affected had changed in ways that decisively affected the propensity to collective bouts of hysteria. Secularization, advances in levels of literacy, the bureaucratic rationalism of the modern state, the scientific revolution and the complex of cultural transformations Keith Thomas terms the 'decline of magic' encouraged the acceptance of naturalistic explanations for medical disasters in lieu of malevolent human agency.[197] And, finally, the abandonment by most European nations after the first pandemic of the draconian public health measures applied to combat the plague de-fused social tension. State sanitary

Table 3.6. *Cholera in Paris, 1832–92*

Year	Population	Deaths from cholera	Deaths per 100,000 inhabitants[a]
1832	785,862	18,402	2,245
1849	1,053,262	19,615	1,861
1854	1,174,346	8,591	732
1865	1,825,274	6,347	354
1866	1,825,274	5,218	289
1873	1,851,792	855	46
1884	2,260,945	986	44
1892	2,447,957	977	39

Note: There are minor discrepancies in the calculations of rates of death in this table. I have reproduced it as it originally appeared in the *Lancet* (April, 1892).

policy ceased to legitimize the belief that outsiders were dangerous and to threaten communities with military encirclement and severe economic dislocation.[198]

For a series of reasons, therefore, the social response to cholera never reproduced the paroxysms of violence against poisoners that so frequently accompanied the plague. Even in the course of the first pandemic when the disease was most mysterious and terrifying, there were no excesses comparable to the genocidal fury of the flagellants or the witch trials described by Manzoni. And thereafter a marked feature of the epidemic history of Asiatic cholera in nineteenth-century Europe was a progressive decline in the mortality it caused and a corresponding abatement in the collective hysterias it generated. Scientific understanding took a quantum leap forward with the establishment of the germ theory of disease through the work of Koch and Pasteur; states adopted major sanitary reforms; levels of literacy rose with broad programmes of compulsory public education; and populations became increasingly accustomed to medical attention and confident of its utility. By the closing decades of the century in the industrialized nations of Europe, cholera was largely contained. Sporadic cases occurred, but whole nations were no longer vulnerable to epidemic disaster. Britain experienced no further epidemics after 1866,[199] and Paris exhibited a steady decline in mortality that was illustrative of a broad European pattern (see Table 3.6). By the end of the century the populations of many of the states of Europe therefore felt a sense of medical security, protected by bulwarks of 'civilization' against sudden death by epidemic disease.

Even when cholera succeeded in breaching the sanitary ramparts and claimed a substantial mortality, it possessed an ever-diminishing capacity to stir the demons of the collective subconscious. An example is that of Paris during the two waves of the fifth pandemic that it experienced in 1884 and 1892–3. On each occasion the French capital suffered approximately a thousand deaths, but reports of the atmosphere suggest calm and a total absence of social conflict based on the disease. Here too is the great interest of Richard Evans's account of Hamburg during the major disaster of 1892–3. In Hamburg, a city of 623,000 inhabitants, the epidemic of 1892 was the most devastating of the century, killing nearly 9,000 people – more than all of the previous outbreaks combined.[200] The city, however, was free of any hint of cholera phobia, poisoning and riot. On this point Evans is emphatic. Referring to the long history of hysteria and disorder during epidemic emergencies, he wrote:

> Yet this pattern of behaviour – from terror released by the arrival of an epidemic through the popular search for a scapegoat (usually the doctors or the authorities), to collective violence and revolt, was conspicuously lacking in Hamburg in 1892. This was not because the habit of collective violence had disappeared, or had been channelled into purposeful political activity through the labour movement: there had been serious rioting in the Alley Quarters in 1890 and it was to occur again in 1897 and 1906 ... The Alley Quarters were severely affected by cholera in 1892: indeed it was widely believed that they bore the main brunt of the epidemic. Yet there was no unrest, not even any small incident of collective hostility to the authorities in these areas during the epidemic.[201]

It is in this context that the Neapolitan tumults of 1884 acquire their particular significance. Chronologically, they formed part of the very same pandemic that passed so uneventfully through Paris and Hamburg. The social and medical attitudes they reveal, however, were radically different. In Naples poisoners lived on in popular belief and despatched the poor to the cemetery. For precisely this reason the events that unfolded in the southern metropolis have enormous meaning for the history of Italy and the comparative history of cholera.

Untori did not emerge from the shadows of Naples as a mere matter of course. Paris and Hamburg clearly demonstrate that by the late nineteenth century cholera and human agency were no longer universally linked in popular imagination. That poisoning played so prominent a part in the epidemic of 1884 reveals much about Neapolitan society and Italian statecraft. The national strategy of relying on coercive prophylaxis by means of land-based quarantine in lieu of costly and extensive sanitary reforms bears a large share of the responsibility, as we have seen. Sanitary cordons were a major difference that set the experience of Italy in 1884 apart from that of France and Germany during the fifth pandemic. The cordons revived the potent mixture of xenophobia and fear of contagion that formed the emotional basis for the search for scapegoats.

At the same time local circumstances in the great Tyrrhenian seaport ensured that, once planted, the seeds of cholera phobia would germinate. The lack of confidence of the people of the city in authorities who won office through dubious electoral practises, who frequently colluded with the criminal underworld, and who carried out no programmes for the welfare of the city made the suspicion of malevolence all too plausible. In conditions where so broad a swathe of the population was malnourished, underemployed, inadequately housed and illiterate, inaction alone led to a silent imputation of ill will. The fact that the governors of the city were the Liberal administrators of a secular regime further confounded their ungodly reputation among a population that was celebrated for its intense, if heretical, religiosity.

It was unfortunate for the authorities at the Palazzo San Giacomo that the sanitary measures they applied were unfamiliar and threatening. After a quarter of a century of *laissez-faire*, the city suddenly invaded the homes of its citizens and intervened in the most emotionally charged matters of life and death. Furthermore, the agents through whom the city acted were the suspect corps of municipal doctors who were unknown in the quarters where they carried out virtual police raids both by day and by night. The medical procedures they called for – the forcible transport of patients to menacing cholera wards from which too few returned and where painful and mysterious experiments were conducted – consolidated the impression of an evil conspiracy, and the symptoms of cholera itself confirmed the idea by mimicking the sudden and agonizing seizures of arsenical poisoning.

Unlike Hamburg and Paris, therefore, the fifth cholera pandemic in Naples led to widespread terror that escalated into violence and desperate resistance against doctors perceived as the agents of a demonic class conspiracy. These tumults were not simply one more illustration of the invariable social consequences of Asiatic cholera. Such events were anachronistic in much of Europe. Their occurrence in Naples was a measure instead of the failure of the Liberal regime to address the 'Southern Question'. The pronounced inequality between North and South had a medical as well as an economic component. Poverty, illiteracy, mass unemployment and the absence of sanitary urban infrastructures ensuring pure water, waste removal and adequate housing established conditions in which cholera could continue to flourish. But, equally importantly, they created an atmosphere of suspicion and hostility of the population towards authority, both political and medical. The inhabitants of the Lower City, far from feeling defended by the sanitary ramparts of the modern state, believed that disease was permanently allowed to ferment in the subsoil of the city by indifferent officials. The sudden emergency of a major cholera outburst seemed plausible as a strategy for eliminating unwanted surplus people. Inequality thus not only bred disease but also transformed the popular response to an epidemic into violent confrontations in which deep-rooted social hatreds were fought out on the streets of the Lower City.

4

Survival and recovery

ALTERNATIVE MEANS OF PALLIATION

Despite so great an ordeal, Naples survived. The plan developed by the municipal *giunta* lay in ruins, but the city nevertheless weathered the crisis. Part of the explanation for this endurance was a feature of the disease itself – one of the great 'cholera mysteries' that characterize the history of this exotic pestilence. For reasons still insufficiently understood, epidemic cholera is self-limiting. Thus in Naples the epidemic began by rapidly and violently destroying those individuals who were most at risk. It then began slowly to subside after the catharsis of mid-September. The circle of its victims narrowed, and the rate of mortality declined. By the end of September it no longer appeared that the city was being inexorably annihilated. The medical crisis was slowly abating. In October the daily bills of mortality were almost comforting, so marked was the contrast with the preceding weeks. Figures that, in August, would have created panic, brought relief after the experience of September. Although the outburst continued into early November, the official daily number of deaths never again climbed as high as ninety. There began instead a slow descent into single digits.[1]

Imperceptibly, tensions in the city followed the downward curve of mortality. With fewer cases a day, conflicts became less frequent, the hospital service improved, the cemetery kept pace with the smaller number of cadavers, and scenes of horror grew steadily rarer. Terror itself began to subside.

The Crosses – White and Red

The spontaneous decline of the epidemic force of the disease, however, is only one aspect of the gradual return to near-normality that occurred in October. Naples rose to the challenge of epidemic cholera because the official anti-cholera campaign launched by Town Hall was not the only resource available. The city coped with the emergency by discovering alternative means of self-defence that both combated the infection and dissipated the social tensions that followed in its

155

wake. Of these resources, the most striking and comprehensive was the voluntary organization officially designated as the Committee for the Assistance of the Victims of Cholera but universally known as the 'White Cross'.

The White Cross was a sort of medical International Brigade. Naples became a symbol of heroic defence against epidemic disease. Its fate stirred the conscience of Europe and mobilized an international force of volunteers who rushed to its assistance. To understand the establishment of such a sanitary crusade in the former capital, one must recall that in 1884 Naples was the only great metropolis in the West to suffer so devastating an outbreak of cholera.[2] Partly for humanitarian reasons, therefore, the travails of Neapolitans were followed with interest by educated people across Europe. The epidemic was a leading topic in the press and in medical journals throughout the late summer and autumn, and the sufferings of the people were portrayed in vivid terms. Queen Victoria, Emperor William I, and Emperor Francis-Joseph all publicly expressed their sympathy with the people of Naples.[3] Open-air concerts to raise funds for the victims of the epidemic were held at Berlin, Paris and Trieste.[4]

More than sympathy was involved, however. As one of the largest cities and principal ports of the West, Naples had intense commercial links with the whole of Italy, the Mediterranean and North America. A violent mass outburst of Asiatic cholera in Naples, therefore, posed a direct menace to every other centre with which it was linked. To contain the epidemic within the great Tyrrhenian seaport was, therefore, not only a matter of humane concern for the fate of its inhabitants but also an issue of enlightened self-interest. Medical students and physicians as far away as Milan and Montpellier saw in the Neapolitan epidemic an opportunity to gain first-hand experience of the most dreaded disease of the nineteenth century. For the partisans of a variety of competing political and religious credos, the return of cholera offered a very public occasion to re-affirm their solidarity with the sufferings of the poor. And for those far-sighted members of the Neapolitan elite who had not taken flight, the launching of a new sanitary initiative provided the possibility of combating not only the disease but also the disorder and class tensions that it left in its wake. For men and women motivated by all of these considerations, the White Cross became the instrument of their faith.

The first step in the establishment of the new volunteer force was taken on 29 August in the Lower City by Neapolitan workers themselves.[5] On that day the most important working-class organization in the city, the mutual aid society founded in 1861 under republican auspices and known as the Società Operaia, launched a new medical initiative.[6] Its intention was to furnish its members with an alternative to the hated visitations of the municipal doctors, guards and disinfecters. For this purpose the Società Operaia, which was articulated in various sub-sections representing the principal crafts in Naples, announced the formation of a 'sanitary company' that would administer to the needs of any members whose families were struck down by the disease and who appealed to the organization for help. The company consisted of a handful of doctors who offered their services and workers who volunteered to assist them as nurses. They had available a fund of 1,000 lire drawn from the reserve fund of the Società to distribute to the families in form of medication, blankets, food and, when urgently needed, ready cash. Unattached to the city or the hospital service, the 'sanitary company' was formed to treat cholera patients exclusively in their homes and to provide a minimum of welfare and sanitary assistance to the survivors.

Unfortunately, it is not possible to explore in detail the functioning of the medical initiative of the Società Operaia as no records of the organization have survived beyond scattered press accounts. It was, in any event, a small-scale operation whose most important contribution was that of catalyst. A week after the founding of the 'sanitary company', Rocco De Zerbi imitated its example on a much more ambitious basis. De Zerbi was a Deputy, a leading figure of the Historical Right in the city, and the editor of the newspaper *Il Piccolo*. He had long taken an interest in the health of the city. De Zerbi had investigated the sanitary problems of Naples and drafted proposals for reform. In 1883 he had played a leading role in organizing relief for the benefit of the survivors of the earthquake at nearby Casamicciola, and in the summer of 1884 he had led the vociferous protests against the establishment of quarantine on Nisida. As the cholera epidemic came to a close, this Liberal deputy was also to play a major part in the campaign for urban renewal.

On Thursday, 4 September he convened an emergency meeting to establish what was in effect a city-wide sanitary company that would replace the faltering attempt of the municipal authorities to assist the victims of cholera. This founding meeting was attended by representatives of the local newspapers, the Società Operaia, the medical faculty of the University, and the local political parties. They agreed forthwith to launch the White Cross; they chose its executive committee; and they issued an appeal for volunteers and financial assistance. The continuity with the workers' initiative of the previous week was demonstrated by the merging of the original 'sanitary company' with the White Cross and the selection of the secretary of the Società Operaia as a member of the executive of the new organization. The workers' associations throughout the city transformed themselves into auxiliaries in support of the initiatives of the White Cross.[7]

In view of the extreme gravity of the danger, the White Cross began to function almost at once. Its executive committee held its first meeting at its new premises in the Via Toledo on Saturday, 6 September. On Monday the organization became fully operational. To reach the people it sought to assist, the new association relied heavily on word of mouth. In this respect it benefited enormously from its origins in the labour movement of the city. Unlike the official medical campaign of the municipality, the volunteer effort of the White Cross possessed enthusiastic advocates in the working class of the Lower City who were above suspicion of participation in the poisoning campaign of the *signori*. And in this time of crisis when cholera was the only topic of conversation in

Naples the news of a new entity offering hope and practical assistance spread rapidly. In addition, the society festooned the walls of all twelve boroughs with posters announcing its existence and purpose. It also relied on an active publicity campaign in the press, taking full advantage of the fact that several editors of the leading Neapolitan papers were represented on its executive, including of course De Zerbi himself. And the commander of the company in each borough under-took an active propaganda campaign on behalf of the association.

For organizational purposes, ten of the twelve *sezioni* of the city were assigned a company of the White Cross, to which were added two further companies for the Vomero and Capodimonte hills and a central reserve force at the head-quarters of the organization in the Via Toledo that stood ready to respond to sudden emergencies that threatened to overwhelm a local company anywhere in the city. The two *sezioni* of Montecalvario and Porto had special arrangements under the overall White Cross umbrella. In Porto the Red Cross acted as the White Cross sanitary company, and in the medically marginal borough of Montecalvario an affiliated benevolent society known as the *Comitato delle milizie* organized medical services on behalf of the parent organization. To facilitate rapid response to appeals for help and to bind the twelve boroughs tightly to the central executive in Via Toledo, the association made use of the most modern technology in the form of the telephone, invented by Alexander Graham Bell in 1876.

Each company possessed its own president, vice-president, secretary, and inspectors in addition to a full complement of volunteer doctors and attendants. The volunteers streamed into the new organization from every borough of Naples, from every region of Italy, and from several foreign countries – Switzerland, France, England and Sweden. They represented all social classes and political persuasions. The White Cross included a delegation of anarchists from Lombardy led by Errico Malatesta, a company of workers from the Romagna, and a group of Garibaldian patriots organized by the radical poet Felice Cavallotti who sought to relive the expedition of the Thousand by wearing red shirts. There were also liberals, clericalists and monarchists. In addition to workers, the volunteers included army officers, aristocrats, financiers, lawyers, physicians, university professors, clerks, members of parliament and local government employees. A team of nurses from the Pharo Hospital in Marseilles brought the experience they had gained in June and July during the outbreak in Provence. The Director-General of the Bank of Naples, Count Girolamo Giusso, served in the organization at the side of the Russian populist Alexandrine Tkatcheff, and in the company of artisans and day labourers. Such was the flood of people that on September 13 the White Cross declared its ranks closed. By that date it numbered 1,084 members, of whom 139 were doctors and 12 were women.[8]

At De Zerbi's instigation, every member of the organization undertook to submit to quasi-military discipline. The executive committee insisted on a unity of approach in every aspect of policy throughout the city. To that end, it bestowed a rank on every volunteer, issued directives and gave, in De Zerbi's words, 'exact and absolute orders'. As he explained, 'When an organization demands of its members that they be prepared to sacrifice their lives, then it must assume the discipline either of an army or of a monastic order.'[9] The military model was congenial to such volunteers as Cavallotti and his red shirts. Offering his services to the Deputy Giovanni Bovio, the Milanese poet wrote on 10 September,

> I am neither a doctor nor a rich man nor a local deputy. I cannot provide the services of science or money or moral authority. I am, however, an Italian with health and good will to offer. I place myself at the service of the committee, and I bring with me squads of Tuscan war veterans organized on a military footing who have kindly asked me to stand at their head. We are ready for any kind of duty – nursing, the transport of patients, the removal of corpses, or whatever the executive requires. I shall probably also lead a Milanese squadron. Inform the executive and the mayor, and telegraph my orders for departure.[10]

The White Cross envisaged the city as a field of battle and regarded itself as a citizens' militia engaged in combat with a deadly but unseen enemy.

The primary mission of the White Cross company in each borough was to respond to urgent calls of help from the families of victims on a twenty-four hour basis. When it received a call, the company would dispatch a doctor and two assistants. Their function was to provide medical and nursing care in the patient's own home until the disease had run its course. In theory, the volunteers in attendance at a sufferer's bedside were to be relieved in shifts of four hours' duration. Under the strain of the emergency as the epidemic approached its peak of ferocity, however, relief was rarely forthcoming. Then the three-man team that first arrived to attend to a sufferer remained in place for an uninterrupted vigil, bearing witness to the suffering of the people.

Like the Società Operaia, the White Cross aimed to provide a service that was broader than medical treatment alone. It also attempted to combat the outbreak of social hysteria and panic. One means of achieving this objective was to break down the barrier of distrust between the medical profession and the population. The White Cross insisted, therefore, that its members not behave like a praetorian guard. The medical teams that it dispatched had no police functions. They entered homes only when summoned and always unarmed. It was no part of their mission to convey patients to hospital or their families to quarantine, and they carried out no programme of compulsory disinfection, fumigation or destruction of property. The White Cross also maintained a stance of total independence from authority, refusing to take part in combined operations with the municipal personnel. As De Zerbi stressed,

> As I remember how many people believed that cholera was a disaster spread by poisoners and that the chief poisoner was City Hall, I am pleased to note that, if our institution had not been created ... , large numbers of sufferers would have died without calling the doctor because, in their misguided thinking, the municipal doctors were murderers. This is the reason that ... I never allowed a merger between our medical service and that of the city. Any such merger would have

made us official and would thereby have destroyed our work ... because the public would have feared and shunned us.'[11]

Under the direction of Professor Mariano Semmola, who commanded the medical service of the White Cross, the physicians who treated patients on behalf of the organization also rejected forms of heroic and experimental medical intervention that multiplied the suspicion and distress that surrounded the cholera hospitals and the visits of some of the municipal medical teams. Under Semmola's instructions, the priority of the sanitary companies was to provide diligent nursing care rather than any specific course of medical treatment. As De Zerbi commented, in Asiatic cholera three-quarters of the hope for saving the patient rested on dedicated nurses rather than physicians.[12] Such an approach made maximum use of the zeal and commitment of the laymen who formed the overwhelming majority of the volunteers, and, as an additional benefit, it made the ministrations of the White Cross medical teams comprehensible to a population that was unfamiliar with medical attention.

Under the difficult conditions of the sudden emergency the sanitary companies regarded it as a major part of their mission to accustom people who had no history of relations with doctors to accept medical attention, care and authority. In this effort to bridge the gulf between the population and the medical profession, it was also significant that De Zerbi's organization avoided conflict with the upsurge of popular religiosity. The adoption of the cross as the emblem of the volunteer force was reassuring and familiar. Furthermore, the White Cross undermined the popular suspicion that doctors had a pecuniary interest in the continuation of the epidemic rather than in its elimination. All of the personnel enrolled in the White Cross were unpaid volunteers.

By their presence and example, the sanitary companies also relieved the panic caused throughout the Lower City by the fear of contagion. Until the arrival of the White Cross, the lesson imparted to the population of the city was that the victims of cholera were a deadly danger. The return of the emigrants from stricken Provence, the flight of the wealthy classes from the city, the establishment of sanitary cordons and lazarettos and the municipal policy of compulsory internment of patients in cholera hospitals were, as we have seen, all measures that vividly demonstrated that those afflicted with the disease threatened the life of the entire community. Superstition, rumour and the example of neighbourhoods that rose up against the passage of stretchers and the opening of hospitals increased the panic and negated all possibility of an effective and rational programme of public health measures. By tending the ill in their own homes and remaining at their bedsides, the sanitary companies of the White Cross began to lower the temperature of the popular cholera hysteria. For Raffaele Parisi, the Vice-President of the organization, this instruction by example was the greatest service that the volunteers rendered to the people. Parisi recalled,

Had it done nothing else, the White Cross would always have the merit of being the means of removing from the masses their fear of contagion. This was a terrible fear that was unlike that of previous epidemics such as those of 1854 and 1873. In this epidemic, panic-stricken sons and daughters abandoned their dying parents.[13]

By combating this anxiety, the volunteers helped to restore order to the Lower City. At the same time they confronted the financial hardship that accompanied the disease. In addition to medical assistance, the White Cross provided welfare. Its teams offered articles of necessity, rations and money to the needy families of victims and to all those who shared their lodgings. During the three weeks that it functioned, the organization provided free medicine to 7,000 patients, delivered soup to 600 convalescents daily, and distributed 50 kilos of meat a day. It also handed out a total of 28,000 lemons, 2,400 eggs, 1,000 wool blankets, 1,500 sheets, 300 mattresses, and untold quantities of disinfectants. Its total operating expenses were 200,000 lire.[14]

The capacity of the organization to carry out such a significant charitable function reflected the sympathy of the nation as a whole for the plight of its largest city. Cities throughout the peninsula voted funds to support the White Cross initiative. Florence provided it with 12,000 lire, Padua and Como 4,000 each. The monarchy donated 12,000 lire, and Palermo supplied shipments of lemons. The Bank of Naples made donations, as did wealthy private benefactors. At the same time more humble contributions greatly assisted the organization. Workers organized collections on its behalf, and pharmacists donated medicine and disinfectants. In the borough of Porto, where the mass epidemic first exploded, the White Cross was flanked by a neighbourhood benevolent association for the assistance of the victims of the epidemic founded by the Deputy representing the *sezione*, Salvatore Fusco.[15]

Thus equipped with manpower and supplies, the White Cross provided a large-scale medical and social service for three vital weeks when the epidemic was at the height of its fury. Between its founding on 4 September and its decision to disband on 26 September when it deemed conditions sufficiently improved for the municipal authorities to resume normal functioning, the White Cross effectively assumed the primary burden of care for the victims of cholera, responding to 7,015 calls for help and treating 5,492 patients.[16]

The volunteer association achieved a strikingly high rate of success by contemporary medical standards. Of the patients its medical teams treated, 2,069 (37.6 per cent) died, while 3,423 (62.4 per cent) recovered – a reversal of the proportions achieved by the municipal hospitals. Such a signal claim to success should not, however, be taken at face value. The White Cross and the municipal doctors confronted very different patient populations. As a result of popular suspicions, the municipal doctors normally saw only serious cases of *cholera gravis*, and often when they were already beyond hope. The White Cross, by contrast, enjoyed the confidence of the people. It was summoned, therefore, by patients who were less severely ill – and at an earlier stage in the course of the disease. But even if the rates of cure achieved by the White Cross were less impressive than they seemed, the appearance of success itself inspired confidence and confirmed the ability of the volunteers to assuage the cholera phobia of the city. The patients transported to the Conocchia, the Piedigrotta and the Maddalena were seldom seen again, but everyone had neighbours and relatives whose encounters with De Zerbi's organization ended happily.

During the desperate weeks of September the White Cross shouldered a large portion of the responsibility for sustaining the city in its encounter with Asiatic cholera. De Zerbi's organization tended the ill, educated the people in the usefulness of medical attention, relieved economic hardship and offered hope where none had existed. In conjunction with the abatement of the disease itself, the volunteers helped the population to cope with the disaster that confronted them. The accomplishments of the White Cross were reinforced by the fact that it did not operate alone. There were other forces at work that helped to reduce the level of tension in the Lower City to such an extent that by the end of the month the volunteers decided to withdraw, leaving the remaining phases of the campaign against cholera to the regularly elected officials of the city. By 3 October, although the epidemic persisted in attenuated form, *The Times* found conditions so vastly improved that it reported that, 'Naples is rapidly regaining its usual aspect.'[17]

Among the factors that assisted the White Cross in its work of restoring the morale of the population was superstition itself. The beginning of the descending curve of the epidemic coincided approximately with the feast day of the patron saint of the city, San Gennaro, on 19 September. For the people of Naples, Gennaro, who had been born in humble circumstances, was the most important of all the saints except the Virgin Mary herself, and never more so than at a time of public calamity. According to the teachings of the Church and popular belief, Gennaro, whom infidels had beheaded at neighbouring Pozzuoli in AD 305, preserved his native city from earthquakes, the eruptions of Vesuvius and pestilence. The Neapolitan martyr was the self-appointed advocate for the city – and especially its common people – in heaven. His statue guarded the entrance to the city at the Maddalena Bridge, where his upraised arm kept disaster at bay.

Twice annually, in May and in September, Gennaro re-affirmed his concern for the Neapolitan people by performing a miracle. The Duomo of Naples sheltered the holy relics of his martyrdom – the saint's skull and an ampulla containing a congealed sample of his blood. On his feast days the saint answered the prayers of the faithful by causing the blood in the phial to liquefy and boil. This biannual event announced his intention to preserve the city from disaster. The miracle took place during mid-day mass celebrated by the Archbishop alternately at the Cathedral in September and at the Church of Santa Chiara on the first Sunday in May. If the blood liquefied, the city was saved; if the miracle failed, Naples was doomed.[18] In this ceremony and in the procession that preceded it the unequal residents of a deeply divided city – Catholic and Liberal, Upper and Lower, rich and poor – came together symbolically to re-affirm their fragile communality.

During the cholera epidemic of 1884 this ritual occasion was charged with an immediate medical significance. In an unmistakable parallelism, the Archbishop knelt in prayer, beseeching the blood in the ampulla to flow, while Cantani and his colleagues anxiously waited at the bedsides of the victims, injecting solution into their bloodstreams to prevent their blood from congealing in their veins. At the Duomo on Friday, 19 September, therefore, it seemed apparent that the saint would provide a collective sign that would reveal the fate of all. For the people of the city, therefore, this day possessed an unrivalled significance: it was the day when Naples would learn its fate. As De Zerbi's newspaper *Il Piccolo* explained, 'The hope of the populace rests entirely on the anniversary of San Gennaro to halt the pestilence.'[19]

On the nineteenth, therefore, the Cathedral was filled to capacity by 10,000 believers, and an even larger throng gathered outside while the Cardinal Archbishop celebrated mass at the high altar and invoked the mercy of the saint. Happily, the miracle of the blood took place on schedule shortly after noon 'amid the cries of women, clapping of hands, firing of mortars, and ringing of bells'.[20] There was jubilation throughout the city as the people learned that their prayers had been answered and that their tribulations were at an end. Everywhere, *Il Piccolo* observed, 'the faithful prostrate themselves, confident now in the mercy of the saint'.[21] Since the disease began concurrently to subside, the popular conclusion was that the avenging Angel of God had sheathed his sword in answer to the intercession of the martyr. 'What hope', asked *The Times* in response to this affair, is there 'for a people so immersed in superstition, ignorance, and dirt?'[22]

From the standpoint of the White Cross and its work, the significance of the miracle of San Gennaro is that it furnished the city with the very hope that *The Times* despaired of, thereby bolstering the morale of the people. Faith and superstition exhibited their psychological power. To many, the volunteers and even the city officials now seemed to operate with a divine sanction. In addition to the intervention of the saint, however, worldly matters promoted the continuing ebb in social tensions within the city. Three sublunary factors are most significant and merit attention – the actions of the King, the Church and the Bank of Naples.

King Umberto and Archbishop Sanfelice

The fact that Naples stood alone among the great cities of Europe in experiencing a devastating epidemic in 1884 had a series of important consequences. One of these consequences, of course, was the great volunteer campaign of the White Cross. Another vitally important result was that Naples became the focus of attention of the monarchy and of the government of Agostino Depretis.

When the sporadic trickle of isolated cases in Italy's largest city burst into a flood in the first week of September, King Umberto decided to visit the poorly prepared and turbulent metropolis. He was accompanied by his brother, Prince Amadeo; by the Prime Minister; and by the Cabinet Ministers Benedetto Brin, Bernardino Grimaldi, and Pasquale Stanislao Mancini. There was nothing new, of course, in the visit of a head of state to the scene of a disaster or national emergency. There were special features, however, that marked this royal journey, transforming it into an international sensation and a major event in the history of the city.

The Italian King's voyage to the former capital was no perfunctory perform-ance of duty. Umberto was a sovereign of limited abilities and no personal charisma. He lacked political vision, read little, and took no sustained interest in affairs of state or the realm of ideas. Having neither the ambition nor the energy to envisage a restoration of absolutism, he was content to reign without govern-ing. What Umberto possessed in abundance, however, was physical courage and sympathy for the suffering of his subjects. Against medical advice, he abandoned his annual hunting expedition in the mountains of his native Piedmont in order to visit the cholera patients of Busca in the last week of August. Busca was the town of 10,000 souls where the disease first burst out in epidemic proportions. The King brought to the sufferers the simple message that they should take heart and trust in God.[23] Deeply affected by the experience, he understood the human consequences of the reports that reached him from Naples barely a week later, and he resolved at once to make whatever contribution he could to relieve the misery of his people.[24]

Arriving in Naples on 9 September, the King and his ministers were immedi-ately escorted by the Prefect of Naples and the Mayor to visit the patients at the Conocchia. Umberto visited every bedside, administering words of comfort, and he held conversations with the convalescents. The tone of this visit contrasted favourably with the example set by the French cabinet ministers who paid their respects to stricken Toulon and Marseilles. In Provence the official visits had proved counter-productive because of the evident fear of the ministers and their all too apparent haste to depart. After hurrying through the wards with their noses covered, the dignitaries left by train on the same day. Rather than strengthening morale in the process, the French ministers confirmed the panic of the populace, lent credence to the fear of contagion, and exposed themselves to ridicule and caricature in the press.

Umberto, who saw himself more in the role of a commander visiting the front, adopted a strikingly different deportment. 'Every inch a king!' was the admiring comment of the *Lancet*.[25] He was unhurried, fearless and visibly concerned for the fate of the sufferers. Taking notes as he went, walking-stick in hand, he inquired into the personal circumstances of each of the victims and the arrange-ments that had been made to deal with the economic as well as the medical consequences of their condition. Setting an example of intrepidity, he refused to make use of the disinfectants urged upon him by the medical staff. Furthermore, instead of hastening back to the station on the day of his arrival, he resolved to remain in the city until the situation showed signs of improvement and to make daily tours of inspection at the cholera wards. Appalled by the inability of the municipal campaign to cope with the magnitude of the crisis, King Umberto and Agostino Depretis determined that their presence should have more than sym-bolic significance. They set to work to render practical assistance. By their orders, the army immediately cleared the Maddalena barracks to provide a second cholera hospital and the navy turned over the military hospital at Piedigrotta to the municipality as the third medical facility. Umberto personally donated 100,000 lire to assist the families of the victims, and he gave instructions that carriages belonging to the armed forces undertake civilian duties transporting patients and bodies in support of the severely overstretched local services. He also maintained his scheduled round of hospital visits even after a member of his entourage was stricken by the disease.

Not content with assisting the sufferers, the Head of State and the Prime Minister made the most momentous decision of their visit. They asked the Mayor and the President of the White Cross to conduct them on a personal investigation into the social conditions that underlay so great a misfortune. Umberto and Depretis together undertook a grand tour of the slums of the city, visiting the worst *bassi* and *fondaci* of the Lower City and speaking to the inhabitants. The King persevered, reported the Parisian newspaper *Le Temps*, despite a firm warning from the Mayor and the city council that the course of action that he proposed would place his life in jeopardy.[26] The tour assumed enormous importance both because of the personal bravery of the sovereign and because the presence of the two most powerful men in the nation focused the attention of the press, the parliament and the government on the 'Question of Naples'. The royal visit thereby marked an important step in the consciousness of the Southern Question in Italian history.

In addition, the royal decision to explore the problems of the Old City was important because the visitors were shaken by the spectacle they witnessed, and they resolved together to launch a national effort to remove the causes of such great misery. In a famous sentence variously attributed both to Umberto and to Depretis, the two tourists vowed, 'We must disembowel Naples!' ('*Sventriamo Napoli!*') Here, in surgical formulation, was the essence of what emerged over the following year as a full-scale programme to rebuild the Lower City – a programme that powerfully conditioned the future course of Neapolitan urban development and of the medical and social history of the city. Fittingly, the great boulevard that was the centrepiece of the rebuilding effort was eventually to be named the Corso Umberto. The renewal project forms the subject of Chapter 5.

In the more immediate term, the peregrinations of the sovereign and his ministers played a major part in assisting Neapolitans in overcoming the crisis caused by the cholera. The visit to Naples proved one of the most successful ventures of a largely undistinguished reign. The *New York Times* informed its readers that, 'The heroism of King Humbert makes the most welcome royal picture Europe has looked on for years.' The Italian people were 'almost crazy with enthusiasm for the King'.[27] Such was the wave of royal fervour that republican and socialist societies throughout the peninsula experienced large-scale resignations.[28] There were spontaneous public demonstrations in favour of King Umberto across all of Italy, and the press indulged in a chorus of adulation that extended even to spokesmen for the Vatican. Here was one of the occasions when this monarch earned his epithet 'Umberto the Good'. 'Never', said *The Times*, 'was Italy so morally united as she is.'[29] A measure of the outpouring of popular affection for the sovereign was the rumour that swept the city that King Umberto had prayed to San Gennaro, promising that, if Naples was saved, he would abdicate, sacrificing his crown to placate the divine wrath.[30]

The highly visible presence of the leading officials in the nation itself provided practical assistance to the beleaguered City Hall, helping it to regain control of events. The royal tour soothed the dread of contagion and dissipated the poisoning phobia. Local officers who had considered deserting their posts reconsidered; notable cholera fugitives stiffened their resolve and returned to the city; and opponents of the Crown swelled the ranks of the White Cross to demonstrate that charity and courage were no monopolies of royalty. Men and women of good will across Europe were moved to make donations to the stricken Neapolitans. People who suspected that a plan had been launched by the city to annihilate the poor now had second thoughts when they witnessed at close hand the concern of the state for the troubles of Naples. Citizens who considered the victims of cholera to be dangerously contagious witnessed the impunity and courage of the King and his ministers, and took heart. It was important to the whole population that, just as the disease reached its furious culmination, the city received a benign distraction from its torment and a powerful source of hope.[31] And even after the departure of King Umberto and Agostino Depretis, the Foreign Minister, Mancini, remained in the city for the duration to continue their work.

Of all the reasons for the extraordinary resonance of the royal visit, however, the one that caused most surprise concerned the Neapolitan clergy. Throughout his stay in the cholera-infested city, King Umberto amazed the nation by the unprecedented presence at his side of Cardinal Archbishop Sanfelice. The surprise resulted from the sudden *rapprochement* between the Liberal state and the Church. The Risorgimento had taken place against the fierce opposition of Pope Pius IX to all of its works. In the course of Italian unification the papacy lost its temporal power, its political influence with the dynasties of the old regime, and much of its land. Pius opposed secularism, liberalism, modernism and nationalism; he feared the anti-clerical current within the ranks of Italian patriots; and he deplored the possible implications of constitutional doctrines for the governance of the Church and the power of the bishops. Refusing, therefore, to accept the newly united state, Pius IX declared himself a prisoner in the Vatican, excommunicated the leaders of the national cause, and forbade Catholics from taking part in Italian political life. He also trusted in the Catholic powers to undo the work of Camillo Cavour.

In the generation since the creation of the Italian state, however, the leading figures of the original conflict – Pius IX, Cavour, King Victor Emanuel – had all died, and the passions of the Risorgimento had cooled. With every year that passed, it also became clearer that the Italian state was not going to be dismantled, but had become instead a permanent fixture with which the Church would have to deal. With the social tensions that erupted in Italy during the course of the agricultural depression in the 1880s and the emergence of a mass-based socialist and labour movement, the Church also learned that it faced newer and more threatening opponents than the Liberals. And in Germany the anti-Catholic campaign of Bismarck's *Kulturkampf* taught thoughtful churchmen the dangers of alienation from the political powers of modern Europe. Furthermore, the Hapsburg Empire, the great Catholic power on whom the Pope relied to reverse the tide, had instead signed the Triple Alliance with Italy in 1882. In this context, there emerged among the clergy a current of clerico-moderates who opposed Liberal Italy in principle but accepted in practice that some form of accommodation was unavoidable and necessary. Pope Leo XIII, who succeeded Pius in 1878, was deeply influenced by this current, and his papacy was to be remembered for its effort to reconcile Catholicism with the modern world. And the Vicar of Naples, Cardinal Archbishop Guglielmo Sanfelice, was an influential advocate of the new course.

When, therefore, in late August 1884 Liberal Mayor Nicola Amore realized the extent of the opposition to the municipal campaign against the pestilence and appealed for assistance to the clergy, he met a sympathetic response from the Archbishop. Sanfelice espoused the biblical theology of cholera as God's punishment for sin, but he refused to draw the conclusion that the Church should limit its intervention to encouraging the faithful to repent and to turn from their sinful leaders. Since the ways of the Almighty were beyond human comprehension, it would be impious to feel confident that one understood the reasons for the unleashing of the scourge. And, in any event, nothing could dispense Christians from the duties of charity. Although he urged prayer and repentance, he also called upon the faithful to take practical, worldly action to combat the sufferings of the city. Most significantly for the fate of Naples, the Archbishop then reasoned that the most useful form of charitable action was to support the recommendations of science embodied in the initiatives of Amore and De Bonis. Far from pursuing the cold war between Church and State of the previous generation, Sanfelice accepted Amore's appeal and issued a pastoral letter instructing parish priests throughout the archdiocese to come to the aid of the embattled City Hall. 'Now', he wrote to the Neapolitan priesthood on 28 August,

> it is your obligation, ... to carry out the duty that is binding on those who care for men's souls in such times. Go among the people entrusted to your care and exercise the charity that Christ Jesus called upon the ministers of the Church to perform ... If God in the inscrutability of His plans has chosen thus to test our dearly beloved people, let us pray that our sacrifice may be accepted by the Grace of God in expiation for the sins of the souls in our care ....
>
> May the priests reassure the faint-hearted and those subject to panic, and may they combat strange and harmful prejudices. Let them persuade the people to welcome with grateful hearts the benign work of the physicians, and to be meek, trusting, and grateful in their attitudes towards the attentive and caring measures of the municipal authorities. And may the clergy, and especially the parish priests, not fail to cooperate effectively with them for the common good of public health.

Curates and priests, teach and inspire calm, confidence, and above all mildness towards those who watch over the health of the people.[32]

Already before the arrival of the King, the Vicar of Naples had launched a major effort to restore order to the city and to re-establish the authority of the municipal authorities in the matter of public health. Setting a personal example of the charity he advocated, Sanfelice began by the end of August to visit the patients at the Conocchia on a regular basis. There he performed the rites of extreme unction and communion, praised the staff for its dedication, and spread words of consolation. He conducted services in the churches in the Lower City and preached his message of cooperation with the municipal anti-cholera campaign. In the neighbourhoods where violence and resistance broke out, he visited the homes of the poor and patiently explained the sanitary measures that were required to save the city. Where the suffering was greatest, he distributed money as well as words of encouragement. He met arriving volunteers for the White Cross and gave them his blessing, not omitting even godless *garibaldini* and socialists. To multiply his influence, he instructed the parish priests to imitate his action and he called on the Catholic laity organized in the 'Leo XIII Association' to cooperate in the effort to calm the terror and assuage the poisoning phobia. Priests began to accompany doctors to patients' bedsides and to vouch for the prescriptions of science. And the Archbishop banned the processions of penitents.[33]

The mission undertaken by the clergy under Sanfelice's direction was not immediately or wholly successful. At the outset the message that the municipal doctors should be trusted caused the Archbishop himself to be hooted and shouted down as a poisoner as well. The processions defiantly persisted in their gloomy and violent progress through the streets. The assaults on municipal personnel continued. Fear was often more powerful than faith, and popular religion was not automatically amenable to the teachings of the official Church. The educational effort undertaken by the clergy, however, was massive, clearly directed, and tenacious. Their authority reached even the remotest alleys and the darkest lodgings of the Old City. And, as in the experience of the White Cross and the King, the very presence of priests in the slums where the cholera germs nestled went a long way to restoring calm and removing the fear of contagion.

The press was unanimous in its assessment that Sanfelice's unstinting courage gradually played a major part in restoring morale and preparing the way for the city to perform its sanitary functions. *The Times* was representative in its summation:

> Great praise is given to the Archbishop of Naples, Cardinal San Felice, for the devotion with which he daily visits the hospitals and the sick in their homes, and the patient care which he bestows upon them. The clergy follow his example, and are active in carrying out his earnest instructions to endeavour to remove the superstitious prejudices of the populace.[34]

Even the radical *Roma*, whose anti-clerical position was evident in its title, agreed that the conduct of the Neapolitan clergy during the epidemic was 'admirable'. The correspondent for the *New York Times* considered Sanfelice 'heroic', and compared him to Saint Carlo Borromeo, who tended the victims of the plague in seventeenth-century Milan.[35]

For Sanfelice, the visit of King Umberto was a continuation of ten days of tireless exertion. There was an obvious rivalry between the prelate and the head of the Liberal state, and each was eager not to be outstripped in public estimation by the other. When the emergency ended, they also resumed their mutual criticism of one another with regard to policies regarding the future of the city. For a week in September at the height of the crisis, however, they set their differences aside in a common humanitarian effort. The King, the Archbishop and the Prime Minister walked together through the hospital wards and the streets of the city. This joint venture created a sensation throughout Italy and gave the combined sponsorship of the anti-cholera campaign the highest possible visibility and legitimacy.

The importance of Sanfelice's intervention was underlined by the contrasting course of events in Sicily, the other Italian region most severely scourged by the fifth pandemic. In Sicily the course of the disease in 1885 and 1886 was marked by a slide into near anarchy as a poisoning frenzy swept the island and the populations of towns and villages desperately improvised sanitary cordons in defiance of the law. In the tumults that ensued, the clergy – a bastion of intransigent Catholicism under Archbishop Celesia – bore a heavy responsibility. Instead of supporting the authorities in their anti-cholera campaign, the Church in Sicily taught its own medical theory of contagionism; urged the people to regard officials as the source of God's displeasure and their misfortune; preached defiance of doctors; and justified vigilantism. The epidemic provided the occasion for an outpouring of legitimist nostalgia for the Bourbon regime.[36] Against the backdrop of disorder on the island, the very different theology of cholera espoused by Sanfelice made a major contribution to restoring both political and medical authority in Naples.

Philanthropy

The municipal strategy to combat the cholera began to falter in the closing days of August. In early September it was overwhelmed by the magnitude of the epidemic and the violent opposition of a frantic populace. But as September progressed, City Hall received powerful reinforcement from unanticipated sources – the Crown, the Church, the White Cross, San Gennaro, and the providential waning of the epidemic. A final additional factor was the influence of philanthropy, which helped the people to cope with the economic collapse that accompanied the cholera.

Donations to the afflicted were both individual and institutional. Individual contributions came from generous men and women of substance who were moved by the ordeal of the population. The most famous private benefactor was the man reputed to be the wealthiest resident of Naples – the financier and urban landlord Matteo Schillizzi. Schillizzi was a personal friend of the Archbishop and, although a Jew, he accompanied the Catholic Primate of Naples to the slums of the Lower City where he opened his purse to the stricken families they encountered.[37]

In the *sezione* of Stella, a group of wealthy ladies, led by the wife of the banker Oscar Meuricoffre, opened a soup kitchen and workshop for the benefit of women afflicted by the economic consequences of the epidemic. The kitchen distributed 1,900 rations of food a day, and the workshop hired 100 unemployed women on a full-time basis, setting them to work sewing linen and fabrics. As their own particular contribution to hygiene and moral uplift, the ladies also organized a daily 'cleanliness prize' for the mother and daughter who arrived to collect their rations in the neatest, cleanest attire and with the best-brushed hair. The winning women collected 10 lire, and their daughters 5.[38]

Such largesse was reproduced in miniature by innumerable and unrecorded single gifts by people of every station who were moved by the plight of neighbours, relatives and fellow citizens. Landlords were suddenly distressed by the fate of their tenants and undertook improvements, whitewashing walls, emptying cesspits, sweeping courtyards and stairways. Such contributions played a part in alleviating distress and hardship. More substantial and better known, however, was the charitable role of the Bank of Naples. Under its Director-General, Count Giusso, the Bank intervened repeatedly and substantially to assist the city and the people, spending a total of 461,452.70 lire[39] – a substantial expenditure both in absolute terms and as a proportion of the gross income of the institution of 9,760,004.72 lire for the fiscal year 1883[40] and of its total assets of 393,922,041.38 lire.[41]

Already in November 1883 after the epidemic had laid waste to Egypt and threatened Italy, the Board had approved in principle the budgeting of 60,000 lire to provide the Mayor with the means of opening a permanent hospital for infectious diseases. The city council, however, proceeded in its traditional dilatory manner. It failed to move beyond the planning stage for the facility until the dramatic outburst of 1 September unmistakably revealed that the Conocchia Hospital alone would not suffice. Nicola Amore and De Bonis urgently arranged for the purchase of land located on the Poggioreale hill on the northeastern outskirts of Naples and commissioned the hasty erection of a wooden shed on the site. On 5 September the Bank credited funds to the municipal account. The Board subsequently allocated a further 100,000 lire to see the work carried through to completion. In this way the Bank provided Naples with the city's fourth and smallest cholera hospital – the Vittoria. Renamed the Cotugno and enlarged, the Vittoria was to play the dominant role as the city's first line of defence when the cholera returned in the new century.

Having financed the construction of a hospital, the Bank, in consultation with the Palazzo San Giacomo, considered other uses for its resources. One intervention was dietary. The best-informed medical opinion of the day held that diet was a vital predisposing factor that put individuals at risk to cholera, and the city posted notices advising the people to eat a diet based on meat, avoiding fruit, vegetables and seafood. The wealthy followed this suggestion, and for the duration of the epidemic suffered atrocious constipation and flatulence as the consequences. For the poor, meat was a rare luxury even in normal times. With the collapse of the economy during the emergency, the idea that the mass of the population should follow the municipal dietary regimen was inconceivable. Hunger instead threatened to prolong the epidemic and to erupt into social disorder. The Bank of Naples, therefore, resolved to subsidize the opening of municipally administered soup kitchens, where the poor would be provided with daily rations of broth and meat. For the purpose it voted 120,000 lire in three separate instalments, beginning on 5 September.

The Bank followed these measures with four additional cholera initiatives. On 9 September the Board voted 50,000 lire to open savings accounts of 100 lire each on behalf of the cholera orphans whose parents had perished of the disease and who had no known source of support. Secondly, it budgeted a further 50,000 lire to underwrite the sanitary measures undertaken by the twelve *sezioni*, the money to be distributed according to need. Mercato would receive 8,000 lire; Pendino, Porto and Vicaria 6,000 each; and the other eight boroughs 3,000 apiece. Thirdly, noting that personal charity was noble but insufficient, the Board of the Bank donated 10,000 lire to the White Cross. And fourthly the Bank of Naples decided to distribute 75,954 lire among those of its own employees who were stationed in Naples and were therefore at risk from the disease. The payments were to be made in accord with a sliding scale that provided the most substantial sums to those employees who not only resided in the city but were also stricken by cholera, either personally or through the illness of members of their families.

Having voted to subsidize the anti-cholera campaigns of the muicipality, the boroughs and the White Cross, the Bank of Naples gave thought on 18 September to the plight of its most impoverished debtors, and it undertook to provide them with relief through the Monte di Pietà, its pawnbroking subsidiary. The economic crisis that accompanied the medical emergency produced a headlong rush to the pawnshops of the Lower City. Most revealing was the distressing proportion of small items pledged for less than 3 lire each. These items were frequently the last personal possessions of those made suddenly destitute by the depression, and their loss contributed to the 'class rage' noted by all observers as a major factor in the disturbances that shook the Lower City. As a contribution to improved social relations, the Bank freely discharged 4,156 pawn tickets for a value of 11,213 lire.

The total contribution of the Bank to the welfare of the stricken city soon extended far beyond these immediate emergency measures to include long-term support for City Hall. The final cost of the anti-cholera campaign carried out by the municipal government was 1 million lire. Unfortunately, this outlay coincided with the collapse of the local economy and with the urgent need to finance additional sanitary precautions to prevent the return of cholera in 1885. Nicola

Amore and his executive found themselves caught in a vice between diminished
resources and the necessity of major expenditures in the interest of public health.
The Bank of Naples intervened to make good the difference. The Board approved
an interest-free, long-term loan to the city of 3 million lire to cover the unanticipated burden of defending the population against cholera. As Nicola Amore
acknowledged in a report to the city council in 1888, this charity extended by the
Bank went largely unnoticed at the time, but it made a vital contribution to the
health of the population.[42]

THE END OF THE EPIDEMIC

The combined efforts of the White Cross, philanthropists, the Church, and the
Crown powerfully supplemented the measures of a municipality that had been
overwhelmed at the start of September. From 15 September, however, the
epidemic itself began to subside, as the daily bills of mortality dropped below 300
for the first time since 6 September. On 24 and 25 September the daily death toll
plunged to 85 and 65 victims respectively.[43] With such visible signs of progress,
the last week of the month produced a vast improvement in morale.

At this reduced level of emergency, the municipal medical and sanitary
activity began to have an impact. As fewer people fell ill and died, the suspicion
that municipal doctors were involved in a plot to destroy the poor seemed less
and less plausible, especially after the testimony in their favour of the King and
the clergy. Furthermore, the city medical teams had learned to moderate their
behaviour, and the four cholera hospitals had abandoned the experimental
attempts to find a cure that had terrified patients without yielding positive
results. The standard of care improved in any case as the wards grew less
crowded and the staff less overworked. The populace was increasingly prepared
to accept official medical attention and even to be hospitalized. By 30 October,
municipal doctors had treated a total of 9,219 cases of cholera.[44]

To explain the decline and end of an epidemic is a 'cholera-riddle' for which
there is no solution, and the Neapolitan outbreak of 1884 is no exception. It is
probable, however, that the much maligned efforts of the city council ultimately
played an important part. The increased cooperation of the population meant
that cases were reported earlier and with fewer attempts at evasion. As a result,
victims could be isolated and their chances of infecting others were greatly
reduced. The reduction in tension itself therefore helped in turn to defeat the
epidemic because an effective programme of public health in relation to Asiatic
cholera depends on the cooperation of the people. As information was increasingly forthcoming, the city was better able to take measures to isolate and
disinfect – measures that limited the further spread of infection.

Other municipal initiatives also played a positive role. Some policies, such as
the lighting of bonfires and the cleansing of sewers, judged by modern epidemiological standards, seem highly unlikely to have made a contribution. Certain
measures, reflecting the emerging germ theory as well as localist strictures, were

timely and appropriate. A first group of important positive steps involved food and drink. The city, imitating the examples set by private philanthropy, opened public soup kitchens where those foodstuffs that are most susceptible to contamination were avoided – seafood, raw fruit, and uncooked vegetables – as the city attempted to provide the population with soup, meat and bread. The municipal soup kitchens first opened their doors on 15 September in the three most afflicted boroughs – Mercato, Pendino and Porto. They were subsequently extended to the whole of the city, so that by the end of the month 18,000 meals were provided daily at municipal expense.[45] The sealing of hundreds of wells after inspection by sight undoubtedly saved large numbers of lives and shortened the outbreak by removing the most polluted water in Naples from consumption.

Another set of initiatives foreshadowed the larger programme of renewing the city that was launched after the epidemic ended. The city authorities considered overcrowding to be one of the major factors in the vulnerability of Naples to epidemic disease. From mid-September, therefore, the anti-cholera campaign sought to identify some of the worst living conditions in the Lower City and to offer the residents alternative accommodation until the crisis was over, when nearly the whole population of the Lower City would be relocated. In pursuance of this policy, military barracks, monasteries and public buildings were equipped as shelters to house the refugees. The buildings and institutions that were prioritized for condemnation under this project were determined by previous experience of cholera and by physical inspection. Examples were the great poorhouse of the city, the Albergo dei Poveri; the provincial insane asylum of Capodimonte; the most notorious *fondaci*; and selected *locande*. These buildings, which had been ravaged in previous visitations of the cholera, were 'thinned out' by the transfer of their excess population to the municipal cholera hostels. The strategy involved was based on the epidemiological history of the city, and it is probable that the preventive relocation of some of the population exposed to the greatest risk of infection helped to prevent history from repeating itself at their expense.

Alfredo Chiaromonte, the Deputy Mayor responsible for the borough of S. Carlo all'Arena, illustrated the strategy of 'thinning-out'. At his instructions, the borough requisitioned the ex-convents of Pacella and of the Maddalena ai Cristallini. Here it housed 400 refugees from the most infected streets of the *sezione*. They were survivors of cholera attacks in their families – widows, orphans, widowers, elderly dependents. After being brought to the newly opened municipal shelters, they were washed and disinfected, and their clothing was confiscated and burned. The borough then housed the cholera fugitives in spacious and whitewashed premises; provided them with a carefully monitored diet at municipal expense; and issued them with beds, fresh linen and new clothes. It was a measure of the success of the initiative that among the relocated survivors, who were among those most at risk in the city, only three cases of cholera occurred.[46]

The threat of the disease slowly receded for other reasons as well. One explanation given by Robert Koch for the decline of all epidemics of cholera is that the whole of the population is not equally vulnerable. Epidemics reach an early peak of ferocity as they strike down those who by reason of occupation, housing, health, dietary habits and individual physical constitution are most at risk. Those who remain unaffected after the first wave of victims are those who possess some degree of resistance. In addition, those who contract the disease and recover are immune for a period and seldom succumb a second time during the same visitation.

Even the weather played an important but immeasurable role. Contemporaries were keenly aware of the seasonality of cholera, which they attributed to the dispersal of the deadly miasmas by the wind and the reduced fermentation of the germs in the subsoil at cooler temperatures. Influenced by the theories of Pettenkofer, the Neapolitan medical profession and the authorities eagerly awaited the arrival of the *scirocco*, the Italian mistral – a strong southerly wind that regularly gathered strength in the autumn. The *scirocco*, they anticipated, would lower the temperature and dispel the poison. The cooling breezes did arrive in October, and deaths from cholera declined still more rapidly. Twenty-five people died of the disease on 4 October, twenty-seven on 5 October, and only eight the following day. The Neapolitan Academy of Medicine, examining the epidemic a year later, received the gratifying report from some of its most distinguished members, including Marino Turchi, that the evidence supported the theory of a close relationship between the course of the disease and the essential data of meteorology.[47] Climatic influence, however, operated chiefly by its effect on the human population rather than on the air or the subsoil. In cooler weather, the people drank far less water, and therefore exposed themselves less often to the greatest source of disease. In a recent work on the history of cholera in France, Patrice Bourdelais and Jean-Yves Raulot also suggest that climate played an important role through its effect on perspiration. Sweat, they argue, is a medium in which the vibrio thrives for an extended period. Cooler temperatures therefore deprived the disease of a favourable environmental factor.[48]

The decline, however, was not smooth and regular, and changes in the weather probably played a part, given the precarious conditions of the Neapolitan water supply. In the second week of October there was a recrudescence. There were sixty-two cholera deaths on the ninth and seventy on the tenth. The ninth and tenth, however, were days of inclement weather with heavy rain.[49] Since a large portion of the population still depended on poorly maintained storage-tanks and wells, abundant rain could have fatal consequences by producing heavy contamination by surface-water. The idea that such a factor was at work is corroborated by a similar correlation between the other period of heavy rainfall between Friday, 13 September and Sunday 15 September, on the one hand, and, on the other hand, the maximum ferocity of the disease which followed immediately thereafter.[50] The correlation was noted and stressed by the municipal officer of health Stanislao D'Alessandro, who regarded the two downpours that occurred during the course of the epidemic as major factors in its progress.[51]

Another factor linked the October recrudescence and the high points of epidemic ferocity that preceded it. This factor was widespread indulgence in celebrations marked by excesses of eating and drinking. The initial outburst of the disease at the end of August followed the premature jubilation that Naples had been spared and the distribution of large-scale winnings in the lottery. The mid-September climax of the cholera came on the heels of the Piedigrotta feast on 7 and 8 September – a 'Bacchanalian fete' that was traditionally celebrated 'beyond the limits of reason in the unlimited consumption of fruit, indigestible food and poor wine'.[52] Although the municipal authorities banned the festival in 1884, the population defied the prohibition. The results, observed the American Consul, 'will be seen in the number of cases and deaths of September 11, 12 and 13'.[53]

In October Neapolitans again ignored an official ban and indulged in the annual *ottobrate*, the local 'pleasure days' on all four Thursdays of the month. On these occasions Neapolitans celebrated the harvest and took advantage of the finest weather of the year to indulge in a bout of open-air carousing in the villages beyond the city walls. In 1884 the high point of the celebrations occurred on the feast of the Nunziatella on 8 October, when the population rejoiced at the end of the epidemic. The revellers sang ironic dirges to mark the death of the cholera and drank deeply from the first supplies of cheap and heavily adulterated new wine. Consumed in quantity, this wine, 'in which the process of fermentation has not been completed', produced widespread digestive disturbances – disturbances that weakened the defences of the body against cholera.[54] The after-effects were clearly visible in the surge in mortality on the following day. On 9 October there were 152 reported cases of cholera and 62 deaths.[55]

After mid-October, the clear weather held; the *scirocco* blew; and, since no further festivals intervened, the people practised a virtuous self-restraint. They were rewarded by the further decline and disappearance of the disease from the city. On 24 October the municipal bulletin again announced deaths in single figures. The last official deaths and cases of the epidemic were recorded in the following ten days, and on 4 November the city published its final cholera bulletin. It would be unwise, however, to attempt to date the last cases of cholera with precision. The last real cases of the disease – as opposed to the last official cases registered by the authorities – are as impossible to trace as the elusive and much debated 'first' case some three months before. Without reliable bacteriological means of diagnosis, physicians could never be certain of correctly identifying victims. In addition, persisting distrust and the mildness of 'cholerine' made it more than likely that not all suspicious sufferers were brought to their attention. On the analogy with epidemics elsewhere, it is probable that what Koch called 'stragglers'[56] continued to occur in the population for weeks, perhaps even months after 4 November. For a relieved and grateful city, however, these cases were unknown and unimportant. Naples resumed its life and went about the business of repairing the losses in its ranks.

(Before the end of the fifth cholera pandemic, Naples was re-infected from

Table 4.1. *Deaths from cholera in Naples, 1886–94*

Year	Deaths
1886	16
1887	373
1893	455
1894	45

outside. There were limited outbreaks in 1886, 1887, 1893 and 1894 as Table 4.1 indicates.[57] On each occasion the city experienced a moment of alarm that rapidly subsided as the disease failed to achieve epidemic ferocity. In the fifth pandemic, only 1884 left a lasting impact on Neapolitan life.)

The significance of the great epidemic of 1884 was not simply a function of the number of victims that it left in its wake. Naturally, the scale of the emergency that overwhelmed the city was an important factor. It is essential, however, to resist the temptation of what might be termed 'statistical sensationalism' in the historiography of the subject – the view that the importance of an epidemic of cholera can be assessed numerically by the length of its bills of mortality: the more impressive the mortality, the more worthy of investigation the epidemic.

The tendency to regard cholera, in the words of one authority, as 'the return of the plague' reinforced this perspective.[58] Since the most prominent feature of the epidemiology of the bubonic plague was the demographic catastrophes it unleashed, scholars found it natural to measure Asiatic cholera in terms of its impact on population. Such an approach has been imbedded in the modern history of the European experience of the disease from the outset. In a seminal essay, Charles Rosenberg implicitly gave his blessing to such an approach. Explaining the reasons that make cholera epidemics meaningful events for the historian, he argued that epidemic disease 'provides an excellent sampling device for studying the numerous yet organically related factors which underline increases in economic productivity. An epidemic, *if sufficiently severe*, necessarily evokes responses in every sector of society.'[59] The implication is that, the more severe the epidemic, the more revealing and worthy of study.

Whether or not 'statistical sensationalism' was Rosenberg's intention, the substance of such an approach has been dominant in shaping the literature on the subject. Because of the dramatic mortality that characterized the first European experience of the disease, the early pandemics in the first half of the nineteenth century have overwhelmingly captured the imagination of historians, to the neglect of the less lethal encounters with the malady in the second half of the nineteenth century and the early years of the twentieth. The major authorities in the field – Michael Durey, Norman Longmate and R.J. Morris on Britain; and Patrice Louis Chevalier, François Delaporte, Ange-Pierre Leca and Jean-Yves Raulot on France – have devoted their attention primarily to the first waves of the disease.[60] Furthermore, the coincidence that British and North American historians have contributed so significantly to the literature of the subject has reinforced this tendency. The British Isles and North America ceased to be afflicted with cholera epidemics after the 1860s. The influential work of Charles Rosenberg on the United States and of Geoffrey Bilson on Canada had no need to confront the later pandemics that continued to affect Continental Europe.[61]

Such an imbalance in the discipline has led to a failure to confront the significant influence of the disease on European society during its later but generally less devastating visitations. *Death in Hamburg* by Richard Evans remains the only extended monograph devoted to either of the final cholera pandemics in any European country.[62] The emphasis on the body count has also led to an almost exclusive emphasis on the history of cholera in major urban centres, where mortality was most dramatic. The history of cholera in the countryside has still to be written.

In the more constricted field of Italian medical history, the same tendency prevails. The sole modern study of any of its aspects – the study by Anna Lucia Forti Messina of cholera in Bourbon Naples – dealt, almost predictably, with the first Italian encounter with the cholera in the 1830s.[63] In a later article assessing the meaning of the Italian history of cholera from beginning to end, she then explicitly weighs the importance of each outburst in statistical terms and concludes that the final pandemic, with its limited mortality, was 'numerically unimportant'.[64]

The Neapolitan epidemic of 1884 demonstrates the impact of the penultimate pandemics, whose importance cannot simply be assessed statistically. There were places in 1884 in Italy – in Calabria and Sicily in particular – where cholera constituted a major local event that precipitated riots, hysteria and economic disruption without causing a single death. In such communities, it was not the disease itself but the fear of its approach that served as the catalyst to severe conflicts and social tensions. For our concern with Naples, however, the point to be stressed is that numbers alone do not explain the importance of the outbreak of that year. Indeed, it is arguable that the 1884 epidemic had by far the greatest lasting consequences for the city of Naples although the outbursts of both 1836 and 1854 were substantially more severe.[65]

The reason for the exceptional influence of the epidemic of 1884 was largely chronological. Italians were horrified that the history of cholera in the greatest urban centre in the nation did not follow the general western European pattern for the severity of cholera to follow a steep downward trajectory over the course of the nineteenth century. It seemed unacceptable that Naples should endure yet another epidemic of the disease when other European capitals – Berlin, Vienna, Brussels, London, Paris – were well on the way to triumph in the battle against cholera and had not experienced major ravages in a generation.

The experience of half a century of cholera had enabled medical men to unravel many of the secrets of the aetiology and propagation of cholera. John Snow, Max von Pettenkofer and Robert Koch, for all the differences that divided them in their understanding of cholera, concurred on a range of preventive strategies that were demonstrably effective and that provided statesmen with the possibility of undertaking measures of prophylaxis such as sanitation, drainage and the supply of pure water. The shock of Naples was that it was still so overwhelmingly vulnerable. In the late summer of 1884 it became the only major city in Europe to experience such a medical crisis due to cholera. Timing rather than the sheer numbers of cases and deaths underpinned the extraordinary impact of the events of 1884. Because the modes of transmission of Asiatic cholera were at least partially understood, the disease mercilessly revealed the hygienic neglect of the greatest metropolis of a regime that claimed to be a Liberal modern state. The Italian Government determined that such a scandal should not recur, and it took steps to revolutionize the sanitary provisions of the city.

To understand the significance of the fifth pandemic in Italy in these terms is to explain the effect of the events of 1884 on Naples. It also accounts for the relative lack of impact of the limited cholera outbursts of 1886–87 and 1893–94. In these years events in Naples were overshadowed by the much greater misfortunes of other cities, and it was still too early to see in such flare-ups a test of the efficacy of the efforts at urban renewal. But there is a further point that the importance of timing also suggests. If chronology more than numbers of victims accounts for the enormous influence of the epidemic of 1884, then it is possible also to appreciate that a still later outbreak with even less mortality could also constitute a major and illuminating experience.

In 1910 and 1911 epidemics that were numerically small in comparison with earlier disasters were nevertheless historically significant. They were important because they occurred at all in an age when cholera was thought to have been vanquished forever: they were in fact perceived by contemporaries as indictments of the modernity of Italian and Neapolitan society. To break with the sensationalism of the statistics of the early nineteenth century is necessary to understand the impact of cholera during the final pandemics and the events to be described in Chapters 5 to 7. There our tasks will be first to consider in Chapter 5 how Naples responded to the experience of 1884 by a major sanitary reform and then to examine in Chapters 6 and 7 how that reform was severely tested and found wanting when the disease stubbornly recurred. Because it took place in the twentieth century, an epidemic of negligible demographic impact produced a major political crisis. Death is unreliable as a criterion of historical significance.

PART III

Risanamento and miasma

5

Rebuilding: medicine and politics

The cholera epidemic of 1884 marked a turning point in the history of Naples. No previous outburst of epidemic disease had ever led to a comprehensive attempt to reform the vulnerability of the population to infection. 1884 was different. In that year the sufferings of the city attracted the attention of the whole country. In the expression of King Umberto, the misfortune of Naples became a national misfortune. The state also correctly appreciated that the insalubrity of Italy's greatest city was a permanent danger to the entire nation. Cholera affected not only health but also public order, commerce and public finance. Furthermore, thanks to the epidemiological advances in the understanding of the mechanisms of cholera that culminated in the work of Pettenkofer and Koch, the disease seemed preventable. Indeed, the local government of Naples and the medical profession of the city claimed to have a plan that would make the City of the Sirens invulnerable to further attacks. After the end of the crisis, therefore, the government of Agostino Depretis attempted to make good the promises that the King and his ministers had made in September to take steps to prevent the recurrence of so great – and so unnecessary – a disaster. Humanitarian sentiment and prudent statesmanship combined to produce a major experiment in preventive medicine.

That experiment involved a major programme of rebuilding and renewal known as *risanamento*. As a result of the events of 1884, Naples joined the ranks of the many European cities that were embellished, enlarged and restructured during the course of the nineteenth century. Sanitary reforms brought sewers and supplies of pure water while renewal projects improved the urban environment and the standard of accommodation. The result was a 'mortality revolution' in western Europe that marked a major advance in the struggle to conquer infectious diseases and a turning point in urban demography. For the first time births exceeded deaths in the great cities of the West.[1] The rebuilding of Paris under the direction of Georges Haussmann is the most famous and spectacular example of urban renewal in nineteenth-century Europe. Milan, which experienced extensive housing reforms in the course of the 1860s, was the Italian prototype.[2]

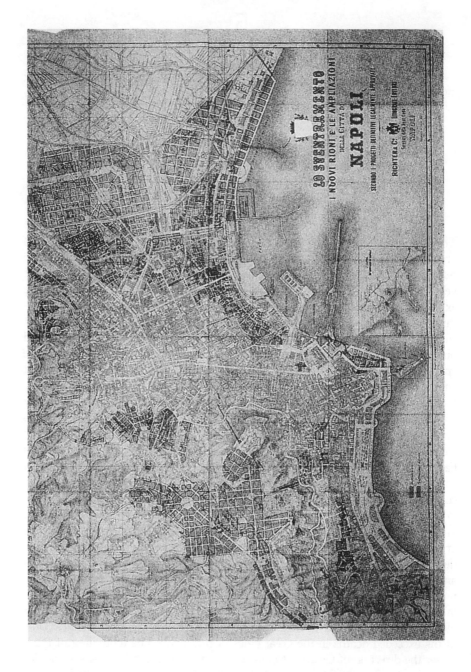

Map 5.1   The renewal and expansion of Naples
source: Franco Della Peruta, ed., *Vita civile degli italiani: società, economia, cultura materiale*
(Milan: Electa, 1990)

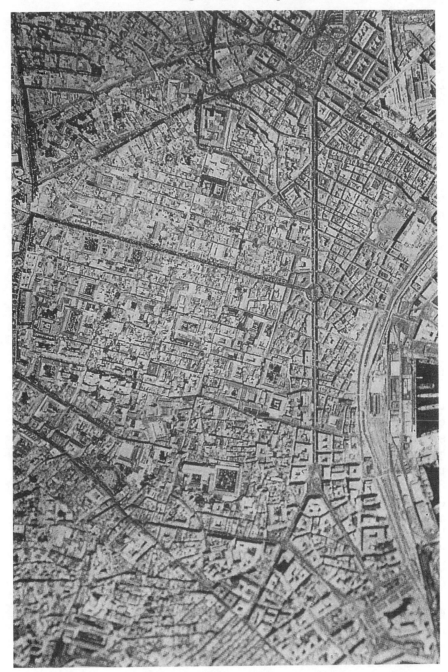

Map 5.2 *Risanamento*
source: Franco Della Peruta, ed., *Vita civile degli italiani: societià, economia, cultura materiale*
(Milan: Electa, 1990)

Naples, belatedly impelled into reform by the catastrophe of 1884, forms part of a larger European pattern. For inspiration and models, the Neapolitan planners examined the experiences of a wide range of Italian and European precedents in the field of urban renewal. Because of the sheer size of Naples and because of the civic pride that led its governors still to view their city as a great capital, the Palazzo San Giacomo rapidly discounted the relevance of all lesser cities and all partial attempts to renew specific neighbourhoods within cities. Within the confines of the Italian peninsula, Neapolitan officials were at pains to regard the experience of their own city as distinctive and pathbreaking because of its scale and expense. Specific areas of Milan, Turin and Rome had undergone renewal, but these earlier cases were dwarfed by the Neapolitan attempt to redeem an entire city. Alberto Marghieri, one of the leading strategists of *risanamento*, explained that,

> What is the point of remembering that Rome, Turin and Milan at their own expense and under their own direction have carried out expropriations? Why bother to lose one's way in such comparisons when the conditions of those cities are unlike those of Naples, indeed are fundamentally different as a result of the law of 1885 itself? Furthermore, the public works projects that have been undertaken until now are of such a limited scale that it is absurd to compare them with our renewal plan.[3]

The Neapolitan planners concentrated their attention instead on those capital cities they considered more worthy and similarly large-scale precedents – Vienna, London, Brussels and, above all, Paris. The French capital was especially influential because the scale, the grandeur and the comprehensive vision of Georges Haussmann's rebuilding programme had endowed it with all the attributes that contemporaries regarded as the embodiments of modernity. Furthermore, the stress that Haussmann had placed on broad boulevards and open spaces, and the example of the new Parisian sewer system meshed perfectly with the medical priorities uppermost in Neapolitan thinking. Not least important, as we shall see, Haussmann's project also embraced a financial rationale to justify so vast an expenditure of public funds. Parisian influences, therefore, can be seen in many aspects of the Neapolitan plan – the architectural aesthetic of the straight line, the breadth of the major boulevard at the centre of the project and the construction of the buildings that lined it on either side, the design and functions of the sewers beneath the streets, and the provisions for the financing of so great a programme of public works.[4]

The specific impetus to renewal in Naples, however, and the medical theory that informed the enterprise mark it as a distinctive and special case. What gives the renewal of the centre of Naples its particular quality and significance is the centrality of the experience of a single disease – Asiatic cholera – to the whole process. Unlike Paris under the Second Empire, the rebuilding of the Lower City of Naples was not undertaken for reasons of prestige, aesthetics and political control. Nor was the overall health of the population of the former capital foremost in the minds of the reformers. *Risanamento* in Naples occurred as a direct consequence of the epidemic of 1884. The plan also embodied a single predominant purpose, that of preventing a recurrence of cholera by means of the 'hygienic redemption of the city'.[5] In presenting the law to the Senate, Depretis stressed its special nature. 'It is', he explained, 'principally, in fact exclusively, a measure of hygiene.'[6] Moreover, the whole direction of the renewal programme was based upon a specific medical theory – the miasmo-contagionist doctrine of Max von Pettenkofer. A unique feature of the rebuilding of the Old City of Naples was that it constituted the translation into stone of Pettenkofer's doctrines. The best place to begin a discussion of Neapolitan renewal, therefore, is the sanitary theory that underlay it.

THE MIASMO-CONTAGIONIST PLAN

The plan put forward by the Palazzo San Giacomo presented a surgical solution to the problem of public health. The medical profession of Naples and the municipal authorities who solicited its advice were divided over the question of therapeutics. They were virtually unanimous, however, in their interpretation of the causes of the frequent episodes of epidemic cholera in the city. Localist medical theory held that the cholera germ arrived from outside by following the main currents of human intercourse. Having gained access to the city, it then thrived like a plant in the subsoil of the city.

The epidemic history of Naples provided a highly plausible demonstration in miasmo-contagionist theory. Here a combination of a temperate climate, abundant rainfall, low altitude, and an alluvial subsoil rich in organic fertilizer provided ideal conditions for the growth of the cholera parasite. Fermenting luxuriantly beneath the city, it emitted lethal exhalations and contaminated the ground water from which the population's supplies were drawn. Pettenkofer taught that a simple algebraic equation captured the essential aetiology of Asiatic cholera: $x + y = z$. The epidemic (z) was caused by the addition of the cholera germ (x) and a porous, damp subsoil heavily polluted with human excrement (y). The extent of the outburst would be determined by the relative degree of predisposition of the population as a result of cleanliness, overcrowding and general health.[7]

Faced with this mathematically expressed dilemma, and spurred on by the Prime Minister's dramatic suggestion of disembowelment, the city council contemplated a radical solution. The Foreign Minister, Pasquale Mancini, abetted the inclination to adopt forceful policies by urging the councillors to 'rip out [*squarciare*] the infected zone'. The strategy that emerged was one of urban renewal by sagittal section. Nicola Amore, advised by Pettenkofer's fellow localist, Teodosio De Bonis, proposed a great incision slicing in a direct line through all four infested boroughs from Via Medina in a northeasterly direction to the railroad station. The planners envisaged a great boulevard – the Rettifilo, later named the Corso Umberto I – 2 kilometres long and 30 metres broad, raised 12.8 metres above sea-level at either end and 8.3 metres in the centre. It would be intersected at right angles and at regular intervals by sixteen wide, straight avenues 10 to 12 metres in width. As a 'great and purposeful street of hygiene and civilization',[8] its function was to purify the city.

The planners rejected all other considerations – aesthetic, economic, and urbanistic – as subordinate to the one great medical purpose of making Naples permanently cholera-free. Adolfo Giambarba, the municipal engineer who drafted the technical specifications for the 'colossal operation', was categorical on this point. In drafting the official municipal plan, he established three leading criteria for the project, all of them 'absolutely hygienic' in their intent. These criteria were:

> [1] Demolition of the *fondaci* and the worst labyrinths. [2] The opening of longi-
> tudinal streets in order to rip out the most unhealthy zone, which will be rebuilt
> with regular and hygienic buildings that allow the free circulation of light and air.
> [3] Elevation of the streets above the present level of the ground-water.[9]

In conformity with these sanitary priorities, Giambarba conceived of the Rettifilo and its network of transverse streets as a great urban lung or bellows admitting air and light to the heart of the Lower City. Neapolitan physicians noted that, in those *sezioni* most devastated in 1884, those streets most swept by the winds suffered many fewer mortalities than the sheltered and poorly venti-lated lanes surrounding them – despite the fact that in other respects the standard of living of the population was identical. E. De Renzi observed that in the Borgo Loreto the lanes running east and west – perpendicular to the direction of the prevailing winds – suffered significantly more than streets running north to south where the breezes gusted freely. Similarly, in the borough of Porto the Via Marinella that ran along the shore and was open to the full blast of the *scirocco* enjoyed a significantly lower death-rate than the protected Via Cosimo located in the interior of the *sezione*.[10]

For this reason, the central boulevard planned by the reformers was to run northeast from the harbour in the direction of the prevailing *scirocco*. Removing obstacles to the free passage of gusts and solar rays, Giambarba arranged for three great open piazzas to be built where before there were only teeming rookeries. There was to be a piazza at either terminus of the boulevard, and one in the centre, with the buildings arranged from one end to the other in straight lines of uniform height. The purifying air and light would then pour unimpeded through the *sezioni* of Mercato, Pendino, Porto and Vicaria, dispersing the foul miasmas and drying out the soil. In Giambarba's explanation, the broad road-ways were, 'the principal means to aerate the zone beyond since the offshore winds from the Gulf are dominant. Channeled in the direction of their flow, they can course not only among the new buildings, but also among the old, which will be redeemed by their action.'[11]

With the bowel of Naples thus laid open by the great incision, the work of purification could proceed further both above and below the ground. Above ground the strategists of the 'sanitary renaissance of Naples' intended the wholesale demolition of the teeming slums where the cholera had run rampant.

The towering tenements, the *fondaci*, and the maze of squalid lanes were all to disappear beneath the redeeming pickaxe of the rebuilders. In their place, well-ventilated, widely spaced new buildings would arise with their heights carefully proportioned to the size of internal courtyards and the width of the streets outside. Detailed regulation by means of a municipal building code would replace the anarchy of old. Most importantly, the population inhabiting the area would be drastically thinned out to eliminate the overcrowding that sanitary theory regarded as the leading factor predisposing Neapolitans to infection.

To achieve the desired thinning, the planners drastically altered the proportions between living quarters and open, public space. The renewal project, which affected a total area of 980,686.76 square metres, particularly targeted the 'deadly zone' of 438,000 square metres in the heart of the Old City. This zone contained 365,325 square metres of buildings where 53,000 troglodytes dwelt in filth and darkness. Renewed, the same area would contain only 225,705 square metres of buildings with the difference filled by air-admitting public spaces. Only 38,000 inhabitants would return to dwell in sunlight and health.[12]

The overall ambition was to reduce the population density of the Lower City from 1,600 people per hectare to 700.[13] To achieve this objective, the city council proposed to abolish a total of 144 streets and lanes and to widen the 127 that were to remain in the zone of renewal. Five hundred and twenty-one blocks of houses and 56 *fondaci* comprising 17,000 dwellings were to be demolished, displacing 87,447 people, 69,198 permanently.[14] The surplus population would be accommodated in a series of newly developed, spacious neighbourhoods beyond the city walls, the most important being the so-called 'industrial quarter' extending to the east beyond the railroad station.

Still above ground, localist theory taught the vital importance of the configuration of the soil. While low-lying cities built on porous subsoil were all at risk because of their location, there were nonetheless enormous differences from neighbourhood to neighbourhood within them. These differences depended on the elevation of each specific quarter above the underlying ground-water. Thus neighbourhoods built on hills were protected by the insulating depth of the ground beneath, while residential districts constructed in declivities suffered more during epidemic outbursts. Pettenkofer examined this factor in detail with regard to Munich, where there were wide variations in mortality from cholera from one quarter to another. These variations closely correlated with differences in elevation. His conclusion was that,

> Where the surface of the earth has an undulating outline it will be found that districts and individual houses which are situated on the summit of the undulation very frequently have no, or only a very small, disposition to the development of an epidemic of cholera, whilst in the hollow of the undulation under like conditions the opposite holds good.[15]

Pettenkofer's followers in Naples noted the applicability of this lesson to the epidemiological pattern of cholera outbreaks in the great Italian metropolis as well. The four regularly devastated *sezioni* were those lying close to sea-level, and the degree of immunity in the other boroughs increased with every metre of altitude. At sea-level, the experience of the boroughs Mercato, Pendino, Porto and Vicaria during the course of five cholera epidemics seemed vividly to substantiate the miasmo-contagionist theory that there was a dangerous circulation of air between the houses and the polluted ground beneath. A favourite image of the localist theorists was that of the burial-ground. According to Pettenkofer, low-lying buildings constructed in perilous proximity to the ground-water below were just as vulnerable to pestilence as if they were sited in a cemetery where bodies were left to decompose in shallow graves immediately underneath them.[16] Explaining the medical purposes behind the municipal renewal plan, Teodosio De Bonis observed,

> Between the subsoil and the bedchambers we live in there is a continuous exchange of gas, just as there is an unceasing transfer between these same rooms and the sewer mains. This exchange is sometimes revealed by evil odours, and sometimes passes unnoticed, but in either event deadly gases and microbes assault our health, and that of our city.[17]

The rebuilders, therefore, gave careful thought to the problem of elevation. An essential feature of the *risanamento* was the strategy of land-fills or *colmate*. Their purpose was to provide an insulating layer of earth corresponding to that of well-regulated grave-yards where the bodies were buried at a suitable and health-preserving depth. The buildings of the new Naples were to rise high above the putrefaction at work in the soil beneath. The existing ground-floor level was to be covered to a depth corresponding to that of one storey of a building. Even in structures that were not demolished, the *bassi* would be interred, and the old first floors above them would open onto the raised streets. A newly enacted sanitary code would then permanently ensure the future. It banned the construction of buildings on sites lying less than three metres above the ground-water table and stipulated that the foundations be laid in impervious materials.[18] Resurrected Naples would be built on a cushion of insulating earth and paving-stone.

At the same time that the rebuilders working above ground sought to protect Naples from the effects of lethal subterranean fermentations, the city fathers sought to attack the problem at its source beneath the soil. It was universally recognized that the antiquated sewers inherited from the seventeenth century were no longer a sanitary asset but a lethal liability. Influenced by miasmo-contagionism, the planners' strategy was to dry out the subsoil, depriving the cholera germ of nutrients and water. To achieve this result, they took advantage of the digging up of the city streets to undertake the colossal public works project of laying an entire new sewerage system. Just as Adolfo Giambarba planned the construction of buildings, thoroughfares and piazzas, the engineer Gaetano Bruno directed the labours that proceeded beneath the streets. Since the main ambition of the city was to drain the soil rather than to remove household waste, Bruno devised a system that was not necessarily linked with individual dwellings.

The first part of the system was a main collector drain to conduct storm-water from the Upper City to the Bay in water-tight conduits that would not allow their contents to ooze into the soil. The second part of the system consisted of two sewerage mains, one for the Lower City and the other for the intermediate boroughs. These in turn were linked with a dense network of secondary pipes beneath every street in Naples. Surface-water was to be deprived of every means of percolating downwards into the earth. Every line was egg-shaped to maximize the strength of the flow in the dry season, and of sufficient diameter to facilitate regular maintenance and cleansing. To prevent infected materials from being poured into the harbour, where offshore winds could blow dangerous miasmas back into the city, both sewer mains were to have outfalls at distant Licola in the Bay of Gaeta where the dumping of their suspect cargo would be of no concern to Neapolitans. Since the collector from the Old City lacked the incline to propel its flow to such a distance, it was to be equipped with a series of pumps. By more modern sanitary standards, the absence of domestic waste pipes linked to the mains was an important omission, but the planners calculated that to drain the subsoil was to render the environment of the city inhospitable to perilous subterranean fermentations. It was sufficient to kill the germ by depriving it of water without worrying about overkill by robbing it of all conceivable nutrient.[19] Localism held as one of its major tenets that a well drained city was exposed to few risks of cholera.[20]

Complementing the underground works was another major component of the Neapolitan sanitary renaissance – the Serino aqueduct that provided the city with a major new supply of pure water.[21] The proposal for a new source of water was far from original as every adult who inhabited or even visited Naples was all too aware that the supplies of the city were inadequate in both quantity and quality. In 1878 a contract to construct the aqueduct was signed with the Naples Water Works Company of London. Budgetary constraints and municipal inertia, however, prevented the idea from being translated into reality. The 1884 epidemic, however, supplied the sense of urgency needed to see pre-existing plans through to completion. In May 1885 the system built by the Naples Water Works Company was completed and in June it was officially inaugurated with a gala celebration at the Piazza del Plebiscito marked by the unveiling of a grandiose new fountain. The aqueduct was designed to supply the city with 100 litres of water per day per inhabitant.

The new supply – that 'immense font of purification'[22] – would fulfill several medically motivated priorities. Its purpose, however, was not primarily to furnish every resident with a pure domestic supply. Cholera as understood by Pettenkofer was uppermost in the mind of the city council. The Munich hygienist taught that, dazzled by the researches of John Snow demonstrating the fatal role of the Broad Street pump in Soho, the English had become unnecessarily obsessed with water as the chief medium for the transmission of cholera.[23] This water-hysteria, Pettenkofer reasoned, had now gained international prominence under the influence of Robert Koch. In the view of the localists, the aetiology of cholera was more complex. Water played a part, but it was less important than poisoned air, and the most important contribution that it made was not the one that so troubled Englishmen and Germans. Water, that is, undermined health less when it was drunk than when it moistened the soil, watered the cholera plant, and – if polluted – provided fertilizer.

Amore and De Bonis were not concerned, therefore, to provide every resident of the city with safe and abundant drinking water. For this reason they were unperturbed that the Neapolitan Water Works Company viewed the Serino aqueduct as a commercial venture. Supplies would be furnished to individual dwellings only if the landlord paid for the subsidiary pipes from the mains to the domestic premises and if the residents paid a yearly subscription that was beyond the means of the majority of the population. As the Saredo Commission reported in 1901, 'The present distribution of the water is incomplete, not as a result of any shortage, but because of its high cost that is beyond the economic means of the majority of the populace.'[24] The abundant Serino water had other purposes in the minds of the localists. It would flush the sewer system, keeping it freely flowing and odourless. Being free of impurities, unlike the Bolla and Carmignano supplies, it would play no part in the manuring of the soil within the city boundaries. And, being readily available at hundreds of public fountains, it would enable the Neapolitans to close their decrepit and notorious wells.

To complete the sanitary renaissance, the city proposed to equip the city with a permanent hospital for infectious diseases in order that the hasty improvisation and disorder of September 1884 would never recur. It was anticipated that sporadic cases of cholera would break out in Naples in the future. *Risanamento* would not isolate the city like a *cordon sanitaire*. Renewal and rebuilding would achieve the very different objective of preventing the disease from taking root and flourishing after it was imported. It was essential, therefore, that the city be equipped on a permanent basis with an infectious diseases hospital where 'sporadic' cases of Asiatic cholera could be properly isolated and treated. The Naples cholera hospital would be designed according to the best-informed and most modern sanitary opinion.

This hospital was based on the Vittoria Hospital, which had been hastily improvised during the September crisis of 1884. The Vittoria was now enlarged to a capacity of 300 beds through the erection of additional wooden pavilions and renamed after Domenico Cotugno, the scientist and benefactor of the Hospital for Incurables. For localist sanitarians, the site of the Cotugno Hospital was ideal, as De Bonis explained to the city council. It was located outside the city on the crest of the Poggioreale hill 150 metres above sea-level to the northeast of Naples. Here the Cotugno was constantly exposed to 'the most active ventilation' by the prevailing winds. The advantages of this elevation were twofold. In the first place, altitude would prevent the contamination of the ground-water below the institution. The hospital would rise above impervious strata of rocks and a soil composed of non-porous pozzolana that together would provide effective insulation. At the same time, the ever-benevolent *scirocco* would dissipate 'mephitic influences', blowing them harmlessly inland and away from the city.[25]

FINANCE

The estimate of the cost of *risanamento*, based on preliminary studies by the municipal engineers, was in excess of 100 million lire – a sum that was far beyond the means of the city. Since the matter was judged to be a question of national urgency, however, the state intervened. While the memory of the disaster was still fresh in the minds of legislators, parliament voted a large-scale subsidy with unprecedented dispatch. Presenting the bill to the Chamber of Deputies, Agostino Depretis explained that in financial matters the Italian practice was to respect a division of labour and expense.[26] It was the responsibility of individual communes to carry out and finance public works projects that primarily affected the interests of their residents. The state assumed the burden only for works that were deemed to be of concern to the entire commonwealth. Normally, therefore, municipalities were responsible for health and welfare because only local inhabitants would benefit.

To make Naples cholera-free, however, was a special case. It would not create a precedent allowing every city in Italy to demand a subsidy from the exchequer. This point needed emphasis because there were Deputies like Pietro Delvecchio of Cuneo who put forward a list of other communes he deemed worthy of state intervention in the national interest.[27] It was significant in its defence that Naples had not asked for assistance: the initiative had come from the Crown and the government. The renewal of Italy's greatest seaport was a national concern, Depretis argued, no less than transportation and national defence because the squalor of the former capital directly threatened the health of every Italian.

Supporting this argument, the Prime Minister explained that the unification of Italy had far-reaching medical implications. As the largest city and busiest port in the peninsula, Naples was constantly exposed to infection. Asiatic cholera had repeatedly invaded the great Thyrrenean seaport before attacking other centres. Before 1861, however, Depretis reasoned, Neapolitan misfortunes were local affairs. Cholera devastated the city, but spread no further. Epidemic outbursts elsewhere were not directly caused by the prior infection of Naples. Unification transformed matters. Improved means of communication and the ever-increasing volume of trade created by economic development linked the medical fate of the former capital city to that of the rest of the country. The leader of the Historical Left informed parliament that,

> Under the conditions that prevailed in Italy in former times, the disease could be largely localized – confined to the city and vanquished there. That is no longer possible. The largest urban centre in the nation is linked to the other leading cities by bonds of family, friendship, commerce, speculation, and industry. Standing open on every side by land and by sea, and emerging as the hub of a major railroad network, Naples cannot be isolated from the rest of Italy, no matter how grave the danger.[28]

In modern Italy, the health of Naples was a national concern. To sanitize Naples was to protect the whole kingdom, and the plan put forward by the Palazzo San Giacomo included no purposes other than public health.

There was a recent precedent for the assumption by the state of financial responsibility for local public works deemed to be a matter of national interest. The state had intervened financially after the Tiber had flooded Rome in 1882. Flooding was due to no fault of the local authorities; the city lacked the resources to control the river that flowed through its midst; and the consequences of a disaster in the capital of the kingdom affected far more than local interests. It was constitutionally correct, therefore, for the government to contribute to the remedy. Cholera in Naples presented a similar principle.

Finally, Depretis suggested that Neapolitans had a special moral claim to national assistance. Bourbon misrule had so crippled the economy of the city that there was an unbridgeable gap between the essential needs of the residents of the city and the means available to meet them. The legacy of the old regime was that the city was caught in a permanent poverty trap. Generating no wealth and lacking an adequate tax base, Naples could not fund essential public services. Subsidies for renewal, therefore, would constitute reparations payments in compensation for centuries of neglect. Depretis, the Prime Minister from Stradella in Lombardy, used the cholera epidemic of 1884 as a means of placing the 'Question of Naples' on the national agenda for immediate attention. The moral unity of the nation would be reinforced.

Furthermore, Depretis argued, *risanamento* was a matter of financial prudence. Epidemics were costly affairs. To erect a sanitary rampart for the defence of Italy against invasion by cholera was a sound investment. A hundred million lire wisely spent in preventive medicine would be swiftly recouped in medical and sanitary savings. Avoiding the necessity to finance the relief of communities stricken by epidemic disease was a great economy. Italy would also experience enormous benefits through uninterrupted commerce and tourism, through undisturbed public order, and through the greater productivity of a healthy workforce.

A practical political consideration was left unspoken. The 'parliamentary revolution' of 1876, which first brought the Historical Left led by Depretis to power, was due in no small measure to the discontents of southern Italians at the neglect of their vital interests by the Liberal state. The Historical Left as a political force was strongest in the provinces of the Mezzogiorno, and it embodied the expectation of reforms and patronage. The elections of 1874, the great seismic shock that preceded the 'revolution', first revealed the extent of southern disaffection. In those elections, the Centre and the North returned 240 deputies loyal to the ministry of the Right and 85 deputies representing the opposition of the Historical Left. In the South, by contrast, the Left triumphed with 152 deputies against the 56 deputies of the Right. The Italian peninsula was starkly divided between Right and Left representing, respectively, North and South.[29]

Despite having risen to power on the discontent of southerners, Depretis as Prime Minister demonstrated few reforming impulses. In particular his government gave little priority to the launching of large-scale public-works programmes south of Rome. The result was the rapid eruption of dissension within the ranks of the new majority. Especially important was Naples, where the Left had its political headquarters and where its electoral victory in 1874 had been most crushing. The Neapolitan parliamentary delegation was also strategically important because of its size and because no critic of Depretis on the Left was more unrelenting than the disillusioned Deputy and former Mayor of the city, the Duke of San Donato. The funding of a major public-works project for the benefit of Naples, therefore, served the expedient purpose of preserving the cohesion of the governmental majority by providing a partial fulfilment of overdue promises. Southern deputies were mollified. In this regard San Donato was a significant weather-vane. Angered by the meager results of the 'revolution' of 1876, the Deputy from Naples had passed into opposition, denouncing Depretis for 'betrayal' and bitterly observing that, 'This is no longer the Left!' San Donato had even proclaimed that Depretis was worse than the Prime Ministers of the Right. Now the ex-Mayor fulsomely embraced the Prime Minister in the Chamber.[30]

To draft the 'special law' providing the needed 100 million lire for the renewal of Naples, Depretis appointed a parliamentary committee of nine deputies, of whom five were Neapolitans, including the Chairman, Giovanni Nicotera; Rocco De Zerbi; and San Donato. They presented their proposals to the Chamber as a matter of urgency on 27 November, only three weeks after the end of the epidemic itself. The bill was approved by the Chamber and the Senate in December and January respectively, and enacted into law on 15 January 1885. Because of its overriding medical purpose, it was popularly known as 'the cholera law'.[31]

Under the provisions of the new legislation, parliament assisted the city by raising the bulk of the funds necessary for the great project – 100 million lire, which it lent to the municipality on generous and heavily subsidized terms. The Italian state raised the capital by issuing redeemable bonds bearing 5 per cent interest in twelve annual instalments beginning in 1886. In each year from 1886 to 1898 Naples would receive a long-term loan – 8 million lire until 1894 and 9 million from 1894 to 1898 – for a total capital sum of 100 million. The intention was that the work of *risanamento* itself would be carried out in stages spread over the same twelve years. Thus by 1898 the impoverished metropolis would have accomplished its great sanitary reform without imposing an impossible burden of taxation on its population.

Until 1899 the only capital expenditure falling on the city treasury would be the payment of any costs incurred by the public works in excess of the 100 million lire provided by Rome. In addition, the city was responsible for interest payments to the bondholders – payments which rose from 206,187.50 lire in the first year to 5,154,650 lire in the twelfth as the outstanding balance increased. Here the state extended a further substantial subsidy. The interest paid by the city was in reality only 50 per cent of the amount owed to the creditors because the state made matching payments, thereby halving the cost to the city. Redemption of the principal sum owing on the bonds began only in 1899, and was then spread over sixty annuities. These terms were sufficiently generous that the city, far from being overwhelmed by the new burden of debt, planned to extend the work of rebuilding to pockets of slums located outside the four *sezioni* contemplated by the government. At its own expense, Town Hall planned the renewal of the neighbourhoods of Santa Lucia and Santa Brigida that had also been decimated in September 1884.

In financial terms, the parliamentary committee that drafted the law calculated that the deferred capital payments made by the city from 1899 after the renewal project had been completed were an expenditure in name only. Indeed, having carefully examined the rebuilding of Paris, the Italian planners invoked the Saint Simonian concept of 'productive spending' that had guided Baron Haussmann. On the basis of this precedent, Depretis and Rocco De Zerbi argued that the project would largely pay for itself. Renewal, that is, would enhance the property values of the city and generate employment, thereby providing the city administration with revenue to meet the costs of redeeming the loan. Writing with regard to Paris, Haussmann had reasoned,

> The theory of 'productive spending', which caused such great astonishment, ... enabled me to demonstrate that the city budget had been balanced without surcharges or additional taxes. The many different undertakings and the very extension of such useful work provided the means. Increased spending brought about a parallel and progressive increase in municipal revenues, just as wise sewing yields a surplus at harvest-time. This theory, although somewhat paradoxical, contains a profound truth, and it has long formed one of the chief articles of my beliefs as an economist.[32]

The concept of 'productive spending' was all the more convincing to Italians because it had been invoked and legitimated by Camillo Cavour, the architect of national unity. As Minister of Finance and then Prime Minister of Piedmont during the 1850s, Cavour had justified major increase in expenditure on public works as instances of 'productive spending'. Railways and roads, he argued in parliament, paid for themselves by generating economic growth and increasing the yield of taxation to the exchequer.[33]

Just as in Paris and in Piedmont, the rebuilders of Naples concluded, public spending on the renewal of the Lower City would spontaneously generate the additional revenue needed to finance the repayment of the debt incurred. Furthermore, the extended period allowed for the redemption of the bonds would permit a significant natural increase of the population of the city. After twelve years of renewal, followed by sixty redemption annuities, Naples would be a substantially more populous commune, although no attempt was made to predict the precise size of its growth. The principle involved was that the larger number of residents would enable City Hall to spread the cost of repaying the municipal debt over a broader tax base, avoiding any further impoverishment of the population. In addition, the city no less than the state would realize major savings by forestalling further epidemic emergencies. In any event, parliament hedged its financial calculations with an additional measure of assistance to Naples. To ensure that the people of the ex-capital were not excessively burdened, the state agreed to provide a measure of tax relief, suspending for ten years the collection of the treasury share of the revenue from the most important tax levied by the city, the *dazio consumo*. It was estimated that the value of the savings created by this relief would total 10 million lire.

Such assistance by the state did not imply control of the project by the central government. On the contrary, having aided the city by providing capital on generous terms, the state agreed to assume only a distant supervisory role during the process of *risanamento* itself. The city would plan and carry out the work, subject only to the requirement that all proposals be approved by parliament through submission to a technical committee of experts appointed by the Chamber for the purpose. Here was a further practical consequence of the localist philosophy of cholera upon which the Neapolitan renewal was based. By contrast, the water-based theory of John Snow and the germ theory of Robert Koch provided a rationale for centralized public health policies. The doctrines of Snow and Koch envisaged that the state would possess all the information necessary to establish a campaign to combat infection. The miasmo-contagionism of Pettenkofer and De Bonis, on the contrary, postulated that the decisive factors in the aetiology of Asiatic cholera were the specific features of the local environment such as topography, soil conditions, elevation, temperature, wind patterns, rainfall, ground-water levels and density of population.

These factors required expert local knowledge, and the application of the necessary remedies was therefore best entrusted to local authorities rather than to distant planners in Rome. It was no accident that in Germany Koch was an agent of centralizing imperial power in Berlin while Pettenkofer worked on behalf of decentralized local authorities in Munich. Similarly in Italy, the adherents of miasmo-contagionism in Naples were jealous defenders of local prerogatives. The constitutional practice of the Italian state of devolving matters of welfare upon the communes reinforced this direction of policy. Despite the pre-eminent role of the state in raising the money, therefore, political precedent and medical doctrine combined to confer upon the Palazzo San Giacomo full authority over the work of renewal and rebuilding. Article 1 of the law of 15 January 1885 stated explicitly that, 'The execution of the work will be entrusted to the municipal government.'[34]

After January 1885, therefore, the discussion of *risanamento* shifted from Montecitorio in Rome to the Palazzo San Giacomo in Naples. What was involved was more than a change of venue. In parliament the emphasis of the discussion of assistance for stricken Naples fell upon the need for humanitarian aid. Depretis, Rocco De Zerbi, and the deputies who played the central part in presenting the case for the law of 15 January were fresh from their direct experience of the worst slums of the city, and they were deeply shocked by what they had witnessed. Their interventions stressed the plight of Neapolitans and the urgent need to improve the conditions of the 'disinherited' of the city.

The priorities of the aldermen and city councillors were different. In part, the change reflected timing. Parliament debated the bill to rebuild Naples in the immediate aftermath of the epidemic. The zeal to prevent further disasters was at its height, and the fear that the following spring would witness a further outbreak unless immediate and radical steps were taken was uppermost in the minds of the deputies. The discussion of *risanamento* at the Palazzo San Giacomo took place later and in less pressing circumstances. A first version of the municipal plan was drafted by the city engineers and approved by the council in October 1885. It was then referred to the parliamentary review committee, which gave its consent in 1886 after a series of minor amendments. The final version was returned to the city council for debate only in 1887 when the events of 1884 were less compelling and the fear of an immediate return of the cholera had disappeared. Humanitarian appeals fell on less sympathetic ears, and the tone of the debate was strikingly different.

Another important factor was specificity. The Chamber of Deputies and the Senate considered the issue of renewal only as a matter of abstract principle. Parliament concerned itself with the overall justifications for the spending of Treasury funds for the benefit of a single city, but it avoided discussion of the details of the public works themselves. For this reason, the interventions of the deputies were brief and high-minded. Depretis and De Zerbi rapidly surveyed the living conditions of the slums they had visited and called upon the nation to correct the outrage of a modern city whose residents were forced to live like troglodytes in urban caves.

The discussion that took place at City Hall observed different priorities. The municipal councillors had no need to consider the general necessity for the programme of public works on which they were embarking. On the matter of principle there had long been unanimity. Mayors San Donato, Giusso and Amore had sponsored thorough investigations of the sanitary problems of Naples, and they had commissioned proposals to rectify them. The law of 15 January 1885 merely provided the municipality with the means to carry out measures that it had already considered and approved. Unlike parliament, City Hall concerned itself with the detailed workings of the rebuilding project as they affected the interests of their grand electors and clients.

Powerful local interests rapidly overwhelmed the humane concerns that first moved the King and his government to intervene on behalf of the Neapolitan people. The gulf between the councillors and the people and even a note of resentment by officials at the popular defiance of September 1884 were evident. An important measure of the difference in emphasis that emerged as vested interests came to the fore is the major speech of Alberto Marghieri, the alderman responsible for public works. On 25 and 27 April 1887 Marghieri presented the final proposal of the *giunta* to the city council, just as De Zerbi had explained the bill of the government to parliament in 1884. In Marghieri's lengthy discussion a harsh tone replaced the reforming zeal of the President of the White Cross.[35]

The alderman responsible for drafting the municipal plan had no solicitude for the Neapolitan poor whom Depretis and De Zerbi had originally designated as the principal beneficiaries of the enterprise. For Marghieri, *risanamento* was not intended for the benefit of any specific social class, and certainly not the undeserving poor massed beneath the respectable proletariat in the social pyramid – the 'under-class' of the 'disinherited'.[36] These were the strata that 'crowd about the others'. 'Imperious, petulant, grasping, and ruthless, they demand that the problems of their existence be solved.'[37] It was vital that the 'living forces' of the city avoid an 'exaggerated philanthropy' that would be 'the great ruin of the rest of society'.[38]

It was significant that Marghieri's keynote speech outlined the effects of urban renewal and rebuilding on every other social class in the city before turning at the end to the position of the poor. The speaker then dealt more succinctly with their interests than with those of such deserving groups as landlords, contractors and industrial workers. It was essential, he suggested, that

> statesmen and local authorities avoid excess and exaggeration. Their feelings must not overcome their reason. They must act, but their actions must walk in leaden shoes, cautious and slow. The alternative is to become like the Gracchi and to share in their downfall.[39]

To explain his viewpoint, Marghieri made a careful distinction between poverty and hygiene. In terms of this distinction, the purpose of the municipal renewal plan was to improve hygiene, which affected the whole of the population, but not to remove poverty, which was the misfortune only of the *plebe*, the undeserving common people.[40] The only aspect of *risanamento* intended by the planners to benefit the poor specifically was the building work that accompanied the project. On the construction sites, the Municipal Director of Public Works predicted, a great moral transformation would occur as shiftless beggars were turned into sturdy proletarians. Here was the city council's vision of their 'redemption'. Labour, Marghieri predicted, ' will make the poor more like us, help them to share our feelings, and enable them to understand our thoughts'. Honourable toil would bring the 'lower orders' (*basso ceto*) into contact with 'modern civilization'.[41]

Labour would also strengthen the social order. The notables of Naples were anxious that despair could ignite the social tensions of the Lower City into a full-scale insurrection. The *giunta* welcomed the rebuilding project in part because it feared that the Neapolitan poor would eventually imitate the example of the Paris Commune of 1871, which they envisaged as the avenging fury of the disinherited and the rabble. Gainful employment would turn the *plebe* away from class warfare, transforming the poor into loyal supporters of the local parties of order. 'Those who work', argued alderman Achille Nardi, who was soon to be publicly exposed as a Camorra boss, 'do not become *communards* but conservatives.'[42] Nardi's theory of the revolutionary potential of the unemployed and the socially stabilizing value of labour was shared by the Mayor. Nicola Amore believed that, without renewal and the employment prospects it offered, the Neapolitan slums harboured the potential for a second Commune.[43] Labour and renewal, however, were not to be confounded with charity.

The intention of the *giunta* was to complement renewal with expansion (*ampliamento*). The city would commission the construction of low-cost and middle-income housing in a series of 'expansion quarters' that would receive the 90,000 people displaced by the demolition of the Lower City. The most important of the quarters intended for the refugees was that of Arenaccia, the so-called 'industrial neighbourhood' to the east of the railroad station, which was to accommodate the working class. Other 'expansion quarters' would rise on the periphery of the Old City or on the surrounding hills – Vomero, Vasto, Orientale, S. Efremo, Materdei, Ponte Rossi and Regina Margherita. The city stipulated that the work of construction in the new neighbourhoods should proceed in phases carefully synchronized with the work of demolition in order to ease the process of adjustment and ensure that it took place without giving rise to homelessness or a worsening of overcrowding in the remaining stock of still-undemolished buildings.

Having arranged for the construction of new accommodation and having stipulated that the new structures rise simultaneously with the issuing of eviction notices, City Hall saw its task as complete. It would not intervene further with arbitrary controls to ensure that the rents charged in the expansion quarters were comparable to those that had prevailed in the Lower City before demolition or that employment followed the migration of people. The laws of the marketplace would be allowed instead to set rent at its 'natural level', and Naples would avoid setting any example of 'socialism of the worst type'.[44] Replying to the accusation that he was indifferent to the circumstances of the poor, Marghieri argued that what was involved was not indifference but adherence to a matter of moral principle acknowledged by all 'civilized nations', namely that the 'economic relationship of supply and demand' must be allowed free expression. He rejected out of hand any suggestion that the city government should interfere.[45] Alderman Nardi, who sat with Marghieri and Amore on the executive committee, stressed that any further provision for the 'disinherited' was the task of charity, not urban renewal.[46]

Such was the lack of attention of the city administration to the specific plight of the poor that Count Giusso, the Director-General of the Bank of Naples, warned of possible catastrophe. A former volunteer in the heroic days of the White Cross, Giusso was a dissenting member of the committee responsible for the drafting of the plan. Marghieri and the majority, Giusso retorted, need have no fear of being accused of socialism. The great weakness of their project consisted of the opposite defect: they had given no thought – and made no provision – for the poor. By such a remarkable oversight, Giusso charged, the city council had both evaded the most pressing problem facing it and avoided one of the chief sources of the disaster of 1884. The only specific remedy for poverty that the executive proposed was that the poor be transformed into workers on the building sites! Such a suggestion, if not intended as sarcasm, was wholly inadequate and inappropriate, the former Mayor argued. The work of rebuilding was temporary and it could never employ more than a small fraction of the 90,000 people about to be displaced. Giusso calculated that the overall effect of eviction and resettlement in the 'expansion neighbourhoods' would be an 'economic disaster' for those affected. The livelihood of the *plebe* in the Lower City depended on a complex 'economy of the street' where the poor eked out their subsistence by providing minor services to more prosperous neighbours and to their fellows. To rehouse them in new quarters was to disrupt this micro-economy without putting anything in its place. The expansion quarters to the east were termed 'industrial' in the plan, but in fact they contained no economic infrastructure and offered no employment to their residents.[47]

Giusso and his fellow critics of the municipal plan illustrated their reservations by recalling the unfortunate consequences of the sporadic past experiences of the city when it had attempted to improve the worst hygienic conditions by condemning and demolishing some of the most obscene *fondaci*. These precedents were far from encouraging. Unable to afford better accommodation, the evicted tenants had simply found shelter in other *fondaci* in nearby neighbourhoods, where they increased the already acute problem of overcrowding. In this way the living conditions of the families affected deteriorated even further. Misguided cures had only aggravated the original malady.[48]

The real concern of the executive, Giusso claimed, was for the landlords about to be expropriated rather than for the tenants about to be evicted. The landlords were electors; the tenants were disenfranchised rabble. The disparity of consideration could be seen in the relative time and space devoted to the two classes in Marghieri's report on behalf of the administration and in the text of the municipal plan itself. The landlords, who numbered 7,000, were dealt with first and at great length. The 90,000 tenants were discussed summarily at the end. In the printed version of Marghieri's report, ten pages were devoted to the effects of the project on the thousands of landlords and only two to the consequences for the tens of thousands of the 'disinherited'.[49] Marghieri's priorities here accurately reflected the perspective of the executive as a whole. The official municipal plan declared that, 'The class that, more than any other, attracted the attention of the executive committee was that of the owners of the properties to be demolished.'[50] Faithfully adhering to these stated priorities, the authors of the plan devoted nine pages to the issue of expropriation and its effects on the landlords of the city and three pages to the plight of the displaced tenants.[51]

In response to the objections of their critics, Marghieri and Amore thought further. The council debates the following year included substantial discussion of the ways in which the city envisaged that the poor would be rehoused, and Article 6 of the contract signed on 3 October 1888 included explicit provisions on their behalf. As a condition for the awarding of the renewal contract, the city stipulated that 40,000 square metres of land be set aside for the construction of low-cost housing. In a move intended to forestall the erection of instant new slums to replace the old, the contract and the building code also determined the types of construction that would be acceptable.[52]

Opponents of the plan, however, were not reassured. Forty thousand square metres of land, they argued, were woefully inadequate. Since the maximum height of the new buildings was set at four storeys and since allowance had to be made for courtyards, stairways, latrines and walls, 40,000 square metres would provide space for only 5,000 rooms of an average size of 25 square metres. Unless the overcrowded conditions of the city centre were to be reproduced in the new quarters, the maximum number of people who could be accommodated following eviction was 20,000. Even in principle, such provision was inadequate for an exodus of nearly 90,000 tenants, of whom the large majority would be poor.[53] Even this measure of attention to the class of tenants, however, was purely notional because, without rent control, most of the people evicted would be unable to afford the rents of the new and improved accommodation they would be offered. Marghieri himself calculated that the probable average for rents in the new buildings would be 15 to 18 lire a month, ranging from a low of 10 to a maximum of 26[54] – all figures well in excess of the rents of 5 to 6 lire prevailing in the slums scheduled for demolition.

From the outset of the debate over *risanamento* in the autumn of 1884, the Catholic paper *Osservatore romano* predicted that the issue of rent would ultimately reveal the underlying reason that the renewal programme would never achieve its objectives – the inherent incompatibility between the laws of the marketplace on the one hand and the interests of the weak and the poor on the other. Private enterprise could not produce an adequate stock of low-cost housing, and the rebuilding of the Lower City would soon reveal itself as a 'businessman's renewal'. The existing dwellings of the poor would be destroyed, and the new buildings would be let at rents the impoverished could never afford. The end result would be an aggravation of their plight.[55] As the chief architect of the municipal plan, Alberto Marghieri attempted to console himself and such critics with a reassuring thought. Although the rent in the new buildings 'would not be low' by the standards of the Lower City, he responded that the expected rises would be offset by the transformation of the poor into construction workers with higher and steadier wages.[56]

In addition to arguing that the city had failed to provide affordable housing, critics charged that the municipal plan spent the money raised by parliament unwisely. Giusso, one of the leading financial experts in the city, conducted a private survey of property values in the boroughs of Mercato, Pendino and Porto where the work of renewal was concentrated. He then compared his findings with the estimates used by Marghieri and the executive to calculate compensation for those whose properties were to be demolished.[57] His conclusion was that the estimates of the market values of the buildings scheduled for expropriation by City Hall had been grossly and arbitrarily inflated. The procedure adopted by the municipal engineers in determining the market value per square metre of the condemned buildings was to take the rateable value of the properties established by the state as a base, and then to increase the figure by 25 per cent. In this manner the city violated the precedents set by all previous expropriations by eminent domain. In the case of the Via del Duomo, for example, the amount of compensation had been determined by adding 6 per cent, not 25 per cent, to the rateable value of the properties. Nevertheless, not satisfied that the results were equitable and politically acceptable, the city increased the 25 per cent to 33 per cent. To cover the cost of administration and possible litigation, the city then added a further 20 per cent – the *decimi di alea* – to the total sum.[58] The final result was to add 40 million lire to the cost of expropriations based on the rateable values alone.[59]

As a result, Giusso reasoned, the compensation money constituted a political windfall rather than a proper commercial transaction. The effect on the public-works programme was severe. The first act of the rebuilders would be to misuse the lion's share of the funds intended for the benefit of the people. Of the 100 million lire provided to the city by parliament, 78 million were to be divided among the landlords of the Old City. Inevitably, therefore, the scope of the renewal project would be greatly reduced. There would be no funds left, Giusso explained, to encourage industry in the 'expansion quarters'; to build schools, orphanages and shelters; to provide the city with a network of canals to stimulate the economy; and to construct new and salubrious markets.[60]

Given the property-based suffrage of the period, the working classes and the poor lacked adequate representation in the deliberations of the city, which made its plans without consulting the residents most directly affected. Only the craftsman Filippo Gattola, elected as an opposition councillor in the Lower City, spoke directly on their behalf. He reminded the council that the idea for rebuilding had originated with the King, who had been shocked by the living conditions of the victims of the 1884 epidemic, four-fifths of whom were destitute people from the slums of the city centre. It was obvious therefore, he suggested, that the original idea of the reform was to improve the housing and hygiene of the poor living in the four devastated boroughs. By its failure to establish the fate of these people as the first priority, the city had subverted the intentions of the sovereign and his ministers. Gattola proposed, therefore, that the city include an adequate area for low-cost housing in its project by at least doubling the 40,000 square metres provided in the contract and that it make the resulting accommodation genuinely available to the poor by instituting rent controls. 'It is unacceptable', he announced, 'that City Hall should be indifferent to these issues, as I seem to have heard alderman Marghieri say that it is.'[61]

Ignoring both Giusso and Gattola, Marghieri and the *giunta* violated the great lesson that emerged clearly from the first major study of the problems of the South – the investigation of social conditions in Sicily by Sidney Sonnino and Leopoldo Franchetti in 1875. The two Tuscan investigators concluded that the 'social question', which included poverty as its primary ingredient, was so pressing in the Mezzogiorno that its solution was the essential prerequisite for all other reforms.[62] It was ironic that the first great public works project in the South set a precedent by paying no heed to this warning.

SPECULATION AND THE NAPLES RENEWAL COMPANY, LTD

Having reformulated the objectives of *risanamento* in less generous terms than the framers of the original bill of 1885 had intended, the city council then turned to the practicalities of its implementation. The question that most concerned the councillors was the issue of who should be responsible for the execution of the programme of demolition and rebuilding.[63] The suggestion that the city itself should carry out the work was the first to be rejected. Experience, the majority concluded, militated against the idea of launching any large-scale programme of municipally administered public works. Municipal projects were slow and encumbered with tedious bureaucratic procedures, whereas the needs of the city were urgent. The record of the city for completing projects that it undertook was discouraging. The principal renewal project undertaken during the San Donato mayoralty was that of the Via del Duomo. It was still unfinished after eighteen years because the work had been suspended when the funds ran out. Similarly, a previously approved 'expansion neighbourhood' – the rione Amedeo – had still not been realized despite the passage of a quarter of a century.[64] By contrast, the only successful public works carried out since unification – the Via Caracciolo, the Piazza del Municipio and the Serino aqueduct – had all been undertaken by private industry.[65]

Reliance on private contractors, the city councillors reasoned, would also facilitate the progress of the local project through legislative scrutiny in Rome. To receive the parliamentary approval required by the law of 1885, the Neapolitan plan would have to provide some guarantee that the work would be securely brought to a conclusion. Marghieri argued that private enterprise rather than a municipal department with a history of unfinished commitments was required. Such a conclusion was all the stronger because even the prompt and satisfactory completion of the project by the municipality could cause political trouble. To bring renewal to such a happy end would be to demonstrate to the electors that City Hall had become absorbed by a single preoccupation to the detriment of its other responsibilities.[66]

The proponents of privatization stressed that the experience of other Italian cities did not constitute binding precedents for Naples. Rome, Milan and Turin had embarked on municipal programmes of sanitary reform. But Naples was a special case. The 'colossal' scale and cost of the work to be undertaken in the Old City and the special financial constraints of the Neapolitan budget had no equivalents elsewhere. Naples was heavily indebted; the estimates of the cost of the work inevitably contained an element of unpredictability; and there was little likelihood that parliament would respond favourably to any further requests for assistance. It was therefore better to minimize the exposure of City Hall to cost overruns by passing on the risk to private enterprise.

In determining the advantages of a private contractor, the city carefully calculated the market value of the project, and the figures it produced reinforced the unwillingness of the executive to carry out the work. The estimates for carrying out the first phase of *risanamento* – the demolition of the slums in the Lower City and the roadworks connected with the new boulevard and the network of crossing streets and piazzas – were a source of concern. The cost of bringing the demolition and roadwork to a successful conclusion was calculated at 133 million lire, divided as Table 5.1 indicates.[67]

Table 5.1. *Expenses of phase one of* risanamento

Item	Cost (in Lire)
Expropriations	94,000,000
Demolition	11,000,000
Roadwork	7,000,000
Administration and Taxes	8,000,000
Sewer lines	1,500,000
Unforeseen expenses	11,500,000
Total	133,000,000

Table 5.2. *Assets available to complete phase one of* risanamento

Item	Value (in Lire)
Sites for development	40,000,000
Materials salvaged	3,000,000
Buildings left standing	12,000,000
Subsidies from public funds	74,500,000
Total	129,500,000

These expenses, the most important of which was the compensation totalling 94,000,000 to be paid to the 7,000 property owners who were to be expropriated, were to be met by sources of income that Marghieri defined as the 'the factors of speculation and the bases of profit'. These were: direct subsidy from the capital raised by the bond issues, the recovery of building materials that could be recycled from the demolished premises, the final rent payments from tenants occupying the condemned premises prior to their destruction, and the sale of the cleared building sites ready for redevelopment. The value of these assets available to the rebuilder for the completion of phase one of the operation was estimated in the manner indicated by Table 5.2.[68] Concern about the financial attractiveness of the demolition contract to a prospective investor arose from the inherent uncertainty of some of the costs involved. The problem was expressed arithmetically in the conclusion that the assets left a shortfall of 3.5 million lire relative to the expenses (129,500,000 lire as opposed to 133,000,000 lire).

Even greater, however, was the uncertainty surrounding the second phase of renewal – the rebuilding proper. The city engineers estimated the cost of constructing the buildings in the plan at 110 million lire.[69] The anxiety of the city council was that the means to cover this outlay of capital was the sale of the 350,000 square metres of building sites, but the proceeds of these sales were inherently unknowable in advance. The project therefore involved a considerable component of speculative risk that City Hall preferred to avoid. The expectation was that the sale would yield a substantial profit or 'surplus value'. In the event of a shortfall, however, the city council could envisage an insoluble budgetary crisis. In the name of fiscal prudence, therefore, the planners preferred to pass the risk of loss – and the possibility of profit – onto private contractors.[70] Contractors could raise part of the necessary capital by the flotation of stock, and the city could facilitate the task of finding the additional further credit by guaranteeing a mortgage on each of the properties to be built and by subsidizing the interest rates. This option of relying on private enterprise was especially attractive because expropriation was a sensitive political issue, and some councillors were reluctant to embark on complex and potentially painful negotiations with their electors. It was to be hoped that, by means of resolute parsimony, contractors would be able to achieve economies that would be impossible for the city.[71]

Having rejected the idea that the city itself undertake the renewal project, the councillors debated at great length the question of whether the work should be divided among a series of contractors or tendered *en bloc* to a single firm.[72] Those who advocated subdividing the work stressed the danger of entrusting the fate of the city to a single entrepreneur. There were no precedents, they argued, for investing a single private citizen or company with such immense power. A contractor acting alone would control the life of the city, setting rents, determining employment, holding the Mayor to ransom in negotiations over the terms of contracts. Naples, argued councillors Francesco Parlati and Girolamo Giusso, would have created 'an immense, monstrous monopoly' that would emerge as 'the master of the city', the 'supreme and absolute lord of three boroughs'.[73] What would happen to Naples, Parlati asked, if the single firm was badly managed and went bankrupt with the project still unfinished? To engage one company to assume responsibility for the entire public works programme was to gamble on the unknown.[74]

A further difficulty, he foresaw, was that the actual building work would be conducted in a shoddy and unsatisfactory manner. The reason was that the scale of the demolition and construction involved in renewing the centre of the Lower City was beyond the means of one construction company. A single contract, therefore, necessarily implied the evil of subcontracting, where builders could turn their undertakings to a profitable account only by skimping on time, labour and materials. It was unlikely, too, that those Giusso referred to as 'mercenary hands' would have the interests of the poor at heart. A Naples rebuilt and expanded by subcontractors, Parlati predicted, would violate the health, hygiene and safety regulations that it had been the ambition of parliament to enforce.[75]

For the executive committee, however, practicalities told decisively in favour of a single contractor.[76] In an operation of the size and intricacy of the *risanamento* of Naples, it was possible for the municipal engineers to estimate the assets and liabilities involved in the global execution of the project. The city could then assure itself that there was sufficient expectation that the project would attract bidders and that the bidders would have the means necessary to see the work through to completion. If the project was subdivided into a multiplicity of small-scale segments, the financial harmony of the whole would be lost. Sections of the plan would prove unattractive to speculators, and the city would find that substantial portions of its plan had to be abandoned.

Furthermore, the success of the Neapolitan rebuilding programme depended upon the complex interlocking of its various components into a single co-ordinated mechanism. The sewer network below ground, for instance, had to be constructed in tandem with the landfills and the streets above ground. Similarly, it was important that housing in the 'expansion neighbourhoods' on the periphery be completed before large-scale evictions began in the city centre if the administration wished to avoid creating a major problem of homelessness. In the same way, the phasing of the financial assistance of parliament over twelve years necessitated synchronization with the work schedule of demolition and construction. Only a single entrepreneur with a vision of the whole could ensure the necessary overall coordination. To subdivide the project was to invite waste, confusion and unending litigation. Unity of approach, Marghieri convinced his colleagues, was indispensable.[77]

The problem of subcontracting was turned by Marghieri into a great advantage of the system that the *giunta* proposed. It was improbable, he reasoned, that the Neapolitan building industry would prove equal to the task of assuming responsibility for the overall renewal project. All of the building firms in the city joined together, he argued, would be unable to supply the capital necessary to obtain the contract for overseeing the whole programme of *risanamento*. Indeed, the Neapolitan building firms had joined together as a consortium to bid for the contract. Although supported by interested local banks, they had succeeded in raising a total capital of only 8 million lire, which the city regarded as insufficient security for so colossal an undertaking.[78] The city stipulated that the capital value of the contracting company be in excess of 30 million lire.[79] Although the major contract would be awarded, therefore, to outside interests, the *giunta* regarded it as important that the greatest public works in the modern history of the city provide a stimulus to local industry and employment for local workers. These results could only be achieved by subcontracting because it was at that level alone that Neapolitan builders were in a financial position to assume responsibility. Only through subcontracting could rebuilding invigorate the local economy.[80]

Having opted for a single contractor, the Neapolitan planners insisted that the proper legal status of the entrepreneur who would play so great a role in the reconstruction of the city was collective rather than individual. It was essential, they argued, that the contractor be a joint stock company. Presenting the conclusions of the executive committee to the city council, Marghieri explained that, as a collective body, a joint stock company would provide the answer to the worry of councillors Parlati and Giusso that a single contractor would possess a dangerous monopoly of power. Through the mechanism of a joint stock company, the power created by the contract would be divided among a multitude of shareholders, including people of modest financial circumstances. By offering the tender to a limited liability company rather than an individual, the city could safely ensure the involvement of a large number of people in the project. 'Thus,' he assured his listeners, 'the monopoly of capital could be avoided with certainty.'[81]

In this manner Naples would enjoy the best of all possible worlds. Alderman Enrico Arlotta painted a rosy picture of the prospects facing the city. On the one hand, the joint stock company, by its financial power, could ensure the completion of the whole project within the ten-year time period agreed in the contract. Its capital assets would stand as security that the interests of the Neapolitan people would be respected. On the other hand, because its financial might was divided among many hands, the company would wield its power democratically rather than behaving as the rapacious overlord envisaged by the critics of the plan. The local economy would prosper as the contractor invested its vast capital in hiring local firms and employing local workers. In this urban idyll the criticisms of Parlati and Giusso were deemed tendentious and misplaced.[82]

On 3 October the city formally awarded the contract for the renewal of the Lower City to a new company to be named the Naples Renewal Company, Ltd (*Società Anonima per il Risanamento di Napoli*) with its headquarters in Naples. The Company was founded by four northern bankers – Girolamo Bassi and Antonio Allievi of Milan, Giuseppe Giacomelli of Udine, and Giovanni Marsaglia of Turin – with a total capital of 25 million lire. The four bankers agreed to sit on the board of directors of their new firm for an initial term of four years in conformity with the municipal vision that it was important to subdivide the power of the great rebuilding firm among a number of hands in order to prevent the emergence of an undesirable monopoly. So pleased was the *giunta* with the bid from the Renewal Company that it drafted a contract that the later investigation led by Giuseppe Saredo described as loosely worded and unjustifiably generous. The city even lowered the previous requirement of a capital sum of 30 million lire, and it avoided any indelicate probing into the Company's financial circumstances.[83]

Even before the Company launched the demolition, however, there were signs that the vision of an urban idyll was seriously flawed in three respects. In the first place, Italian commercial law expressly negated the democratic division of responsibility within a joint stock company so strenuously invoked by Marghieri. The law stipulated that members of the boards of directors of joint stock companies bore no direct personal legal responsibility for the activities of the companies themselves, and that all responsibility of the founders of a concern ceased at the moment of its legal incorporation.[84] When the contract was signed in October, therefore, it was already possible to discern the image of a monopoly overlord in the person of the Managing Director of the Company, Giovanni Abignente, who emerged as the effective tsar of Neapolitan renewal.

Secondly, although the matter did not become public knowledge for some years, it was inauspicious that the founding of the Company was marred by fraud. The 25 million lire that the Company claimed as its capital value and the guarantee of its good performance was fictive. When the Company was formed, it raised capital by a bogus stock issue whose subscribers were the employees of the banks with which the founding directors were associated, each of whom claimed to have acquired 250 shares. As security for the performance of its commitments and as the democratic stake of large numbers of shareholders in the activity of rebuilding, the money was nonexistent. The shareholders were ghosts.[85] Nardi warned the council that the city lacked a sufficient guarantee that the Company would honour its contractual obligations.[86]

Finally, the organizational structure that the Company established in the city did not suggest a vigilant regard for the welfare of Naples. The operational decisions affecting rebuilding were to be made by a Technical Committee that reported directly to the Managing Director. This committee, as its name suggested, was responsible for taking engineering and architectural decisions in conformity with the building code and for enforcing safety regulations. It was a reasonable expectation, therefore, that it would be composed principally of experts in the building profession. As an indication of its priorities, the Company for the Renewal of Naples, however, appointed financial experts to its Technical Committee and only one engineer. His background, moreover, was in the laying of railroad lines rather than the construction of buildings. It was immediately apparent that the new Company would possess neither the will nor the expertise to promote quality or even safety in the work it commissioned.[87] It was not long before a disillusioned Mayor would find that the Company for the Renewal of Naples was 'a financial institution rather than a building firm'. It paid far more attention to its accounts than to the technical specifications of construction, despite the enormous importance of its mission.[88]

Although the city made a festival of the first blow of the demolishing pickaxe, which fell on 29 June 1889 in the presence of the King, there were early hints that renewal was not being launched in the way that the sanitary reformers had intended. A first shift in policy concerning the rebuilding of Naples had already occurred when the responsibility for renewal moved from parliament to City Hall. Now there was a second and no less decisive shift as responsibility migrated again, this time from Palazzo San Giacomo to the boardroom of the Company for the Renewal of Naples.

REBUILDING WITHOUT IMPROVING

The pickaxe had barely fallen when controversy over the conduct of renewal erupted. By the autumn of 1889, when approximately 8,000 bricklayers were at work transforming the centre of the Old City into a giant building site, public opinion was already turning against the Company for the Renewal of Naples and its subcontractors. Signs of popular discontent were apparent in a series of autumnal demonstrations by workers and tenants protesting against eviction. Still clearer was an important political shock that struck the city in November. In the local elections of that month the two men most closely associated in the public mind with the rebuilding project – Mayor Nicola Amore and Alderman Alberto Marghieri – both lost their seats on the city council. The restricted property-based franchise prevented the *plebe* from being consulted. What is all the more striking, therefore, is that even at this early date disillusionment with renewal had spread among the relatively privileged ranks of the grand electors of the city. Rocco De Zerbi's newspaper *Il Piccolo*, interpreting the unexpected defeat of Amore – a defeat it called 'the assassination of the Mayor' – had few doubts about the cause of Amore's discomfiture. 'He seems', the paper commented,

> to have become a victim of renewal, of the masterpiece of his career. The voters of Porto, Mercato and Pendino – the three boroughs to be rebuilt – have not forgiven him for imposing cut-rate expropriations upon them and forcibly evicting them from their homes. What has occurred is the vengeance of offended self-interest.'[89]

This theory was supported by the sweeping successes of the two most prominent critics of the municipal plan, Giusso and Parlati. Both were returned with increased majorities in the sections where the rebuilders had began to drive large numbers of people from their homes.[90] For De Zerbi's paper, such ingratitude was a sign that the *plebe* was still 'too uncivilized' to understand the long-term advantages of the project. Giusso and Parlati had taken advantage of the 'ignorance' and 'misery' of the boroughs of the Lower City to turn public opinion against the Mayor and his unpopular alderman.[91]

Events soon disclosed, however, that more was involved than the spleen of the ignorant. Even *Il Piccolo* reminded its readers that the rebuilding contract stipulated that low-cost housing was to be built in synchronization with the demolition of the slums so that the evicted tenants would have the offer of alternative accommodation. The rebuilders, however, took no notice of this provision of the contract. They found it convenient instead to evict sitting tenants and demolish the buildings they occupied as rapidly as possible, proceeding only much later to construct the alternative lodgings that had been the subject of such lengthy debate in the city council. Tens of thousands of residents were thus thrown onto the streets without provision. The newspaper commented sardonically that, although the purpose of *risanamento* was to provide the people with light and air, no one had anticipated that the Company in its generosity would furnish them with so much of both.[92]

The quality of the building work further inflamed opinion. In the autumn *Il Piccolo* observed that, 'Hardly a day passes without the notice of the collapse of a building.'[93] The theme of falling buildings soon became a regular staple of the paper's account of municipal events.[94] Mariano Semmola, one of the heroes of the anti-cholera campaign of the White Cross, rose in the Chambers of the city council to protest against a new threat to health. All too frequently walls under construction suddenly collapsed, killing or maiming builders and menacing the lives of passers-by. He demanded an explanation from the *giunta* and wondered what such occurrences indicated about the practical effects of the course of renewal on which the city had embarked. Semmola speculated, however, that accidents were the unintended byproducts of a well-intentioned effort. After only six months of experience with *risanamento*, his view was that the instability of the buildings probably resulted from the influence of the new drainage system on the ground-water beneath the city. As the subsoil dried out, he reasoned, sanitary benefits could be anticipated in the long run, but the immediate unhappy side-effects were subsidence and collapsing[95]

Then in February 1890 Arlotta, one of the most vociferous proponents of the municipal renewal project and the alderman in charge of the Department of Public Works, stunned the council by announcing the occurrence of a major disaster. On a building site under the direct supervision of the Company, a section of wall nine metres wide had fallen from a height of two storeys, crushing twelve stone-masons to death. Had this tragedy been an isolated event, it would have caused immediate dismay but not enduring alarm. Unfortunately, however, Arlotta reported that such collapses were becoming 'a system', and that they raised serious questions about the practices of the Company and its subcontractors. In particular, he reported publicly, there were indications that the builders were systematically employing illegal methods, substandard materials and lethal haste in their zeal to minimize costs. 'Is it a fact', he asked, 'that, as some are now beginning to claim, all of the buildings belonging to the Company for the Renewal of Naples, have been faultily constructed?'

Drawing back from the radical and self-accusatory conclusions that an affirmative answer would suggest, Arlotta exculpated himself and reassured his listeners by insisting that any such imputation was outrageous libel. What interest could the Company have in sinking capital in unsafe buildings? Indeed, the Company had at once assured the city that it was taking steps to prevent further mishaps. At this early date, therefore, Arlotta chose to believe the rebuilders and to hold two hapless municipal officials responsible – the Chief Inspector of the renewal works and the author of the detailed specifications of the municipal plan, Adolfo Giambarba, and his subordinate, the City Engineer Enrico Albarella. He demanded, and obtained, their immediate dismissal.[96]

Other councillors drew less sanguine and more far-reaching conclusions. Arlotta's disturbing report and disciplinary actions were not followed by an abatement in the rate of accidents on building sites in the Lower City. According to the Prefect of the city, the renewal operations were causing unprecedented numbers of injuries and deaths, due not to the negligence of the workers themselves but through the frenzied pace demanded by the contractors.[97] Against this background, Salvatore Fusco, the Deputy and veteran of the White Cross campaign, informed his colleagues of his own informal investigation into the reasons for the latest disaster. Fusco's preliminary sounding uncovered a widespread pattern of abuse. What particularly shocked him was the evidence that the Company ruthlessly and illegally exploited its monopoly position to dictate impossible terms to its Neapolitan subcontractors. It was common knowledge, Fusco reported, that the market value of buildings in the 'industrial quarter' where the twelve workers had been killed was estimated at up to 400 lire per square metre. To obtain business, local firms were compelled to sign contracts on piece-work terms that were without precedent in the Neapolitan building trade, agreeing to run up the Company houses for 220 lire per square metre. For that price, the only way to make the contract pay was to violate the building and hygiene codes, to ignore the safety of the workers, and to trim wages to the minimum. The inspectors of the Company closed their eyes to such practices because they allowed the parent firm to achieve a usurious rate of profit. The Company bought the buildings cheap by squeezing the subcontractor and then sold them dear. Far from having a long-term interest in the welfare of Neapolitans, the Company, Fusco reported, commissioned the construction of buildings today solely in order to sell them tomorrow.[98]

On the site of the accident, the contractor had built the wall that collapsed of materials taken direct and uninspected from a recently demolished structure, had employed mortar of dubious quality, and had erected upper storeys before the mortar on the supporting walls below had dried. Here was criminal negligence, but the blame went beyond that of the contractor. Why was the Company, which had overall responsibility, not effectively overseeing the practices of its subcontractors? Why were the city's own engineers not conducting rigorous and frequent inspections to enforce the building code? Fusco suspected, but could not prove, a web of complicity that linked the city Public Works Department and the Company for the Renewal of Naples in a tacit conspiracy to advance profit at the expense of the public welfare.[99]

The outraged Republican Councillor Matteo Renato Imbriani had already heard enough to call in October 1890 for the termination of the contract between the city and the Company. He argued that the firm had obtained its contract by fraudulent means, claiming as shareholders people who in fact possessed no stocks and no interest in the Company. It had then broken its obligation to enforce standards of quality and safety. The low-cost housing that was rising under Company auspices consisted of 'new slums' to replace the 'old caves' that had been demolished. Anxious to cut costs and raise profits, the contractors blatantly ignored the specifications in the plan, building tenements with illegal storeys rising above courtyards that were disproportionately small. In addition, the Company had systematically defrauded the owners of the expropriated properties. Its strategy was to offer them far less than the 33 per cent above rateable value established as the norm by the city, relying on the fact that the majority of landlords would accept the modest sums they were offered rather than go to court. Indeed, Imbriani charged that, instead of 94 million lire in compensation, the Neapolitan property owners would be fortunate to receive 50 million. The remainder, subsidized by public money, formed an additional but illegal speculative profit.[100]

Imbriani then explained that the methods of the Company directly contributed to the death of twelve builders. The immediate cause of the disaster, he revealed, was the corruption of signor Martinoli, the Chief Engineer of the Company and a member of its Technical Committee. As a private initiative of his own, Martinoli owned a brick-making firm that supplied the fifty-three subcontractors engaged by the Company for the Renewal of Naples. Such a proceeding clearly constituted an unethical conflict of interest. More severe, however, was Imbriani's charge that Martinoli supplied substandard bricks made of pozzolana, an inferior material known to crumble under pressure. It was a wall made of Martinoli's pozzolana bricks that had crushed the twelve construction workers.[101]

What was unknown to most of the councillors and to the public was that the relations between City Hall and the Company in the spring of 1890 had already reached an impasse. On 1 May the Mayor sent Abignente, the Managing Director, a bitter letter castigating him for his indifference to the welfare of the city. 'The continuous run of disasters', the Mayor wrote, 'has produced two very serious results. It has both morally discredited the operation and revealed the responsibility of the individuals in charge.' The specific faults of the Company that angered the Mayor were the failure to carry out technical inspections of the work as it progressed and the refusal to respond to the repeated warnings of the municipal engineers.[102]

The results of such negligence compromised the integrity of the entire rebuilding project. Leading objectives of *risanamento* were the purification of the workers' quarters by ventilation and the admission of the sun, the resolution of the chronic problem of overcrowding, and the enforcement of new sanitary standards. In the 'expansion neighbourhoods', however, the new buildings conformed no more closely to the municipal standards of hygiene than the slums they replaced. For the workers in the strict sense of the term, the Company constructed new soaring tenements that ostentatiously violated the city codes; they narrowed the width of the streets where the air was intended to flow unimpeded; and they skimped on the space intended for courtyards, stairways, and even the rooms themselves.[103] Saredo wrote of the quality of the new accommodation that emerged in the 'expansion neighbourhoods'. The new dwellings contained, he observed,

> a quantity of dark or poorly lighted rooms, so arranged as to make necessary the use of skylights known as *vanelle*. The courtyards are tiny in proportion to the height of the buildings; the latrines for the most part are located in the kitchens and lack any means of ventilation; the ground floor rooms are dark and unpaved; the roofs are irregularly built; and there are many, many other unhygienic conditions.[104]

Furthermore, the laws of the marketplace, upon which the city had placed such emphasis, negated the intention of the reform to improve overcrowding and sanitation. By the turn of the century, 21,733 refugees from the demolitions in the city centre, together with new arrivals as the population of Naples continued to expand, had found accommodation in the low-cost houses purpose-built for workers in the new neighbourhoods located in the northeastern and eastern periphery. Unfortunately, the demand for housing was intense. Without taking into account the growth of the population of Naples, the 21,733 refugees were more than sufficient to fill the 5,000 rooms that the rebuilders had provided, especially since the new buildings rose at a far slower pace than the demolitions and evictions. Evictions began immediately in the summer of 1889, but the first of the new dwellings became available only in 1891.[105] Demand, therefore, far outstripped supply and rents soared to rates far above the levels that had prevailed in the Old City and well beyond the means of most evicted tenants. The result, the Saredo Commission reported, was that the inhabitants normally reduced their rent burden by sharing their dark and poorly constructed apartments with other families. The average occupancy was four people to a room.[106] In this way they survived by reproducing the overcrowding that Depretis and the King had intended to abolish. The new quarters such as Arenaccia, Ottocalli and S. Maria delle Paludi instantly became unhygienic modern slums.

To live in Arenaccia, however, denoted a position of relative privilege. For the undeserving poor – Marghieri's 'disinherited' – the consequences were still worse, as Giusso and Parlati had predicted. A number of paupers facing eviction described their predicament in appeals that they sent to the Prefect, imploring him to intervene to mitigate the harsh treatment that they were receiving at the hands of the Company for the Renewal of Naples. Some of these appeals have survived in the files of the Prefecture. An example is that of a petition from the inhabitants of the Via Alta Carmignano. Writing on 11 April 1890, they explained,

> The Disembowelment Company [*sic*] has ordered that, as of 1 May, the inhabitants of the buildings facing the above street be evicted. They are therefore giving notice that their circumstances are such that, if they leave, they will be forced to spend night and day in the open streets because there are no dwellings available with rents as low as those they pay at the moment. And this is all because of a whim of the Company that says that it needs the buildings in order to demolish them and supply materials for the construction of another building in Via Carriera Piccola. For this reason the petitioners ask, please, that ... this operation be suspended until such time as the workers' houses are offered for rent. Your Excellency can see for himself the condition of these poor tenants, the misery of their lives, and the fact that none of them can pay more than 10 lire a month in rent, and some of them still less.'[107]

Another illustration is that of a letter from a tenant writing on behalf of the illiterate members of his community. The unsigned letter stated,

> All the residents of the Borgo S. Maria della Fede, and in particular the tenants of the Case del Macello, who total more than 400 people, have received notice to quit within the week.
>
> Sir, there ... is not a family among us that does not contain three or four ill people, stricken with the current sickness. There are rather hundreds of people, all poor, and where will they find shelter in so short a space of time?

For this reason these unfortunate people do not intend to disobey the order they have received, but they prostrate themselves at the feet of Your Excellency, and they beg the grace of Your Excellency to kindly grant them a little time until the buildings in the Arenaccia quarter are completed and the poor people can find lodgings at a low rent.[108]

The ordeal of such people after eviction was painful. They were unable to join the migration to Arenaccia because accommodation was lacking, rents were astronomical and employment was unavailable. But they received no helpful response to their petitions. The city failed even to monitor the effects of renewal upon the most vulnerable of its inhabitants. No statistics were kept, no studies were conducted, and no measures were taken to alleviate the harsh consequences of eviction by assisting those affected in the process of relocation. City Hall did not even enforce the contractual obligation of the Company to build low-cost accommodation contemporaneously with the demolitions.[109]

At the turn of the century the Saredo Commission, unlike the municipal Department of Public Works, examined the fate of the poor who had been given notice to quit the centre of the Lower City. In 1901, when Giuseppe Saredo reported the findings of the Commission, the work of *risanamento* was still limping forward with drastically reduced objectives and an indefinite time schedule. By that date, a total of 56,737 residents had been forcibly removed from their dwellings in the Lower City, of whom 35,658 were included in Marghieri's category of the 'poor'. Dividing the total exodus into the two categories of 'rich' and 'poor', the Commission charted the flow of population affected by *risanamento* as Table 5.3 demonstrates.[110]

Saredo's statistics are not free of ambiguity. The figures do not include people removed from their homes during the course of the series of smaller renewal projects under municipal auspices that supplemented the great work of *risanamento*, such as the reconstruction of the neighbourhoods of Santa Lucia and Santa Brigida. A second problem is that the report confines itself to the movement of population from one borough to another. It does not make finer distinctions between various neighbourhoods within the various *sezioni*. But the most serious difficulty is that the categories of 'rich' and 'poor' are unhelpfully broad and unspecific. Fortunately, the context provides some clarification. Elsewhere in the report the Commission uses the term 'poor' as an equivalent for those Marghieri classified as the 'disinherited'. The general argument suggests this conclusion and its corollary, which is that the designation 'rich' includes everyone else, from full-time workers to wealthy aristocrats and merchants. The orders of magnitude involved support such a view. That it seemed useful to investigators to make the possession of a full-time, steady job the basis for classifying a person as 'rich' is itself an eloquent commentary on social conditions in the slums of the Lower City.

In any event, two striking conclusions emerge from the chart. The first concerns the destination of the poor after their eviction from the demolished slums. Saredo provides support for the now familiar view that the principal effect

Table 5.3. *Flow of the population evicted by* risanamento, *1889–1900*

Sezioni	Increase		Decrease	
	Rich	Poor	Rich	Poor
S. Ferdinando	0	0	921	6,781
Chiaia	4,025	1,390	0	0
S. Giuseppe	0	0	0	381
Montecalvario	0	0	5,737	0
Avvocata	0	0	2,784	0
Stella	146	0	0	0
S. Carlo all'Arena	3,055	1,677	0	0
Vicaria	6,538	18,663	0	0
S. Lorenzo	0	0	5,059	0
Mercato	0	3,078	0	0
Pendino	0	0	2,914	13,134
Porto	0	0	3,654	15,362
Villages				
Posillipo	1,185	423	0	0
Fuorigrotta	0	6,372	0	0
Vomero	6,130	2,866	0	0
Miano	0	787	0	0
Piscinola	0	442	0	0
Total	21,079	35,698	21,069	35,658

of the demolition of the tenements in the *sezioni* of Porto and Pendino was that the tenants moved the shortest distance possible, adding to the press of population in the neighbouring boroughs of Mercato and, above all, Vicaria. A trickle found its way to the suburban villages. For both the people evicted and the residents of the boroughs to which they migrated, the effects of *risanamento* were to make the problems of poverty and sanitation worse rather than better. In the tenements of Mercato and Vicaria overcrowding increased and competition further fuelled the upward spiral of rent. Saredo quantifies this process by tracing the movement of 18,663 evicted paupers to Vicaria and 3,078 to Mercato. Since they were unable to afford housing in the new buildings in the 'expansion quarters', the inescapable result was they further overburdened the existing stock of tenements and added to the numbers of the homeless. Summarizing the results of the process, the Ligurian Commissioner found that,

> With regard to the inhabitants of the quarters that were demolished, some crowded, beyond all means of containing them, into the [official] low-cost housing; others, such as the residents of Santa Lucia, were forced to leave the centre of their own city and to settle in distant Fuorigrotta; and the others, finally, occupied the unhealthy *bassi* of new constructions or squeezed into those of the Old City that were not included in the demolition.[111]

The second conclusion was that the numbers of people evicted during the course of the rebuilding program were significantly fewer than the municipal plan had anticipated. The demolition schedule for which the Company contracted called for the displacement of 90,000 people. The effect in practice, however, was the removal of 'only' 56,737 residents. Given the foreboding of Giusso and Parlati before the work began and the dismal fate of the people who were dispossessed of their homes, such a result seems almost reassuring, as if the critics of *risanamento* had exaggerated the magnitude of its negative social consequences. Unfortunately, this superficially reassuring result was instead the effect of a major scandal that had profound consequences for the overall objective of making Naples cholera-proof. Only 60 per cent of the scheduled evictions were served because the Company for the Renewal of Naples pocketed all of the public money but left a substantial portion of the great sanitary work undone.

The reason that the project was aborted was that by the early 1890s the Company possessed all of the monopoly power that its critics had feared, and it exploited its position to maximize profits rather than welfare. The Managing Director and the financial experts on the Technical Committee that advised him manoeuvred with great skill. On 23 September 1893 they abruptly presented the city with a memorandum explaining that the Company was facing bankruptcy. Regrettably, therefore, there were only two possibilities, they argued. Either the Company could go into dissolution, leaving the centre of Naples as a building site, or it could continue the work on the basis of additional subsidies and a renegotiated contract that imposed fewer and much less onerous obligations than the original terms of October 1888.

In effect Abignente and his fellow directors demanded the right to pursue exclusively commercial objectives if they were to resume construction, regardless of the consequences for the humanitarian and hygienic ambitions of parliament and of the city council. Specifically, the Company proposed to persevere with the great central boulevard, the piazzas along its length, and its major intersecting streets. Here the plan agreed upon in 1888 called for the building of expensive commercial premises and elegant private residences. The construction and sale of these properties constituted the speculative heart of the rebuilding scheme. Since these buildings would be at a premium, a substantial profit was almost assured.

In accord with the speculative logic that was coming to overshadow the demands of public health, the Company listed thirty-four 'cuts' or *stralci* that it proposed to eliminate from the contract because they posed the greatest commercial risk. It was the misfortune of the city that the zones to be sacrificed included some of the worst slums in the whole of Naples – *bassi* and *fondaci* at the centre of the boroughs of Porto and Pendino where the population had paid a great tribute of death in 1884. Among them were the infamous vicoli della Duchessa, piazza Francese, Lavinaio, Santa Maria della Scala, Santa Caterina Spina Corona, Portanova and Mezzocannone. Councillor Arlotta, a leading proponent of renewal now dismayed by its mutilation, reminded his colleagues that these names were well known to every Neapolitan as places of desperate poverty and disease.[112] Here, if anywhere, were the very 'bowels of Naples'. To exclude them was to negate the whole purpose of *risanamento*. The great surgical operation had failed to remove the cancer.

From an entrepreneurial perspective, however, the zones listed as candidates for elimination were not commercially profitable. They included quarters where the work stipulated in the contract was particularly intricate and expensive, as well as secondary streets where property values would never soar to the heights of the Rettifilo and its principal crossings. By refusing to undertake work of any sort in these zones, whether of demolition, roadwork or rebuilding, the Company could save 29 million lire in reconstruction costs and avoid a poor investment. It also laid claim to several million lire in outright subsidies. The subsidies arose from two rights in the liquidated zones that the Company demanded – the right to keep for eventual sale those buildings whose owners had already been expropriated and the right to salvage materials from buildings already demolished.

For the hygienic objectives of renewal, the adoption of commercial priorities had serious repercussions. The most obvious problem was that the Company for the Renewal of Naples intended to leave some of the most foul slums of the city standing instead of razing them to the ground as the King and Depretis had envisaged. Foci where the cholera parasite had nestled in every previous epidemic were to survive, ready to harbour the vibrio again if ever it returned. When the issue of *risanamento* was raised in the city council early in the new century, the alderman in charge of public works, Carrelli, observed that the work that had been carried out to that date was completed in reverse order of sanitary priority. As a result, the slums that remained were the 'ugliest part of the project, the most uncivilized and unhygienic quarters that exist in a great city like Naples'.[113]

A second disturbing implication was that such a severely abbreviated renewal project would provide only a fraction of the promised work for Neapolitan building firms and their workers. In addition, industries allied to the building trade would be thrown into disarray, creating a crisis for companies that supplied wallpaper, tiles, bricks and fittings. The anticipated stimulus to the local economy and the 'redemption' of a portion of the poor by the transforming power of labour would never materialize. It was revealing that in 1902 the great industrialist and city Councillor De Luca remarked, just as observers of the nineteenth century had regularly pointed out, that, 'Nothing can give even the most approximate idea of the ... frightful problem of unemployment in our city.'[114] Far from having been corrected by the opportunities created by renewal, the official rate of unemployment in that year approached 40 per cent.[115] Pauperism was growing, and the consumption of the necessities of life was steadily declining.[116]

The most serious difficulty resulting from the *stralci*, however, was that they aborted not just a part but the whole of the renewal project. The *stralci* posed two great threats, one affecting the timing of the work and the other the overall integrity of the programme. The issue of timing was that the Company demanded an alteration of the agreed order of the work, allowing it to proceed with the financially attractive Rettifilo before it built additional low-cost housing for the evicted workers. Such a modification of the contract of 1889 undermined the whole of the public-works scheme. The synchronization of the various aspects of renewal was an essential part of the programme. To allow demolition to precede rebuilding was to generate homelessness, overcrowding and human misery – the very vices of Neapolitan life that *risanamento* was designed to remedy.[117]

More was involved, however, than timing alone. The contractual modifications demanded by the Company destroyed the overall harmony that bound the various components of renewal into a single coherent and harmonious vision. To remove major parts was to wreck the entire mechanism, to the detriment of the city as a whole. An example was that of the landfills called *colmate*. To cancel the *colmate* in the zones eliminated from the contract would have severe reverberations throughout the Lower City. The miasmo-contagionist strategy of the planners was that the raising of the street-level of the Lower City by three metres would provide a thick layer of insulation protecting the population from the poisonous emanations from the contaminated subsoil beneath. Without such protection, all of Naples would remain vulnerable to the lethal cholera-gas.

A second danger to the entire city was that the lack of *colmate* would compromise the new sewer system. Unless the elevation of the streets was increased, the sewer mains beneath would lack the necessary incline to ensure that the whole system flowed freely and that the linkages between conduits from different neighbourhoods would be secure. Under the reduced contract put before the council in 1894, blockages and seepage could be anticipated, adversely affecting drainage and contaminating the subsoil. In addition, the ability of the system to pump the waste of the Lower City to the distant Bay of Gaeta would be jeopardized, and Naples would once again require outfalls in the waters of the harbour.

At the same time that the *stralci* contravened the whole localist strategy of public health by their effects on the ground-water and subsoil beneath Naples, they also nullified the grand medical purposes of the work above ground. The towering rookeries and labyrinthine streets left in the wake of an abbreviated renewal would block the free passage of light and air that was at the heart of the project. The soil would not be dried out; the dwellings would not be ventilated and purified; and pestilential miasmas would not be dissipated by the gusting *scirocco*.

In its self-defence, the Company made the case that the force of changed circumstances made it impossible to honour the terms of the original contract. Since 1889 the renewal project had been overtaken by a major crisis of the national economy in general and of the banking system in particular. In their wake, the financial projections of the original plan had been overturned. Because the property boom had collapsed, the value of the development sites and the buildings that the Company had to sell had fallen disastrously. Furthermore, renewal itself had damaged the local property market in an unforeseen manner.

The simultaneous completion of a large stock of buildings had created a glut that drove prices down. As a result, the planners' calculations of profit and loss had proved to be completely unrealistic. In the economy of the 1890s, rebuilding on the terms of 1888 was not commercially viable.

In addition, the Company argued, the cost of credit had soared. Two particular circumstances affected the ability of the Company to raise capital at affordable rates. The first was that the legal context had been altered by a law of 1891 that banned the granting of mortgages on privileged terms such as those that the city had guaranteed as a form of subsidy to the rebuilders. The second new circumstance was that the banks represented by the four original founders of the Company for the Renewal of Naples – the Banca Generale, the Banca di Credito Mobiliare, the Banca di Torino and the Banca Subalpina – had all been dragged into the vortex of the banking crisis. The result was that credit had become prohibitively expensive at the same moment that the Company's assets had depreciated.[118]

The response of the city to the Company's September memorandum required time. The implications of the new proposals had to be considered by the municipal engineers and lawyers, and the final decision had to be taken by a vote of the full city council. The subject was the main item of business at the regular spring session of the council in 1894. The stormy debates in the Palazzo San Giacomo took place against an eerie silence in the surrounding streets. To make its position unmistakably clear, the Company had suspended nearly all of its operations. The workforce it employed now numbered only 750 builders – down from a high of 8,789.[119] For the first time since 1889 there was virtually no noise of demolition and reconstruction in the Lower City. The landscape outside the council windows was one of total chaos, prefiguring the consequences of rejecting the terms offered by the firm. Parlati described the scene as follows,

> a city abandoned with its streets in disorder amidst piles of rubble and sudden differences in level; communications made difficult or completely severed; hygiene turned into a mockery and an insoluble problem by the ruin of such a large part of the city; and sewerage interrupted with the old mains buried or broken. How much longer will all of this last?[120]

The discussion that took place among the councillors was no repetition of the debates of 1888 when the initial contract was voted on. In March 1894 the enthusiasm for joint stock companies, privatization, monopoly and subcontracting had vanished. The Company for the Renewal of Naples no longer had many avowed friends among the councillors. The difference in the atmosphere was most dramatically demonstrated by the impassioned intervention of a political revenant, Nicola Amore, who had returned to City Hall as a councillor after the humiliation of defeat in 1889. The former Mayor and leading figure in the municipal rebuilding scheme now argued that renewal was a failure and that the council should reject the terms offered by the Company as blackmail. Even if the city capitulated, the work that remained was hardly worth having, and there was no reason to expect that even the truncated contract that was negotiated would be performed with any better faith than the first version that the Company had so cynically broken.[121]

Amore argued that the financial description of its position that the Company used to justify its grasping demands of the city was entirely mendacious. Most disturbing was the flagrant contradiction between the evidence that the directors of the firm presented to the city and the reports they provided to their own shareholders. In every annual report since 1889 the board of directors had informed its stockholders that 'the building work was proceeding under the happiest possible circumstances, and that the demand for properties and the value of rent exceeded all expectations.'[122] Here, Amore informed the council, was a 'stubborn and irreconcilable contradiction.'[123] Similarly, Salvatore Fusco contended, the argument based on the banking crisis was untrue. The banks that had been affected by the crisis were irrelevant to the Company's ability to raise capital on viable terms because they were not the sources of credit for its building operations. The argument was merely a pretext.[124] Finally, Arlotta, another disillusioned proponent of rebuilding, reported to the council that the complaint about changes in the profitability calculations on which the contract had been originally based was inaccurate. The calculations of the municipal engineers had stood the test of time, and the experience of the Company in practice conformed the municipal estimates. The Company had not encountered unexpected losses.[125]

Retrospectively commenting on the performance of the Company in the 1890s, the Saredo Commission found that there was substantial evidence as well of waste and corruption. One reason that the funds made available by parliament in 1885 for the great Neapolitan public-works programme proved insufficient was that subcontracts for various portions of the contract were regularly granted not on the basis of open competition for the tender but rather as a result of political favouritism. The Company cultivated amicable relations with members of the administration by rewarding important clients with subcontracts. Often the terms were negotiated in informal, private discussions where the contractors profited more by exerting their influence than by carrying out the work itself. For the Company such uneconomical arrangements were lucrative in the long run because they helped to ensure that the decisions made by City Hall in all matters affecting its interests would be favourable. Such corruption became a pervasive system in the latter years of the decade during the infamous mayoralty of the camorrista Celestino Summonte.[126]

Despite the revelations of Amore, Arlotta and Fusco, the council was persuaded by the view, most strenuously defended by Parlati, that the alternative to the acceptance of the terms demanded by the Company for the Renewal of Naples was to leave the work disastrously and permanently incomplete. Unlike Mayor Amore, the full council concluded that a truncated renewal was far better than none at all. Accordingly, it voted to accept the *stralci* and to draft a new contract, which was signed on 24 October 1894. The project envisaged by the King and financed by parliament was never to be realized.

In the years that intervened between the 'cuts' of 1894 and the renewed threat of cholera from the East in 1910, modifications to the contract of 1888 twice more became the subject of extended debate in the Council Chamber at Palazzo San Giacomo. In 1897 the Company demanded and obtained further financial subsidies from the city, but without additional modifications to the building project. Then, in the light of the recommendation of the Saredo Commission that renewal could not be brought to a satisfactory conclusion without contributions from the state, parliament voted the law of 7 July 1902 that provided substantial supplementary funds. In each case, however, in Marghieri's words, the result was simple – 'less building and more expense'.[127] The *stralci* of 1894 were never restored, and the unofficial violations of the contract introduced by economizing subcontractors were never rectified.

A CITY STILL AT RISK

In the summer of 1910 the sixth and final pandemic of Asiatic cholera to decimate Europe reached Italy, claiming its first victims at the coastal towns of Barletta and Trani in Apulia. There was reason to fear that the anti-cholera defences of the city of Naples, now swollen to a population of 731,000 people,[128] would soon be tested. The unhappy premonition of some well-informed observers was that, despite the expenditure of vast sums of public money, the city was no less at risk than it had been in 1884. Considering the effects of renewal from the perspective of the return of cholera, Alberto Marghieri concluded that *risanamento* had failed. The project that Nicola Amore and he had championed in order to make Naples safe from the disease had been mutilated and transformed. The city, the disappointed Marghieri argued, remained dangerously vulnerable.[129] A marble statue had been erected to the memory of Nicola Amore, but his stone effigy surveyed the negation of his life's work. The great Rettifilo had been built, but its double line of stone buildings served only as a curtain to conceal the squalor of the slums on either side. Marghieri wrote,

> With regard to housing and hygiene, a very substantial part of the city remains in dreadful condition, despite the work of demolition and reconstruction. Dark, narrow streets, teeming *fondaci* and filthy *bassi* still play host to many thousands of impoverished people. These teeming slums provide the material for macabre reports that all too accurately describe the many foci of infection ... .Nicola Amore's marble statue still contemplates ... urban caves, rat-holes, alleyways, tenements, and rookeries that the pickaxe never destroyed. Today, more than twenty years on, they still cause visitors to tremble in horror. Here Neapolitans live out their hard lives, or are struck down by consumption, typhoid, gastro-enteritis, and the comma bacillus.[130]

Writing in 1905, Matilde Serao also concluded that *risanamento* had perpetrated a cruel and expensive fraud. The Rettifilo, she argued, had no more substantial reality than a 'stage-set' because all around it the disastrous conditions that had given rise to the epidemic of 1884 remained unchanged. Only a short walk from the Corso Umberto I, Serao wrote,

A large portion of the population of the city lives in filth and poverty, in slums and urban caves. These are the people for whom the renewal and sanitation programme was intended, for whom 100 million lire were spent. Now, having lived through the rebuilding, these people reside just behind the new structures while they continue to die from every manner of disease. It is this fact that fills me with pain and regret. The majestic façades of the new buildings seem like a sardonic joke because they serve only to shield the eye from the squalor and canker of our city.... Just like before! Worse than before![131]

In 1912 the local government carried out an investigation into the hygienic conditions of the city. Its findings, gloomily reminiscent of the nineteenth century, abundantly confirmed the misgivings of Marghieri and Serao. At the height of the Giolittian era there was no sign of a 'sanitary renaissance'. Affordable accommodation, 'thinning out' and spacious dwellings were nowhere in evidence. All of the symptoms of urban pathology targeted by the great renewal project were still present, including the marked disparities between the Upper and Lower Cities. The major change was that, in the wake of the demolitions in the boroughs of Porto and Pendino, the worst conditions were now concentrated in the *sezioni* of Mercato and especially Vicaria.

No differently from Mark Twain in 1867, the investigators of 1912 were most struck by the frightful overcrowding of Naples. So teeming were the boroughs of the city centre that the report chose to express its statistics for density of population in terms of residents per square decametre rather than per square kilometre, as Table 5.4 illustrates.[132] The 'terrible press of population' revealed in these figures, the report suggested, was 'rather worrying'.[133] But of even more concern was the overcrowding within the still-standing rookeries of the Lower City. Far from disappearing beneath the redeeming pickaxe, the notorious *bassi*, the *locande* and even thirty *fondaci* had survived into the new century;[134] 27,224 *bassi* – 'authentic charnel-houses' – accommodated 126,254 tenants, with a result-ing average of 4.6 people sharing a sordid all-purpose single room. The con-clusion of the municipal authorities was far from reassuring:

> If one considers these figures, and if one takes into account the fact that often these single rooms serve all the requirements of a dwelling, a kitchen, and a workshop, then it must be recognized that Naples is uninhabitable. This is a most serious problem that affects the economy, the health, and the morals of the population.
>
> Much has been done, but much more remains to be achieved before it will be possible to claim that this great city ... has provided for the needs of a civilized people.'[135]

Nowhere else in Europe, the administration reflected, did ordinary people live in such squalor.[136]

The Neapolitan daily paper *Il Mattino*, its concern aroused by the return of the cholera-scare, undertook its own examination of the living conditions of the population. Its conclusions, illustrated with lurid photographs, were published in instalments from the last week in September until late October. They provided little comfort for anxious readers. Naples, despite *risanamento,* remained

Table 5.4. *Naples: residents per square decametre, 1912*

Sezione	No. residents per decemetre^2
S. Ferdinando	10.9
Chiaia	9.5
S. Giuseppe	8.8
Montecalvario	17.7
Avvocata	15.0
Stella	14.8
S. Carlo all' Arena	11.3
S. Lorenzo	10.0
Porto	10.4
Pendino	13.0
Vicaria	24.7
Mercato	28.5

'without air, without light, and without water.'[137] The *sezioni* of Mercato and Vicaria were singled out as demonstrating a 'state of truly deplorable neglect'. [138] Here the residents of lanes like the Vico Guardia inhabited 'innumerable *bassi*' that were 'the shame of Naples'. Human beings lived, worked and died in 'pigsties' fouled with waste of every description – damp, stinking lairs that were 'unworthy of a civilized nation'.[139]

The poverty of the families who occupied these tenements was the negation of every possibility of public health. The average Neapolitan worker in 1910 earned 3.5 lire a day. Typically, this worker was a man with an unemployed wife and four children, one of whom was old enough to supplement the family budget by working as an apprentice for 0.8 lire a day. The total family income for a month, therefore, was 129 lire. Since the minimum rent for a *basso* in the Lower City was 18–20 lire a month, and since the essential outlays for light, washing, and clothes averaged 30 lire a month, only 79 lire a month remained for food – 2.65 lire per day for six people. This money was spent by a representative family as Table 5.5 indicates.[140] The unavoidable consequence stressed by the paper was that the average Neapolitan 'can live only by having just one meal a day, when he eats macaroni and fills his belly with rotten fruit'.[141] Meat was unknown, and heat in the winter was a prized luxury.

The pattern of mortality in the borough of Mercato, with its population of 102,645 in 1912, was consistent with such impoverishment and such an urban environment. In 1909, a 'normal' year when there were no outbreaks of epidemic disease, 1773 people died. The ten leading causes of death – those which claimed fifty or more lives – are shown in Table 5.6.[142]

Even if one makes ample allowance for changes in diagnostic fashions and for inaccuracy in diagnosis, such a pattern of death is highly suggestive of poverty,

Table 5.5. *Daily food budget of an average Neapolitan family, 1910*

Item	Expenditure
1.5 kg of macaroni	1.15 lire
1 kg of bread	0.6 lire
1 litre of wine	0.4 lire
1 kg of fruit	0.3 lire
Total	2.45 lire

Table 5.6. *Leading causes of death in Naples, 1909*

Cause of Death	Number of Deaths
Pneumonia	268
Gastro-enteritis	247
Bronchitis	173
Senile marasmus	140
Endocarditis	125
Cerebral haemorrhage	83
Eclampsia	72
Nephritis	71
Meningitis	64
Tuberculosis	50
Total	1,293

malnutrition, overcrowding and filth. In Lower Naples adults died in the winter of respiratory diseases when they skimped on clothes, heat and food. Children and infants instead perished primarily in the summer from diarrhoeal disorders classified as gastro-enteritis, which resulted from dietary deficiencies and poor sanitation.And the fourth cause of death in early twentieth-century Naples was 'senile marasmus' or starvation, which claimed its victims primarily among the homeless and destitute elderly, who still died on the public thoroughfares.

Also indicative of severe overcrowding and omnipresent filth was the prevalence of trachoma. Transmitted by the chlamydia parasite, which spreads through physical contact with soiled bedding and unwashed bodies, trachoma or granular conjunctivitis is the foremost cause of blindness in the Third World today. An infallible indicator of unsanitary conditions, it was widely reported by the medical press to have assumed epidemic proportions in early twentieth-century Naples, where it spread misery and economic ruin. Its incidence among the poor of the city was constantly increasing.[143]

Table 5.7. *Expenditure on hospitals per 1,000 inhabitants in 1910*

Piedmont	4,455 lire
Venetia	5,143 lire
Liguria	5,362 lire
Romagna	5,487 lire
Tuscany	5,582 lire
Lombardy	6,273 lire

In the face of the advancing threat of cholera, a particularly ominous aspect of the incompleteness of the renewal program was the defective state of the Cotugno Hospital. Established on the site of the Vittoria, one of the four hospitals involved in the anti-cholera campaign of 1884, the Cotugno was conceived as the solution to the chaos that had overwhelmed Naples when the epidemic first struck the city. Since the city then lacked a hospital for infectious diseases standing in permanent vigil, the medical profession was caught unprepared for the emergency. The results were uncertainty in the diagnosis of suspect cases, delay in the isolation of victims, and the inability to provide timely and appropriate care.

The Cotugno Hospital was intended by the administration of Nicola Amore as the long-term answer to the enduring menace of a reappearance of the cholera at the gates of the city. The intention of the programme of *risanamento* was that the Cotugno would be located on a site selected in accord with localist theory, constructed in harmony with the pavilion design that was favoured for hospital architecture, equipped with the most modern facilities for the management of cholera patients, and manned by a specialist staff. The new hospital was central to the strategy of making Naples immune to a new disaster.

In practice, the new hospital perpetuated in microcosm the chronic deficiencies of the Neapolitan hospital system, fully illustrating in particular the effects of inadequate local funding. Prospero Guidone, Professor of Surgery at the University of Naples, analysed in the pages of the local newspaper *Roma* the financial constraints that had long undermined the ability of the hospitals of Naples to serve the needs of the population. Guidone calculated that the hospitals in the city received, on average, 1,600 lire of expenditure for every thousand inhabitants of the city – a figure that contrasted starkly with the official estimates for expenditure in the most favoured regions of Italy (See Table 5.7).[144] Because of such lack of funds, he continued, the wards were overcrowded and badly equipped; the doctors skimped on medication; administrators allowed the buildings to decay; the nurses were poorly trained; and 'every service is badly organized'. Guidone was discrete about the quality of the medical care dispensed by his colleagues on the wards of the Neapolitan public hospitals, but he noted that the salaries were inadequate to attract the best physicians and that morale was low.

The Cotugno illustrated every point of Guidone's analysis. The buildings first erected on the site in 1884 and 1885 were five temporary wooden sheds. Unfortunately, as financial exigency overtook medical considerations, the provisional sheds were neither replaced nor adequately maintained. By 1910 they were decrepit buildings with leaking roofs, unvarnished floors that were difficult to clean, and a problem of infestation by rats. Illumination was provided by oil lamps described by the City Councillor Ettore Epifania as 'filthy and indecent', and baths were administered in portable metal tubs sheltered by curtains in the middle of the wards.[145] Orazio Caro, who directed the Office of Hygiene, described the buildings as 'unserviceable' – 'crumbling old huts built without the least understanding of the rules of modern hygiene.'[146] Councillor Corsio Bovio, who inspected the facility in September 1910, was appalled by the conditions he encountered. The wards, Bovio wrote, were

> shacks of primitive construction that resembled a gypsy encampment and presented the same appearance of sadness and misery. What can one say of the furnishings? Dreadful beds with blankets that are soiled and torn, tattered sheets, and bare mattresses. One sees such poverty only in the *bassi* of the lower-class neighbourhoods. The renovation of the hospital has always depended on appropriations that are never voted.[147]

Alfonso Montefusco, who directed the establishment, lamented its 'deplorable conditions',[148] and Bovio wondered if perhaps the poor were better off if they were left to die in their own homes. The people of the city, Councillor Altobelli reported, viewed the cholera hospital with 'an unconquerable revulsion'.[149]

The nursing staff, so vital to the recovery of patients in a time of cholera, lacked the qualifications for the practice of modern medicine. Pressed by a lack of funds, the Cotugno relied on untrained sisters of mercy, who cost little, and young women whose only qualifications to attend seriously ill patients were literacy and the willingness to work for little reward. As the cholera returned, the Neapolitan Hospital for Infectious Diseases staffed its wards with 14-year old-girls, such as the nurse Agata Troia, who at the age of 16 in 1910 had two years of experience on the Cotugno wards and was said to be devoted to her duties.[150] A city then numbering nearly three quarters of a million people had been cheated of the means required to protect its health, and was soon to endure a further disaster.

PHYSICIANS IN THE NEW NAPLES

The vision of a great sanitary renaissance in Naples led in reality to results that fell far short of the intentions of the original planners. The sewer system; the interrelated projects of demolition, rebuilding and expansion; the Serino water supply; and the modern hospital for infectious diseases all suffered from fundamental defects that undermined their usefulness and disappointed their advocates. There was one domain, however, where results surpassed expectations – the position of the medical profession itself. Here the legacy of the epidemic of 1884 effected a lasting and important transformation.

Miasmo-contagionist doctrine provided a convincing explanation for the epidemic catastrophes of the past and a seemingly precise, infallible programme of action to guarantee that there would never be a recurrence. By thus elaborating the implications of localist philosophy for the permanent protection of Naples, physicians like Teodosio De Bonis persuaded the municipal council that medical science provided a powerful instrument for the resolution of some of the most urgent problems facing the city. In a recent article exploring the 'social construction' of medical knowledge, Roger Cooter suggests that the preoccupation with filth and excrement represented by miasmatic medical theory had a subconscious basis as a response to anxiety about social control and disorder.[151] In Naples, where the events of the epidemic itself had powerfully underscored the potential for rebelliousness of the 'dangerous classes' of the Lower City, the medical profession advanced the soothing message that the local elites could effectively control and re-shape the urban environment. As a metaphor for control, cleanliness was psychologically reassuring.

More was involved, however, than emotional reassurance. Cleanliness also provided an authoritative underpinning for the claim by the elites of the city to manage the lives of the poor. Localist doctrine, as it was interpreted in Naples, had clearly hierarchical implications. Danger, the miasmo-contagonists asserted, rose up from below, literally as a deadly stench from beneath the foundations of the city. Salvation was to be imposed from above as the city government, armed with superior scientific knowledge, dug up and purified the earth, cleansed the citizens, 'thinned them out', and moved them. Translated into the project of *risanamento*, the medical philosophy of localism provided the ideological underpinning for a vast exercise of social and political power as the dominant classes in the city claimed a medical right to appropriate the whole urban space of the city. Science was like a moral and legal trump card that overrode the prior claims of existing property rights, customs, contractual obligations and the *laissez-faire* strictures of Liberal thought, allowing the elites in City Hall to redefine urban space and to relocate its inhabitants as they saw fit.[152] Here was a sinister and authoritarian reading of the ancient precept *salus populi suprema lex esto*.

Medicine as an ideology also demonstrated its power beyond the narrow confines of local issues. In the broader context of national politics, Pettenkofer's doctrines, as elaborated by Neapolitan doctors, legitimated the city's request for a 'special law' redistributing wealth between North and South by means of the first great public works programme in the Mezzogiorno since unification. Medical theory thereby ennobled a giant venture in patronage politics by lifting it above the sordid terrain of contending vested interests and into the lofty sphere of the people's health.

In the age of Pasteur and Koch, the ideology of science conveyed a new authority as the neutral arbiter of social problems. The new knowledge was particularly persuasive because the rulers of the new, secular Italian regime were eager to be convinced. Indeed, the success of Agostino Depretis and Nicola Amore in so rapidly securing the allocation of 120,000,000 lire owed much to the prestige of science and the medical rhetoric with which they framed their case. For this very reason, the seemingly irresistible passage of the *risanamento* programme through the Chamber of Deputies, the Senate and the Palazzo San Giacomo in quick succession demonstrated important ways in which medical men could be of use to holders of power. Rebuilding and renewal therefore established the claim by the medical profession to a more influential position in society. And the physicians of Naples were rewarded for their labours in three instalments.

The first reward was embodied in modifications made in 1894 to the original programme of rebuilding. This was the moment when tens of thousands of humble Neapolitans had just been evicted from their homes without provision for their rehousing, and when the Company for the Renewal of Naples was dictating enormous cuts in the scope of the overall programme. At this seemingly unpropitious juncture, Filippo Masci, the Vice-Chancellor of the University of Naples persuaded the city council to divert 1,500,000 lire from the stated purposes of renewal in order to realize a special project intended to enhance the dignity and status of the medical elite and of the students in the Faculty. They occupied premises that had fallen into a 'deplorable state' of dilapidation. Now the profession was to be provided with facilities worthy of the new century. On 24 October 1894 the city signed a contract with the Renewal Company for the 'grand work of the expansion and modernization' of the Faculty of Medicine. Three former convents – S. Andrea delle Dame, S. Patrizia, and S. Aniello – were confiscated and refurbished, while a fourth – the Sapienza – was demolished to allow six new buildings to rise on its site, which was located appropriately on the great Corso Umberto I (the renamed Rettifilo) that was the centrepiece of the whole rebuilding scheme. By these means the medical profession acquired 50,000 additional square metres for library facilities, spacious offices for the professors and administrative staff, and accommodation for the institutes of obstetrics, anatomy, pathological anatomy and legal medicine. At the same time the University reached an agreement with the city regularizing and increasing the supply of cadavers for instruction in anatomy. Furthermore, the endowment of the former College of Medicine, a corporation of the *ancien regime* abolished by the Risorgimento, was placed at the disposal of the University to provide scholarships for its students. As Masci's successor, Luigi Miraglia, announced in 1896,

> Not one request or desire of the directors of the clinics has been unanswered, because the funds have always been found. We have even installed an amphitheatre and administrative offices, modernized the lavatories on every floor in accord with modern standards of hygiene, restored the lecture halls, painted the benches and corridors, cleaned the statues, and renovated the fire hydrants.'[153]

At the expense of other components of an already truncated *risanamento*, the Faculty of Medicine acquired premises that proclaimed its new standing in the city. The fact that these facilities were located on the sites of expropriated monasteries and convents was the symbolic proclamation of an era. The Liberal local authorities, who marked the occasion by evoking the memory of Giordano Bruno, envisaged themselves as clearing away obfuscation and prejudice and replacing them with progress and science.[154]

If renovated and expanded facilities constituted a first sign of the enhanced prestige of the profession, the second was a large-scale organizational offensive to 'medicalize' and 'sanitize' the population. The central instrument for this purpose was a new municipal institution – the Office of Hygiene. Created in the 1890s at the instigation of one of the medical veterans of the 1884 disaster, Orazio Caro, this agency became the most powerful operational arm of the municipal Department of Health. The Office of Hygiene assumed responsibility for the direction of a series of public health initiatives, all of which involved increased power and employment for doctors.[155] An important aspect of this campaign was an enhanced scale of the free medical service for the poor, now centralized under the control of the Director of the Office of Hygiene. Each borough of the city was now to open a neighbourhood clinic staffed by four public health doctors and placed directly under the control of the central Office.

Painfully aware of the barriers of distrust between municipal physicians and the public that had been revealed during the cholera epidemic, Caro regarded it as a principal mission of the Office and its borough clinics to create the bases for regular and continuous contact between the *medici condotti* and the poor. Caro was highly conscious of the heavy responsibility 'not only for one of the most densely populated cities in Europe, but also one of the most neglected and mistreated cities in the world.'[156] For the purpose of ministering to this city, Caro conceived of the neighbourhood clinics as highly visible and accessible institutions staffed by rejuvenated, better qualified and better paid physicians. Furthermore, since women were especially alienated from the profession, Caro's vision included a strategy of providing benefits of immediate interest to them. In particular he conceived of childrearing as the Trojan horse with which to breach by stealth the ramparts of female hostility to doctors. Thus every clinic was to employ a midwife, to operate a dispensary for the provision of free milk and medicine for children up to the age of 8, and to provide a 24-hour obstetrical service equipped to attend to deliveries in women's homes. Infants and children would provide the means for doctors to gain access to a sceptical and illiterate population. Commenting retrospectively on this aspect of the Office of Hygiene, Caro wrote that,

> It is in fact of interest to note the moving joy of so many poor mothers, and the expressions of gratitude of all of those unhappy children for the care they received. It is also worth observing the meekness and trust with which the mothers accept all of our daily advice on matters of cleanliness and hygiene....
>
> Now it is obvious that all of this, repeated and multiplied by thousands of people, must necessarily in time have an influence and serve as an effective means ... for the spread of a sanitary consciousness among the masses.[157]

In addition to operating clinics in the twelve boroughs, the Office of Hygiene created a new bureaucracy of trained sanitary personnel to enforce the municipal sanitary and housing codes. Caro's institution hired teams of engineers, veterinarians and inspectors to visit markets, butcher shops and foodstalls; to superintend building sites; and to enforce sanitary standards for dwellings throughout Naples. Thus equipped with legal authority and trained personnel, the medical profession assumed police powers in matters of sanitation and hygiene. And to make its power visible, the Office of Hygiene opened premises in the Palazzo San Giacomo itself and in the city hall of each *sezione*. Caro's Office became a key instrument for the benign exercise of 'professional imperialism' as a resurgent and newly confident medical profession claimed new spheres of influence in the life of the city.

This second important reward was accompanied by a third – permanent inclusion of a representative of the profession in the deliberations of the executive committee of City Hall. From the time of unification physicians had always been elected members of the Naples city council, and in the persons of doctors Trisolini and Barbarini had even held departmental responsibilities and sat on the executive. Initially, however, doctors who undertook such political functions did not do so *as* physicians. While attending sessions at the Palazzo San Giacomo, they in effect ceased to be doctors, and were seldom asked to represent the profession or give opinions based on their medical competence. A turning point arrived in the 1870s with the entrance of the psychiatrist Giuseppe Buonomo into the *giunta*. As he explained in a speech to the city council in 1874, he regarded himself as the first physician in Liberal Naples to have been asked to serve on the executive specifically because he was a doctor and to represent the profession in the deliberations of the municipality.[158] After the emergency of 1884, the precedent created by Buonomo was regularized and made permanent. Doctors had demonstrated the usefulness of their skills for the exercise of power, and the Department of Health, invariably directed by a physician, became one of the most important offices in the city and the power base for such important politician-doctors as Giulio Rodinò, who was as influential as any figure in the city during the Giolittian era. The epidemic of 1884 had significantly assisted the Neapolitan medical profession in its coming of age.

The fact that Neapolitan physicians and ruling elites made such use of the medical philosophy of Max von Pettenkofer does not, of course, imply that the Munich hygienist endorsed their efforts or indeed that their reading of his work was part of an international orthodoxy at the time. On the contrary, the Neapolitan medical profession reformulated his theories and extrapolated from them in ways that fit their own scientific and political agendas. Pettenkofer's sanitary views could be put to very different social and political purposes in other contexts, as Richard Evans demonstrates in the case of contemporary Germany. Elsewhere in Europe, moreover, the divisions of opinion regarding the aetiology of Asiatic cholera at the time of the fifth pandemic ran along still different fault lines. Pettenkofer's hegemony within the shadow of Mount Vesuvius was a particular case that is intelligible only in the context of the ability of his ideas to make sense of the epidemiological history of the city, to support certain therapeutic initiatives and to further the interests of powerful elites. Methodologically, the Neapolitan case confirms the need to situate ideas in their precise social context, where alone they acquire meaning and force.

Events in Naples clearly suggest that it is necessary to revise Erwin Ackerknecht's influential view that anticontagionism as a medical doctrine was associated with radicalism and the political Left.[159] Even in the British context, which was the particular object of his enquiry, Margaret Pelling has suggested that the political contours of anticontagionism were not so clearly delineated as Ackerknecht had supposed.[160] In Italy, the uses made of miasmo-contagionism, a direct successor of anticontagionism, indicate that a further qualification is needed. Neapolitan medical and political authorities used the stance of anticontagionism as a vehicle for conservative and authoritarian purposes.

Furthermore, the history of Naples in the closing decades of the century does not imply that miasmo-contagionism possessed any inherent qualities that enabled it to function as the ideal philosophy of a rising medical profession. On the contrary, even in Naples, where localist ideas had served physicians so well, Pettenkofer's views suffered a rapid decline during the course of the 1890s as Koch's germ theory established an international ascendancy. Koch's triumphant assertion of contagionism, Evans rightly suggests, was ultimately even more useful in validating the 'scientific' status of the doctor.[161] The point here is simply that, at an important turning point in the history of both the city and its medical profession, Pettenkofer's theory of cholera played a major role in allowing the physicians of the city to speak with a united voice, to persuade City Hall that medicine had the power to resolve the problems of Naples, and to lay claim to a new place in the governing of the metropolis.

PART IV

The secret epidemic of 1910–1911

6

The return of cholera: 1910

PROLOGUE: THE INVASION OF APULIA

By the time of the renewed threat to Naples in 1910, the local and national authorities had long anticipated the return of Asiatic cholera. The sixth pandemic began its ravages in 1899 in Bengal. It then moved relentlessly westward along two established bacterial highways. To the north the disease followed the trade routes to the Punjab, Afghanistan and Persia. Crossing the Caspian Sea, it journeyed up the Volga to Moscow and the west. At the same time the cholera moved in a second, more southerly direction, travelling overland to Bombay and Madras; then by sea to Ceylon and Jeddah. It then accompanied the pilgrims to Mecca in 1902 and dispersed with them across the Red Sea to Egypt, the Middle East and North Africa.

The Department of Public Health in the Ministry of the Interior anxiously followed this westward movement and sounded the alarm in 1904, when cholera invaded the Russian Empire and developed into a full-scale epidemic. In the summer of 1905 the Ministry recorded outbreaks in Poland, Germany and the Hapsburg Empire, and observed that Italy was in clear danger. The authorities identified the Austrian border, Apulia and the ports of Naples and Genoa as particularly vulnerable. In September 1905 the Ministry of the Interior declared that Italy was now on a sanitary war-footing because the arrival of the disease on Italian soil was 'not just probable, but imminent'.[1]

As the Ministry had feared, the *Vibrio cholerae* reached Italy in the summer of 1910, claiming its first victims on the Adriatic coastline of Apulia that the authorities had identified as a locality of special risk. The 1,000 kilometres of shore between Venice and Brindisi lacked all maritime vigilance. Small craft were free to dock without regulation or inspection.[2] Wise after the event, the inspectors of the Department of Public Health established that the cholera was imported by the long-distance fishermen of Trani and Barletta. These fishermen departed in the autumn for voyages that lasted from six to nine months. During this lengthy absence, the seafarers plied the waters of the Aegean, the Levant and North

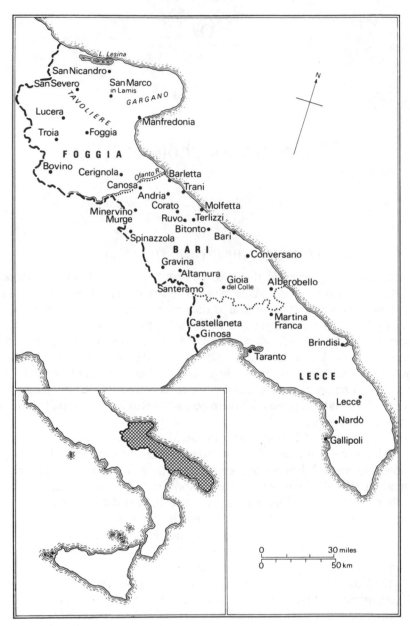

Map 6.1   Apulia

Africa, calling at harbour after harbour and encountering their fellows from the Balkans, Russia and the Middle East – areas where cholera was already epidemic. The Romanov domains above all were the epicentre of contagion in Europe: in the eight months from May 1910 cholera slew 100,982 people in the Russian Empire.[3]

Just as Muslim pilgrims had aided the vibrio in its westward progress by carrying it as they travelled from Mecca, and as French sailors had conveyed the infection from Tonkin to Toulon in 1884, so Apulian fishermen enabled the bacillus to complete its voyage in 1910.[4] Returning in the late spring to Italy, they brought the contagion with them. The risk to health was all the greater because of the squalor of the fishermen's ageing vessels. On the seamen's return, in the inspectors' words, 'their rejoicing women rush up with their carts. Then, after long embraces and loud chatter, they unload mattresses, cushions, sheets and an infinite variety of other objects that bear the encrusted filth of months and years.' In the two months of July and August 1910, 208 boats returned to Barletta amid such scenes. Popular wisdom had it that the first person to die of cholera in Italy during the new epidemic was the fishing captain Savino Nenna, who landed at Trani on 5 June and died on 18 June – officially of a cerebral haemorrhage.[5] In both Barletta and Trani the first mysterious deaths occurred in the fishermen's quarters.

At Barletta a focus of contagion was established long before Rome was informed. The statistics for mortality rose sharply in Barletta from the late spring, but the death certificates remained bland and reassuring – enteritis, fulminant diarrhoea, arsenical poisoning. Only the sheer volume of death alerted the resident Deputy Prefect. On 11 August he cabled his master in Bari, who in turn alerted the Ministry on 12 August. There the Director-General of Public Health was Rocco Santoliquido, a cholera expert and a veteran of the Neapolitan epidemic of 1884. Santoliquido felt that there were serious grounds for suspicion. He therefore ordered that specially trained army laboratory technicians under the direction of the military doctor Bartolomeo Gosio be immediately despatched from the capital. On 16 August Gosio confirmed the diagnosis of Asiatic cholera. The young peasant woman Rosa Quarto became the first Italian officially to contract cholera during the sixth pandemic and die of it.[6] The news was made public on 17 August.

What happened next was dramatic, violent and unexpected. Medical events in Apulia signalled a national emergency. Cholera was well established in a substantial town whose authorities had demonstrated their inability to take effective action. The disease threatened both the economy and public order. An epidemic of Asiatic cholera would halt trade, tourism and emigration – and just at a time when the nation was in the grip of a recession. Such reverses would raise storms of protest from the propertied interests and the deputies who represented them. There was the parallel danger of increasing unemployment and social tensions. Gasperini, the Prefect of Bari province, warned Rome of the economic and political complications of declaring the province an infected area, and he urged a policy of concealment. It would be wise, he cautioned, to diagnose the disease as meningitis. This deliberate subterfuge would allow the authorities to take sanitary measures, but without risking quarantines and the boycott of Apulian goods.[7] Gasperini wrote with regard to the scattered cases in Apulia that,

> The limited number of these cases, the fact that they have not assumed epidemic proportions and the speed with which measures are taken have led me, in agreement with the state technicians, to refrain from declarations that would undermine the most vital interests of this city. I was confirmed in this conviction by the fact that the diagnosis of cerebro-spinal meningitis issued by the attending physicians on various occasions permitted the adoption of the most rigorous sanitary measures without causing alarm and without the necessity of publicly explaining their purpose.
>
> Given the ruinous economic conditions of this city and province, I believe it to be essential to spare the people this new misfortune while at the same time carrying out the most careful preventive measures.[8]

The greatest cause of concern, however, was the threat to Naples. An epidemic in Bari province directly menaced the southern metropolis because of the massive trans-oceanic emigration which linked it to Apulia in a continuous chain of infection. Over a thousand emigrants, drawn from the very classes of workers and peasants who were most susceptible to cholera, departed every month from Bari province alone for the New World.[9] In 1910, 26,061 people emigrated overseas from the whole of the region.[10] The majority, bound for North America, left via the port of Naples. Cholera in distant Barletta and Trani therefore posed an immediate danger to the health, the commerce and the economy of the capital city of Campania. The United States Surgeon-General accurately identified the direct risk that Apulia posed for Naples. Apulia, he noted, 'is in most intimate commercial relations with Naples both by land and by sea, and from the moment of the appearance of cholera in Bari and the rest of Apulia, the more or less rapid infestation of Naples ... became a foregone conclusion.'[11] Naples, in turn, had innumerable links by rail, road and sea with the whole of the peninsula and by sea with the islands of Sicily and Sardinia. The Apulian emergency, as a result, was a menace to all of Italy.

In the summer of 1910 the state was especially fearful because the government was a weak coalition under the conservative elder statesman Luigi Luzzatti. Luzzatti governed on the basis of a temporary parliamentary alliance between the deputies of the radical Left and supporters of Giovanni Giolitti to the Right. In the long run, the experiment could not be sustained; in the short run, it resulted in a policy of zig-zags to left and right to satisfy the contradictory aspirations of the two wings of the majority. An epidemic of cholera that afflicted Italy alone in western Europe could seriously embarrass his government. How seriously Luzzatti regarded cholera was made public in October. The Secretary of State for the Interior, Teobaldo Calissano, presented Luzzatti's parliamentary programme in a major speech in his constituency at Alba. Cholera was the first and chief item on the agenda.[12]

In mid-August, unhappily summoned from his Alpine holiday, Luzzatti resolved to act decisively to crush the threat. He gave the task of containing the epidemic to the most dependable instruments of the Italian state – the army and the police. Inspector-General Serafino Ravicini was ordered to Apulia to occupy a position without precedent in Italian history or law. He was named in effect health dictator with full emergency powers. He took up office on 18 August, with the mission of policing the sick.

Under orders from Rome, Ravicini instituted a reign of terror hardly suggestive of a modern Liberal state or mindful of the advances of scientific medicine. The essence of state policy was coercion. By Ravicini's edict, at Barletta all cholera victims were to be transported alone and against their will to an improvised pest-house set up in the open countryside on the road to Foggia. At the same time all who lived with the sufferers fell under suspicion of contagion. They were to be dragooned for observation to the city castle, now hastily converted into an internment camp. Meanwhile, in the homes the poor left behind, their personal effects were burned and the premises disinfected.

The paradox was that the Italian state resorted in 1910 to coercive measures of public health that had demonstrated their futility in 1884. Indeed, with the advances in diagnostic procedures accomplished by Robert Koch and the microbiologists who further refined his techniques, such a strategy had become utterly anachronistic. Only on the basis of mutual confidence between the authorities and the public could information be obtained, preventive measures taken, and cooperation elicited. The authoritarian Barletta regime was reminiscent instead of the cordon sanitaires, the quarantines and the lazarettos that had served Italy so poorly a generation before and that informed medical opinion unanimously rejected.

When cholera first appeared in two communes in a single province, however, the authorities in Rome undertook a desperate local gamble. There was no question of applying the coercive strategy on a national level. The calculation was instead that a sharp shock of local repression might kill the infection before it spread from Bari province. A rigour that would no longer be attempted nationally or in a major city was applied in Apulia.

As Morana had learned in 1884, the reaction of the populace to authoritarian public health was resistance and evasion. Terrified of the lazaretto, outraged by the internment castle, and threatened with ruin as their possessions were consigned to the flames, the labourers of Barletta and Trani undertook desperate measures. Families tended their ill in secret or, fearing discovery, abandoned them to die alone while they undertook midnight removals of their belongings. Neighbours and relatives also gathered to protest and protect. On several occasions medics and troops were driven off, only to return with reinforcements and drawn weapons.[13]

The army responded with further repression. Heads of families were ordered to report all illness in their households, under pain of savage fines.[14] Still fearing non-compliance, the army divided the city of Barletta into six military districts.

Each was patrolled day and night by armed platoons of infantrymen, *carabinieri* and vigilantes. The vigilantes were bounty-hunters paid piece-work rates for every cholera victim they carted away and every healthy relative they interned.[15] This work of sanitary squadrism had no legal sanction. Nevertheless, the hunt continued without pause from 18 August until 2 September. In Ravicini's words, 'The present exceptional moment explains this holy violation of the law.'[16]

Not surprisingly, tension in the city mounted daily. Vito Lefemine, Secretary of the Bari Chamber of Labour, visited the city. There he described the atmosphere as 'social hysteria'[17] – a view reiterated by the Department of Public Health.[18] The hysteria was stoked by the authorities, who clumsily attempted to divert attention from the reality of sanitary conditions in the peninsula by blaming the gypsies for the outburst. Gypsies, together with Jews, had long served as scapegoats for large-scale misfortunes. A prominent illustration of the wide-spread anti-gypsy phobia in Italy was the commentary of the criminal anthro-pologist Cesare Lombroso. He wrote of the travellers that,

> They are the living example of a whole race of criminals, and have all the passions and all the vices of criminals ...
>
> They are given to orgies, love a noise, and make a great outcry in the markets. They murder in cold blood in order to rob, and were formerly suspected of cannibalism. The women are very clever at stealing, and teach it to their children. They poison cattle with certain powders in order to get the credit of curing them, or perhaps to get their flesh at a low price ... They all excel at some form of rascality ... As the name 'Jew' with us is synonymous with usurer, so in Spain *gitano* is synonymous with rascally cattle trader.[19]

The association of gypsies with poison and the fact that, in popular culture, the cholera was known as *lo zingaro* – the gypsy – were points that were not lost on Luzzatti and his subordinates at the Ministry of the Interior. In the summer of 1910 they sought to exploit this latent xenophobia. The strategy was to create a state-sponsored wave of anti-gypsy terror. The Prime Minister himself gave 'urgent orders' to the police to prevent all gypsies from being admitted to Italian territory – orders that were interpreted to apply not only to gypsies but also to anyone with 'habits similar to those of the gypsies'.[20] Here there was a bitter irony. Although Luzzatti was Jewish, he did not refrain from making use of the racialist sentiment of his countrymen against a despised minority now that it was expedient to do so.

In pursuit of this strategy, the Prefect of Bari announced that the medical emergency in Apulia was due to the arrival in the province of caravans of gypsies. They were, he announced, infected Russians, who were spreading poison by washing their filthy linen in public wells. To protect the populace, the police ordered the arrest and internment of all gypsies on Italian soil, pending their disinfection and expulsion from the kingdom. Within days the press, the deputies and the authorities at every level were in full cry against a people that *Avanti!*, to its shame, denounced as 'those Russians with rough and unkempt beards whose ignorance and filth fit them for classification in lower spheres of the animal kingdom'.[21] In a similar vein, *Messagero* reminded its readership that travellers were not only a medical risk, but also a threat to public order as they stole 'animals, property and even children'.[22] For *Resto del carlino*, the gypsies were 'like bottle-flies, wolves, and locusts – one of the many scourges of the country-side'.[23] Even after the emergency Luzzatti's leading collaborator in internal affairs and the Secretary of State at the Ministry of the Interior, Teobaldo Calissano, justified his actions in the Chamber of Deputies. Calissano reminded the nation that gypsies were the cause of 'constant crimes against property and the person, and of the absolute disregard of sanitation ... Our rigour was just and timely'.[24]

In Barletta, the official explanation of the epidemic was outlined by the unrepentant Calissano. He reasoned that the disease had arrived in Italy with a caravan of thirty-seven gypsies from the Caucasus who had crossed the Black Sea and boarded an Italian ship at Constantinople bound for Brindisi. Dis-embarking in Apulia in July, they had made a pilgrimage to the relics of St Nicholas at Bari and then they travelled to Trani and Barletta in the first week of August. With their arrival and their evil ablutions the epidemic began.[25] This scurrilous mythology has become a standard part of the account of the origins of the sixth pandemic in Italy, and was repeated without criticism by the official World Health Organization history of cholera written by R. Pollitzer in 1959.[26]

It was of no avail that investigations by the Ministry of the Interior revealed that the unfortunate gypsies at Barletta were not from Russia but Corfu; that the gold they carried on their persons established that they were not poor; that in the matter of personal hygiene they were indistinguishable from the other arrivals at the port of Brindisi; and that not one of them had taken ill.[27] They were all herded into a barbed-wire encampment on the shore near Trani for the duration of the outbreak, and then repatriated in the autumn. Reports such as those of the Prefect of Bari, who informed Rome that all of the people interned in tents were 'healthy and harmless', were not made public.[28]

A racist manhunt had begun. Gypsies throughout Italy were arrested by the police, whose work was facilitated by the anti-gypsy provisions of articles 74 and 75 of the Italian Public Security Laws of 1889, which specifically provided for their forcible repatriation.[29] Prefects called upon municipal officials to cooperate in the great work of stopping gypsy caravans and detaining their members for medical examination and interrogation.[30] At the same time, warned by the state of the diabolical plot of the travellers, mobs of angry citizens attacked gypsies or 'innocent' vagabonds and street vendors whom they mistook in their zeal for the accursed race of poisoners. From cholera-stricken Trani the outraged citizen Lorenzo Cortellino expressed a widespread sentiment that the state had encour-aged. He wrote to the Prime Minister explaining how disaster had been brought to his city and urging Luzzatti to take vigorous action before it was too late. Of the gypsies Cortellino said, 'Woe to those who live where they pass. Microbes fall from their foul garments and lay waste to the population.'[31] At Pontedera in Tuscany, a group of homeless men was set upon by a crowd and beaten, while at the village of Santo Felice di Roccella in Palermo province a beggar was stoned to death by frightened residents who believed that he was malevolently spreading the contagion.[32] The misfortune of all tramps in the inflamed climate of 1910, commented the paper *Resto del carlino*, was 'to be expelled when they arrive and hunted when they depart'.[33]

Despite the exceptional rigour of state policy in Apulia, however, the hope that extreme measures and a xenophobic manhunt could halt the spread of cholera, absolve the government of all responsibility and calm the anxiety of the populace proved illusory. In the microcosm of Bari province, the Italian authorities re-learned the lessons of 1884 when the attempt to combat disease with coercion and to evade responsibility by blaming returning emigrants proved to be fatally counter-productive. Similarly in 1910 as the troops and vigilantes carried out their work of purification and destruction, fear gripped the population and provided the means to spread disease. Indeed, the official mythology of a wholesale poisoning conspiracy heightened popular anxiety. Just as in 1884, the result was a mass exodus from the stricken towns of Barletta and Trani. Families of substance escaped to distant Rome and Naples. Lesser members of the middle classes sought refuge in nearby Spinazzola, which was known for its supply of pure water. Shopkeepers and artisans contented themselves with setting up tents and bivouacking in the surrounding countryside. Within days Barletta became a ghost town of twenty thousand people – farm labourers, peasants and builders unable to flee.[34]

At the same time public order, strained by the terror, began to break down. In Barletta and Molfetta widespread evasion and resistance to official measures taken against the disease escalated into full-scale riots.[35] At the same time in the smaller surrounding towns citizens set up improvised and highly illegal sanitary cordons to protect themselves, repelling refugees from the affected communes. Crowds, sometimes enjoying the support of municipal officials and local doctors, overturned carts and either burned their loads or dumped them into the sea. There was, remarked the health inspectors at the Ministry of the Interior, 'an instinct among the masses to personify the cholera, so that they can hope to keep a careful vigil and repel it with a shotgun'.[36]

Just as in 1884 the Italian army had failed to defend the nation from the *Vibrio cholerae*, so in 1910 hastily improvised local cordons were unable to protect the towns of Apulia from infection. Cerignola, Molfetta, Canosa and Grumo, where sanitary cordons manned by armed residents were established with exemplary rigour, were attacked by the disease no less than towns such as Andria, which did without them.[37] Transported by fugitives and by the sanitary militiamen themselves, cholera broke out in a series of communes located in a semicircle around Barletta and Trani and linked to them by road and railway. The disease was spreading in two provinces: Andria, Bisceglie, Bitonto, Corato, Molfetta, Ruvo and Spinazzola were affected in Bari province as well as Cerignola, Ortanova, S. Margherita di Savoia and Trinitapoli in Capitanata. Between 17 August, when the presence of the disease was first made public, and 3 September, when a new course in policy was adopted, cholera infected all of these localities. More alarmingly, mysterious reports began in early September to emanate from Naples, where terrified veterans of the Apulian emergency had fled. The eventuality that Luzzatti had so desperately attempted to avoid was coming to pass. The logic of continuing to apply the shock prophylaxis was rapidly losing its *raison d'être*, and was even becoming counterproductive as hysteria enabled both disease and social disorder to spread. On 3 September the Ministry quietly abandoned the policy of coercion, dismantling the sanitary dictatorship and allowing the hunt for scapegoats to lapse. The second phase of the epidemic, concentrated above all in Naples during the autumn of 1910, had begun, and it ran its course under different auspices.

In Apulia the early events of the outbreak in August bore all of the hallmarks of the social cataclysms that took place during the 1830s across Europe and of the Italian experience in 1884. In the twentieth-century epidemic cholera once again abundantly demonstrated in the province of Bari its ability to create terror, poisoning phobias, mass flight, assaults on doctors, concealment and full-scale riots. Even *untori* reminiscent of the plague appeared in the form of gypsies. These social tumults, moreover, occurred despite a very limited mortality from the disease. In an era when the mechanisms of the malady were well understood by the medical profession and when the modern state possessed workable strategies of prophylaxis to forestall wholesale disasters, cholera nevertheless clearly retained the ability to generate panic and violence.

The history of the disease, however, suggests that the social consequences that it evokes are enormously variable. Under certain conditions the outbreak of cholera causes the social tensions of a society to erupt into open and violent tumults. Apulia in 1910 was such a case. There the circumstances that favoured sharp conflicts even though the mortality was limited included the following: profound and bitterly resented social inequalities; a widespread distrust of authority; mass illiteracy; lack of contact between the people and physicians; and a military policy of preventive health. Such a combination of materials was highly combustible, and it rapidly degenerated into an atmosphere of hysteria, riot and flight.

Unlike 1884, however, in 1910 the state rapidly abandoned the experiment at coercion. The contrast is striking. From the announcement of the first cases of cholera in Provence in June 1884 until late in the autumn, Agostino Depretis grimly persisted with the strategy of containing cholera by military means. Despite widespread evasion, resistance and the collapse of social order as well as the spread of the disease itself, Depretis continued to rely on sanitary cordons and lazarettos. In the late summer of 1910 Luigi Luzzatti responded differently. After the debacle of repression in Apulia, Luzzatti turned to liberalism when the disease broke out at Naples in September. Riots at Barletta and Molfetta, together with the clear inability of the army to contain the disease, prompted the state to change its sanitary policy. From September the Department of Public Health pursued an anti-cholera campaign based on the scientific procedures most closely associated with Prussia under the sanitary direction of Robert Koch. Prussian defensive measures, now applied in Naples after the failure of coercive anti-plague measures in Apulia, were dependent not on soldiery, but on laboratory diagnostic techniques and the voluntary cooperation of the population.

This major change in sanitary policy affected the subsequent course of the entire epidemic. With the end of a strategy that fostered both terror and the belief in demonic plots, hysteria never held sway in the imagination of the population of Naples. There were scattered incidents of concealment and of protests at the intervention of public health officials in the Lower City in September and October; and a substantial proportion of the wealthier residents of the Upper City took flight. But a poisoning frenzy and mass uprisings of the sort that marked the onset of the disease on the Adriatic coast and that had formed such an important feature of the 1884 crisis did not materialize.

Naturally, the more circumspect direction in public health policy was the most conspicuous but not the only factor involved. Four other significant considerations were: the level of mortality; improved relations between the population and the medical profession; developments in the theology of cholera; and a local sense of protection behind a rampart of 'civilization'. The first of these was mortality. In 1910, and even in the more violent outburst of 1911, there was no repetition of the dreadful days of the fifth pandemic when it literally seemed as if the whole of Naples was doomed to die. Barletta, Trani and Molfetta, of course, demonstrated that terror can take root even in the presence of a limited mortality. It was soothing, however, that the disease seemed relatively containable, and that the state and municipal bureaucracies had not lost control of events.

Apart from the reassuringly small numbers of deaths, a second calming factor was the newly prominent position of the medical profession in the city. Since the epidemic of 1884 the Office of Hygiene had undertaken a diligent effort to 'medicalize' the Lower City, accustoming the population to medical care and breaking down the barriers of distrust and unfamiliarity of the past. After a generation of solicitous penetration into the homes of the poor with advice and assistance, the strengthened corps of municipal doctors was no longer a body of strangers whose arrival spread alarm. In Gramscian terms, the Office of Hygiene had formed a new medical 'common sense' that provided the profession with a greatly enhanced authority in a time of crisis. Caro expressed this point clearly, writing,

> We have given the people the security of knowing that their health will be protected by the responsible authorities, and we have demonstrated to them on a daily basis our concern for their welfare ... In this way we have made the citizens rather more careful to carry out our sanitary precepts, and at the same time we have taught them to trust us, which is the only way in times of crisis to guarantee order and to achieve victory.'[38]

This new medical authority was enhanced by the more visible and active presence of physicians in positions of influence in the city in the years since the last epidemic and by the fact that by 1910 the profession spoke with a more united voice in the matter of cholera. Koch's germ theory provided an almost universally accepted consensus, and the sense that doctors were more confident and unanimous in their advice lowered the level of apprehension. In Orazio Caro's view, a revealing measurement of the difference in attitudes between the epidemics of 1884 and 1910 was the fact that by the latter date sufferers sought medical attention voluntarily and at an early stage in the course of the disease.[39]

In Catholic Italy, a factor which played a role in reducing the alarms and tumults of cholera was a progression in the theology of epidemic disease. During the nineteenth century the doctrine that cholera was the sword of God unsheathed to scourge the sinful and to demonstrate the inferiority of the Liberal state to the old regime immeasurably heightened the terror that accompanied epidemics. Religious belief encouraged the search for scapegoats and the suspicion of officials. This factor was apparent in the panic of the populace when the disease approached Naples in 1884, but was de-fused by the determined stance of the Cardinal Archbishop. In Sicily, where the clergy instead exploited the disease to encourage legitimism, religion became the ally of social tumults and violent resistance to physicians.

In the generation that separated the fifth pandemic from the sixth, Catholic teachings with regard to epidemic disease accommodated themselves to scientific advances and to the permanence of the Italian state. A clear measurement of the distance travelled is the position of *Civiltà cattolica*, the mouthpiece for extreme Catholic opposition to the public health measures of the Depretis government in 1884. By the time of the return of cholera in 1910, the Jesuit review expressed no independent position on the epidemic in opposition to the sanitary policies of the state. On the contrary, it acknowledged that the prophylactic measures announced by the Department of Public Health were appropriate and deserved the cooperation of the faithful. Commenting on the outbreak in Apulia, it stressed that the state had taken the necessary sanitary measures to defend the nation; it criticized those foreign powers that adopted excessive quarantine against uninfected Italian ports; and it praised the clergy for its collaboration in the work of defeating the disease and aiding its victims.[40] Although popular religion moved at a pace different from that of the Church, the alliance of the clergy with the state on the issue of public health was a substantial factor in the relative calm that marked the final Italian experience of epidemic cholera.

Finally, as an explanation for the absence of pronounced disorder in the fifth pandemic, there was also a fragile but nonetheless important sense of civic pride that had developed among many Neapolitans as a result of *risanamento*. As we shall see, there was a widely publicized current of opinion in the city that the Serino water, the sewer system and the renewal of the boroughs of Porto and Pendino constituted impregnable defences guaranteeing the city against all possibility of a new epidemic invasion. Events were to suggest that some of this confidence was misplaced and that the anti-cholera fortifications of the city were a sanitary Maginot Line that failed to hold when an emergency struck. But Maginot Lines, both military and sanitary, generate a psychological sense of security, and this factor diminished terror when cholera reappeared. Many Neapolitans felt safely defended, and there were powerful interests vociferously at work to proclaim the message that all was well. Here was a factor which undoubtedly had a parallel and a precedent in the similarly striking calm displayed by Parisians during the invasions of cholera in 1884 and 1892–3. In the aftermath of the rebuilding projects of the Second Empire, many Parisians felt that the modern state had actively and effectively intervened to guarantee the hygienic safety of the city and that it was no longer vulnerable to epidemic catastrophe.

Thus while tumults raged in the cities and towns of Provence, Paris preserved its self-confidence. On 15 November 1884, for instance, in the midst of the Parisian outburst of that year, the *New York Times* reported of the atmosphere in the French capital that, 'The epidemic shows little, if any, effect upon the pleasure-seeking proclivities of the people. The theatres and other places of amusement are well filled every night.'[41] Indeed, a local apothecary was disappointed with the effect of the outbreak upon his trade. He had hoped to do a thriving business as a result of popular anxieties, but found instead that the epidemic 'was not half so profitable for him as a period of weather when cold-catching was prevalent'.[42] The paper commented that, despite the spread of the disease throughout the city, 'the people show no signs as yet of panic'.[43] It was indicative that *Le Temps*, which devoted a daily column to the outbreak of 1884, made no mention of such occurrences of the past as panic, tumult, mass flight or violent resistance to authority. In 1892 the sense of security within the city walls was further enhanced by the geography of the outbreak. The cholera raged in the communes of the *banlieu* – Nanterre, Saint Denis, Suresnes, Colombes, Aubervilliers, Courbevoie – but largely spared the Haussmannized capital itself.[44]

In a similarly renovated context, the impact of the cholera outbreak in 1910 and 1911 in Naples was far removed from that of previous epidemics in the city and from the tumultuous outbreaks of the disease elsewhere in Europe that have been discussed in the literature. The course of events in this final epidemic was *sui generis*. The historiography of Asiatic cholera has been preoccupied with the capacity of the disease to produce social tension and disorder in its wake. The pioneering figures of the field – Briggs, Chevalier and Rosenberg – set an enduring pattern of investigation by stressing the way in which cholera served as a catalyst causing pre-existing social tensions to erupt into violent clashes. Following Chevalier's lead, Briggs regarded cholera as a 'social irritant' that above all deepened the class antagonisms between rich and poor. Thinking of the possible links between the epidemic history of Paris and the parallel events of the 'rebellious century', and quoting Chevalier, Briggs wrote:

> Cholera, if only because of its mode of communication, ... was predominantly a disease of the poor. In metropolitan Paris not only did inequality of life and inequality of death move together, but reactions to the epidemic were closely associated with social conflict. '*Le choléra précise les fondements biologiques des*

antagonismes de classe.' Contemporaries recognized this: cholera thereby exacerbated class hatred.[45]

Working within the same analytical framework, Rosenberg stressed the social tensions that marked the history of epidemic cholera in the United States. In a recent reflection upon his early work *The Cholera Years*, Rosenberg argues that the distinguishing feature of North America was the nature of the conflicts that occurred. While class conflict was dramatically revealed in Europe during the recurring cholera visitations, in the United States the same underlying stresses found expression in a different form. In his words, 'The antagonisms of class ... that marked the English and French urban experience with cholera were recreated in a rather different style in America's cities; religion and ethnicity were rather more prominent on this side of the Atlantic.'[46]

More recently, studies by Michael Durey on Britain; Roderick McGrew on Russia; Patrice Bourdelais, Ange-Pierre Leca and François Delaporte on France; and Vincent Bernard, Antonio Fernandez Garcia and Esteban Rodriguez Ocana on Spain[47] have charted disturbances of all sorts stretching over the whole continent. These disturbances are complex in their origins and cannot be reduced to the single paradigm of class conflict. The essential point, however, is that historians have described a rich and variegated pattern of riots, assaults, demonstrations and flight. Naples in 1884 and Apulia in 1910 conform to this pattern, providing further illustrations of the capacity of cholera to unleash civil disorder. Thus, surveying the historiography of the European experience of cholera, Richard Evans considered it logical to raise the question of whether cholera should be considered a major contributory factor in the coming of revolutions. Although his conclusion was not affirmative, the question is indicative of the direction of the literature to date.[48] The issue of the role of epidemic disease in fostering social revolution has even been taken up by Pule Phoofuto as a starting point for the analysis of the epizootic of rinderpest in Southern Africa at the close of the century.[49]

Here, in an examination of the experience of a single city, it is impossible to resolve such a general issue for the whole of Europe. Clearly, however, the recent investigation of the later cholera pandemics suggests that the disease has a more complicated history than conclusions based on the stormy early decades of the century indicated to some of the early investigators of the subject. On the contrary, Hamburg in 1892 and Paris in both 1884 and 1892–3 demonstrate that, especially in the late nineteenth century, cholera visitations did not ineluctably result in large-scale upheavals.

Against this background, the Neapolitan experience in 1910 and 1911 provides a distinctive variant. In 1910 the city demonstrated once again that cholera was a significant event. It did so, however, without giving rise to major disorders or expressions of violent opposition to authority, political or medical. The return of cholera intersected politically with the specific local history of *risanamento* and economically with the interests built on the export of labour. In political terms, the renewal and rebuilding scheme had involved enormous cost, given rise to mass evictions, created vast expectations and raised allegations of corruption and misgovernment. With such a background, the onset of a fresh epidemic produced a severe political challenge to the authority of the ruling elites associated with the scheme and its ambivalent legacy. Cholera took its place at the centre of Neapolitan political life, but not as a fomenter of impromptu and leaderless tumult. Here one must avoid being categorical. There were scattered incidents, but these never matched the frequency, the scale or the ferocity of the clashes that marked 1884 and the Apulian events of 1910. On the contrary, in 1910 at Naples the disease became the basis for a highly organized attempt by the opposition republican and socialist parties through legal and electoral means to cashier the ruling Catholic party that had risen to power when the Liberals had been discredited by a major political scandal at the turn of the century. In the twentieth-century context of a liberal state with organized political sub-cultures, cholera placed public health and the ability of the ruling elite to protect it at the centre of a major electoral challenge.

Economically, the arrival of Asiatic cholera, even in the form of a minor outbreak, presented the port of Naples with a serious danger. The economy of the city in the Giolittian period was overwhelmingly dependent on a single activity – the export of migrant labour from the southern provinces of Italy to North America. In an era when the germ theory of disease had made contagionism the medical orthodoxy in the matter of cholera, however, the international community had established rigorous measures of prevention by maritime quarantine. These measures had been agreed upon by the International Sanitary Convention of 1903 to which Italy was a signatory. To admit the presence of cholera in Naples, therefore, was to threaten the city with the closure of the harbour and the diversion of the steamships to another port.

Such a menace produced an anti-sanitary backlash unique to the city of Naples. The opposition of merchants in European seaports to official acknowledgement of the presence of Asiatic cholera, of course, had a long history. At the initial outburst of cholera in Britain, for example, the merchants of Sunderland in 1831 pressed for concealment to protect their trade and their profits. And commercial interests in other major ports, including Marseilles and Hamburg, reacted in a similar fashion throughout the history of cholera invasions. The anti-sanitary movement in Naples, however, was very different, and not only because the instigators of the protest were not merchants but boarding-house owners and Camorra bosses. More significant was the fact that the campaign was a mass movement, uniting the Chamber of Commerce and organized labour in a common front against the sanitary policy of the state. The campaign successfully mobilized the city with a populist political rhetoric of defending the exploited South against a rapacious northern plot to ruin Naples and advance the fortunes of Genoa. And the weapons the movement deployed were clearly modern – the industrial lockout and the general strike.

Cholera in Naples therefore gave rise to two powerful movements in 1910 – one directed at the electoral overthrow of the ruling political elites in the city, the other at the sanitary policy of the state. Together they played a major part in destroying the ministry of Luigi Luzzatti, and they persuaded his successor, Giovanni Giolitti, to initiate what, so far as is known, constituted an unprecedented policy in the history of epidemic cholera – a sustained national campaign of secrecy and denial. This chapter explores the two movements, and Chapter 7 investigates the conspiracy of silence. The point at which to begin an account of the cholera years 1910 and 1911 in Naples, however, is with two 'official' mythologies regarding the course of the sixth pandemic. These mendacious versions of events have distorted the historiography of the subject ever since.

THE EPIDEMIC THAT DISAPPEARED

The fears of the Department of Public Health about the possibility of a new large-scale epidemic in Italy were rapidly realized. After reaching the fishing towns Barletta and Trani, cholera spread to the interior of Apulia. In quick succession it then invaded the two great seaports of Naples and Palermo that were linked epidemiologically to Bari and Foggia provinces by the ideal vehicle for long-distance transmission of infection – mass trans-oceanic emigration. In these two cities the disease established an enduring presence. In the autumn of 1910 cholera produced a limited outbreak, causing several hundred deaths in each seaport. The epidemic then subsided during the winter of 1910–11, only to flare up with much greater force and dispersion in the spring, summer and autumn of 1911. After first reaching peaks of ferocity in Naples and Palermo, where it killed thousands in each of the two centres, the cholera spread across mainland Italy and the whole of Sicily. As in previous epidemics, including 1884, the disease caused only scattered deaths in most of the provinces it attacked, but it broke out with considerable fury in many Sicilian communes and in the vulnerable ports of Genoa and Livorno. The disease then abated in the winter of 1911–12 and erupted only once more with an outburst at Cagliari in the summer and early autumn of 1912. The last known case occurred in Sardinia on 17 October 1912.[50]

This epidemic carried with it a heavy indictment of both Neapolitan and Italian sanitary conditions. As a result of the medical knowledge, the hygienic provision, and the bureaucratic vigilance of the modern state, epidemic cholera was widely deemed to be an anachronism in the industrial nations of twentieth-century Europe. Indeed, Italy was the only industrial nation to be afflicted during the course of a pandemic that otherwise raged only in the underdeveloped world. By 1910 an important aspect of the epidemic was that it was experienced by Italians not just as a misfortune but as a stigma that raised questions in their minds about the modernity and civilization of the regime. The return of cholera remorselessly exposed unacceptable shortcomings in living conditions in large areas of the peninsula, and nowhere more than in its most populous and expensively reconstructed city.

The return of Asiatic cholera therefore unleashed a major psychological and political crisis. Its presence challenged the authority of the national government and of the ruling elites in Naples by raising in dramatic fashion the question of whether they were capable to defending the most elementary interest of the population – its security from sudden and tormenting death. Confronted with a challenge on this ground, neither the national authorities nor the executive of the Naples city council were prepared to acknowledge the extent of the epidemic of 1910–12. Instead, they fabricated two medical lies.

The first was intended for public consumption at the time. According to this invention, which produced a mythology of the Italian triumph over infectious disease, the nation experienced no epidemic but only a minor outburst in September 1910 that was successfully contained. The events of 1910 were minimized, and the tragedies of 1911 and 1912 were concealed. In total, the sixth pandemic was asserted to have claimed a few hundred Italian lives in the space of two months. The sombre truth that thousands – perhaps tens of thousands – perished during the course of three successive years was concealed from contemporaries. The official account was sustained by means of censorship, political pressure and the threat of violence. Cholera demonstrated much about the nature of statecraft in the Italian Liberal regime.

The second misrepresentation of the events of 1910–12 was produced for a different audience. Foreign governments, and especially the United States, kept a watchful vigilance over the state of public health in Italy because of its potential international repercussions. It proved impossible to conceal the existence of a widespread epidemic of Asiatic cholera from the American authorities when Italian emigrants repeatedly arrived at Ellis Island suffering from the disease. For the particular benefit of the United States Public Health and Marine Hospital Service (USPH&MHS), the Italian state embarked upon a highly secret policy of half-truths that flagrantly contradicted all public discussion of public health but that stopped well short of a full and frank disclosure of the reality concerning cholera. In exchange for public silence, the Department of Public Health furnished American consular officials with daily bulletins of health purporting to disclose all cases and deaths from Asiatic cholera throughout the peninsula. In reality, these bulletins contained a carefully edited and misleading version of the course of the disease intended to reassure the American authorities that the Italian government was in control. If Italian officials could persuade the American Surgeon-General that the disease could be contained, then there would be no need for American health officials to disrupt trade, tourism and emigration.

This second account of the course of the disease was subsequently embodied in the official statistics of the sixth pandemic in Italy. These figures, which acknowledged the existence of a cholera epidemic but greatly understated its extent, were made available to the public only after the disease had departed from the peninsula and the issue was no longer of burning concern either to Italians or to foreigners.

The combination of the two mythologies – the original categorical denial and the subsequent half truth – has distorted the historiography of the European encounter with Asiatic cholera and the history of modern Italy. With the collusion of the American Government, Italy in 1911 and 1912 successfully suppressed all public discussion of a major cholera epidemic. Without explanation for the contradiction, the state later provided mortality figures, although the statistics it furnished significantly understated the magnitude of the event. With such falsified statistics and without the usual array of sources in the press, medical periodicals and official documents, the Italian experience of the sixth pandemic of Asiatic cholera has fallen victim to an almost total collective amnesia. Leading experts on the history of cholera in Europe, such as Richard Evans, Patrice Bourdelais and Jean-Yves Raulot, have uncritically accepted the official version of events. Evans argues that the last epidemic of Asiatic cholera in western Europe took place in Hamburg in the 1890s during the course of the fifth pandemic. In his account, the Italian experience of the sixth pandemic has vanished.[51] Bourdelais and Raulot conclude in the same vein that,

> At any rate, as a consequence of the latest advances in the understanding of the pathogen responsible for cholera, the westard progress of the sixth pandemic came to a halt in October 1910 at the island of Madeira. The pandemic affected Europe only marginally, and left the American continent untouched.[52]

In analogous fashion, cholera has virtually disappeared from the historiography of pre-war Italy. General histories, collections of documents, monographs on modern Naples and Campania, studies of the period, works on Italian mass emigration, and biographies of Giolitti make no mention of the medical emergency created by the return of cholera. Here Giolitti himself established a precedent by ignoring its existence in his autobiography, just as he did in his parliamentary speeches and public lectures.[53] Unaware of the care with which the Prime Minister personally directed first the campaign against the disease and then the suppression of all record of its passage, scholars have neither corrected the omission nor examined its significance.[54] It is characteristic that Alan M. Kraut's important recent history of disease and mass immigration to the United States – *Silent Travelers: Germs, Genes, and the Immigrant Menace* – makes no mention of the Italian cholera epidemic of 1910–11. The omission is striking because cholera is central to Kraut's account, because Italians as the most numerous immigrants to America between 1880 and 1921 are necessarily at the heart of the analysis, because the epidemic was a central preoccupation of American public health officials, and because the *Vibrio cholerae* was a 'silent traveller' that repeatedly reached New York Harbor and even the American mainland during the outbreak.[55]

The principal alternative account, which is only marginally revisionist, is that of Anna Lucia Forti Messina. Forti Messina is the author of both the only modern monograph on cholera in Italy and of the chapter on cholera for the Einaudi *Storia d'Italia*. Unusually, she acknowledges the existence of an outbreak of Asiatic cholera in Italy during the sixth pandemic. Unfortunately, however, she succumbs, not to the contemporary categorical denial, but to the later half-truth.

Relying on official mortality figures for the period without critically examining the manner in which they were compiled, Forti Messina dismisses the events of 1910–12 as unimportant. The disease, in her words, was 'numerically insignificant'. Furthermore, as an explanation for such severely limited mortality, she speculates that 'perhaps in truth it is reasonable to believe that the thousands of popular instructions on how to protect oneself from cholera had not gone unheeded'.[56] Ironically for a historian of cholera at Naples, Forti Messina failed to discover that the disease ravaged the city in the summer of 1911. Her version of the last European experience of epidemic cholera – that it was an event of no consequence – ends by repeating the misleading accounts contained in the history of Asiatic cholera written for the World Health Organization by R. Pollitzer[57] and in the report of the United States Surgeon-General.

At the heart of the official cover-up is the experience of Naples, which was the storm-centre of the last Italian cholera epidemic. When health bulletins were issued for the United States Public Health Service and later published for posterity, the Italian strategy was to admit a widespread outbreak in the peninsula, but to deny a major calamity in any great urban centre. According to the Italian authorities, the outer ramparts against the disease had been breached at several points, but the defences in depth had held firm. Only a series of limited outbreaks had occurred, and Italy had been spared a serious epidemic. In pursuit of this logic, it was particularly prudent to deny the existence of an epidemic in Italy's largest metropolis, where massive sums of public money had been spent to make the city immune. Naples, therefore, became the centre first of the disease and then of an elaborate fiction.

This fiction was fully and authoritatively stated by Dr Orazio Caro. As Director of the Office of Hygiene, Caro headed the municipal anti-cholera campaign. His Office was responsible for taking the measures necessary to combat the emergency under the overall authority of the Department of Health, which was led by Alderman Giulio Rodinò. Because of his broad mandate in time of medical crisis, Caro was known as the 'supreme *duce*' of public health in the city.[58] In 1914 he published a great falsehood that has misled all discussions of the subject ever since.[59]

Caro's narrative, corroborated by the perjured testimony of Rodinò, his direct superior, is the ideal version of the epidemic as officials in the city wished that they had experienced it. According to Caro's narrative, the arrival of cholera in Apulia confronted Naples with a great challenge. It was the first test of the defences that were intended to make the city free from epidemic cholera. These defences consisted of the prophylactic outer rampart of the bacteriological laboratory of the Office of Hygiene located on the top floor of the Palazzo San Giacomo, and the inner fortifications represented by the achievements of *risanamento* – Serino water, the sewer mains, the improved housing of the population, and the closer contact between the people of Naples and the medical profession. It was only because the anti-cholera bulwarks of the city had never been put to the test that 1910 was a time of great anxiety.

In Caro's account, the city succeeded beyond all expectations in meeting the challenge. The Neapolitan triumph was apparent in the contrast between the course of events in 1910–11 and all previous invasions of the enemy from Bengal. In the sixth pandemic, Caro asserts that the cholera was rapidly and correctly diagnosed, swiftly isolated, and promptly eliminated. Naples, like other cities in modern Europe, had been made cholera-proof. In the wake of the rebuilding programme, there were no longer any sanitary differences between the Upper City and the Lower. *Risanamento* had brought about the sanitary unity of the metropolis by 'the progressive elevation of the poorer classes'.[60] Nowhere was the transformation more evident than in the *sezione* of Vicaria, which had been thoroughly and effectively renewed. Here the people no longer lived in urban caves but in modern houses; here the impoverished *plebe* had been converted by industry into a sturdy and healthy working class.[61] The results were apparent to all. Caro wrote that, 'In our day, cholera remains a frightful and exotic diseases that kills more than half of those it strikes. But we now possess the means to combat it with the necessary vigour and to snuff it out before it spreads.'[62] 'Our city', he reassured his readers, 'was ready to confront any epidemic invasion':

> From the first day of the appearance of the disease in Apulia, we had a clear and precise idea of the measures needed. We acted with rapidity and rigour ... There were no uncertainties or hesitations because everything had been foreseen, studied and arranged, down to the smallest details. In a word, we were ready for the battle.... We can only congratulate ourselves and our city.[63]

To substantiate his case, Caro fabricated a table (Table 6.1) contrasting the outbreak of 1910 with the havoc of 1884.[64]

Apart from the arbitrary figure of 6,971 cholera-deaths in 1884, when the municipality officially recorded 7,143 fatalities and many authorities believed the real total to be significantly higher,[65] the table is intentionally misleading on two grounds. The first is that the estimate that 282 Neapolitans died of cholera in 1910 is far too low, and was achieved only by halving the unpublished official estimates. The Department of Public Health at the Ministry of the Interior recorded the significantly higher figures of 860 cases and 684 deaths, and it noted that the outbreak lasted for a longer period than Caro's notion of immediate victory suggests. According to the Department of Public Health, the disease began in August and lasted until November.[66]

The most deceiving aspect of Caro's table, however, is different. It was pointless to claim victory by contrasting 1884 with 1910 rather than with the far more significant and revealing epidemic year of 1911 that Caro never mentions. The real comparison with the summer of 1884 is the summer of 1911 when thousands perished.

Concluding his specious argument, Caro turned to the atmosphere of the population when cholera reappeared in the city on 25 September. In 1884, the news had produced hysteria manifested in the poisoning frenzy, the dread of physicians, the phobia of disinfection, violent resistance to isolation and every

Table 6.1. *Deaths from cholera in Naples, 1884 and 1910*

	No. of cases	
Sezione	1884	1910
San Ferdinando	138	9
Chiaia	133	10
San Giuseppe	182	3
Montecalvario	212	4
Avvocata	102	15
Stella	176	16
San Carlo all'Arena	161	40
Vicaria	947	74
San Lorenzo	125	4
Mercato	1,507	41
Pendino	876	5
Porto	885	3
Villages	146	38
Hospitals and non-residents	1,381	20
Total	6,971	282

manner of excess. In 1910, the people had full confidence in the defences of their city. They responded, he wrote in a description that has all the hallmarks of mythology,

> like a well drilled army. Every infected residence was carefully disinfected. These disinfections were calmly endured, and often sought by the tenants. The transportation of the sufferers to the hospital for infectious diseases caused no uproar but only a sense of pity. It was possible to isolate thousands of people from every social class in an atmosphere of order and discipline that was absolutely unprecedented and unexpected. The population never lost its serenity and went about its usual business![67]

Rather than correct Caro's observations, Rodinò took the opportunity to honour the memory of Nicola Amore, the true architect of the great sanitary victory. The factors that prevented the recurrence of an epidemic, he stated, were the works achieved by *risanamento* and the splendid organization of the Neapolitan medical services.[68] To honour Caro and Alfonso Montefusco, Director of the Cotugno Hospital, for their efficient and rapid containment of the outbreak in 1910, City Hall held a banquet of triumph at the end of October. And in the new year, it passed a resolution commending them for their conduct.

Caro had every reason to exult. His legend of an impregnable city that heroically saved the nation from epidemic cholera by swiftly repelling the enemy when he appeared in 1910 has stood, unquestioned, as truth. In histories of Liberal Naples the epidemic of 1910–11 in the city has entirely vanished. The authors of the recent history of Naples edited by Giuseppe Galasso, for example, avoid all consideration of cholera after 1884.[69]

Another revealing and very recent example is the study of cholera in Naples by Dr Ugo Fusco and Dr Mario Soscia, who succeeded one another as Medical Directors of the Cotugno Hospital. Without explicitly raising Caro's account in order to test it, they confirm his findings with two minor qualifications. There was a higher mortality from cholera in Naples in 1910, they argue, than is normally thought, and in 1911 there were scattered minor outbreaks in various cities of Italy although 'the phenomenon did not assume vast proportions'. They agree with Caro on the two main points, however. The first point is that in 1910 the disease flared up on 26 September but was rapidly contained so that by 25 October it had been eliminated from the city, never to return until 1973. The second point is that in 1911 Naples 'was not affected' and Italy was spared a major tragedy.[70]

A further instance of the triumph of mythology is the uncritical history of the rebuilding and renewal of Naples by Giuseppe Russo.[71] Although published in 1960, Russo's account of *risanamento* is similar to that of Orazio Caro in charting the triumph of a far-sighted municipal government over poverty, insalubrity and disease. The critics of the project, Russo argues, are motivated by a prejudice against Neapolitans. The Saredo report, he asserts, had a 'libellous character', 'unleashing the most pernicious storm of calumny ever to afflict an entire city, an entire population'.[72] The truth instead is that 'from the sanitary and hygienic point of view the work of *risanamento* fully achieved its purposes'.[73]

If the 'official' version of the events of 1910–12 has completely concealed the truth, what was the real course of the sixth pandemic in Naples? What are the sources for a revisionist account of the ravages of the disease? What were the motivations that led the authorities at both the local and the national levels to conceal reality from the population, from the international community, and from posterity? Why were they so overwhelmingly successful? The intention here is to answer these questions by turning, in the remainder of this chapter to the limited outburst of 1910 and then in Chapter 7 to the substantial but covert epidemic of 1911.

1910: EPIDEMIC DISEASE AND THE THREAT TO LOCAL POWER

When Asiatic cholera returned to Naples in August 1910, it could hardly have appeared at a more inopportune moment for the local authorities. The Catholic administration under Mayor Francesco Del Carretto was under assault by the 'Popular Bloc' – a left-wing alliance of socialists, republicans, syndicalists and radicals, who were seeking to destroy its authority on the specific issue of public health. *Risanamento* and its legacy had come to haunt Del Carretto and his executive committee.

The Catholic majority had governed Naples for a decade – ever since, at the turn of the century, the Left had launched an earlier campaign concentrating on the theme of moral fitness for office. Initiated by the socialist newspaper *La Propaganda*, the moralizing offensive of 1899–1902 resulted in the disgrace and downfall of the Liberal administration of Celestino Summonte and Alberto Casale.[74] In a city with a small, dispersed and poorly organized working class, the Italian Socialist Party (PSI) could never expect to gain electoral success on the basis of class-based issues and the traditional promises of socialism. The strategy devised by the socialist leaders Arnaldo Lucci, Ettore Ciccotti and Arturo Labriola focused instead on corruption, favouritism, and the collusion of the government of Naples with the Camorra. Joining forces with the radicals and republicans, the PSI mounted challenges to the most tainted officials in the elections of 1900, carefully documenting a series of sensational allegations of criminal corruption.

In the summer of 1900 Naples experienced a seismic political shock when the ruling political machine suffered a series of unexpected electoral defeats. In a wave of public outrage against the Camorra, reform candidates such as Ciccotti and De Martino were elected in the boroughs of Vicaria, Mercato and Porto – the previously impregnable fiefdoms of the notorious Liberal Deputy and *camorrista* Alberto Casale and his associates. These first victories were consolidated in the autumn when Casale, publicly accused by *La Propaganda* of electoral fraud, favouritism and graft, unsuccessfully sued the newspaper for libel. The revelations produced by the defence in the trial – one of the most famous in modern Italian history – were substantiated by the testimony of members of parliament, prefects, cabinet ministers and high-ranking police officers. The case made by the socialist paper was accepted as proven by the court, the libel charges were dismissed and Casale was ordered to pay all the costs of the litigation. The result was a national political sensation that forced the state to dissolve the municipal government and to appoint the commission of enquiry chaired by Giuseppe Saredo. The Saredo Report, published in 1901, comprehensively discredited the Liberal parties of Naples. In the local elections of 1901 they were swept from office. The clerico-moderates formed a new majority on the city council, and the Left was rewarded by the election of a substantial cohort of opposition councillors.

A decade of Catholic administration failed, however, to produce the anticipated moral reform. The clerico-moderates in office conformed to the familiar local pattern of favouritism, inertia, and clientage politics. *Avanti!*, the socialist newspaper, described its disappointment in the spring of 1910, writing that,

> Certain figures who were thought to have disappeared forever, who had not set foot in the corridors of city hall since the Saredo enquiry, have returned. Acts of complicity that one assumed had been permanently eliminated are once more in vogue. The operating methods of the Summonte regime can be seen again. Above all, the representatives of companies exposed in the Casale trial have regained their courage, and are again arranging contracts and applying for licences.[75]

In the summer of 1910 the Left returned to the offensive. Sensing that, like his Liberal predecessors, Del Carretto might be vulnerable to a moral challenge, the

'Popular Bloc' launched a new campaign to coincide with the July elections, which took place just weeks before cholera reappeared. Under the existing electoral law and with the political traditions of the city, there was no realistic hope that the Popular Bloc with its strength among workers, students at the University and enlightened professionals would win a majority of seats on the Neapolitan city council. The immediate aspiration of the Popular Bloc was instead to form a substantial and truculent opposition in the Council Chambers, with the hope that the vigorous exposure of the problems of the city in the months that followed would further erode the strength of the administration. If, as already seemed likely, parliament passed an electoral reform that significantly broadened the franchise, the prospects for the opposition would significantly improve and in due course a second stunning victory might be won.

Led by Lucci and Ciccotti, the victorious strategists of Casale's downfall, the *bloccardi* charged that the record of the Catholic administration in the field of public health destroyed its moral mandate to govern. In a keynote speech in the campaign, the opposition councillor Ettore Epifania reminded the voters of the disappointed expectations of the administrative 'revolution' of 1901. 'The clerico-moderates', he charged,

> took office under exceptionally favourable moral and financial conditions. The moral campaign initiated by the socialists and supported by all the popular forces of the city had crushed the Casale machine ... But the Catholics have taken no advantage of the opportunity, or of the cleansed moral climate.[76]

On the contrary, the executive committee had fallen into inertia and business as usual. Naples was still waiting for its political and moral redemption.

The central accusation made by Epifania and the Bloc against the municipal majority led by the triumvirate of Del Carretto, Arlotta and Rodinò was that it had failed to complete the great task of urban renewal. Renewal was the key to the resolution of all the great issues that affected the lives of Neapolitans – employment, accommodation and health. The new Catholic regime, moreover, had not been denied the opportunity to carry the mutilated programme to a more satisfactory conclusion. To enable the new Neapolitan administration to rise from the ruins of the Casale era, the state had voted substantial new funds in 1902 and 1908 to restore the municipal budget to health, to ensure economic development and to guarantee the belated completion of *risanamento*. Unfortunately, the new regime displayed no more zeal in matters of public welfare than the old, and the results of the money spent were nowhere apparent – only the 'usual swindling', Epifania informed the electors. The budget by 1910 showed a deficit of 15 million lire; 'disastrous contracts' had been signed with dubious contractors; public services had reached a state of dangerous disorganization; and 'every vital interest' of the population had been neglected, from housing to diet.[77]

In a public debate with Giulio Rodinò at the height of the campaign, Arnaldo Lucci argued that the Catholic administration had held power long enough to have assumed the responsibility for the failure of renewal. Naples, Lucci declared in his peroration, 'is uncivilized because of its filth and squalor. It has the appearance of a peasant village rather than a great city. And all of this is the fault of the present administration!'[78]

The charges levelled by the Bloc coincided with a period of depression in the local economy. As a result, the accusations made by Epifania and Lucci fell on fertile soil. Neapolitans were anxious and restive. There were angry demonstrations in the spring and summer of 1910 about housing, the cost of living, health and unemployment. Indeed, the spontaneous protests of the people in the streets may have provided the incentive for the opposition to launch a great electoral offensive. In this tense climate the campaign rapidly assumed apocalyptic tones reminiscent of the elections at the turn of the century. The Catholic candidates were clearly defensive and frightened that history could repeat itself – that Lucci and his colleagues could engineer a second municipal revolution. The tone of Catholic rhetoric demonstrates a considerable unease. Although the Popular Bloc avoided issues of class, the electoral organizations representing the administration – officially designated as the 'United Associations' – were known as the 'parties of order' as if their mission were to defend religion, civilization and property against red revolution and social levelling. Raising the temperature of the campaign to a fever, the Catholic candidates referred to their opponents as 'anarchists' and 'subversives'.[79]

The results of the election vindicated Lucci's strategy. Del Carretto, as anticipated, returned as mayor, but he and his clerico-moderate colleagues now had to contend with a strengthened and more aggressive opposition. Furthermore, Catholic fears were deepened by their much poorer performance in the simultaneous election held for the renewal of the provincial council. There the outgoing clerico-moderates standing for re-election were all defeated, with the single exception of councillor Carola in the constituency of Porto.[80]

Appropriately for the times, the first meeting of the eighty members of the city council began with fisticuffs between the Catholics and their enemies. The Catholic paper *La Libertà* warned its readers that, 'The rabble sits in the city council!' With the representatives of the 'Popular Bloc', it asserted,

> The council chamber of Naples has been invaded by all the lower depths of Mercato and the borough of Vicaria. They have arrived with the unworthy intention of making noise, of preventing free discussion, of insulting the most notable personalities of the majority. People like Epifania, Lucci and Altobelli, who call themselves intelligent, unleash the uproar, shout and hurl themselves upon their colleagues. They defend the mob and exalt the Camorra.[81]

The issue was drawn, and the question was whether the Left could again find a weapon that, like the Casale trial or the Saredo enquiry, would deliver a mortal blow to the ruling party. If a new electoral law was passed extending the suffrage, the political landscape of Naples would prove ripe for transformation. Such was the pressure, moreover, that suffrage reform was a dominant public issue. In November 1910 Luzzatti, as had been widely expected, presented a bill to make literacy the only requirement for males over the age of 21, thereby removing the property qualification and raising the electorate from 2.9 to 4.5 million.[82] Luzzatti's ministry collapsed before passage of the bill into law, but in June 1910 his successor, Giovanni Giolitti, presented a still more radical and ultimately successful proposal for nearly universal male suffrage.[83] The expectation of an extended electorate, therefore, already formed part of the political calculations of the Popular Bloc.

It was in this charged atmosphere that cholera arrived. Just days after the election, the first mysterious cases occurred, raising the spectre that the opposition would find a sanitary equivalent of the Casale or Saredo episodes – a dramatic and authenticated revelation of the deficiencies of local government. A medical emergency would give substance to the charges levelled by Lucci and Epifania. The socialist doctor Giuseppe Tropeano, writing for *La Propaganda*, the instrument of Casale's political demise, gave a sample of what could be expected. Tropeano argued that the sanitary negligence of the Carretto regime was such that, 'If cholera were to break out in Naples, ... the father of every family that lost a child would have the right to hold the Mayor of Naples liable for criminal and civil damages!'[84]

Under the pressure of such a menace, the representatives of the incumbent administration greeted the early reports of cholera in the city with scorn. Giulio Rodinò responded to the anxiety of an opposition councillor by demanding that he not insult the administration. To question the immunity of Naples was 'unpatriotic': unfounded accusations of cholera would ruin the city.[85] Exploring a line of argument that Orazio Caro would soon make his own, the officers of the city assured the public that a return of cholera was impossible because the success of *risanamento* and the medical services provided by the administration had made the city permanently cholera-proof.

Alfonso Montefusco, Medical Director of the Cotugno, was politically correct when on 17 September he discussed cholera in an interview for *La Libertà*, the Catholic newspaper and friend of the Del Carretto administration. By that date cholera had already broken out in the city and Montefusco, as the Director of the Cotugno Hospital, was necessarily more aware of this fact than anyone else. Nevertheless, hoping that the disease would be contained without the need for a public admission of its presence, he resolutely denied that Naples could ever be vulnerable to Asiatic cholera. 'First of all,' he reasoned,

the cholera in Apulia can be said to be over. The admirable organization of our national Department of Public Health immediately conquered the infection, and there is no reason to doubt the health bulletins of the day. But in any case Naples ... has nothing to fear. In our city we are too inclined to criticize everything, to despise everything that is ours.

Of course no one would dare to say that the organization of the Neapolitan sanitary services is perfect, but they are by no means inferior to those of other cities. ...

It is sufficient for you to know that Naples is in no danger. In our day an epidemic of cholera in Naples is impossible because of the great works of hygiene that have been carried out – the aqueduct, the sewers, the *risanamento* – and because of the fine organization of our medical services.[86]

'Our water,' he noted in conclusion, 'is the best in the world.' *La Libertà* loyally supported Montefusco's analysis of Neapolitan conditions, editorializing that, 'There is no cholera in Naples, and never has been since 1884. Nor is there any possibility ... that it can ever return.'[87]

Other interested and informed observers took a less optimistic view of the medical condition of Naples. One such person was Dr Henry Downes Geddings, Medical Officer in Command of the USPH&MHS stationed at the American Consulate in Naples. Geddings was an authority on Asiatic cholera who had represented the United States at the International Sanitary Convention at Paris in 1903. Because of the large numbers of Italian emigrants departing from Naples to New York, the city was a strategic posting, and H. D. Geddings had been entrusted with the delicate task of following the course of infectious diseases in Naples in order to determine whether ships sailing from the port should be cleared for passage to North America. In accordance with practices that dated from the seventeenth-century anti-plague regulations, his instructions were to issue ships with bills of health that were of three sorts – 'foul', 'clean' and 'suspect'.

From 24 August this representative of the USPH&MHS became convinced that many of the cases formally diagnosed as 'gastro-enteritis' by Neapolitan health officers were in fact victims of Asiatic cholera. Between 24 August and 18 September – well before the official Italian announcement on 25 September – Geddings recorded seventy-two deaths that he regarded as cholera, despite the resolute denials of Neapolitan officials.[88] The USPH&MHS received confidential information by secretly cultivating relations with a prominent Professor of Medicine at the University. The informant was subsequently revealed to be Professor Vincenzo De Giaxa, an authority on cholera and a member of the Royal Hygiene Society who was well connected with municipal doctors. He was paid a retainer fee by the American Consulate.[89] Through De Giaxa, who provided reliable information throughout 1910–12, Geddings learned that the symptoms of cases officially diagnosed as 'gastro-enteritis communis' were identical to those of Asiatic cholera and that death frequently followed within hours of seizure.[90]

On 7 September the American doctor informed Washington that he was convinced of the presence of authentic cholera in Naples. Seeking confirmation for his suspicions, he obtained interviews with the Prefect and the officials of the Office of Hygiene. Prefect De Seta insisted that there was no cause for alarm or for doubts about the accuracy of the prevailing diagnoses. Meanwhile municipal health officials refused the American's requests for additional information, instructing Geddings that in future he should address all official queries to the American Ambassador, who could contact the Ministry of the Interior in Rome. These interviews suggested duplicity. More darkly, Geddings began to suggest that the atmosphere surrounding the officials of the USPH&MHS in Naples was becoming hostile and full of menace.

As Alan Kraut reminds us, reports from the USPH&MHS cannot be accepted uncritically because the service was born in part of a fear of foreigners, and especially of such impecunious and diseased immigrants as southern Italians.[91] In American immigration policies, science and xenophobia were intertwined. Even after allowance is made for the anti-Italian rhetoric of Geddings and his colleagues, however, the conditions they encountered were clearly dramatic. Describing a situation that was soon to lead to death-threats directed against himself and his subordinates, Geddings wrote cryptically to the Surgeon-General that,

> it is impossible to adequately inform you of the difficulties by which the situation is surrounded here, and the terms in which to express it would be out of place in an official communication. I can only say that .... I am at a loss whom to trust, and have gotten to the point where I doubt every statement made to me, which is not accompanied by documentary verification.[92]

For an authority on cholera whose anxieties had already been thus aroused, Neapolitian figures for 'gastro-enteritis' in the week from 18 September were unacceptably suspicious, especially since 90 per cent of the cases ended in death. The official records of gastro-enteritis for that week are shown in Table 6.2.[93] On Sunday, 26 September Geddings unilaterally reported to Washington that Naples was in the midst of an epidemic of Asiatic cholera. The French, British, Spanish and Portuguese Consuls also began to issue foul bills of health that proclaimed the city an infected port.[94]

Geddings's explanation for the sudden flare-up of cases on Friday, 21 September was in line with the epidemiological experience of 1884. Just as in 1884, he reasoned that the disease had simmered slowly for a month before breaking out in epidemic force. Since late August, Geddings maintained, cholera had been continuously present in Naples in the form of a slender but unbroken chain of 'sporadic' cases. Many of these cases, he argued,

> have been stricken upon the streets of the city, where the lower classes of Neapolitans spend most of their time. Naturally the streets have been more or less soiled by the dejections and the vomiting of these cases, and as in some of these streets the sun never penetrates, there has been little opportunity for the germicidal action of sunlight.[95]

For several weeks the consequences for public health remained slight – until two developments provided favourable circumstances for a sudden upsurge in the disease. The first was a change in the weather. During August and the first half of September the weather had been dry and hot without relief. Then on 19 September torrential rains began and lasted for a week. The result was that, 'while some of the filth of the streets was washed into the sewers, much also was distributed more widely and carried to points more or less remote from its point of origin'.[96] Wells, cisterns and the harbour were abundantly contaminated.

At the same time that rain exposed the population to danger, dietary excesses associated with the feast of San Gennaro on 19 September lowered resistance to

Table 6.2. *Cases of gastro-enteritis in Naples,*
18–24 September, 1910

Date	Cases
18 September	11
19 September	3
20 September	4
21 September	11
22 September	44
23 September	20
24 September	94

the cholera bacillus. On that day, Geddings explained, there was 'much feasting and carousing, with the probable consumption of many tons of foodstuffs of all kinds, much of which was in all probability unfit for consumption'. The results were apparent in the sharp upturn in mortality on the 22nd, 23rd and 24th, and in Geddings's unambiguous warning of the 26th, when he condemned the 'policy of concealment' of the Neapolitan authorities.[97] 'Other bacteriologists,' Geddings concluded,

> and some of great repute, have all along had no doubt of the nature of the disease prevailing in Naples, but Prof. Caro has been unamenable to reason, and is believed by many who are informed to have received instructions from superior authority to persist in his ruinous policy.[98]

In addition to Henry Geddings, another anxious and suspicious observer of Neapolitan affairs was the alderman who directed the Department of Health of the city of Rome, Dr Tullio Rossi-Doria. He was concerned that travellers arriving from Naples could infect the capital. On 15 September – two days before Montefusco's public reassurances – Rossi-Doria wrote in alarm to the Ministry of the Interior,

> Because I have personally conducted investigations by means that I am not at liberty to reveal, it is known to me that Naples is infected with authentic Asiatic cholera.
>
> I know this despite the repeated denials of the Ministry to our public health officer.[99]

Despite the fact that he received no satisfactory reply to his enquiry, Rossi-Doria ordered that all railroad passengers from Naples be medically examined upon arrival in Rome and that their personal effects be disinfected.

The suspicions of Geddings and Rossi-Doria were also raised in the Naples city council by Altobelli and Moresca on 26 August. They informed their colleagues that insistent rumours of suspect cases were sweeping Naples, that there was a mysterious flurry of activity at the Cotugno Hospital and that the filthy state of the streets was spreading anxiety.[100]

Concern that cholera had already invaded the metropolis was voiced from early September by local newspapers opposed to the ruling clerico-moderates. They were unmoved by a systematic municipal campaign of disinformation and pressure to refrain from reporting accurate medical news. On 18 September the ever vigilant *La Propaganda* raised the question of whether Naples was already in the grip of a cholera outburst. Without reaching a definitive answer, the syndicalist paper observed that the Neapolitan people no longer had any doubt that the disease had broken out.[101]

More audacious still in its medical reportage was the republican paper *Roma*, which on Friday 26 August revealed a first suspect case, which it recorded as having occurred two days earlier – on the same date mentioned by Geddings as the beginning of the Neapolitan outbreak.[102] Thereafter *Roma* carried almost daily accounts of possible cases of Asiatic cholera. Intriguingly, its correspondents' descriptions of popular responses to the disease bear no resemblance to the stoic and confident heroism that Caro later depicted. In late August and September 1910 *Roma* reported an atmosphere resembling 1884. As in the fifth pandemic, the wealthy classes fled the city for safe havens while the poor violently resisted the municipal doctors. *Roma* recorded 'savage scenes', 'rebellions', 'assaults', 'threats', 'menacing demonstrations', 'disorders' and 'serious ferment'.[103] With its evident mission of disgracing the Del Carretto regime, the republican daily was not entirely free of sensationalism.

There were, however, scattered and authenticated examples of violent tumult. One instance was the uproar in the borough of Mercato that greeted the arrival of the disinfection team at the home of Maria Grazia Camilli, the 40-year-old wife of a worker in the *sezione* who died at the beginning of the first week of September. *Roma* described the events that ensued in the following terms:

> This time as well the lower classes began to raise a furore instead of assisting the arriving officials. Disgusting scenes took place. A municipal vehicle was stoned and its front windows were smashed. And the unreasonable, brutal mob would have done far worse if municipal guards, carabinieri and a platoon of sailors had not intervened.
>
> After infinite difficulty and in the midst of an indescribable tumult, the body of the deceased Camilli was loaded onto a car and carried away, accompanied by a large police escort.[104]

Such events validated the suspicion of some residents that the twentieth century had arrived in Naples without effecting a fundamental transformation in the urban environment or in social attitudes. This suspicion was articulated by the Popular Bloc. The accounts in *Roma* of violent clashes, however dramatized by the rhetoric of a political campaign, were not inventions. Proving an enduring distrust for authority, they are confirmed by a confidential and unimpeachable report prepared for Rocco Santoliquido, the Director-General of Public Health, on the health of Naples. This document acknowledges that in the autumn of 1910 there were 'frequent riots' in the city when officials arrived to remove cadavers, disinfect apartments or transport patients to the Cotugno.[105] In addition, the reports in the republican paper were corroborated by the surprising candour of one of the dominant figures in the Neapolitan establishment – the Deputy Arlotta, a veteran of 1884. He declared that, although the outbreak of 1910 was mild and brief, it gave rise to more terror than the great disaster of 1884. So acute was the fear that 80,000 Neapolitans fled the city.[106] Arlotta spoke in order to denounce the policy of secrecy, on the grounds that it led inevitably to rumour, distrust and panic.

Although it is important not to accept blindly the accounts of the Popular Bloc press, the critical comments of Arlotta, or the occasional alarms of the Department of Public Health as objective assessments of the atmosphere of the city, they provide an important corrective to the triumphant claims of the ruling party and its spokesmen. At both the national and local levels, the public statements of officials were far from candid. Their mendacity is demonstrated by the direct testimony by the highest state authority in Naples. In a confidential telegram already labelled 'the return of cholera', Prefect De Seta on 10 September informed his superiors at the Ministry of the Interior that,

> Both in my correspondence with foreign consuls and in my relations with the press and the general public I have not failed to observe the secrecy necessary in my position. The silence of the Neapolitan newspapers with regard to the disease that has broken out here is due to my influence and persuasion. But I cannot exercise the same influence over papers that are published elsewhere, especially if they are not supporters of the government.[107]

De Seta assured his masters that he could maintain the secrecy observed by the Prefecture and the Police Department. He was worried, however, about City Hall, which was more porous because of the many temporary employees in its service – people whose willingness to lie could not be guaranteed.

A week after De Seta expressed his belief that he could contain the situation in Naples, the Italian Foreign Minister, San Giuliano, cabled Luzzatti with the outline of a new diplomatic offensive. San Giuliano's plan was to dissuade foreign powers from taking public health measures against steamships sailing from Italian ports. The means would include both persuasion and coercion. Persuasion was to be carried out by the Italian diplomatic service that would be instructed to lavish assurances on governments abroad that Italy was 'absolutely free from cholera'. To make the argument more convincing, the Italian Government would threaten countries taking unfriendly sanitary measures with reprisals against their imports into Italy.[108]

Just as San Giuliano's telegram was reaching its destination, however, his scheme to preserve the fiction of a cholera-free Naples became obsolete. As the number of deaths from the disease rose sharply, and as rumours and press accounts grew ever more insistent, further concealment became impossible. On 25 September, therefore, the municipal government belatedly announced that Asiatic cholera was prevailing in the city. Commenting on the outbreak, Orazio Caro explained in an interview with the local paper *Il Giorno* that the breach in the sanitary defences through which the disease had invaded the city was the unfinished sewer system, which still poured untreated waste into the waters of the harbour.[109] Here, Caro reported, 'is the source of all our troubles'. Bacteriological tests had determined that the Bay of Naples was contaminated with the cholera bacillus. The most likely explanation for the outbreak was that the dejecta of the initial cases imported from Apulia had polluted the Bay, which in turn compromised the health of all who used its waters. The early cases broke out, Caro continued, among residents who had contact with the sea – bathers, fishermen, sailors and consumers of local shellfish. The first recognized Neapolitan case was Ernesto Vigilante, a cobbler and professional thief from the quarter of Santa Lucia, the neighbourhood of fishermen.[110]

On the nefarious role of the waters of the harbour, if on nothing else, Henry Geddings and Orazio Caro agreed. Geddings believed that the waters of the Bay had been polluted by unrecognized cases among Apulian cholera-fugitives and emigrants. The unifinished Neapolitan sewer network poured raw waste from the Lower City, where the emigrant lodging-houses were located, directly into the harbour. The first four cases of cholera for which he had received reliable information occurred during the last week of August and the first week of September among people who had been in contact with harbour water in the vicinity of the sewer outfall. These cases were those of an elderly female ragpicker who had sorted through waste on the city beaches, two street urchins who had gone swimming in the Bay, and a fisherman. It was the further misfortune of the city, Geddings reported, that 'in one corner of this same harbor are beds for the propagation of mussels, a favourite article of food among the lower Neapolitan population'.[111]

Vigilante, the cobbler and part-time burglar, was taken to the Cotugno Hospital, where he recovered; his family and closest contacts were detained for observation; his home was disinfected and the building was isolated by a line of police. In the aftermath of this first recognized case, conditions in the city were starkly described in the *New York Times*. On the day of the public announcement, the New York paper estimated that Naples already had 100 new cases and 80 deaths[112]. Under large headlines announcing '100,000 Flee from Cholera in Naples' and 'Persons Die in Streets and the Inhabitants of the City are in a Panic', the *New York Times* reported:

> With the removal of the censorship, startling news in regard to the cholera epidemic in Naples is being received.
>
> A number of persons have died in the streets, and the popular excitement is such that the police have great difficulty in maintaining public order.
>
> It is reported that 100,000 of the better classes have already fled from Naples. . . .
>
> Most of the cases are in the most squalid quarters of the city – in the Vicaria and Mercato districts . . .
>
> The authorities, who long concealed the truth from the public, until the press made known the real state of affairs, are now doing their utmost to relieve the situation.[113]

Unlike 1884, in 1910 the confirmation that Naples was an infected city was not followed by a season of official candour. City Hall had resisted making a statement until silence had become counter-productive, enlarging rumour and spreading incredulity. After the announcement, the strategy adopted by the Palazzo San Giacomo was to reassure the population by minimizing all public assessments of the danger. In a meeting on 28 September, the *giunta* decided that, in the interest of prudence, it would fabricate 'official' figures relating to the disease. Prefect De Seta reported the event by declaring that, 'With regard ... to the compilation of bills of health, the administrators of the city decided in a meeting yesterday that it was advisable to publish *statistics that approximate the truth*, just as I did this morning.'[114] To reinforce this policy, the administration ceased after the first week of the outbreak to publish official bulletins.[115]

In the columns of the semi-official *La Libertà*, the results of the municipal policy were sometimes unintentionally amusing. The Catholic paper refrained, for example, from all acknowledgement of cholera until 28 September. On that date – supposedly the first day of the epidemic – the paper launched its coverage of the disease with the announcement that conditions had 'improved'.[116] Thereafter *La Libertà* devoted scant space to public health, and its columns provided a sustaining diet of optimism. An illustration of its *modus operandi* was the premature headline of 1 October proclaiming that, 'The disease is abating'.[117]

Don Marzio, the scourge of the 'Popular Bloc', took a more truculent stance. During the weeks of silence preceding the announcement of 25 September, the newspaper of the Neapolitan Right had taken an uncompromising line on issues of public health. Its argument was that, in matters of hygiene, 'Naples has no grounds to envy any city in the world'![118] Throughout August and the first weeks of September *Don Marzio* steadfastly repeated that, 'There is no cholera!'[119] The editors even made medical diagnoses, declaring that various cases of severe diarrhoeal illness were only benign gastro-enteritis.[120] Within the framework of this uncompromising position there was no room for extended discussion of the unwelcome malady from Bengal or of the problems of sanitation that it laid bare. During the entire month following the official municipal admission on 25 September, *Don Marzio* printed only five articles on cholera, and these were so worded as almost to constitute denials of its presence. The first article proclaimed the good news that the 'little epidemic' was 'almost over', and the remaining reports informed the population that the news was 'constantly improving' (28–9 September) and that the outbreak was 'almost at an end' (2–3 October).[121] By the reckoning of this optimistic daily paper, the disease lasted only ten days.[122]

At the Cotugno Hospital, which he had recently declared to be in deplorable condition, Alfonso Montefusco even had a rush of therapeutic optimism. On 28 September – just three days after the first acknowledged case – he announced that the cholera hospital was achieving a remarkable recovery rate of over 60 per cent. Such an early announcement suggested that the Cotugno was curing victims of *cholera gravis* almost before it admitted them. Contradicting his own recent description of the institution, Montefusco went on to claim that the experience of patients on the Cotugno cholera wards was so positive that grateful convalescents were the best possible agents to overcome the irrational fear of the hospital among the *popolino*.[123]

The defensiveness of leading members of the local administration is understandable. As the Catholic majority had feared, the left-wing opposition eagerly seized on the disease to castigate the authorities of the city. Thus the onset of cholera initiated a season of acute schizophrenia in the Neapolitan press with regard to sanitary matters. On the one side, Catholic and Liberal newspapers virtually ignored Asiatic cholera while, on the other hand, republican and socialist journals charged City Hall with criminal negligence. With an epidemic to support its charges, *Roma* restored the vexed question of *risanamento* to the centre of political debate. 'In essence,' the republican paper reasoned, 'the present epidemic, that they [i.e. the local authorities] tried at all costs to keep secret in order to hide responsibilities and omissions, places the issue of *risanamento* back on the political agenda.'[124]

While the opposition press launched its offensive, the labour movement, led by the Borsa del Lavoro, organized rallies and demonstrations to protest at the sanitary neglect revealed by the return of cholera. Addressing an audience of local workers, for instance, the republican Corsio Bovio and the ubiquitous socialists Lucci and Ciccotti castigated the administration for failing to safeguard the proletariat by means of adequate urban renewal. 'If the programme planned by Amore had been carried out in its entirety,' *Roma* echoed the day's oratory, 'today the boroughs of Mercato and Vicaria would not have the lion's share of the cases of cholera and gastro-enteritis.'[125]

The revolutionary *La Propaganda* called for 'the identification of those responsible' for the disease. 'Only now', it protested, 'are the Prefect and the Mayor discovering Vicaria.' Ever available to the paper for interviews in which to attack the ruling classes, Dr Giuseppe Tropeano made the most of his opportunity:

> What we see today in the boroughs of Porto, Mercato, San Ferdinando, Vicaria and Chiaia is the darkest and most painful spectacle that the human mind can conceive.
>
> For two hundred thousand Neapolitans, air, light and water are luxury items, as are unadulterated bread and meat that is not in a state of putrefaction.
>
> It is shameful, gentlemen, to be a Neapolitan in these circumstances!
>
> The truth is this: Naples must be rebuilt! And we must not allow a few incompetent administrators to rebuild it.[126]

Under such intense pressure from the opposition, the administration determinedly avoided any admission that would give credence to the charges levelled by the 'Popular Bloc'. This policy led the executive and its supporters first to deny the truth and subsequently to minimize the danger. But considerations of power and fear of the Left were not the only considerations in the calculations of the Mayor and his aldermen. In addition to posing a political challenge, cholera threatened to undermine the Neapolitan economy by halting emigration, the most important local industry. Here was a second great incentive to secrecy.

1910: GERMS, EMIGRANTS AND THE THREAT TO THE LIFE OF A SEAPORT

Long depressed and vulnerable, the Neapolitan economy received a major fillip at the turn of the century. The new source of dynamism was mass trans-oceanic emigration, which began in the 1880s and lasted until the outbreak of the First World War. This vast exodus of southerners to the New World was a response, first of all, to 'push' factors that drove impoverished peasants off the land. As an economically backward region, the Mezzogiorno was unable to provide more than precarious employment for the growing mass of its population. Industry was virtually non-existent except in isolated pockets in Naples and its hinterland. At the same time the fragility of the all-important agricultural sector was demonstrated by primitive crop rotations, an absence of animal husbandry, a lack of irrigation and fertilizers, an archaic technology and low yields per acre that fluctuated wildly in accordance with the elements. The mass of the population, which depended for its living on the land, was therefore condemned to poverty, illiteracy and permanent under-or unemployment.

Already vulnerable because of its backward productive structures, southern agriculture was further weakened by a series of severe dislocations in the closing decades of the nineteenth century. These dislocations included population growth and pressure on scarce resources; high and regressive taxation; the relentless privatization of common land and the resulting extinction of the collective rights on which peasant subsistence depended; the worsening of the terms of agricultural contracts; phylloxera and the destruction of Italian vineyards; the completion of a unified world market system and the competition it entailed from more capitalized and rational producers; protectionism and the resulting pressure on consumers; and low wages. The accumulating pressures of economic hardship persuaded millions to emigrate overseas.

Charting the overseas migration of Italians as their great exodus began in the 1880s, the American consular service correctly attributed the phenomenon to widespread economic hardship in the countryside of the Mezzogiorno. B.D. Duncan, the Consul at Naples, observed that German emigrants took flight to avoid the military conscripter; Italian peasants, by contrast, sought to evade the tax collector. Emigration, he informed Washington,

> is owing mainly to heavy taxation which renders labor unremunerative either to employer or employed. In parts of Italy and especially in the poorest parts the taxation for Government purposes ... amounts to 40 to 50% and even more of the agricultural hands. It is no wonder then that the laborer is poorly remunerated, that his life is a terribly hard one, and that he should seek relief by emigration.[127]

The American official was overly selective in isolating taxation, but he was accurate in attributing the decision to emigrate to poverty – a conclusion on which contemporary observers and subsequent students of Italian emigration have agreed.[128]

For this reason, the social profile of the typical emigrant was that of an impoverished peasant or farm labourer. Duncan's successor, Edward Camphausen, wrote in 1888 that,

> The persons emigrated from this country to the United States during the last two years belong to the poorest and most ignorant classes; they are without any school education and with few exceptions are unable to write their names; they have no conception of our institutions and form of Government.... Their sole aim is the amelioration of their pecuniary condition.... The average fortune of this class of people at the time of landing at New York does not exceed twenty lire or four dollars.
>
> Of the persons emigrating to the United States from here 85 or 90 per cent are farm hands and the balance journeymen mechanics, mainly tailors, shoemakers and carpenters. They are not as a rule first class mechanics or artisans.[129]

Camphausen neglected to add that the steam revolution in trans-oceanic transportation effectively created a single international labour market by providing speedy and reliable journey times, and by reducing the cost of trans-Atlantic fares, which oscillated between 175 and 220 lire for the whole period down to the First World War. These rates enabled residents of Calabria and Sicily to reach North America more cheaply than Germany.

The economic impetus behind the emigrant flood from the Mezzogiorno to the United States was exhaustively examined by the Immigration Commission under the chairmanship of Senator William P. Dillingham that reported in 1911.[130] The wages for Italian farm workers in Italy varied widely, the Commission found, according to region and the season of the year. The year-round mean national daily wage for adult male farm hands, however, was only $0.40 to $0.50 (2 to 2.5 lire) in 1905. In parts of Calabria and Sicily the remuneration for a ten-hour day in the fields was only $0.14 to $0.20.[131] Such pay necessarily implied hunger.[132]

Indeed, it was the very fact that poverty caused emigration that generated the enthusiasm of Francesco Saverio Nitti. Nitti concluded that the enormous rural exodus had a great transforming power of unrivalled importance for the Mezzogiorno: it drew impoverished and disaffected peasants from their native villages and converted them upon their return into sturdy and contented small proprietors, the social base for a new 'rural democracy'.[133]

At the same time that economic hardship drove peasants from the South of Italy, the recovery of the international economy; industrial advance and urbanization in the United States; and the bringing into cultivation of vast tracts of virgin land in Latin America created an insatiable demand for unskilled manual labour. Italy, of course, took a modest part in the international economic spurt, but the industrial take-off between 1896 and 1914 involved the North rather than the whole of the peninsula. In a classic case of economic dualism, the South remained backward, agricultural and poor. For this reason the Mezzogiorno could not sustain its people, but at the same time northern industry failed to expand with sufficient dynamism to absorb the surplus population. Southern Italian migrants, unable to find work at home, therefore filled the demand in North and South America. In one of the great population movements of modern

European history, millions of southern Italians emigrated overseas between 1880 and 1914, the majority of them with the intention to return to their native country when they had accumulated sufficient savings to buy land. Men from Calabria, Sicily, Apulia, the Abruzzi, Campania and Basilicata worked as railroad navvies, mill hands, street-sweepers, miners and builders in New York, Boston, Chicago and Philadelphia. By 1910 New York alone contained more Calabrians than any city in Calabria and more Basilicatans than the two largest cities in Basilicata combined.[134]

After the United States, the second great destination for Italian emigrants was Argentina. In the Argentine Republic the 'pull' factor was not, however, the development of industry but rather the settlement of the immense territory of the interior and its conversion to terraculture.[135] Until the foundation of the Argentine Republic in 1859 and the establishment of a strong general government, the vast expanse of the pampas had been devoted to the grazing of sheep and cattle. Despite the fact that the land was among the most fertile in the world, the barriers to cultivation had been insurmountable – remoteness, lack of security, shortage of labour and the absence of means of communication. In a country with an area of 2,000,000 square kilometres, only 1,000,000 acres of land were under cultivation at the time of unification and Argentina lived through the import of breadstuffs. The establishment of a strong general government committed to economic development through the modernization of the countryside transformed the situation. The Republic created political stability, built railroads into the interior, and encouraged a vast immigration of Italian peasants to till the soil. The Argentine Government subsidized passage, offered vast tracts of land for purchase and undertook a great publicity and recruitment campaign. By 1881 the American Consul at Buenos Aires could already report that an agricultural revolution was in full progress on the South American frontier, and especially in the provinces of Buenos Aires and Santa Fé. The breadth of agricultural land had doubled in the previous decade, and the nation had become a net exporter of agricultural produce and a limitless importer of unskilled labour. Once despised by *gauchos* and ranchers, agriculture had become the pillar of the economy and the key to its development.

If economic factors underlay the exodus of Italians to North and South America, the movement was greatly magnified by the activities of an army of 'emigration agents', 'sub-agents' and 'representatives' of the steamship companies. 41,000 of them operated in Italy, and especially its southern provinces, in 1911. The agents and sub-agents were local notables – merchants, municipal councillors, teachers, shopkeepers, lawyers, bankers, pharmacists and parish priests – prepared to use their influence and prestige in the interest of profit. Since the movement of cheap Italian labour overseas was one of the most profitable of contemporary business investments, the great navigation companies worked tirelessly to ensure that the flow continued. For this purpose they employed agents working on a commission basis. The agents earned an average of 65 lire for every steerage passenger they recruited, plus bonuses if they succeeded in filling a designated ship to capacity. Motivated by the generous fees to be made from every increase in their productivity, the agents earned an evil reputation for the misleading portraits they painted of the opportunities available for Italians in the Americas, and for the ruthless ingenuity with which they exploited the vulnerability of an ignorant and illiterate clientele. Virtually unregulated by the state, they employed every means, both legal and illegal, to increase the numbers of bodies they delivered to the docks.

In the midst of the great spurt in the international economy, the demand for cheap manual labour was so great that the agents frequently also worked directly on the behalf of North and South American employers – mine owners, railroad companies, mill operators and planters. Like the steamship tycoons, these entrepreneurs paid the agents a fee for every labourer they delivered. Most profitable of all was the highly illegal system of 'prepaid' tickets and 'contract labour', which constituted a modern form of indenture. Industrialists and farmers instructed the agents to pay the fares of Italian labourers in advance, on the agreement that the first claim on their wages in the New World would be a deduction to reimburse the employer for the price of the ticket, plus a usurious interest charge. Here was a form of 'debt labour' that tightened labour discipline and held wages down. Steamship companies also found in the advance of 'prepaid' passages a means of artificially generating traffic during the off-season and of filling their ships during economic recessions.[136]

With such major interests involved in stimulating the supply of low-paid manual labour, mass Italian emigration must not be regarded as solely a spontaneous response to disembodied 'push' and 'pull' factors in the economy. A massive recruiting effort by agents prepared to misrepresent conditions in the New World was an essential component in the movement.[137] Indeed, one American authority, quoted at length in the *Bollettino dell'emigrazione* published by the Ministry of Foreign Affairs, estimated in 1911 that two-thirds of the Italian emigration to the United States was 'artificial' in the sense that it was not driven by the informed decisions of Italian workers aspiring to better their economic conditions. The vast majority of emigrants made the journey as a result instead of an unrelenting advertising campaign carried out by powerful interests at the expense of an illiterate and vulnerable population.[138] Although the attempt to quantify the proportions of 'spontaneous' and 'artificial' emigration is suspect, it is impossible to understand the vast exodus without underlining the role played by a thick network of tens of thousands of agents and sub-agents. The resulting outward flood from 1876 was charted by the Italian Bureau of Statistics (*Direzione Generale della Statistica*) as it gathered momentum. The Bureau recorded the statistics (shown in Table 6.3).[139]

These facts are well known. What needs to be stressed here is the enormous local consequences of this development for the city that served as the gateway to North America. For the most part, Italian emigrants bound for South America embarked at Genoa, whereas the vast majority of those destined for the United States and Canada sailed from Naples or, to a far lesser extent, from Palermo.

Table 6.3. *Annual average number of*
trans-oceanic emigrants, 1876–1910

Quinquennium	Emigrants
1876–80	26,596
1881–5	58,995
1886–90	131,283
1891–5	147,444
1896–1900	161,901
1901–5	309,242
1906–10	393,694

Table 6.4. *Shipping tonnage in 1910*

Port	Tonnage (millions)
Hamburg	12
Antwerp	11
Rotterdam	11
Marseilles	9
Naples	8
Genoa	8
Palermo	3

In the Giolittian era, as the Neapolitan deputy Arlotta explained, the export of people became the great dynamic sector in the economy of his native city – the foundation for all of its economic life. On its strength, Naples became the fastest growing port in the world. By the outbreak of the cholera in 1910, Naples had become, in terms of tonnage, the greatest port in Italy and the fifth in Europe. The comparative position of Naples relative to other major ports was as shown in Table 6.4.[140] The distinguishing feature of Naples among European ports, however, was its overwhelming dependence on the movement of passengers rather than goods. Naples specialized in the shipment of people – a category in which it led the seaports of the Mediterranean and of Continental Europe, as indicated in Table 6.5.[141]

This massive movement of people affected every sector of the economy of the city.[142] Emigration, in the words of one councillor, was the 'river of gold' in which every Neapolitan entrepreneur slaked his thirst. The effects were apparent in all branches of economic activity. The shipping industry and the port are the most obvious examples. On the crossing from Naples to New York, an average steamship of nine to twenty tons carried from 1,500 to 2,500 third-class passengers. Since the steerage fare for the journey cost from 180 to 210 lire (see

Table 6.5. *Passengers handled by leading
European seaports in 1908*

Port	Passengers (1,000s)
Naples	787
Le Havre	531
Marseilles	436
Genoa	369
Palermo	167
Venice	67

Appendix, Table A5), the voyage yielded 300 to 500 thousand lire in steerage fares alone, plus whatever the vessel carried in cargo and its complement of cabin passengers. Here was an opportunity for substantial profits which formed the life-blood of the sixteen companies involved in the emigration industry such as the White Star Line, the Fabre Line, the Navigazione Generale, the Lloyd Sabaudo and the Anchor Line, as well as for the stevedores who loaded and unloaded their ships.

Shipping, however, was only one of the many Neapolitan activities directly affected by emigration. Financial ripples radiated outward from the port to affect the entire city. The wholesale trade, for example, depended heavily on demand generated by the emigration industry. Each ship that docked in the Bay of Naples en route to New York spent 60,000 lire on supplies for the crossing. During the peak months in the spring, when the demand for seasonal outdoor labour in the United States reached its high point, as many as forty-five steamships departed from the harbour every month. Neapolitan suppliers received lucrative commissions to provision the vessels.

Retail businesses also drank deeply in the waters of this flood. The reason was simple but significant. Before embarking, emigrants inevitably made their final purchases of necessities for the journey and returning veterans of the New World, with substantial savings in their pockets made their first purchases on Italian soil – shoes, hats, umbrellas, trunks and scarves. The estimates for the average amount spent per person vary from twenty-five to fifty lire. Even adopting the more conservative estimate, Arlotta calculated that emigrants and returnees spent from 6 to 8 million lire a year in the city. The real figure was perhaps considerably more.[143]

Emigration was also a boon to the hotel trade. Luxury hotels like the Excelsior benefited because the steamships, calling in the Bay of Naples to board emigrants, brought with them first-and second-class passengers who would not otherwise have visited the city. The sector of the trade to profit most, however, was its suspect lower depths in the vicinity of the harbour. In the tenements of this quarter were located the notorious *locande* where Asiatic cholera had made its first appearance in the city in 1884 and where departing migrant workers from Apulia became the first victims of the disease in August 1910. The *locande* enjoyed an evil reputation, and in 1910 they achieved a national notoriety. The local paper *Il Mattino* labelled them 'the true sources of moral and hygienic infection'. The Italian press, it continued, had painted them in a lurid light, but nothing written ever fully captured the evil that they embodied.[144]

They were workers' hostels that catered to a captive clientele of nomadic labourers who arrived in the city disorientated, unorganized and in transit to a destination abroad, where there was no recourse for complaints about their treatment in Naples. The proprietors, known as *locandieri*, knew how to make the most of their market advantage. They charged 2.5 lire a night for room and board, but economized by crowding their customers into poorly ventilated barracks where they slept ten strangers to a room, by neglecting all civilized norms of sanitation, and by defrauding the travellers of the meals for which they had contracted. Many a migrant found that, no matter how he arranged his timing, he mysteriously always arrived just too late or too early to be served. An inspection of the hundred boarding-houses involved in the emigration industry by the police estimated that only eighteen were in condition to deserve a licence.[145]

Public outcry about the conditions prevailing in the boarding-houses had led in 1905 to a first attempt at closer supervision and regulation.[146] The Commissariat of Emigration ordered that, in order to obtain licences to let rooms to the public, *locande* were required to satisfy certain legal standards. They had to pass inspection to verify that each boarding-house possessed bathrooms, a dining room, a sick-room and a storage-room for baggage, and that it observed the minimum standards of the local sanitary code. In practice, however, enforcement was slack, and in the autumn of 1910 Foreign Minister San Giuliano could still report that the hygienic conditions of these unhappy institutions was 'truly deplorable'.[147]

Although the proprietors protested bitterly that the new regulations constituted a regime of 'oppression' in which they were financially ruined while their customers lounged in luxury,[148] the Deputy Director of Public Health reported in the spring of 1911 that the *locande* bore no trace of improvement and gave no indication that the required inspections had ever been carried out.[149] Giolitti himself complained to the Prefect of Naples about a widely practised ruse to evade the sanitary rules. The abuse he identified was the system by which the *locandieri* maintained a few boarding-houses in reasonable sanitary condition to please the inspectors. These model establishments functioned only as a façade, however, because the emigrants were sent to them only in the final hours before departure. For the remainder of their stay they were diverted to the same 'lurid and unregulated hostels' of the past.[150] Thus buildings in the final stages of decay continued to yield profits that made their slumlords as wealthy as the hoteliers engaged in the luxury trade. The average keeper of an emigrant boarding-house, the newspaper *Il Mattino* reported, earned twice the income of the owners of the most sumptuous local hotels, The Palace and the Excelsior.[151] The Neapolitan *locandieri* were substantial local businessmen with a powerful voice in the Chamber of Commerce and influence on City Hall.

The profitability of the boarding-houses did not result simply from their charges for rooms and services, however exorbitant. The Commissioner-General of Emigration, Pasquale Di Fratta, complained that they lived by 'small extortions and petty swindles' that made their very existence a scandal.[152] The socialist Deputies Filippo Turati and Angiolo Cabrini explained the 'unofficial' workings of these institutions. As long-term campaigners on behalf of the rights of migrants and as members of the Commissariat of Emigration established in 1901 for the protection of Italians overseas, they were well placed to observe the mechanisms of the trade. In an interpellation in March 1911 they reported to the Chamber that the Neapolitan *locande* were strategic institutions in the world of organized crime that viciously exploited a uniquely vulnerable sector of the population.[153] In the *locande*, emigration accommodated itself to one of the guiding principles of economic life in Naples – monopoly pricing. The movement of goods into the city was almost universally subject to a substantial and illegal levy, which was the original meaning of the word *camorra*. Emigration was subject to the same factor.

Cabrini argued that the *locanda* was the 'key agency in the exploitation of the emigrant'. It acted as a 'connecting link' between the emigration agent, who recruited the migrant in his native village, and his employer across the waters. The agent, who often acted through the intermediary of subcontractors, was the active recruiting sergeant who first persuaded young men to make the journey. It was then his business to book the trans-Atlantic passage and the onward railroad ticket from New York to the final destination in America; to lend money to clients struggling to meet the fare; to gather those departing from a single locality into groups; and to deliver them directly to the hotelier in Naples. The *locandiere*, who also worked on contract to the shipping companies, had the strategic task of arranging the final consignment of this human cargo to the docks, then 'squeezes his victim for all he is worth' and 'delivers him to his exploiter across the Atlantic'. In Cabrini's words, 'The truth is that the emigrant is accompanied to the port by the representative of the steamship company; ... he is then delivered to the boarding-house, where he is auctioned to the highest bidder.'[154] In a string of surprising metaphors, Turati described the *locanda* as 'the nest, the womb, the hearth' of the most abusive practices of the trade.[155] He also described it as the directing centre of a new International that enmeshed the worker in its coils on both sides of the Atlantic.

The *locandiere* was typically a Camorra boss who used his position to conclude a series of highly profitable business arrangements that the paper *Il Mattino* called 'criminal'.[156] According to the socialist paper *Avanti!*, the proprietor of a boarding-house often had a police record, and he worked at the centre of a 'thick Camorra network' that 'lives exclusively by exploiting emigrants'.[157] The *locandiere*, the paper continued, operated in concert with an entourage of 'thugs, con

artists and pimps' and moved in the midst of 'a seedy underworld of parasites'.[158] His associates included priests like Ciro Vitozzi, the chaplain of the
cholera cemetery, who became a celebrity during the Cuocolo trial. Vitozzi, who
had not conducted a mass in years and carried a revolver under his tunic, was the
adviser of the Camorra bosses in the borough of Porto. The *locandiere* also
worked with corrupt physicians like Carmine Striano, who was disgraced during
the Casale trial, and with dishonest shopkeepers, porters, and the boatmen who
ferried the emigrants to their ships.[159] Frequently he offered his good offices as
an employment broker, using his contacts to place his clients with jobs in
America – jobs that paid little, that sometimes involved breaking strikes, and
that entailed mysterious deductions from wages and the expectation of 'favours'
at a later date. Often, to facilitate the deal, the emigrant was encouraged to part
with his money to join an association that would increase his chances of
employment – a so-called masonic lodge, for instance, or a putative religious
association, depending on the beliefs of the traveller.

Another service was that of assistance in handling the emigrant's eventual
savings and remittances. Naturally, the hotelier never recommended the Bank of
Naples, but directed his guests to the nearly 3,000 *banchisti* operating by 1910 in
the United States. The *banchisti* – unregistered and unregulated emigrant
bankers – kept convenient hours and spoke their customers' language. They
charged heavily for their services, however; they paid no interest on the savings
they collected; they kept no written record of transactions; and they all too often
disappeared with the money entrusted to their care. In the description of the *New
York Times*,

> They bear little resemblance to our regular financial institutions. They are without
> any real paid-up capital, have little or no legal responsibility, and, for the most part,
> are without legal responsibility ... Immigrant bankers, as a rule, conduct some
> other business in connection with their 'banks'. Consequently the 'banks' are
> conducted for the most part in saloons, grocers, bakers, fruit stores and other
> establishments...[160]

The scale of the profits involved was indicated by the Immigration Commission
in the United States, which calculated in 1908 that over $130 million in remit-
tances and savings passed through the hands of the *banchisti*.[161] The treasurer of
the Camorra in the borough of Porto, the notorious Giovanni Rapi, who also
specialized in gambling and prostitution, ran a series of these emigrant banks in
New York and they made his fortune.[162]

In addition to employment and banking, which were the main sources of
irregular income, the *locandieri* through their contacts provided a variety of other
minor 'services'. Of these the most lucrative was the sale of insurance to cover
the cost of a return passage in the event that the emigrant was refused entry to
America at Ellis Island. Here the agents tapped a rich vein of anxiety because
deportation from New York Harbor for medical reasons was both frequent and
inherently unpredictable. The instructions of the medical officers who examined
arriving immigrants were both economic and eugenic. Rejection was automatic in

the event that mental and physical examination revealed that the applicant was likely to become a charge on public welfare because he or she was unable to work, or was likely to breed physical or mental degenerates. Mental conditions that were to be eliminated were feeble mindedness, epilepsy, insanity, alcoholism and 'constitutional mental inferiority'[163].

More menacing to arrivals from southern Italy were the physical disqualifications, which included three major categories that frequently and capriciously applied to large numbers of impoverished peasants. The three categories were: (1) 'contagious diseases' of which the most significant was trachoma, the major cause of deportation,[164] followed by pneumonia and tuberculosis; (2) 'loathsome contagious diseases', of which the most important were gonorrhoea, syphilis and ringworm; and (3) 'poor physique', an inherently subjective assessment based on such criteria as inadequate body weight relative to height, insufficient muscular development, curvature of the spine, flat feet and hernia. [165]

On the basis of these criteria, of which 'poor physique' was necessarily the most unpredictable, the Ellis Island physicians ordered the deportation of 3,500 prospective immigrants in the first three months of 1911.[166] Under these circumstances, rejection upon arrival was the greatest of all anxieties of the departing labourer – an anxiety that it was the professional interest of the *locandiere* to magnify. Deportation insurance covering the cost of the return passage to Naples was a precaution that was reassuring to the traveller and profitable to the insurer, who earned $1.50 per immigrant in 1911 against a rejection rate of about 2 per cent. The profits were all the greater because the premiums invariably contained detailed exclusion clauses that virtually eliminated the real liability of the insurers.[167]

In addition, the *locande* furnished false documents, medical certificates, religious charms that were said to prevent seasickness, instruction in English and the company of women. These were the 'little extortions' and 'little swindles' which, as the General Commissioner for Emigration explained, 'generate some not inconsiderable sums for the *locandieri* and their employees' while plunging the emigrants into a 'deplorable existence'.[168] With good reason Herman Stump, the United States Superintendent of Immigration, reported in 1894 that, 'It can be safely said that a large portion of the Italian immigration into the United States (men, women, and children) have been and are at the present time imported under conditions of servitude.'[169]

In 1910 and 1911 the significance of emigration to Neapolitan business interests was underscored by economic recession. The course of the downturn was outlined by the Bank of Naples in its annual reports on the state of affairs in the city. According to the Bank, Naples had been badly affected by the national economic crisis of 1907, and as late as 1911 had still not recovered. The financial community had anticipated an upswing in 1910, but a series of three unexpected setbacks had disappointed its hopes and prolonged the hardship. The local economy was seriously affected by the bad harvest of the summer of 1910 and the poor performance of all of the leading crops of the nation – wheat, olives and grapes. Recovery was then undermined by an unfavourable balance of trade and the resulting necessity for a squeeze on credit. Then in September the medical emergency seriously disrupted business. The epidemic itself was limited, but its repercussions for the economy were important.[170] Workshops and shops closed as employers and wealthy customers fled the city; the tourist trade collapsed; unemployment soared; and municipal finances were heavily burdened by the expenses of the anti-cholera sanitary campaign. In the resulting climate of 'general malaise', the hopes for recovery hinged on the stimulus of the emigration business. After four years of lingering hardship followed by the sharp September crisis, Neapolitan businessmen were desperate for the profits from the export of people to revive their fortunes.

Important as it was, emigration was not the only economic factor that hinged on the question of public health. A second important issue centred on a further round of negotiations between Rome and Naples on the question of public works. Cholera arrived just after Ettore Sacchi, the Minister of Public Works, had announced that the economic renaissance of Naples was a matter of 'the greatest national interest'. Visiting the city in June, he outlined an ambitious program of state investment for the benefit of the local economy, including improvements to the port, an express train service between Naples and Rome, a customs-free zone for the stimulation of industry, and a package of subsidies for industry and the local administration.[171] Parliament was preparing to vote in December on a special law providing funds for these projects and for further steps to bring renewal nearer to completion. To reveal that the money appropriated by parliament in 1885, 1902 and 1908 on behalf of Naples had achieved little effect because of corruption and incompetence – as the opposition argued that the return of cholera conclusively proved – was to jeopardize the allocation of the additional funds for public works that Sacchi had outlined.

Furthermore, the funds voted by the state were intended to form part of a larger partnership between public and private funds in the development of the city. The national funds were intended as an investment in infrastructure that would entice outside companies to the city. In line with this objective, Del Carretto had launched a publicity campaign to convince foreign and Italian businessmen that a 'new Naples', modernized and reformed, had been created where far-sighted entrepreneurs could make handsome profits.[172] Public health formed a major part of the Mayor's sales effort. Addressing the American financial community through the *New York Times*, Del Carretto, used the already dated metaphor of infectious diseases as a process of fermentation by terming them 'zymotic diseases'. In other respects his assurances in an interview during the summer of 1910 were resolutely forward-looking:

> Tell America ... that to-day we have a new Naples; that to-morrow we shall have a still newer city. You have been all over the city, and you have seen for yourself what has been done to modernize it, without destroying its picturesqueness.
>
> Water, do you say ... ? Vienna is the only European city which has a water supply to compare with ours. ... This and our newly completed sewerage system,

which cost about 5,000,000 dollars are two of the municipal improvements of which modern Naples is duly proud. Deaths from zymotic diseases in Naples are less than in Rome, London, Paris, Berlin, or Vienna. That is the best testimony I know in favor of Naples's sanitary condition, and should confound all its traducers.[173]

'There is', he concluded, 'no finer business opportunity in the world for foreign capital than right here to-day in Naples.' To expose the reality of conditions in the slums of Mercato and Vicaria would refute the Mayor's claims, destroy his propaganda effort and undermine his overtures to investors. Cholera could endanger the economic future of the city and offend the Mayor's sense of civic pride.

THE ANTI-CHOLERA CAMPAIGN

With so much at stake in the export of people and the attraction of outside funds to the city, the Neapolitan business community did not welcome the sanitary campaign undertaken jointly by the local Office of Hygiene and by the Department of Public Health in Rome. The measures taken to defeat the disease inevitably entailed major disruptions in the emigration industry and unhelpful public revelations of insalubrity. For this reason, vested interests in the city pressured the administration not to acknowledge the cholera. Most energetic of all were the *locandieri*, described by *Roma* as 'the new barbarians'. They lobbied the press not to report the outbreak,[174] and they violently denounced Tullio Rossi-Doria for the precautions he instituted in Rome against Neapolitan travellers.[175] In November they also launched a campaign to force the authorities to rescind the initiatives designed to protect the health of the public.

To understand their position, one needs to consider the measures undertaken by the municipality and the state. A full account of the means adopted to defeat the invader in 1910 also sheds light on the otherwise mysterious undertakings of the city in the unacknowledged epidemic of the following summer. One means to demonstrate the scale of the undeclared emergency of 1911 is the similarity of its policies to those it undertook during the course of an 'official' epidemic.

The sanitary policy of City Hall deserves careful scrutiny for an additional reason as well. The actions of the authorities when confronted with an emergency provide an unspoken commentary on living conditions in the city. It was possible for Caro and Rodinò to publish a myth, but what they did can be decoded as bearing a different and more authentic message. For all of these reasons, the specifics of the anti-cholera campaign of September and October 1910 merit attention.

As in 1884, the preparations of the city to meet the danger passed through several stages. The Ministry of the Interior had called for sanitary vigilance in every major centre in Italy from 1906 and especially those communes that it identified as high-risk localities, including Naples. In early 1910, as the disease advanced closer, Rome renewed the alarm, calling on municipalities to prepare health staff, laboratories and hospitals for a crisis; to conduct public-health courses in town and countryside; to instruct the public in the measures necessary for its protection; and to identify possible sources of contamination of food and water supplies for remedial action. Several Italian cities – Milan, Florence, Turin, Novara – responded vigorously and early to the appeal from the Department of Public Health.[176]

In Naples, however, the *giunta* and the Office of Hygiene followed familiar dilatory procedures, postponing action until late August when the outbreak in Apulia provided irrefutable proof that the danger was direct and immediate. The city then launched a flurry of activity that, by contemporary medical standards, was unimpeachable except in the vital respect that the effort had begun far too late – when Asiatic cholera was already present in the city. In August and during the early weeks of September the local authorities reinforced the medical personnel available to combat the disease, hiring additional doctors, nurses, laboratory technicians, street-sweepers and gravediggers. The Town Hall also instituted surveillance procedures at the railroad station to identify and examine travellers arriving from Apulia; it set up sanitary teams to visit all hotels, rooming houses and *locande* to observe the state of health of their inhabitants; and it inspected the Serino aqueduct from its source to ensure that it was pure and that no repairs were required that might interrupt the supply during the course of an eventual emergency. By virtue of the denial of the presence of the disease, there was a tentative, preparatory quality to the actions of City Hall.[177]

An indication of the leisurely approach of the city to the renewed threat was the fact that, as late as 18 August, the local councillor Luigi Palomba protested to Rodinò that events in Apulia demonstrated that the menace to Naples was too serious to be ignored, and that the time had come for the local administration to set aside 'its usual torpor'. 'Never has Naples been so filthy as it is now,' he concluded, 'and never has public hygiene been so badly neglected.'[178] Far too little, observed the Naples correspondent for the Rome daily paper *La Tribuna*, was done to prevent the arrival in the city of a disease that all informed opinion agreed was inevitable.[179]

With the declaration that the affliction of Ernesto Vigilante was an authentic case of Asiatic cholera, the priorities of the city became suddenly urgent. City Hall hoped that the still limited outbreak could be prevented from becoming a major epidemic. In Caro's words,

> The chief aim of our action was to respond with the greatest secrecy and energy in order to snuff out the epidemic at its outset. And since the essential condition to combat the disease is to uncover the initial cases as soon as possible, we employed the maximum care to achieve this result.[180]

In pursuit of this aim, the new science of bacteriology allowed the authorities a certain precision in their objectives that had not existed in 1884. In the last epidemic of the nineteenth century, the municipality had reacted to the arrival of cholera by a frenetic effort to clean and disinfect the whole of the city and its atmosphere. By contrast, in 1910 advances in the understanding of the disease allowed officials to concentrate their efforts on a more clearly delineated range of targets that were directly and unmistakably implicated in the spread of infection.[181]

In accordance with the priorities dictated by Koch's discoveries and confirmed by the success of a series of western nations in halting the advance of the disease, the Office of Hygiene began its offensive by an intensive effort to find and isolate sufferers as rapidly as possible before they could infect others and contaminate the water. For this purpose the city recruited a thick network of informants as its forward eyes and ears. The authorities notified private physicians, employers, hotel managers, urban landlords, school teachers, priests and the superiors of convents and monasteries that they had a legal obligation to report all cases of serious illnesses at once. Employers were required to keep records of attendance at work and to make daily reports of all absences. The city also established a clandestine service of the municipal guard whose function was to trace suspect cases that had gone into hiding to avoid internment at the Cotugno. To speed the lines of communication, the city ensured that its potential informants were linked by telephone to the Office of Hygiene and that they were reminded of the serious legal penalties that would be used to punish non-compliance.

By decentralizing the burden of sanitary surveillance, the city also demonstrated that it had learned a significant lesson from the travails of 1884. In the fifth pandemic the reliance on teams of municipal guards and physicians to locate and isolate the ill had all too visibly linked municipal authority and the medical profession with the work of repression. The sudden incursions of these 'medical police' teams had all too frequently set a spark to the inflammable apprehensions of the Lower City. In 1910 municipal officials acted indirectly and with far more circumspection.

A logical corollary of the search for timely information was the ability to act quickly on reports of suspicious illness. The objectives of City Hall were to transport sufferers to the Cotugno, cadavers to the cemetery at Poggioreale, and samples of their faeces for bacteriological analysis in the laboratory of the Office of Hygiene; to isolate relatives and neighbours who had been in contact with the victim; and to carry out a programme of disinfection of premises and personal effects. To meet these objectives, Caro and Rodinò stationed rapid response teams of health officials, disinfecters and gravediggers on twenty-four hour duty in the Palazzo San Giacomo and each of the town halls of the twelve boroughs, and equipped them with horse-drawn carts and conveyances.

Having identified suspect cases as rapidly as possible, isolated them and their contacts, and diagnosed the illness with certainty by means of laboratory tests, the city intended to break all possible links in the chain of infection between those already infected and the still healthy inhabitants of the city. One such link was the market, where contaminated produce could spread the disease. To prevent such an eventuality, the city enforced rigorous inspection of all markets, ensuring that all produce was kept under glass, free from contamination by flies and dust from the streets.

Another aspect of the danger posed by vegetable markets was the result of sewage farming. This practice, carried on by the market gardeners or *padulani* had played a significant part in propagating the epidemic of 1884. To prevent a recurrence, the Office of Hygiene decreed that untreated human waste had to be stored within the city borders for a week before being transported to the countryside for use as fertilizer. The strategy here was a product of laboratory experience in the cultivation of the *Vibrio cholerae*. In such a favourable medium for bacterial growth as raw sewage, the vibrio proved to have a competitive disadvantage. In the space of a week hardier and faster-breeding germs monopolized the environment, eliminating the cholera bacillus. To protect consumers from the unsanitary practices of the peasants in the surrounding province, the city prohibited the use of the carts that conveyed waste from Naples to the sewage farms from being re-used for the return trip to town bearing produce. Each sewage cart was marked with a seal that identified it as a conveyance banned from the transport of edible produce. Enforcement was entrusted to the customs guards who manned the barriers at the gates to the city where the consumption levy was collected.

Sanitary inspectors also sealed all the wells and cisterns in the city, arranged for the emptying of cesspits throughout the Lower City, and ordered the removal of waste and the disinfection of walls, courtyards and stairways that were visibly fouled. Public latrines were disinfected on a daily basis. Caro regarded the work of the inspectors as one of the most important activities in the municipal campaign, and he reported that the scale of their efforts was without precedent in the history of the city. 'The sanitary teams in question', he wrote,

> were kept in continuous service from August 1910 until December 1911, thanks to the orders of signor Rodinò, the alderman in charge. Thanks to their effort, we were able to intervene effectively on an unequalled scale. Thousands and thousands of *bassi*, courtyards, stairways, back streets, cesspits, waste-pipes and latrines were cleaned, disinfected and, where necessary, repaired. Hundreds of wells and cisterns were closed at the same time.[182]

With the same end in view, every building in Naples that was tenanted was issued with a covered metal bin for the collection of all the waste of the residents. The municipal dustmen, reinforced in number for the duration of the emergency, were entrusted with the daily emptying of the bins and their disinfection.

Aware that the waters of the Bay were heavily implicated in the outbreak, the city undertook to limit the danger. One means to achieve this goal was by disinfecting the sewer mains themselves in an effort to destroy the vibrio before it entered the harbour. Other measures attempted to prevent the recycling of germs that successfully reached the port. For this purpose a ban was imposed on swimming and fishing in the Bay, and on the sale and consumption of shellfish. The links between the sea and the city were severed.

The city also attempted to interrupt the pathways by which cholera could spread sporadically, from person to person. Municipal disinfection teams patrolled the back streets of the Lower City in search of dirty linen, which they promptly disinfected. All laundry received by washerwomen was subjected to the same procedure. For the same purpose of preventing 'sporadic' cholera, the city sought to isolate those 'closed institutions' that in previous epidemics had demonstrated a particular susceptibility to infection – prisons, hospitals and insane asylums. Visits to the inmates of these facilities were prohibited until the city was again declared free of the disease. Lastly, to reduce the danger of infection through contact, the city forbade assemblies, demonstrations and public gatherings of all sorts. As in 1884, the *ottobrate* were celebrated only with difficulty as the authorities had ordered the closure of all bars and taverns.[183]

Finally, there were municipal measures that sought in a broad manner to raise the resistance of the whole population to Asiatic cholera by regulating and improving diet. The people were informed of the risks involved in the consumption of fruit and vegetables, and the municipality, supported by the contributions of Cardinal Archbishop Giuseppe Prisco and of private charity, opened soup kitchens throughout the Lower City. Their purpose was to make a wholesome and affordable regimen universally available. With the intention of encouraging the consumption of produce that was free of all suspicion of encouraging indigestion and inducing diarrhoea, the city also instituted price controls and distributed financial subsidies among the unemployed so that quality produce would become affordable during the sanitary crisis.

Italian sanitary law entrusted the municipalities of the nation with the task of 'sanitary vigilance'. Respecting the division of labour between Rome and Naples intended by the existing legislation, the national authorities at the Department of Public Health exercised primarily a distant supervision, exhorting the Neapolitan officials, advising, and ensuring the observation of laws and regulations. In the field of emigration, however, the state was bound by international treaty to intervene in order to avoid the export of the disease to other countries. In accordance with international law, therefore, on 25 September Italy declared Naples an 'infected' port, required all ships sailing from the city to be issued with a *patente brute* or dirty bill of health, and ordered the yellow flag to be flown over the harbour.[184]

Under pressure from foreign governments, the Italian authorities went further. All emigrants who had contacts in Naples were to be detained in quarantine for a period of five days prior to departure aboard the ship *Marsala*, which was anchored in the Bay for the purpose. Meanwhile, all further emigrants hoping to embark at the port of Naples were to be met at the railroad station and accompanied directly to an isolation station 'without their having any contacts or entering the city'. They were to be housed instead in a single large publicly managed hostel outside Naples 'where they could be easily and conveniently held in observation'. Finally, there was to be an embargo on the shipment of foodstuffs of all kinds from the port of Naples.[185]

Any definitive assessment of the effectiveness of the various measures adopted by the city and the Italian state in combating the cholera is impossible. The outbreak did not lead in the autumn to a major epidemic. Municipal officials proclaimed that this happy result vindicated both the long-term salubrity of the city as a result of *risanamento* and the wisdom of the sanitary campaign adopted by the Office of Hygiene. It is difficult, however, to share such an optimistic interpretation of the course of events. One reason, of course, is that the facts on which the 'official' view is based can no longer be accepted. The outbreak of 1910 was of far greater magnitude than official figures suggest, as the Prefect of Naples acknowledged and as the unpublished statistics collected by the Department of Health clearly indicate. The difference matters because an outbreak involving nearly 1,000 cases and almost 700 deaths – the magnitude suggested by the unpublished records of the state – was a substantial event that, far from confirming the idea that Naples was immune to Asiatic cholera, suggests instead that there were serious sanitary deficiencies that remained to be addressed.

Furthermore, the city declared that the epidemic was completely finished by the end of October, and the Department of Public Health officially concurred in this judgment. The information gathered by the Department in private, however, indicated that the disease continued well beyond its 'official' termination in October. The severity of the outburst abated, but scattered 'sporadic' cases were confirmed well into November. Indeed, such informed sources as the American, British and French consuls believed that 'stragglers' continued to occur throughout the winter of 1910–11. In December the government of Norway issued a quarantine proclamation declaring that cholera still prevailed in the province of Naples.[186] Concurrently with the Norwegian decision, Geddings reported that he once again believed that cholera was causing scattered cases that were being suppressed by municipal authorities. 'I have no hesitation in informing you', he wrote to the Acting American Consul in Naples on 30 December, 'that I have long since lost all confidence in the integrity of the municipal health authorities, in the matter of the declaration of infectious diseases.'[187]

On the basis of the conclusions of various informed foreign sources, therefore, it is possible to argue that the anti-cholera campaign was not a success at all but a failure. It is entirely probable, in other words, that it lowered mortality but failed to eliminate the disease, allowing the cholera instead to persist in an unbroken chain of infection until the following spring, when it exploded with much greater epidemic force. A categorical decision on this speculation is impossible, in large measure because the municipality and the state suppressed all information relating to the real state of public health in 1911, but the circumstantial evidence suggesting the more pessimistic version of events is persuasive and suggestive.

Indeed, the executive committee demonstrated an extreme sensitivity about the events surrounding the 'end' of the outbreak in the autumn of 1910. Italian law stipulated that it was obligatory for the city council to hold two annual sessions, one in the spring and the other in the autumn. Precedent also demanded that the conclusion of a public health emergency be followed by an explanation of the action of the city, when the authorities would make themselves available for questioning and could be held responsible for their policies in the interest of the population. Between 30 August and 10 December 1910, however, the executive violated both law and precedent, initially by refusing to convene the city council and subsequently by declining to present a full report on the course of the disease despite the insistent demands of the opposition, which made urgent representations to the Prefect and to the Ministry of the Interior. When discussion of the issue of public health finally began in the New Year, it took place in secret sessions where the public and the press were banned.[188]

A veil of secrecy also descended in November over the Cotugno Hospital. In the month of the acknowledged outbreak, city councillors made inspection visits to the cholera wards and made public reports on their findings. From the time that the city declared that the outbreak was over, however, it became impossible any longer to verify the real state of public health. The Cotugno was declared out of bounds, and visits inside the gates were banned. Councillors Palomba and Epifania, whose earlier inspections had caused much embarrassment, now protested that they were not allowed access.[189] Such a denial of the possibility of public scrutiny both in the Council Chambers and at the infectious diseases hospital raises doubts about the reliability of the account of events given by the administration.

In addition, even if one accepts some variant of the 'official' history of the outbreak, there are reasons to question the extent of the contribution of the municipal and state anti-cholera campaign in bringing about the desired result. Suppose, for example, the relatively favourable view that the outbreak actually came to an end in November and that there was no direct link of infection binding the autumnal outbreak of 1910 and the larger conflagration of the following year. Even with that most favourable supposition, it is important not to accept without question the claim made by the Office of Hygiene that the victory over cholera was the result of its own policies rather than of other, more fortuitous circumstances. In strict logic, it is essential not to confuse *post hoc* with *propter hoc*: 'after' and 'because of' are two very distinct propositions. It is all too likely that the epidemic declined, perhaps without ever disappearing, for reasons unconnected, or only partially connected, with the official campaign. The weather, of course, was one such imponderable. In the history of Naples, even before the development of scientifically reliable strategies to combat Asiatic cholera, the disease always abated or disappeared with the advent of the winter. The vibrio suffers a reduction in vitality in cold weather, and – more significantly – the population of the city was much less at risk as cold weather lowered the consumption of possibly contaminated water, reduced the numbers of flies, and ended the season of bathing in the waters of the Bay and of the highly polluted Sebeto River. In the case of infectious diseases, moreover, allowance must always be made for sheer serendipity. It may be the case that Neapolitans escaped a major epidemic in the winter of 1910–1911 through plain good fortune rather than through the debatable effectiveness of their governors at defending the city. If that was the case, the least that one can conclude is that their luck ran out in 1911. The balance of probability, however, is that the cholera persisted, unacknowledged, all through the winter, ready to erupt again when circumstances favoured its recrudescence.

The purpose of a critical assessment of the campaign against cholera waged by the Neapolitan authorities in the autumn of 1910 is not to impugn the Office of Hygiene and the work of Orazio Caro. Indeed, the variety of interventions undertaken by the Office indicates a prodigious effort guided by a coherent strategy. The very scale of the battle, however, suggests a number of conclusions. The magnitude of the sanitary operation carried out under Caro's direction clearly confirms the suspicion that the urban environment in the Lower City was seriously contaminated, its sanitation undermined by multiple deficiencies in the work of *risanamento*. The activities of the Office of Hygiene are intelligible only on the assumption that the 'official' assessment of the rebuilding programme is seriously flawed. The policies of the city in the time of cholera are consistent instead with the following observations: that overcrowding and substandard housing were pervasive; that the sewer system was so defective that the streets and courtyards of the Lower City continued to function as the receptacles for waste of all types; that the water supply furnished by the Serino aqueduct was so inadequate to the needs of the modern city that a large proportion of the population still drank from lethal cisterns and wells; that filth was omnipresent; that sanitary regulations were comprehensively ignored in the marketplace; that the diet of large numbers of Neapolitans was seriously deficient; and that the waters of the harbour and the market gardens of the province were constant perils to the welfare of the people.

Actions, the proverb informs us, speak far louder than words. Judged by this criterion, the deeds of the municipality during the course of the emergency belie its rhetoric about the successful transformation of the city into a 'new Naples', modernized and hygienic. Perhaps Caro's Office of Hygiene failed to eradicate cholera because the task it confronted in the field of sanitation was overwhelming. Naples had inherited too many sanitary dangers.

There were two aspects of the 1910 anti-cholera campaign, however, that were inherently suspect and for which the authorities bear responsibility. The first defect was timing. The executive committee of Town Hall undertook a serious defence of the city far too late – after the disease had already invaded. As a result, the project undertaken was not one of preventive medicine but of remedial sanitation. Only after the disease had established a widespread presence in the city and its harbour did the work of the Office of Hygiene begin. Valuable time was squandered, and lives were lost in the process.

The second avoidable weakness of the defensive campaign of the Palazzo San Giacomo was its dishonesty. The constant effort to deny the presence of the disease or to minimize its extent had the dire consequences of diminishing the vigilance of the population and the medical profession, of severing the lines of communication between City Hall and the informants on whom it depended. The Office of Hygiene could not reasonably expect both to affirm that the city was free of cholera and at the same time to receive accurate and prompt notification of suspect cases.

Secrecy is antithetical to scientific medicine, and no steps were more dangerous than the postponement of an official acknowledgement of the disease until late September and the premature announcement at the end of October that the outbreak was over and that the city was entirely free of the disease. Such a policy was the sanitary equivalent of removing the sentinels from their posts, and the probable consequence was that the enemy infiltrated the city unobserved. Unmolested, the vibrio prepared the ground for a renewed assault. As early as 24 September, *Roma* forthrightly explained the necessity of candour in the matter of public health. Repeatedly mixing its metaphors, the republican newspaper nevertheless made an important point. It argued that,

> Those in charge of public health did not have a clear sense of the responsibilities that they bore. They thought that it was admissible, even useful, to keep silent, to understate and to disguise facts, concealing the gravity of the situation.... The unpardonable error was made of denying the danger in the hope that this was the way to avoid it.
>
> Once again men have imitated the ostrich....
>
> By this means we have achieved this painful result: the disease that first arrived timidly among us has been allowed to grow. Safely concealed, it spread and grew in vigour....
>
> Hidden wounds cannot be treated.[190]

The practical result, the paper concluded, was that the campaign against the disease was 'uncertain, confused and inconsistent'.

This criticism was not raised only by the political opposition. The Italian military was deeply concerned about the lack of official candour because concealment carried the risk of disastrous consequences. Because their normal operations required drafting soldiers, transporting them from one part of the peninsula to another and sending them home on leave, the armed services were aware of the heavy responsibility they bore to avoid transmitting the disease throughout the peninsula. The chief medical officer of the army explained, however, that the military was unable in 1910 to take effective sanitary precautions because it received no reliable information on the real geography of the epidemic. The doctor was uncertain about the issue of whether 'one can regard those localities officially designated as free from cholera as really free of the disease', and the truth was especially difficult to obtain in the city where it was most important – Naples.[191] The result was that the army did not know whether to suspend recruitment, transfers and leaves, and in what places.

THE INSURRECTION OF THE *LOCANDIERI*

If the effect of the anti-cholera campaign on the disease is difficult to assess, it is much easier to evaluate the impact that it had on the economy and on those residents of the city with business interests. At a time when the city was already suffering from a painful recession, the hoisting of the yellow flag over the harbour brought a halt to the greatest resource of Naples in the Giolittian era – the emigration industry. Faced with cumbersome public health regulations and with the potential hazard of an outbreak of cholera at sea, the steamship companies decided to avoid the city entirely. The port of Naples, on which the wealth of the residents had come to depend, came to a standstill as the steamships re-routed their Neapolitan sailings via Genoa and Marseilles.[192] And, in the words of the Catholic monthly *Civiltà cattolica*, 'a blow to the port is a stab to the heart of Naples'.[193]

It was with the needs of the economy foremost in their thoughts that the officials in the Palazzo San Giacomo hastened the declaration that the outbreak of cholera was at an end. Their chosen date of 30 October was premature, but the logic of their reasoning was that a little cholera was less harmful than a major depression. Unfortunately for Neapolitans with an interest in the port, the steamships received information from sources other than the Palazzo San Giacomo. Foreign Consuls, for instance, took a far from sanguine view of sanitary conditions in the city. In November the USPH&MHS still insisted that vessels sailing from Naples would have to carry a dirty bill of health. The American Consul openly contradicted the declarations of the local government of Naples, while the French and British Consuls greeted municipal statements on the subject with wry smiles and witticisms.[194] The caution of the American authorities was increased by the outbreak of the disease at New York in mid-October, when six arriving Italian immigrants fell ill with Asiatic cholera.[195] The impact on trans-oceanic emigration of a sanitary announcement by a municipal government that no one believed was nil and the docks remained idle.

In this dilemma Luigi Luzzatti invented an ingenious compromise for the benefit of the becalmed southern seaport. Luzzatti's solution was to extend the existing sanitary regulations by diverting arriving emigrants from the *locande* of the city to the state-run hostel – the *Casa degli emigranti* – in the Via Santi Cosma e Damiano on the outskirts. While not an open disavowal of the Neapolitan sanitary announcement, the position taken by Luzzatti constituted a tacit admission that the disease had not yet been eradicated. Indeed for the newspaper *Roma* the idea of a single great hostel was contradictory. It would be more logical, it reasoned, to suspend emigration completely until the sanitary conditions in the city had returned to normal, especially since such a facility, concentrating large numbers of indigent travellers on a single site, risked spreading rather than combating the disease.[196] A further illogical aspect of Luzzatti's hostel, which began to function on 2 October, was noted by Nitti in a parliamentary speech. The sanitary contradiction was that Apulian emigrants from infected *comuni* could still depart without hindrance from Genoa and possibly convey cholera to South America. Sanitary vigilance applied only to Naples, and this loophole caused the plan to be treated without respect.[197]

On the other hand, by severing the links between the emigrants and the infected city, the hostel would allow Naples additional time to combat the disease without having to suffer all of the consequences. Departing emigrants could be allowed to embark, and the steamships could safely return. While not being able to assure foreign governments that Naples was free of cholera, the Ministry of the

Interior could plausibly give an assurance that the emigrants who successfully embarked were in good health. As Luzzatti explained in parliament, the object to be achieved by sanitary measures had shifted during the course of the outbreak. At the outset, the priority had been to defend Naples from contamination by cholera-bearing emigrants from Apulia who passed through the city en route to America. From the autumn, the priority was precisely the reverse – to protect the emigrants from the infected city. If the state failed to act, the United States intimated that it would turn away ships arriving from Italy. Almost reluctantly, therefore, Luzzatti felt compelled to take energetic measures.[198]

The fatal problem for Luzzatti's compromise was that he was too widely associated with the protection of emigrants to reassure the vested interests involved in the trade. He had acted as *rapporteur* for the 1901 law for the protection of emigrants – a law that included provision for the phasing out of the private *locande* and their replacement by state-operated hostels. As a declared enemy of the *locandieri*, Luzzatti seemed to many in 1911 to have found a new opportunity to advance his cherished but never-implemented reform.[199] In any case, the Prime Minister's compromise provided scant consolation for the myriad interests that depended on the physical presence of the emigrants in the borough of Porto. Emigrants not safely ensconced in the local boarding houses could not patronize Neapolitan shops and brothels, purchase accommodation and board, make financial arrangements for the repatriation of remittances, arrange employment or secure insurance. The extent of the losses sustained by the local economy can be gauged by the numbers of people diverted under police escort from the railroad station to the *Casa degli emigranti* in its four and a half months of effective operation (see Table 6.6[200]).

In mid-November, the association of boarding-house managers – the 'Co-operativa dei locandieri' – launched a campaign to protest against Luzzatti's initiative and against all other sanitary measures that suggested to interested parties that Naples was infected and therefore was no longer eligible for a major role in the emigration trade.[201] The first step in the offensive against the public health measures of the state was a rally initiated by the *locandieri*. Held at the Umberto Theatre on 13 November, the rally demonstrated that the boarding-houses and their political stance enjoyed widespread support. Three thousand people gathered to listen to speeches by Domenico De Martino, the Secretary of the *Cooperativa*, and Carmine Striano, a physician for the Fabre Line and a municipal Councillor. The demonstrators included Luigi Schioppa, one of the leading figures of the Naples Chamber of Commerce; representatives of the steamship companies; the municipal and provincial councillors elected from the borough of Porto; five members of the Neapolitan parliamentary delegation; and representatives of the wholesale and retail trades in the city. More surprisingly, an event sponsored by the most rapacious of Neapolitan entrepreneurs also attracted representatives of the labour movement affected by the crisis of the port – the stevedores, porters and coachmen, together with a member of the executive of the Società Operaia.

Table 6.6. *Emigrants detained at the* Casa degli Emigranti[202]

Month	Emigrants detained
October, 1910	1,769
November, 1910	14,114
December, 1910	10,009
January, 1911	13,688
February, 1911	12,164
Total	51,744

In their speeches De Martino and Striano inveighed against the state hostel. Although they clearly represented special interests, the two orators took a high-minded and public-spirited tone. Striano, a notorious *camorrista* and the son of a *locandiere*, claimed that, as a doctor, he had been scandalized by the conditions emigrants sleeping at the public facility were forced to endure.[203] Declaring his solidarity with the 'poor emigrants', he termed the state hostel 'indecent' and called for its abolition. The lawyer De Martino took a similar line. A former socialist candidate and leader of the moralizing campaign against the Casale political machine, De Martino had left his radical past behind. Called a 'former socialist' by *Avanti!* and accused of selling his political convictions, he now represented some of the leading Neapolitan *camorristi*. Despite such dubious paymasters, De Martino proclaimed that his sole concern was humanitarian and that he unreservedly favoured all effective measures to defend emigrants. The problem, he argued, was that the existing facility was a scandal and that the sanitary regulations imposed by Luzzatti were more damaging than helpful to the interests of emigrants. Like Striano, therefore, he urged a return to *laissez-faire*.[204]

The November rally was the opening gambit in an offensive that was to play an important part in bringing down the government. In November the *locandieri* and their allies could afford to be patient because the emigration business was in the depths of the winter off-season. In the three-month period from November to January of every year, the demand for outdoor manual labour in North America was scant. Emigration, therefore, was negligible, and the chief business of the port was the much smaller and less lucrative trade of return migration as veterans of the New World returned to Italy in time for Christmas. It was only in February that the great outbound movement gathered momentum, and that an idle port would seriously affect Neapolitans. Lucci noted this seasonality in the trade, which he illustrated by monthly figures from the preceding year, when the difference between winter and spring – the low and high seasons respectively – was as shown in Table 6.7.[205]

Given this chronology, it is understandable that the opposition to Luzzatti's emigrant hostel gathered force as 1911 began. In February the issue erupted into

Table 6.7. *Monthly emigration from Naples, 1909–10*

Month	Emigrants
November	8,571
December	3,377
January	5,101
February	10,648
March	26,990
April	29,410

open warfare as the high season began and a wave of bankruptcies swept the city.[206] Sanitary regulations, chief among them the state hostel, were the source of contention. The emigration facility stood accused of radically reducing the flow of traffic from the port. Since the facility had a capacity of 1,200 occupants, under the most favourable circumstances only one steamship a day would sail, in contrast with the three to four daily departures of the high season in normal times. Furthermore, even this seriously depleted trade would completely bypass the city itself, threatening nearly every sector of the local economy. Emigrants arriving at the railroad station were met by the police and taken to the hostel. There the travellers were detained in quarantine for three days; their personal effects were disinfected; and finally they were escorted directly to embarkation stations in the harbour.

The Italian government was reluctant, however, to rescind the offending health measures and to close the hated hostel. With the commerce of the nation as a whole to defend, Luzzatti was unwilling to yield to the protests of the city of Naples alone. His hesitation was increased by the findings of Dr Geddings. An authority on tropical diseases, Geddings travelled extensively throughout the Mezzogiorno to determine the extent of the infection. On the basis of his own independent enquiries, he declared in February that the epidemic in the city of Naples had still not run its course, and in the American press he publicly warned his compatriots planning holidays in the city to stay away.[207] In March the American doctor informed his government that the disease was increasing, and that the city would be in serious peril when the heat returned in the summer. The Italian authorities had failed to take the disease seriously, he reasoned, and they had neglected to institute adequate sanitary measures.[208] The conclusions of Geddings suggested that 'sporadic' cholera persisted throughout the winter of 1910–11. Geddings's views resulted in warnings in the American press such as the article 'Italian Cholera Lingers' in the *New York Times*.[209]

Isolated cases and the anxieties of Americans were of no importance, however, to Neapolitan entrepreneurs threatened with financial ruin. As the high season approached, their resolve hardened. The movement of resistance initiated by the Cooperative of *Locandieri* broadened and acquired more effective organization.

The *locandieri* were too closely associated with a series of squalid interests to lead a successful political cause. The Cooperative therefore gave way to a new pressure group called the 'Association for the Interests of the Twelfth Electoral District' (i.e., the borough of Porto). The 'Association' united all the economic, political and business interests with a stake in the issue of emigration into a campaign demanding that Naples be declared free of cholera and that, as a consequence, all the sanitary measures introduced to fight the epidemic be revoked in order that emigration be allowed to resume its normal course.

The 'Association' enjoyed the support of all of the most powerful political and economic figures in Naples – the entire Neapolitan parliamentary delegation, the majority of the members of the city council and its executive committee, the leaders of the Chamber of Commerce, and the wealthiest entrepreneurs of the city, including representatives of the De Luca company, the steamship lines and the hoteliers. Among its members were arms manufacturers, retail merchants, fishermen, tour guides and *locandieri*. Orazio Caro, the director of the Office of Hygiene and the theorist of the invulnerability of Naples to cholera, was a prominent figure in its deliberations.[210]

The campaign also enjoyed the backing of the Borsa del Lavoro, whose members were being made unemployed by the crisis affecting the port. In January and February the workers of the city had begun their own independent agitation against the high cost of living and rising unemployment with rallies, demonstrations and rent strikes by tenants. Against the background of three years of economic hardship followed by a sudden sharp crisis, tempers reached boiling point. *Avanti!* reported that the situation was in urgent danger of escalating into open rebellion.[211] Some of the demonstrations ended in street brawls with the police.[212] With experienced ex-socialists like De Martino and former radicals like Luigi Palomba (now in the employ of the steamship company Transatlantica) among its organizers,[213] the Association succeeded in reaching the dockers and porters of the harbour and in convincing them that the real source of their discontents was the stagnation of the port under the anti-cholera regime enforced by the state.

Ironically, the agitation of the Popular Bloc on the issue of public health inadvertently prepared the ground for the orators of the right-wing Association. The Popular Bloc position, as presented in the new year by the socialist Dr Tropeano, was that the economic conditions of the city and the medical crisis of cholera were inseparably linked. Tropeano's conclusion was that more, rather than less, state intervention was needed to resolve the problem.[214] For many members of his audience, however, it was possible to accept Tropeano's diagnosis while rejecting his cure. It was logical, in other words, for them to see the link between poverty and cholera as the reverse – to believe that poverty was the result of anti-cholera measures, as De Martino and Palomba argued. Populist rhetoric about a vast plot by Genoese capitalists, foreign exploiters and northern cabinet ministers gave the new movement a radical veneer and disguised the conservative interests involved. The call for direct action in the streets even suggested a robust political radicalism that suited the mood of rage that was so widespread among the people of the *sezione* Porto. The anger of redundant stevedores thus found a new outlet. This suspect alliance between the Borsa del lavoro and the *locandieri* was denounced by the socialist party and the national trade unions. On the local level, however, a deal was struck, and the militancy of workers gave the Association a dynamism it would not otherwise have possessed.

The vision of the crisis presented by Association orators and the solutions they offered were apocalyptic and violent. According to their analysis, the city of Naples had been condemned to death by the sanitary initiatives of the government. 'Naples is dying!' was the theme of a rally called by the movement in the last week of February, and the chants shouted by the assembled crowd were 'Down with Luzzatti!' and 'Down with the enemies of Naples!'.[215] The newspaper *Il Mattino*, sympathetic to the cause, proclaimed that Naples was fighting for its life with its back to the wall.[216]

As an explanation for the crisis, Association speakers eliminated the possibility of infection out of hand. There was afoot instead, they claimed, a vast international plot of northern Italians, socialists and foreigners to strangle Naples to death in the interest of the rival port of Genoa. The northerners, it was asserted, were led by Rocco Santoliquido, the Director of the Department of Public Health. The radical municipal councillor Palomba, who was retained as a physician by the steamship company Transatlantica, argued that Santoliquido had 'taken it into his head to destroy Naples once and for all'. In the pursuit of this objective, the doctor responsible for Italian public health policy 'made fools of us', proclaiming 'asinine statements' and 'utter scientific heresies'.[217] And by means of sinister machinations, Santoliquido had persuaded the Prime Minister to consider Naples an infected port.[218]

If Santoliquido acted unabashedly on behalf of Genoese merchants, the Association continued, the socialists disguised their intentions behind the humanitarian rhetoric of the Commissariat of Emigration. Hijacked by such northern socialist leaders as Turati and Cabrini, the Commissariat had become a 'tyrannical socialist state within the state', a private 'fiefdom' that they used and abused at their pleasure. While the Commissariat claimed to defend exploited nomadic workers, its real mission was to advance the interests of the North at the expense of the Mezzogiorno. To achieve this evil objective, it employed the devious means of burdening the Naples harbour with such onerous public health regulations that commerce became impossible. According to Giovanni Marino, the President of the Cooperative of *Locandieri*, the Commissariat pressed the owners of boarding-houses to undertake reforms that had no genuine hygienic function and served only to treat the workers to unnecessary and costly luxury.[219]

After the evil Santoliquido and the hypocritical socialists, the third agent of the conspiracy to destroy Naples was the American 'phenomenon of Geddings', the great slanderer of the Neapolitan people.[220] The arms manufacturer and municipal councillor De Luca, a member of the Association, vehemently denounced

Geddings at a session of the city council. Geddings, De Luca claimed, had a comfortable and well-paid position at the American Consulate, where he earned 3,000 lire a month. To keep his position and justify his salary, he had to appear to perform useful work. It was in his interest, therefore, to invent problems and to busy himself with non-existent matters of public health. Geddings, De Luca protested, 'has behaved very badly. He has slandered Naples and exaggerated every issue. But the root of the problem is here with us, with our own officials who promote the interests of Genoa by holding Naples down under the pretext that sanitary measures are necessary.'[221]

Opinion concerning the American doctor ran high. At a meeting of the Naples Chamber of Commerce, Girardi, the senior Deputy from the city, demanded that the government expel Geddings from the country. No one seemed to recall that as recently as 1902 the Italian state had decorated Geddings for his contribution to Italian medical research. In recognition of his work on yellow fever, Italy had named him a Knight of the Order of Saints Maurizio and Lazzaro.[222] Now the President of the Chamber, Luigi Petriccione, wrote to the Prime Minister, urging that 'there be an end to international hospitality for anyone who abuses his freedom to cause direct and serious harm to the nation that hosts him.'[223] Less charitably, Luigi Palomba shouted during a session of the city council that the American should be lynched.[224]

The storm unleashed by the Association was violent. The organization held an emergency plenary session on the evening of 22 February, and its leaders – De Martino, Striano, De Luca and Palomba – presented a resolution calling for extreme measures that would cause total chaos in Italy's largest city. If the Luzzatti government and the Department of Public Health failed to close the emigrant hostel and to revoke its sanitary regulations by 27 February, the Association called for the employers of the city to begin a general lockout and for the members of the city council to resign en masse. The motion was adopted without dissent. This action was followed on 24 February by simultaneous meetings of the Chamber of Commerce and the Borsa del Lavoro, where resolutions were presented and unanimously passed to support the initiative of the Twelfth Electoral District. The Chamber of Commerce resolution called for its members to resign in protest if the demands of the Association were not met, and the Borsa del Lavoro called for a general strike by all of its affiliated labour organizations.[225]

Not by accident, the city council convened at the same time as the Borsa and the Chamber of Commerce. Although brief, the session was possibly the most tempestuous in Neapolitan history to that date. The planned resolution announcing the mass resignation of the members of the council no longer satisfied the rage of the city's representatives. They also voted a motion of no confidence in the national government – a measure that was constitutionally *ultra vires*, but that conveyed their sentiments. In addition, the more ardent councillors urged more resolute measures. Luigi Palomba called for a Neapolitan insurrection. 'I invite the entire council', he announced, to join with the people in protest against a government that has forgotten that Naples is Italy's largest city and that it has a right to the protection of the law. Therefore the representatives of the city must unite with the people and resign if the state fails to revoke the measures that are so harmful to the interests of our city.[226]

It was no longer sufficient, Palomba shouted, for councillors to pass resolutions: the time had come for them to take to the streets and to make common cause with the people of Naples. 'We shall build barricades,' he asserted.

This proposal was enthusiastically endorsed by Witting, the Harbour Master, who declared, 'If the lock-out is not enough, we shall resort to whatever means necessary, with nothing excluded.' 'On Monday,' he continued, 'we shall begin the lock-out. And, if the lock-out is not enough, we shall have a rally. And, if the rally is not enough, we will do everything that needs to be done and we shall know what that means.'[227] The Council chambers echoed to stormy applause greeting the call for an armed uprising.[228] 'It's a fact', Witting concluded the meeting,

> that the Mayor and the Chamber of Commerce have been saying for a month now exactly what we're saying today – that the Government is ruining Naples, that the Government has always laughed at our protests and made light of our interests. If it moves today, it is because it sees before it the danger of an insurrection.[229]

To drive the point home, the city sent its foremost representatives to Rome to present the Prime Minister with an ultimatum. On the eve of the coordinated meetings of the Borsa del Lavoro, the Chamber of Commerce and the city council, the Neapolitan parliamentary delegation, which included Mayor Del Carretto, met at the Palazzo Braschi with Luzzatti and his most important political advisers with a responsibility in the relevant fields – the Foreign Minister San Giuliano; the Secretary of State at the Ministry of the Interior, Teobaldo Calissano; the Director of the Department of Public Health, Rocco Santoliquido; the Minister of the Treasury, Francesco Tedesco; and the director of the Commissariat of Emigration, Pasquale Di Fratta.

From Luzzatti's standpoint, the threat from Naples seemed entirely credible because the course of state policy regarding cholera from the time of the initial outbreak in Bari province to the end of 1910 had been punctuated throughout with violent protest. In the early weeks of the infection there had been riots first in the town of Barletta and then at Molfetta. The most important precedent, however, was that of the major Apulian city of Taranto on 30–1 December. There public health measures, particularly those affecting the cultivation and sale of shellfish, had caused widespread economic hardship and unemployment. On 30 December, the accumulating tension exploded when the authorities sought forcibly to remove the body of a cholera victim against the will of his family. A clash ensued, and it rapidly developed into a major confrontation when thousands of people from the dead man's neighbourhood poured into the streets. They converged on the barracks of the hated *carabinieri*, who had been charged with enforcing the sanitary regulations of the state. The crowd stoned the barracks, and the police responded by opening fire, killing three demonstrators and wounding dozens. Public order was restored only by a large display of force by the army, and by a series of concessions by the state – subsidies to workers unemployed by the closure of the oyster beds and fishmarkets; a commitment by the authorities that there would be no further sackings; and the opening of soup kitchens.[230]

With this background, Luzzatti arrived at the meeting already convinced that a dangerous defiance of authority had begun at Barletta, had gathered momentum at Taranto, and was about to culminate in an all-out insurrection at Naples. Naples was uniquely dangerous not only because of its sheer size and the variety of interests affected but also because of the fact that the protest would no longer be spontaneous. In Apulia the rioters had lacked leadership and political direction. An insurrection at Naples, by contrast, threatened to have the full support of the labour movement and of the local authorities. The potential consequences were incalculable. Unfortunately, there are no records of the discussion between Luzzatti and the irate Neapolitan delegation. The conclusion, however, was a total capitulation by the state. Faced with the revolt of the southern metropolis, Luzzatti agreed to send representatives to Naples to take the necessary measures to restore free trade.[231]

The public humiliation of Luzzatti, however, was left until 26 February – the day before the expiration of the Neapolitan ultimatum. On that day, as arranged in Rome, Luzzatti's representatives – Santoliquido; Di Fratta; the Minister of Post and Telegraph, Augusto Ciuffelli; and the Secretary of State at the Ministry of Justice and Grace, Alessandro Guarracino – met at the Prefecture in Naples with the leading authorities of the city. There they officially announced that the state hostel was to close; that all *locande* were free to re-open; that the steamship *Marsala* was to be withdrawn from the harbour; that the city was to be unambiguously declared cholera-free; and that City Hall rather than the state was to assume responsibility for all matters affecting public health. In exchange, the local authorities agreed to call off the insurrection and to withdraw the mass resignations.[232] Declining to be interviewed or to explain their actions in public, Luzzatti's unhappy messengers hastily departed for the capital.

Anarchy in Naples had been averted, but the repercussions were serious for Luzzatti's already fragile government, which had just survived a vote of confidence on 2 February.[233] In the wake of the announcements made by his ministers at the Prefecture in Naples his political authority was irreparably compromised. The display of the Italian government capitulating to an ultimatum initiated by *locandieri* and *camorristi* created a major outcry. National newspapers denounced the deal that had been made. The socialist paper *Avanti!* unambiguously described the agitation in Naples as 'the uprising of the Camorra'.[234] In the Chamber of Deputies fourteen members immediately tabled interpellations demanding an explanation of the sordid bargain that had been struck on the issue of public health, and a much publicized debate began on 7 March and lasted four days.[235]

The tone of the questions gave a measure of the incredulity of the Chamber. The radical Deputy from Varese, Carlo Bizzozero, asked if the revocation of the measures to defend the nation against cholera signified that the state proposed to consider emigration primarily as a business venture; Enrico Arlotta bluntly declared that the 'prestige and the authority of the State have been undermined'; and Ettore Ciccotti remarked caustically that Luzzatti's willingness to contradict himself and to give in to every threat demonstrated his 'innate kindness and sweet disposition'.[236] Turati protested against the 'sordid interests' involved. The measures adopted by the state were originally intended as both 'a moral and a physical prophylaxis – a prophylaxis against cholera and a prophylaxis against the Camorra'. Luzzatti had abdicated on both counts, the socialist Deputy from Milan charged. In the wake of this surrender, the nation was left wholly defenceless, while both the disease and the Camorra lay in wait.[237] Angiolo Cabrini condemned the 'weakness' and 'vacillations' of the ministry.[238] In a more literary vein, Nitti observed that, 'At first the Right Honourable Luzzatti appeared before us in the guise of Saint Michael with his flaming sword unsheathed to slay the dragon of the Camorra. Then, after looking the dragon in the eyes, he decided that it was better to come to terms in private.'[239]

Luzzatti's discomfiture was completed by an inept and incoherent reply on 10 March. Having no reasonable explanation to offer in defence of his policy, the Prime Minister made such transparently feeble excuses that they unleashed a torrent of ridicule. Luzzatti began implausibly by insisting that his policy had been unwavering on the question of public health; only circumstances had changed. Furthermore, to general mirth, the Italian premier claimed credit for a great success: his policies had successfully defeated the disease and prevented its spread from Italy to other countries. Defending his record, Luzzatti exclaimed that, 'We have contaminated no one! This is a great thing, and other nations are grateful to us.' From the Chamber benches there were shouts that the government would need foreign votes because it would find itself lacking at home.

Pretending that the return to *laissez-faire* in matters of public health was due to the victory over cholera and making no allusion to the pressure of Neapolitan vested interests, Luzzatti then made an effort to convince the Chamber of a position that was logically inconsistent. His argument was that, with the great triumph over the cholera, the state could remove sanitary restrictions; at the same time, however, he asserted that there was need for constant vigilance and that his government was taking every precaution. There would be constant vigilance over arriving emigrants with physicians manning health inspection posts at the railroad station, with teams of municipal doctors carrying out watchful interventions in the *locande*, and with detectives assigned to special duty in the port to prevent the emigrants from being exploited. Having taken all of these measures, therefore, he challenged, 'Now let the Chamber condemn me if it wants to!'; and his remark was greeted with a chorus of 'No! No, never!'

Finally, Luzzatti reasoned that under the 'new regime' that his government had introduced in Naples, it would be possible for the emigration trade to have the best of all possible worlds. The private *locande* would function once more, while the state hostel would remain open on a purely voluntary basis. In this way, he argued, 'the emigrants will be able to see and compare the advantages and disadvantages of both systems, with full freedom of choice'. At the end, as throughout, the speech was greeted with peals of laughter.

After the premier had resumed his place, the Deputies who had tabled inter-pellations intervened. Turati and Cabrini declared that their questions had not been answered, and they called for a clearer policy from the state. Bizzozero shouted that the conduct of the government was simply 'incoherent'. The final word of the day, however, belonged to Nitti, who mordantly invited Luzzatti to travel abroad with him because he would soon have ample free time. The Chamber, the press reported, reacted with 'prolonged hilarity'.[240] The humili-ation of the Government was capped by the prominence that the Italian news media gave to the debate on public health and emigration. For three days in succession Luzzatti's actions in Naples became the chief item of news in the national press, with banner headlines and nearly the whole of the front page devoted to the Prime Minister's embarrassment. The press sensed that the government was collapsing, and it rushed to record the event.

Less than a week after Luzzatti's parliamentary speech on cholera in Naples, his government fell. The radicals announced that Luzzatti no longer had their confidence and that they would vote with the opposition. Public health was not the only issue that brought about the dissolution of the ministry. Luzzatti's coalition of Left and Right was inherently unstable, and it proved impossible for it to agree on terms for the resolution of the great political issues of the day. Above all, the questions of electoral reform and of state subsidies to the steamship companies divided the two currents that provided the conservative financial expert with a parliamentary majority. Cholera proved, however, to be a key factor in the final unmaking of a fragile ministry.

In the spring of 1911, therefore, Giovanni Giolitti returned to power, bringing with him a lesson that affected public health profoundly and rapidly. Giolitti had witnessed the pillorying of Luzzatti. He understood the explosive potential of cholera and anti-cholera in the former capital of the South, and his conclusion was that such matters were best kept far from public scrutiny. Even without causing vast mortality, Asiatic cholera had demonstrated once more its capacity to sharpen social and political tensions, disrupt public order and undermine trade and commerce.

7

Concealment and crisis: 1911

Almost unnoticed, Asiatic cholera persisted throughout the winter of 1910–11 – despite resolute denials by Italian and Neapolitan officials. As we have seen, occasional 'stragglers' attracted the attention of anxious American officials for months after Italian authorities had declared the autumn outbreak finished. In January 1911 Henry Geddings informed Washington that the continuing existence of foci of infection and 'the inertness of the authorities' warranted a 'gloomy prognosis' for the spring and summer. On the basis of this information, Surgeon-General Walter Wyman published in the sanitary bulletin *Public Health Reports* an official warning to Americans contemplating 'the usual tour of southern Italy in the spring and summer'. The abiding presence of the disease in the city, he argued, suggested that there was a grave danger that the return of warm weather would unleash a new and possibly even larger epidemic. American citizens would be wise, he cautioned, to consider alternative destinations.[1]

Between February and May, a sharp divergence developed between the public pronouncements of Italian authorities and the confidential files of the Department of Public Health. Stunned by the Neapolitan revolt, state officials categorically repudiated all suggestions that there was any danger to public health. The outbreak that caused such alarm first in Apulia and then in Naples, they claimed, had been totally vanquished. Signor Cusani, the Italian Ambassador to Washington, specifically protested to the American Government about the offensive, unjustified and – above all – public musings of the Surgeon-General and his subordinates. 'Italy', Cusani informed the Secretary of State, 'is entirely free from cholera and public health is excellent.'[2]

The files of the Department of Public Health clearly establish, however, that such claims about the freedom of Italy from cholera were disingenuous. The Department kept a vigilant watch on the progress of Asiatic cholera throughout the winter and spring. All of the records were carefully stamped 'secret' in bold red lettering, and at the bottom of each page there was the careful reminder,

'N.B. No official bulletin was published.'[3] Although the news was never made public, the Department monitored an unbroken chain of cases confirmed by laboratory diagnosis stretching from the end of 1910 through the spring of 1911, when the infection erupted once more with epidemic force.[4]

Unfortunately, however, even these confidential files do not allow a precise estimate of the extent of this lingering contagion. One reason is 'innocent': the state was unlikely to be aware of all of the cases that occurred. As in previous epidemics, a suspicious and frightened public was certain to conceal suspect illness from the authorities. In the important industrial centre of Torre Annunziata in the province of Naples, for example, inspectors from the Department of Public Health concluded that, 'From the onset of the epidemic, a very large number of cases was concealed. This policy was favoured by doctors from the communes near Torre Annunziata. They were consulted by the stricken families and did not make the required reports.'[5] Between the beginning of the epidemic and the middle of July, the Department estimated that approximately a hundred cases successfully evaded detection by the authorities in this manner at Torre Annunziata alone.[6]

Furthermore, regardless of the intentions of the state, the integrity of government statistics was inevitably undermined by the policy of silence. The declaration that Italy was free of cholera lowered the vigilance of physicians and increased the likelihood that cases would be misdiagnosed and never reach the attention of officials. In Sardinia in 1912, for instance, the Prefect of Cagliari explained that governmental records of the outbreak were not to be relied upon for precisely this reason. In a lengthy report on the outbreak, he argued that,

> In addition to the known cases, it may be that many other cases occurred but were never recognized as such by the victims or even by the physicians. The patients were motivated by the fear of being taken into isolation, and the doctors were misled by ignorance. Like their patients, the doctors were inclined to believe that there was no question of authentic Asiatic cholera.[7]

Beyond such unintentional sources of inaccuracy, however, official records are untrustworthy because the Department deliberately and systematically underestimated the prevalence of the disease. The concern in Rome was that even confidential sanitary files could eventually form the basis for published statistics or for bulletins to be furnished to foreign governments or international bodies. It was always prudent, therefore, to maintain records that significantly understated the magnitude of the crisis.

In its caution, the Department of Public Health employed a recordkeeping ruse that broke with the statistical methods employed in all previous cholera epidemics. This stratagem consisted of recording only those cases in which the clinical diagnosis of cholera was 'bacteriologically confirmed' by laboratory examination. As Italian health officials were well aware as a result of the Apulian outbreak of 1910, practitioners, especially in the Mezzogiorno, suffered from a severe shortage of laboratories, trained technicians and microscopes. In such conditions, only a strictly limited proportion of suspected cases would ever be diagnosed with the scientific rigour of Robert Koch's procedures. Entirely to exclude cases diagnosed on the basis of clinical symptoms was therefore an effective means of minimizing the statistical record of the disease.

In a letter to Luigi Luzzatti, Giovanni Raineri, the Minister of Agriculture, Industry and Commerce, explained the extent to which the stipulation of bacteriological confirmation could lower the statistical profile of a cholera epidemic. Since the Department of Statistics operated under the aegis of his ministry, Raineri's assessment is especially important. For the outbreak of 1910, he explained, the number of deaths from cholera recorded on the basis of clinical diagnoses or post-mortem examinations was 1,815. The number of these cholera deaths that were 'bacteriologically confirmed', however, was only 805.[8] The latter category, therefore, was highly efficient as a means of reducing unpleasant mortality statistics. Indeed, Raineri claimed credit for first noting the extent of the difference such a bookkeeping device could make. Gratified by his discovery, Raineri ordered the publication only of 'rigorously confirmed figures'. As he slyly noted in his letter,

> I too was convinced of the advisability of avoiding the spread in the Country of exaggerated and conflicting statistics regarding cholera, which still causes great alarm and which is the source of formal commitments towards the nations adhering to the Sanitary Convention of Paris of 1903. I therefore gave immediate instructions to suppress the publication of the former figures [based on clinical diagnoses and post-mortem examinations].[9]

During the first five months of 1911, the disease lingered in the form of scattered cases with no established epidemic foci. Since mortality, therefore, was almost invisible, cholera descended ever lower in the hierarchy of public concerns. In these circumstances, the combination of public reassurances and the private doctoring of the statistical record sufficed to assuage ministerial concern that the situation was under control. Compiled under such conditions, the statistics contained in the files of the Department of Public Health and in the subsequent publications of the Department of Statistics are of limited utility. Despite their inaccuracy, however, the state figures provide incontrovertible proof of two important points: (1) that cholera persisted without interruption in Italy from the summer of 1910 until the eruption of the disease with epidemic force in the summer of 1911; and (2) that the Italian state, despite its vociferous public denials, was fully aware of this fact.

From 1 January 1911 until May the undisclosed cases were stubbornly clustered in Apulia at a distance from the great population centres of the nation. In January, when the government loudly declared its victory over cholera, fresh 'bacteriologically confirmed' cases were secretly recorded on every day of the month except the 30th. In February, March and April, when cholera officially no longer existed on Italian soil, the state tested, confirmed and recorded at least one new case on average every other day. In the words of the indefatigable and anxious Henry Geddings,

Cholera was officially declared to be extinct in the Provinces of Bari, Foggia and Lecce on the 5th of February 1911, yet I know most positively, and could prove it were my information not confidential, that there was not a week, and hardly a day, that there were not sporadic outbreaks of the disease, requiring the most energetic measures to control . . .[10]

In this unbroken sequence of cases, May Day marked a new and disturbing departure. On 1 May the first bacteriologically authenticated case outside Apulia since January was recorded when Vincenza Esposito was stricken at Pianura in the province of Naples. To preserve secrecy and to avoid 'widespread alarm', the Ministry of the Interior ordered that Esposito be transported to hospital silently and in the dead of night.[11] This first case in Campania was then rapidly followed by three additional cases at Fuorigrotta and Bagnoli in the immediate environs of Naples. Then on 9 May eight cases were confirmed in the province on a single day. Ominously, the city itself figured among the infected communes. A new epidemic was beginning.

In May 1911, therefore, the foreboding of Henry Geddings and the United States Public Heath Service proved correct when cholera flared up in Naples with menacing force. It is impossible to know whether the disease had persisted, in the form of unnoticed stragglers since the last documented victim in January, or whether the history of 1910 had repeated itself as Naples was once more infected by people arriving from Apulia. Whatever the path taken by the vibrio, however, it is certain that by the second week of May 1911, both of the two lies invented by Italian officials – the contemporary assertion that no cholera existed anywhere in the peninsula and the later retrospective account that at least no epidemic had occurred in the city of Naples – were being contradicted on a daily basis.

Neither at the time nor subsequently was there ever any public disclosure of the true state of public health in Naples. The United States Public Health Service, however, having detected Asiatic cholera in May, surmised that the disease had probably never disappeared from the city since the end of 1910. Surgeon-General Wyman had identified a recurrence of cholera in southern Italy as potentially the greatest external health threat to the United States.[12] Thus alerted to redoubled vigilance, American public health authorities in Campania discovered cases among the crew of a ship sailing from Naples to Reggio Calabria. Gedding's subordinate, Passed Assistant Surgeon W. W. King, reported the event. 'On May 16th,' he wrote,

the brigantine *Giovanni Costa* sailed direct from Naples to Reggio Calabria. A few hours after arrival, two seamen were taken ill with suspicious symptoms. One died within a few hours, the other after four days, and I am credibly informed that the bacteriological examination made at the University of Catania demonstrated the presence of cholera bacilli. This vessel took $3\frac{1}{2}$ days for the trip, hence these cases were presumably of Naples origin.[13]

As the unhappy Luzzatti's successor, Giovanni Giolitti was determined to avoid any similar misadventure. Giolitti's caution with regard to possible complications in Naples was reinforced by the continuing pressure of the Association for the Protection of the Interests of the Twelfth Electoral District, which had played such a major part in Luzzatti's downfall. Throughout the summer of 1911, led by its President, the lawyer Francesco Montefredini, the Association organized rallies of industrialists, tradesmen and workers. On these occasions Association spokesmen announced that Naples was completely healthy. 'There is no cholera, and never was!', proclaimed the paper *Il Mattino* in support of an Association rally in July.[14] The assembled crowd on that occasion voted resolutions demanding that freedom of trade be unencumbered with unnecessary and harmful sanitary restrictions.[15] In mid-July the spokesmen for the Association further claimed that the absurd sanitary measures imposed by the United States were costing the city 100,000 lire a day in lost revenue by driving the steamship companies, as in 1910, to call at Genoa instead of Naples. A committee consisting of influential businessmen, politicians and trade-union leaders was elected to carry the protest to Rome and to exercise careful watchfulness lest the interests of the city once more be compromised.[16] And once again the threat was made of a combined lockout and general strike unless the anti-cholera measures affecting emigration and the port were revoked.[17]

Rather than confront the wrath of a volatile city that had humiliated his predecessor, Giolitti implemented the strategy demanded by Neapolitan interests – a national policy of concealment. In his desire to placate a large and strategic parliamentary delegation and to avert anarchy in the great metropolis, Giolitti resolved to suppress all information regarding the real state of public health. Here it is important to stress the magnitude of the decision that his government took in May. Misleading statements and laundered statistics marked Italian policy for the whole period from the start of the year. May, however, marked a quantum leap in the process. Until May the state failed to disclose a troubling but small-scale infection consisting of one or two cases a day in remote Apulian communes. Between mid-May and early June, however, the infection exploded into a full-scale epidemic in Italy's leading seaport. The decision to conceal this new threat therefore involved responsibilities of a wholly different order of magnitude. It necessitated the wholesale violation of international treaty obligations; and it required the use of authoritarian police methods that were familiar in other spheres of Italian state policy, but that had never before been deployed at the national level in the field of public health. As the Liberal regime entered upon its turbulent final crisis, cholera provided the occasion for an ominous display of unaccountable power by the executive in violation of both domestic and international law, and to the detriment of both civil liberty and the health of the nation.

Pressure from the southern metropolis first led the Italian Prime Minister to the policy of secrecy. He was confirmed in this course, however, by other considerations, as the American Ambassador, John Leishman, carefully explained to Philander Chase Knox, the United States Secretary of State.[18] One such concern was patriotism. The summer of 1911 marked the fiftieth anniversary of Italian unification, and major international exhibitions to mark the occasion were planned at Turin and Rome, where millions of tourists were confidently expected. A major medical emergency would destroy the festivities and halt the arrival of foreign visitors, just at a time when their stimulus to a national economy in recession was eagerly awaited. In such an eventuality, Italy would also lose its reputation for modernity and salubrity. A second anxiety was commercial. Knowledge of a large-scale outbreak would cause other nations to apply restrictive measures against Italian goods, especially those highly perishable exports of grapes and olives on which the Italian economy depended, and against Italian immigrants, whose remittances were so important to a successful economic recovery. Finally, cholera and the announcement of measures to combat it posed severe problems of public order. The experiences of Giolitti's recent predecessors – G. Morana as Minister of the Interior confronting the epidemic of the 1880s and Luzzatti as Prime Minister combating cholera in Apulia and Naples in 1910 – both demonstrated the potential that cholera possessed for creating panic, flight and rebellion. Giolitti intended to avoid their travails.

A policy of secrecy on a vast scale presented two great practical difficulties, one domestic and the other external. The domestic obstacle was that to suppress information was to negate the possibility of taking effective measures to combat the disease. If the state failed to declare the presence of epidemic cholera, it would deprive itself of all legal means to take effective sanitary counter-measures. A solution to this difficulty had been first suggested by the Prefect of Bari during the summer outbreak in Apulia. At that time he urged concealment behind a fictive diagnosis of meningitis that would allow the authorities to take preventive measures of isolation and disinfection without causing terror or risking inter-national repercussions. When the disease broke out at Naples in September, the authorities adopted this astute suggestion, but they replaced the façade of meningitis with the alternative diagnosis of gastro-enteritis. As the recurring scourge of the Neapolitan summer, gastro-enteritis had the advantages of plausi-bility and familiarity.

No degree of diagnostic skill, however, could have concealed reality if the progress of the disease had been marked by large-scale tumults. Events of the kind that occurred in Apulia in 1910 would have alerted the nation, particularly if they took place in such a highly visible and important centre as Naples. A silent precondition for the success of Giolitti's strategy was the assumption that alarm could be contained and order preserved. Here the Neapolitan outbreak of the previous autumn was encouraging because it suggested that, with circumspect public health policies, cholera need no longer be accompanied by violent disorder.

The external difficulty was international law. Because of its dependence on the export of agricultural goods and people, Italy had long been a leading force in devising an international sanitary framework that would minimize the disruption that the great epidemic diseases of cholera and plague caused to international trade. Italian efforts bore fruit at the Paris Convention of 1903, which was attended by twenty-four nations. The delegates at Paris abolished the anarchic sanitary world where every state was free to impose health regulations of its own devising and where the absence of reliable information often caused anxious nations to impose quarantines and embargoes of an exaggerated and harmful rigour. The Convention established instead a uniform global system that hinged on two essential agreements. The first was the commitment, embodied in Articles 1, 2, 4 and 5, of all the signatories to provide full, immediate and continuous disclosure of the presence of cholera or plague anywhere within their territories.

Article 1 provided for urgent disclosure in its declaration that, 'Each government should immediately notify other governments of the first appearance in its territory of authentic cases of plague or cholera.'[19] Article 2 then specified the information to be submitted when notification was provided. It required that,

> This notification is to be accompanied, or very promptly followed, by the following circumstantial information:
>
> 1. The neighborhood where the disease has appeared.
> 2. The date of its appearance, its origin, and its form.
> 3. The number of established cases, and the number of deaths.
> 4. For plague: the existence among rats or mice of plague, or a pronounced mortality.
> 5. The measures immediately taken as a subsequence of its first appearance.[20]

Article 4 stipulated the provision of a steady stream of progress reports on the subsequent course of the disease. The text of the article stated that, 'The notification and the information prescribed in Articles 1 and 2 are to be followed by further communications dispatched in a regular manner in order to keep the governments informed of the progress of the epidemic . . . at least once a week.'[21] Finally, Article 5 underlined the significance of Articles 1 to 4 and added a note of moral exhortation. This Article urged that, 'The prompt and honest accomplishment of the provisions which precede above is of the very first importance.'[22]

If the Articles on notification comprised the first essential component of the system devised by the Paris Convention, the second was global uniformity. The Convention established standardized measures of public health that were to be taken by the signatory nations receiving notification of an outbreak of cholera. Land-based quarantines, sanitary cordons and lazarettos reminiscent of the Italian experiment of 1884 as well as total embargoes on goods and bans on travellers from infected countries were forbidden.

Maritime quarantine, however, was preserved as an integral part of the international system of defensive measures. But the stringency of the quarantine procedures was limited to those practices that scientific understanding of the life-cycle of the *Vibrio cholerae* confirmed as rational public hygiene. In the case of Naples in 1911, the crucial issue was the restrictions that, under the terms of the international agreement, the United States was authorized to impose on steamships, passengers and cargo bound for New York Harbor. The Paris Convention stipulated that, upon the declaration of a foreign port as infected, the

United States Public Health Service could decree the isolation of all steerage passengers and crew prior to embarkation for a period of five days during which they would be subject to the bacteriological examination of their faeces, the disinfection of their personal effects and the confiscation of all foodstuffs in their possession. American officials were also allowed to prohibit the loading of cargo originating in Naples or in other infected centres, ban the use of water from the port for the washing of decks and require that ships be issued with foul bills of health that would alert officers of health at Ellis Island to redoubled vigilance.[23]

In addition to measures to be taken before sailing, the Convention regulated sanitary procedures during the crossing and after arrival in the New World. On the high seas the masters of vessels were obliged to isolate all suspiciously ill passengers, to disinfect their possessions, and to require that the ships' doctors maintain detailed clinical records.[24] When an arriving immigrant vessel docked at New York Harbor, the examining physicians of the United States Public Health Service could impose an additional period of quarantine, require all steerage passengers to submit to disinfection and bacteriological examination, and detain any suspect cases on Hoffman and Swinburn Islands. Cabin passengers, considered people of quality unlikely to present a medical risk, were free from the restrictions affecting their impecunious fellow travellers.

The rationale for these sanitary provisions of the Paris Convention was the incubation period for Asiatic cholera which contemporary medical opinion set at a maximum of seventeen days. Five days of quarantine in the port of departure, twelve days for the average crossing to New York, and a further five days of quarantine in New York Harbor were thought to be sufficient to prevent fresh cases from gaining admission to North America. At the same time, bacteriological examination on Ellis Island would provide the United States with a defensive shield against asymptomatic carriers, while the disinfection of all personal effects and the destruction of foodstuffs would eliminate all other sources of contamination. In the event of a fatality among the detainees, there were strict instructions for the rapid cremation of the body.

As a final precaution against the possibility that a case of cholera or a carrier should slip through the defensive net, the Quarantine Regulations of the United States authorized the Public Health and Marine Hospital Service to issue final destination cards to all passengers arriving from an infected port. The destination cards were forwarded to the health authorities in the states to which the immigrants were bound. State Boards of Health would then assume the responsibility of monitoring the health of newly arriving immigrants, of alerting local doctors to be aware of suspicious symptoms, and of eliminating all immigrants from such medically sensitive employment as work on the filter-beds or reservoirs of public water supplies.[25]

Since rational public health policies involve information and public awareness, the Convention also stipulated that all measures taken to combat plague and cholera be immediately published. The course of the disease and the sanitary means employed to defeat it were to be matters of public record available to governments, the press, shipping companies and international sanitary bodies.

The requirements imposed on the Italian Government by the Convention of Paris were explicit. When the first cases of Asiatic cholera occurred in 1911, Italy was obliged at once to inform the international community, to undertake preventive measures and to publish an account of its success or failure. Any possibility of ambiguity was eliminated by the double coincidence that the Director-General of Public Health in Italy was Rocco Santoliquido, who had served in 1903 as the Vice-President of the Convention and as the Italian signatory, and that the American representative and signatory had been Henry Geddings.[26] How the Italian Government reacted was especially important because the epidemic in Italy in 1910 and 1911 provided the first opportunities for the provisions of the Convention to be tested in practice.

In Rome, worries about public order, economic interest and political expediency triumphed over treaty obligations and the requirements of public health. When cholera broke out menacingly in Naples in 1911, Giolitti immediately took two important decisions. The first was to centralize the direction of the renewed anti-cholera campaign. In 1910 Luzzatti had relied in Naples on the efficiency of the Neapolitan Office of Hygiene and on the zeal of its director, Orazio Caro. For Giolitti and Santoliquido, the recrudescence of the disease indicated that Caro and his Office had failed. In 1911, therefore, the Department of Public Health, an agency of the Ministry of the Interior, was entrusted with operational direction of the war against cholera. Professor Loriga was despatched to Naples as a virtual sanitary Prefect with full powers to direct the work of the municipal health officials. The Office of Hygiene was instructed merely to implement policy determined by central government. Like a Prefect, Loriga was also given authority in medical matters throughout the province as well as the city of Naples. Only in this way, it was reasoned, could a coherent strategy be devised to prevent the spread of the disease from the city to its hinterland as occurred in the preceding autumn.[27]

The decision to centralize control of public health was also a means to facilitate the second policy, which was secrecy. Concealment of course was not new as a temptation, as the Palazzo San Giacomo had amply demonstrated when confronted with the need to acknowledge the presence of cholera in 1910. Procrastination, denial and invention were weapons that the administration of Ferdinando Del Carretto and Giulio Rodinò had deployed to avoid the consequences of full public knowledge of the return of epidemic cholera. The silences and duplicity of 1910, however, were local initiatives. The great innovation of 1911 was the deployment of the full resources of the nation-state to prevent all knowledge of a major cholera epidemic. Giovanni Giolitti immediately adopted this course of action when the first confirmed cases of cholera in Naples occurred in May.

On 13 May – three days before the sailing of the brigantine *Giovanni Costa* that initially attracted the attention of the American Consulate – Giolitti was already seriously concerned by medical events in Naples. In dealing with the emergency, the Prime Minister urged the Prefect to take action, but in such a way as to avoid the need for official acknowledgement of the crisis. Giolitti was moving rapidly in the direction of total concealment. With this policy in mind, Giolitti was displeased with the Prefect's initiative of establishing soup kitchens under state aegis. It was useful, Giolitti suggested, to provide the poor with nourishment in time of cholera, but to do so openly was to admit the presence of the disease and to attract unwelcome attention. As the Prime Minister informed his subordinate,

> This Ministry must explicitly stress that you must act with all possible vigour, but also with all possible care in order, no matter what, to avoid causing alarm. Act therefore with the greatest caution … and avoid all public displays, such as are involved in the operation of proper soup kitchens. The private delivery of food supplies to people's homes, for example, can be carried on by means of benevolent associations. This is a normal activity that could be much intensified now without giving rise to any need to change appearances.[28]

Within a week of this first suggestion of secrecy, the strategy was more systematically developed. On 20 May Giolitti sent a lengthy and highly confidential telegram to the Prefect of Naples with instructions to implement a comprehensive policy of silence, even though the failure to notify foreign powers entailed the risk of allowing the epidemic to spread abroad. It was one of the ironies of 1911 that Rocco Santoliquido, the Director-General of Public Health, was now employed to direct a sanitary campaign in flagrant violation of the treaty that he had been instrumental in creating in 1903. With respect to secrecy, the premier's orders stated that,

> The seriousness of the situation developing in Naples and emerging from the growing number of daily cases in the city and the nearby villages demands the energetic and uninterrupted deployment of all the means at your disposal. It is essential, whatever the cost, to suffocate the infection. At the same time, this work must be carried out without any unnecessary publicity. Make use of all the contrivances and expedients that, given your experience and wisdom, I have no need to specify. The aim is to obtain and maintain the greatest possible secrecy …
>
> Make certain that all functionaries are aware that they must carry out all of their duties without making any noise, and that the Government will be merciless [*severissimo*] with all those who are slow or negligent in carrying out your orders or who are unable to keep the necessary discretion.[29]

This cable marked a watershed in Italian public health policy against Asiatic cholera. In 1911 the Giolitti government broke new ground by making Italy the first and only European nation, as far as is known, to conceal a major epidemic of the disease. Asiatic cholera ravaged Naples, invaded most regions of the peninsula, devastated Sicily, and finally reached distant Sardinia in 1912. In so great a misfortune Naples renewed its unhappy national primacy in the history of epidemic cholera. Nevertheless, there has been no recognition by historians of this display of the power to suppress information; there has been no extended study of the epidemic itself, which has been thought to have constituted a minor, inconsequential outbreak; and there has been no discussion of this final chapter in the Neapolitan experience of cholera. So completely was Giolitti able to conceal the events of 1911 in the great southern metropolis that his efforts enabled Orazio Caro in 1912 to publish his mythology of the invulnerability of the modern city to infection without fear of contradiction. Such was Giolitti's legacy, and our task is to reconstruct the record of this secret epidemic.

OFFICIAL SILENCE

The press

Evidence of the success of the state-sponsored conspiracy is abundant. From the date of Giolitti's telegrams in May until the final week in August 1911, the press, both national and local, almost completely ignored the issue of Asiatic cholera. It is important to avoid categorical statements because no comprehensive study of the Italian press in 1911 with regard to epidemic disease has ever been undertaken. On the other hand, to examine a selection of the most influential national papers is to gain the distinct impression that Italy escaped almost entirely unscathed after the alarm of the previous year. *Il Corriere della sera, Avanti!, La Nazione, Il Giornale d'Italia, Il Messaggero, Il Resto del carlino* and *La Tribuna*, for example, all failed until the end of August ever to mention the cholera prevailing on Italian soil. Thomas Mann was strictly accurate when he observed in *Death in Venice* that it was impossible for his protagonists to obtain news of the cholera epidemic of 1911 in Italian newspapers.

Finally on 29 August – three months after the onset of the epidemic – the principal national newspapers very partially lifted the veil of silence by reporting the violent incident of a cholera riot in the Calabrian village of Verbicaro. There the local shepherds, fearing that the disease was a mass murder perpetrated by the authorities, took desperate and bloody revenge on the men they regarded as ruthless killers. To the cry of 'Kill the poisoners!', they rampaged through the centre of the village, killing innocent people, pillaging dwellings at random and setting buildings ablaze. While disclosing these dramatic events, the press made no effort to link them with the prior history of the epidemic. The state had finally lifted the censorship, but only to a limited degree and at a carefully chosen time. By late August the disease was rapidly receding, and Giolitti felt confident that the sanitary situation was once more in control. The outbreak in Naples, the most sensitive centre, was nearly over. The patriotic celebrations commemorating Italian independence, the tourist season, and the peak period for emigration to North America were past. Furthermore, in the gathering international crisis that was taking the country to war in Libya, revelations concerning public health were unlikely to capture public attention.

In any event, partial disclosures of sanitary developments in Italy had grown so numerous abroad that it was becoming increasingly problematic to expunge the word cholera entirely from the Italian media. Seepages first began in foreign papers and medical journals. The Vatican press is a special case. Because of its dense network of parish priests and its contacts throughout Italy, the Church learned of the presence of cholera at an early date. Safely beyond the reach of state pressure and jaundiced in its view of the patriotic festivities of the year, the papal newspaper, *Osservatore romano*, was also relatively free to voice its misgivings. In the first week of July it published its first article of the summer on public health, demanding that the state set the many rumours of cholera to rest by providing accurate and honest information – a demand that it repeated at intervals for the rest of the month. Without definitively asserting that Italy was in the midst of a major epidemic, the paper assumed a cautious note, reminding the authorities of their duty rather than making specific allegations of mendacity.[30]

In August, *Osservatore romano* took a different and more combative position. Without attempting to provide a detailed account of sanitary conditions in Italy, the paper specifically charged that cholera was present at Naples and Livorno, and it charged the government and the press with a derelection of duty in maintaining an 'irresponsible and, by now, ridiculous silence'.[31] Giolitti in particular, it claimed, had taken a grave moral responsibility for placing the success of the tourist industry and the jubilee celebrations above the health of the nation.[32] Unfortunately, the editors argued, *Osservatore romano* had only been preaching in the desert. Its message was dismissed as an outpouring of Catholic venom against the Liberal regime. Only the universal acknowledgment of the 'scenes from the *Decameron*'[33] that transpired at Verbicaro on 29 August gave credibility to the Vatican's position on cholera and encouraged the newspaper to take a still more militant stance. From 30 August until the end of September, therefore, *Osservatore romano* provided specific details of the epidemic in several centres apart from Calabria, and above all at Livorno. The papal newspaper also accused Giolitti of responsibility for the outbreak of cholera north of Rome because the vast movement of people throughout the peninsula in conjunction with the festivities had provided the disease with an ideal means of spreading. Only with the absorption of the whole nation with events in North Africa did the issue of public health disappear from its pages.[34]

From the greater distance of the British Isles, the *Lancet* and the *British Medical Journal* published several articles of increasing awareness on the Italian epidemic and the policy of secrecy. Beginning in June, the *Lancet* hinted at 'cholera shadows' in the peninsula and it questioned the wisdom of tourists who planned to attend the Exhibitions at Turin and Rome. By September, the 'shadows' had been transformed into a certainty that the disease was prevalent in large areas of the country, despite official denials that were 'not in harmony with the truth'. Lacking accurate information, however, the Italian correspondent for the *Lancet* mistakenly viewed the port of Livorno as the centre of the contagion.[35] Finally, in December the *Lancet* belatedly printed news of the Italian epidemic, which was no longer present on the mainland.[36]

With its headquarters in the immediate vicinity of New York Harbor, where Italian cholera victims began to arrive at the end of June and where the disease even reached the mainland, the *New York Times* had a strategic vantage point from which to be alerted to the existence of a medical emergency in Italy. The issue assumed local prominence after the deaths in mid-July of recently landed immigrants at Auburn, Brooklyn and Staten Island in New York State. Wild rumours began to circulate that seriously ill and malevolent Italians had eluded the medical examiners and were at large in New York City, indulging themselves in an evil cholera-spreading spree. *Untori* as well as disease had reached the New World.[37]

From that time, although the *New York Times* had no access to conclusive or comprehensive information, it was evident to its editors both that cholera was prevalent in Italy and that it posed a danger to public health in the United States. In the second half of July, therefore, the paper published a series of tentative and circumspect articles suggesting that cholera had broken out in Italy. Initially, the *New York Times* made no effort to quantify the cases and fatalities, but it hazarded the view that the disease had probably been imported from Russia and that it had claimed victims at Palermo, Naples and Venice.[38] On 17 July the newspaper also relayed a report that appeared in the French press that 2,300 people had died of cholera in Palermo.[39] It also correctly concluded that Naples was the 'centre of Italy's present cholera-infected district'.[40]

The New York paper had succeeded in penetrating the mystery. Lacking detailed information, however, its coverage of the issue was sporadic, limited and highly speculative. With approximately ten, mostly brief, articles devoted to the issue between mid-July and December, there was no parallel with the extensive accounts of Italian and Neapolitan public health that appeared in its pages during the fifth pandemic. Italian events, in any case, were considered principally in terms of the possible risk they posed to the United States and no attempt was made at a comprehensive or detailed assessment of conditions on the far side of the Atlantic. By the end of July, moreover, the apparent danger to Americans posed by the emergency in Italy had not materialized as the early cases were successfuly contained. With the end of the immediate crisis, the interest of the paper in Italian public health waned. At the same time, the cholera cases on which it depended as a readily available source of definite information ceased. Not until the easing of the censorship in Italy at the end of August, therefore, did the paper return to the issue. With access to more reliable sources in September and October, the *New York Times* then printed three dramatic articles on the occurrence of violent cholera-riots in the regions of Apulia and Latium.[41] An interest in the sensational replaced the theme of the danger to America.

On the strength of such glimpses into the reality of public health in Italy, the Italian state began in June to receive a stream of correspondence from careful epidemic-watchers who had traced the cholera to Italy. Throughout the summer and autumn they wrote to offer advice on prevention and treatment or to market remedies. Some were cynical speculators who sought to profit from Italy's misfortunes by peddling specific remedies and infallible cures. An example is the

Vice-Consul of Guatemala, who claimed to have developed a chemical guaranteed to restore sufferers to health. He urged the government to order his product in bulk for the Italian army. Similarly, Rudolph Dotterweich of the Red Seneca Rock Oil Company of New York advertised an oil 'discovered by the Indian before the white man came to America' that was certain to cure cholera; G. Avogardo of the Chioselli Company urged the Ministry of the Interior to order his cholera-destroying yoghurt; Alex Kerr of Spokane, Washington wished to sell the King large supplies of 'Kerr's cholera cure'; Nicola Vanacore of Aversa offered 'Vanacore's anti-cholera pills'; and a representative of the 'University College of Africa' advertised a secret medicine developed by 'our chemical laboratory'. Others wrote without financial motive, hoping to save lives by informing the Italians of exotic cures for epidemic disease. From Sandringham, Australia, for instance, came a note explaining to King Victor Emmanuel that the writer could save sufferers by surgical means, pouring a strong tincture into a deep incision made in the shoulder with a 'clean scalpel'. Alternatively, Mrs Augusta Anderson of Salt Lake City recommended peppermint tea and strong coffee; James Griffin of St Petersburg, Florida urged the administration of a beverage of chloroform and water; and Charles Meighan of Chicago suggested a mixture of pulverized rhubarb and spearmint tea. Bernardino Pisa of Cagliari asked only for access to the cholera wards of the mainland, where he proposed, *pro bono*, to test his own secret substances on the patients.[42] The variety of sources for this correspondence from every continent during the summer suggested that interested parties were penetrating the secret.

Finally at the end of August, as the prevalence of the disease rapidly contracted, the state lifted its medical censorship sufficiently for public discussion of the issue to appear for the first time. In Naples itself, the local press, like the national media, had avoided all discussion of public health throughout the summer of 1911. In a city where thousands of people perished, not one newspaper broke ranks by reporting the issue. Strikingly, the ban on the forbidden cholera-word did not affect only those conservative and Catholic papers that supported the ruling clerico-moderate administration – papers such as *Il Mattino, Don Marzio*, and *La Libertà*. More noticeably, the prohibition on discussion of public health and disease in 1911 also silenced the combative organs of the Popular Bloc – the republican *Roma* and the anarcho-syndicalist *La Propaganda* – despite the fact that these two papers were the very ones that had seized so eagerly on the outbreak of 1910 as a weapon to scourge the Carretto regime.

The first and most informative article on cholera to appear in any Neapolitan paper during the course of the epidemic appeared on 29 August, when the daily *Roma* followed the example of the national daily papers by printing an account of the turbulent events at Verbicaro.[43] This article and its timing reveal the severely limited audacity of the editors. Breaking months of absolute silence, the republican paper went beyond the standard, anodyne account that appeared in the pages of other Italian newspapers. Almost alone in Italy, *Roma* hinted at a broader national context and chastised the Giolitti ministry for its policy of secrecy. Because the comments of *Roma* are almost the only discussion of the conspiracy to appear in any newspaper in Italy, they merit analysis. 'There is no one', the republican daily observed,

> who is so blind as not to see that the responsibility for what took place rests with the central government. The state has always abandoned the South, where it favours local camarillas and undermines society. The government has left the population in brutishness and ignorance, and it has failed in its civilizing responsibilities....
>
> But in addition to these general failings and generic responsibilities, the painful events of Verbicaro reveal a recent and immediate wrong. This is the injustice committed by the present government, which decided the keep the sanitary conditions of the country a secret in order to evade its responsibilities for the defence of public health ...
>
> Thus the disease was able to spread and to ravage various regions of Italy from deepest Calabria to Liguria and Venetia. Everywhere the sanitary intervention of the government was weak, poorly coordinated and ineffective.[44]

Thus *Roma* roused itself to a clear and specific indictment of the Giolitti government. There were two significant limits, however, to the courage of the paper. The first was the tardiness with which *Roma* confronted the issue of cholera, delaying publication until the epidemic had almost concluded, the patriotic festivities of the summer were over, and the high seasons for emigration and tourism were past. The second major limit was the refusal to admit that the disaster had ever involved the city of Naples itself. On the thorny issue of local events, for which it had a special responsibility, the paper lost its nerve and meekly repeated the official line. 'This time,' it reassured potentially hostile readers in positions of power, 'Naples was able to escape the danger. Because its means of self-defence were ready, ours is the city in which the state of public health is the best.'[45] There were clearly major constraints on journalistic freedom, and they operated with such force as to blunt what began as a bold and forthright condemnation of Italian public health policy. For even the boldest of Neapolitan papers, discussion of the summer epidemic was confined to the experience of Calabrian shepherds.

Parliament and City Hall

The press was far from alone in its obedience to state policy. The two political assemblies where previous epidemics in Naples had been debated and the conduct of the authorities presented – parliament and the city council – were either silent or became sounding-boards for the presentation of the official version of events. On 17 July the city council received its only opportunity to discuss public health and to question the administration about cholera. On that occasion Councillor Alessandro Elefante, a supporter of the administration, quizzed Mayor Del Carretto. In Berlin, Elefante reported, the government had stated in an official public health bulletin that cholera was present in Naples.

Various German newspapers had taken up this item of news, he declared, tendentiously and maliciously exaggerating it, 'even declaring that cholera victims were dying in their hundreds in the streets of the city'. 'Therefore,' Elefante continued, 'I ask the Mayor to declare formally and explicitly what the real conditions of public health are in the city of Naples.'[46] The question and its preamble suggested that Elefante's was a 'friendly' question rather than a probing one. It seemed that he was not seeking information but attempting to provide the administration with a public and well-rehearsed occasion to confront troubling reports and rumours.

In a lengthy reply, Del Carretto explained that, from the time of the outbreak of 1910, the executive committee had acted energetically but 'without making loud noises' to guarantee the health of the city. In recent months the central government had intervened, but it was motivated by the desire to protect emigration rather than by any worries about the sanitary condition of Naples. As a result of the vigilance of the local authorities, public health was 'completely satisfactory'. The real concern of the administration, therefore, was not disease, but rather the many malicious rumours about disease. Del Carretto promised that his intention was to confront such reports one by one and 'to deny them in the fullest and most categorical manner'.[47] For this reason, the need for further discussion of epidemic disease did not arise: cholera was non-existent.

Consistent with this vision of a Naples that was cholera-free, the executive committee of the city council expunged all mention of cholera from the written record of its deliberations.[48] The reason for such caution was that the resolutions passed by the *giunta* were communicated to a wide circle of councillors, members of municipal departments and the employees of contracting firms. Their discretion could not be guaranteed. Only prudent self-censorship, therefore, could ensure the desired secrecy. In order to maintain this confidentiality, the executive also altered its normal procedures for the conduct of business. For purposes of carrying out medically related public works, the aldermen were authorized to award contracts by means of private negotiations rather than by holding public competitions.[49]

Despite such careful precautions, the minutes of the deliberations of the executive are revealing because its actions in practice contradicted its bland public reassurances. The concerns of the *giunta* in the summer of 1911 differed radically from those of 'normal' years when there was no cholera. From May until November public health suddenly became an urgent preoccupation for the aldermen of the city. Sanitary measures became the principal item on the agenda of meetings, and medical necessities became the reason for onerous appropriations that are intelligible only in the light of a major sanitary campaign against Asiatic cholera.

In June 1911, for example, the executive took action to ensure the supply of pure water for the surrounding villages; to fund orphanages; to establish disinfection stations; to provide free public baths for the indigent; to inspect markets and water supplies; to hire additional municipal physicians, nurses and gravediggers; to provide the Cotugno Hospital with emergency supplies and personnel; and to convert both the former Maddalena barracks, used in 1884 as a cholera hospital, and the New Castle facing City Hall into isolation barracks for the quarantine of people who had been in contact with infected people.[50] On 3 June, the *giunta* voted unanimously to hire the following personnel on an emergency basis under the direction of the Office of Hygiene: three health inspectors, six doctors, two clerks, five guards, four porters, sixteen nurses, six orderlies, thirty manual labourers employed for services of disinfection, and eight gravediggers.[51]

The disease that so heavily demanded the attention of the local authorities and that claimed such major allocations of public funds was never mentioned by name. Urgent matters of public health, therefore, were discussed only by means of elaborate but largely transparent circumlocutions. The resolution to provide Serino water to the neighbouring centres of Fuorigrotta and Bagnoli, for example, was taken on the basis that 'there are imperative necessities, primarily of a hygienic nature, that require urgent measures'.[52] In a similar tone and on the same day, a decision was taken to enlarge the central disinfection station and to equip it with additional carts, horses, stables and electric lighting on the grounds that,

> the execution of the forementioned works admits of no delay, and it is essential to begin them as rapidly as possible as a measure of hygiene. Therefore, it is out of the question to hold a public competition for the building contract, and the matter will be resolved by private negotiation.[53]

Equally revealing was the obscure language used to justify the granting of a subsidy to a local orphanage. Referring to the epidemic of 1910 but without mentioning the word, the Neapolitan aldermen decided that the reasons that had justified the subsidy the previous autumn now applied again. 'There is therefore', the resolution stated, 'no reason to deny the charitable institution the same aid that it received in 1910 and for which it has an urgent and absolute need if it is to perform its mission of mercy.'[54]

With regard to the hiring of additional municipal doctors, disinfection teams and veterinarians for the inspection of markets, the executive noted that their employment by the city was essential under the prevailing circumstances and that the normal emergency rates of pay for such personnel had to be substantially increased due to the 'onerous labour that these officials must bear at the present moment'. Physicians engaged in the municipal campaign against disease were to receive 8 lire a day because the demand for their services was so great that they were compelled to work 12-hour shifts day and night 'at serious personal sacrifice and to the neglect of any other professional interest or concern'.[55] On every front the city found itself confronted with necessities of 'an extraordinary nature', 'exceptional circumstances', 'emergencies' and conditions that 'admit of no delay'.

Nevertheless, the executive committee of the city of Naples used the words 'cholera' and 'epidemic' only once – on 17 October, in the context of a decision to provide the Office of Hygiene with additional funds.[56] It is plainly evident that the *giunta* took elaborate precautions to edit its language in order to conceal the truth with regard to matters of health.

The Cotugno Hospital

The archives of the Cotugno Hospital are also compatible with the theory of a well-organized cover-up, although the evidence is only circumstantial rather than conclusive. Patient records at the public hospital for infectious diseases for the cholera years of 1910 and 1911 have survived. There are, however, two large and suggestive gaps in the files. These gaps encompass the very months when cholera prevailed in the city and when the Cotugno was one of the major instruments in the defence of the city. No patient records exist for the autumn of 1910 or for the period from 1 May to 1 November 1911. There are no documents in the Cotugno archive, therefore, that could be used, with their compromising notation of cholera, to contest the official interpretation of the Neapolitan experience of the sixth pandemic – that a successful campaign against a strictly limited outbreak in 1910 was followed by total immunity in 1911. The only clinical records for cholera patients treated at the hospital during the course of the sixth pandemic date from November 1911. In that month the Cotugno admitted nine men to its cholera ward, but they were Italian sailors who contracted the disease in Tripoli and therefore posed no troubling problems for the myth of a cholera-free city.[57]

Apart from a possible 'disinfection' of the medical records, there are two other possibilities. The first is that the Cotugno generated no records during the contentious months because the city was free of infectious disease. With regard to the autumn of 1910, there is no dispute, however, that cholera existed and that patients were treated at the Cotugno Hospital. The controversial issue at that time was the more limited one of whether the disease had actually followed the course claimed by the administrators of the city. Did the outbreak really begin only on 25 September? Were there only a few hundred cases as Orazio Caro claimed? Did the infection terminate before the end of October? Clinical records could have shed light, perhaps in an unwelcome fashion, on these issues. Conveniently and perhaps not entirely by chance, the charts compiled in 1910 have not survived.

With respect to the summer of 1911, even the expurgated official records of the municipal *giunta* demonstrate that there was a serious epidemic of contagious disease in Naples. The executive committee of the city council repeatedly voted emergency funds to finance treatment at the infectious diseases hospital. On 21 June the executive committee voted the urgent allocation of 3,000 lire for the institution and revealed that 150 patients 'in critical condition' were undergoing treatment on its wards. Their numbers and those of the attendants required to attend them, moreover, were 'increasing day by day'.[58]

The money was voted in urgent response to a report of Giulio Rodinò on the financial plight of the hospital.[59] In existing circumstances, Rodinò explained, 3,000 lire would allow the Cotugno to operate for only a fortnight. The money would be absorbed by food, medicine and ice 'in large quantities' for the patients; and for the wages of a quintupled staff of orderlies and nurses. Such was the gravity of the medical condition of the sufferers that they required greater care and expenditure than the 'ordinary' patients managed on the Cotugno wards. The Medical Director, Alfonso Montefusco, was working on 24-hour call in response to the crisis; the doctors on night duty never rested; and the nurses were said to be 'in danger of fainting from exhaustion and sleep deprivation'.[60] Rodinò revealed that the emergency that was overwhelming the Cotugno had begun on 4 May, which should, therefore, be taken as the beginning of the 1911 epidemic in the city.[61] One of the most powerful officials in Naples, the alderman responsible for public health did not forget himself by discussing the nature of the malady that was causing such anxiety and expense. He never provided the committee with a specific diagnosis, and his colleagues appropriated funds to combat and treat a mystery disease. Clinical records that could have resolved this issue conclusively have disappeared from the Cotugno archives.

Since the records of the *giunta* demonstrate that the hospital was operating at full capacity, there is no doubt that files once existed. Logically, therefore, the second 'innocent' possibility is that the patient files were lost through deterioration or misadventure. Such an outcome cannot be disproved. On the contrary, the surviving Cotugno records for 1910 and 1911 are in a very poor state of preservation, and additional files could well have succumbed to time, moisture and poor maintenance. Furthermore, the archives of the Cotugno Hospital were moved and rehoused during the 1960s when the facility was rebuilt on a new site. The removal was a propitious moment for accidental loss. A theory of conspiracy, therefore, cannot be conclusively established by the absence of patient records alone. What suggests such a possibility in the case of the Cotugno is the combination of two additional factors. The first is the fact that the gaps in the hospital archives during the cholera years are highly selective. Is it by chance that records for the politically sensitive months of the summer disappeared, but not for the remainder of the year? The second suspicious consideration is that cholera patients did not disappear only from the archives. In addition, they vanished without trace from the journal *Rivista di Malattie Infettive* published in Naples under the auspices of the hospital and edited by its Medical Director, Alfonso Montefusco. In 1911 there is no reference in this journal specializing in communicable disease to such obviously pertinent issues as the presence of Asiatic cholera in the city, the treatment of cholera patients, or the public health campaign undertaken to defeat the disease. It is tempting to speculate that the same hand that censored the journal may have 'laundered' the archival records, especially since the hand in both cases was that of Montefusco, who served as one of the principal architects of the 'official' municipal position on epidemic disease in Naples.[62]

The cemetery

The care with which officials avoided all acknowledgement of cholera was apparent, therefore, in the secrecy that concealed the diagnosis and treatment of patients. Official prudence also shrouded the bodies after death. Secrecy followed the funeral carts on their journey from the Cotugno Hospital to the Cemetery of Pity. Here indigent Neapolitans who had to be buried at public expense were laid to rest in unmarked graves at a respectful distance from the monumental cemetery for their betters at Poggioreale. Unlike Neapolitan practice in previous epidemics, the cemetery register for 1911 contains no troubling indiscretions. The contrast with 1884 is striking. In the earlier epidemic the cemetery made a notation of cholera beside the name of all those who died of the disease. It also recorded the names of the cholera victims in a separate volume labelled *'Colerosi'*. Indeed, the size of this volume gives eloquent expression to the magnitude of the disaster that overtook the city.[63]

In 1911, by contrast, there is no indication of the cause of death, and no separate record was kept of the victims of cholera. The only suggestion of the presence of epidemic disease emerges indirectly from a long-standing bureaucratic practice. In its register the Cemetery of Pity made a notation of the *sezione* from which the bodies of the deceased were removed – except for corpses arriving from the Cotugno Hospital. For them 'Cotugno' was recorded as the borough of origin. This notation provides further definitive proof that the hospital was engaged in combat with a major epidemic. A comparison between 1911 and the 'normal' year 1912, when there was no cholera, makes the point. In the months of June, July and August 1912, the Cemetery of Pity recorded respectively 10, 13 and 14 burials of bodies originating at the Cotugno, for a total of 37 for the whole of the three-month period. This figure contrasts sharply with the 531 Cotugno burials listed for the period 1 June to 31 August 1911.[64]

Alfonso Montefusco, the Medical Director of the Cotugno, provided grounds for additional speculation. In 1912, when the disease was safely past, he published a lengthy treatise on the latest developments in the treatment of Asiatic cholera. In that work he barely mentioned the events of Naples in which he played such a leading part. But it is surely no coincidence that cholera was at the centre of his professional concerns and that he had found new grounds for reflection on the 'rational' system of treatment that he had first practised at the Conocchia Hospital in 1884.[65] Furthermore, in the course of his account of various systems of treatment, he referred, without elaboration, to the Neapolitan epidemic of 1911 and to the methods he had adopted on the cholera ward at the Cotugno.[66]

Medical journals

Montefusco, however, did not stand apart within the medical profession for his reticence on the issue of Asiatic cholera. The leading medical journals both nationally and locally almost completely avoided the epidemic of 1911 in Italy.

The argument here is similar to that regarding the press. Just as in the case of newspapers, it is important not to be categorical when considering Italian medical periodicals. But a sample of the leading reviews published in Naples leaves no room for doubt. *Gazzetta di medicina pubblica*; *Giornale di clinica, terapia e medicina pubblica*; *Medicina contemporanea*; *Rivista internazionale di clinica e terapia*; and *Rivista di medicina pubblica* all adhered by their silence to state policy on cholera. In the same spirit, the Royal Neapolitan Academy of Medicine failed to debate public health in the city during the year 1911.

At the national level, the two specialist journals in the field of public health – the *Giornale della Reale Società Italiana d'Igiene* of Milan and *Igiene moderna* of Genoa – adhered to Giolitti's position that there was no cholera in Italy. *Igiene moderna* simply ignored the medical crisis. The Royal Hygiene Society took a more combative stance. In the pages of its journal, the Society proclaimed that the state of public health in Italy was excellent, and it suggested that those who stated otherwise were guilty of the 'sanitary defamation of Italy'. The slanderers, the Society, argued were assorted malcontents – clerical extremists who used every opportunity to attack the Liberal regime and to ruin the anniversary of Italian unification; traitors who saw a chance to malign their fatherland; and speculators who encouraged a climate of anxiety in order to peddle the specific remedies of charlatans. Fortunately, in its view, a wave of healthy and truthful patriotism was sweeping the nation, and the baseless accusation of cholera was being forgotten.[67]

The tempting but impressionistic conclusion that the medical profession faithfully repeated the official sanitary line is confirmed by consulting the most complete available index to the contemporary medical periodical literature – the index compiled by the Surgeon-General of the United States. For all previous epidemics of Asiatic cholera, this work contains extensive listings under the two entries 'Cholera, History, Italy' and 'Cholera, History, Naples'. For 1910 and 1911, however, the Surgeon-General's index contains few references to Italian medical journals under either of these entries, and those few deal almost exclusively with the events of 1910. Only the *Rivista critica di clinica medica* of Florence broke the silence concerning 1911. In October the *Rivista* published an article on the cholera epidemic that had devastated the city of Livorno since July. Giacomo Lumbroso and Cesare Gerini, the authors of the article, however, treated the matter with great circumspection, announcing the existence of the epidemic but failing to provide any specific information about its origins and course, the numbers of deaths and cases, the policies of the sanitary campaign, the reactions of the populace, or the methods of treatment.[68] It was sufficiently controversial merely to announce that an epidemic of cholera had taken place.

EVIDENCE OF INFECTION

In the midst of so much silence, what is the evidence that the epidemic did afflict the city and the nation? How many people perished during its course?

Here it proved impossible for so large an emergency to obliterate all traces. The epidemic of 1911 inevitably left documentation in spite of the best efforts of the authorities and the interested silence of the press. Municipal records provide an illustration. The minutes of the executive committee of the city council, as we have seen, commit at least one major indiscretion in allowing the phrase 'cholera epidemic' to be entered as part of the permanent record of the year. Another indirect indication is the allocation of large sums of money to furnish ice and snow for the treatment of patients. Current orthodoxy in the management of cholera patients was that liquids were contra-indicated because they led to increased vomiting, but that the sucking of ice was a useful instrument in the alleviation of the unrelenting thirst that was one of the agonies of Asiatic cholera. The repeated delivery of large consignments of packed snow to the Cotugno Hospital was a clear and unmistakable sign of the presence of cholera patients on its wards.[69]

Extensive records for the epidemic also survive in the archives of the USPH&MHS, and scattered reports on the state of health in individual provinces have been preserved in the files of the Ministry of the Interior. With regard to US sources, American authorities did not become aware of the Italian epidemic through the official channels stipulated in the Paris Convention. But, by breaking the Convention of 1903, the Italian Government took the calculated risk of spreading the disease abroad, and especially to the United States, which received tens of thousands of steerage passengers from the infected Mezzogiorno during the summer of 1911.

It was from this latest instalment of the Columbian Exchange that the United States public health officials learned of the epidemic in Naples. On 20 June the SS *Berlin* arrived at Ellis Island. It had set sail from Naples with a clean bill of health that 'no cholera or other pestilential disease existed in Naples or vicinity'.[70] In mid-Atlantic, however, the Calabrian infant Giuseppe Colella was seized with violent convulsions and died on 11 June. The ship's doctor performed a bacteriological examination and confirmed that the cause of death was Asiatic cholera. On 19 and 20 June two members of the crew – the firemen Melchiorre Raffo and Vincenzo Passaro – fell ill and died in quarantine on Swinburn Hospital Island in New York Harbor. Laboratory tests for cholera were positive.[71]

The *Berlin* was the first of a series of ships stricken with cholera to arrive in New York Harbor during the summer of 1911. The most unfortunate was the *Moltke*, which suffered a serious outbreak aboard and caused a brief cholera-scare in New York State in mid-July.[72] The Surgeon-General noted in his annual report that, 'During 1911 the United States was seriously threatened by the extensive prevalence of the disease in Italy, and during the summer months cases of cholera and cholera carriers repeatedly arrived at New York from Italian ports.'[73]

Confirming this view, George W. Stoner, the Chief Medical Officer at Ellis Island, recalled the arrival of thirty-five cases of cholera and twenty-seven asymptomatic carriers. Stoner's figures and dates differ slightly from those

Table 7.1. *Cases of cholera among Italian immigrants at Ellis Island, 1911*

Ship	Number of cases	Date of arrival
S.S. *Berlin*	1	13 June
S.S. *Europa*	1	14 June
S.S. *Duca degli Abruzzi*	7	20 June
S.S. *Laura*	2	21 June
S.S. *Carpathia*	1	26 June*
S.S. *Moltke*	14	5 July
S.S. *Perugia*	2	15 July
S.S. *Venezia*	1	11 August
S.S. *King Albert*	2	17 August
S.S. *Re d'Italia*	3	18 August
S.S. *Europa*	1	25 August
Total	35	13 June–25 August

Note: * The report lists the arrival date for the Carpathia as 6 June, but since the arrivals are ordered chronologically, that notation was clearly a clerical lapse and the correct date was 26 June. Such a correction is supported by the course of events.

provided by Geddings, probably because he wrote from memory a year after the events. Stoner, for example, listed only one case aboard the *Berlin*, and he inaccurately remembered its date of arrival as 13 June rather than 20 June. Nevertheless, Stoner's report on the experience of cholera among Italian immigrants at Ellis Island is the most complete and authoritative available. His statistics are shown in Table 7.1.[74] In addition to fully developed cases of cholera, the laboratory under Stoner's direction detected cholera carriers among arriving Italian steerage passengers (see Table 7.2).[75]

The gravity of the danger posed by the Italian policy of secrecy was fully revealed in June 1911 after the docking of the SS *Duca degli Abruzzi* of the steamship company Navigazione Generale Italiana on 20 June. Since the Italians had provided no notification of cholera, the United States Public Health Service was taken by surprise and had not yet deployed the strategy of routinely conducting laboratory examinations of the faeces of all arrivals. Since suspicious symptoms had developed among several of the steamer's passengers at sea, the authorities detained all steeragers in quarantine for five days. Those who showed no signs of disease were then released. Within two weeks, two of them developed cholera ashore and died in New York State, one at Auburn and the other in Brooklyn, together with a New York Harbor hospital attendant who fell ill at his home on Staten Island. These cases created the cholera-scare that first alerted the *New York Times*. The local health officials isolated all people they could trace who had been in contact with the victims; they fumigated the premises they had occupied with formaldehyde throughout and washed the floor with bichloride of mercury; they burned all the personal effects of the victims; they boiled all eating

Table 7.2. *Cholera carriers among Italian immigrants at Ellis Island, 1911*

Ship	Number of carriers	Date of diagnosis
SS *Moltke*	18	18, 21, 22, 23 July
SS *Carpathia*	1	17 July
SS *Amerika*	1	18 July
SS *Pennsylvania*	2	18 and 19 July
SS *Duca di Genova*	2	5 August
SS *Venezia*	1	15 August
SS *Koenig Albert*	1	20 August
SS *Re d'Italia*	1	20 August
Total	27	17 July–20 August

utensils they had used; and they destroyed all foodstuffs in the apartments they occupied. By good fortune alone, none of the victims became the centre of a larger outbreak in the United States.[76]

After the death of several Italians, and an orderly who attended them, aboard ship, at Ellis Island and on the mainland, it was impossible for the Italian government any longer to conceal the presence of authentic Asiatic cholera from American health officials. Surgeon-General Wyman rapidly reached the conclusion not only that cholera existed in Italy but also that the disease was widely prevalent. Only an extensive and severe epidemic, he reasoned, could cause so many cases in New York Harbor. The American government protested about the absence of notification as specified by the Paris Convention.

Accurate information about the real state of public health reached Washington almost simultaneously from a different source – the American Consulate at Palermo. There the first case of cholera, in the person of the lamplighter Carmelo Bennincasa, occurred on 20 May, and the clinical diagnosis of Asiatic cholera was confirmed by laboratory examination on 22 May.[77] Sporadic cases then broke at scattered locations in the city, causing nineteen cases to be reported prior to 8 June, when the disease assumed epidemic proportions.[78] By 23 June the Palermo epidemic had reached its height of sixty-three cases a day, and it stayed at this level until the middle of July.[79] It then began a slow decline, which persisted until its final disappearance with the last known case in late September. At Palermo as at Naples, however, the authorities insistently denied the existence of the disease. The American Consul in the city, Hernando de Soto, reported that, 'Since the beginning of June there had been persistent rumors of cholera having re-appeared in this city, but every effort made by this Consulate to secure definite information from the local authorities was unsuccessful. The existence of the disease was obstinately denied, and the press remained silent.'[80]

De Soto had become particularly concerned after news reached him of the case aboard the *Giovanni Costa* as well as a series of rumours from Messina and

Palermo itself. His anxiety became a near certainty as a result of the behaviour of the provincial physician, who was his personal friend and informant, occupying the same role that Professor De Giaxa filled in Naples. Clearly frightened and under external pressure, the provincial physician refused to confirm or deny the various rumours and he insisted on being excused from providing any further information.[81]

On 18 June, however, an unusual bureaucratic mistake confirmed De Soto's suspicions and considerably embarrassed the Prefect. On that day the Palermo Bureau of Health forwarded to the American Consulate a confidential health bulletin intended instead for the Prefect. Covering the week 11 to 18 June, the bulletin reported to the Prefect that there had been 41 deaths from cholera and 135 from gastro-enteritis, 'the greater part of the latter being undoubtedly also cholera'. Despite all official denials, Palermo was in the midst of an epidemic that was already claiming nearly thirty lives a day. The American Public Health Service had been accidentally notified.[82]

The turning point in Palermo coincided with the docking of the *Berlin* at Ellis Island on 20 June. From that date, the United States unilaterally instituted the defensive measures contemplated in the Paris Convention. Italian emigrants intending to embark at Naples were to be quarantined for five days in the Bay of Naples and bacteriologically tested for cholera; their effects were to be disinfected; and all foodstuffs in their possession destroyed. This series of procedures was then to be repeated upon disembarkation at New York Harbor.[83]

The Italians responded with a secret proposal that they presented through four separate channels simultaneously. The Prefect of Palermo contacted the American Consul in the city; the Department of Public Health in Rome approached the American Ambassador, John Leishman; the Italian Ambassador in Washington conferred with the Surgeon-General; and the Italian Foreign Minister, Antonio Di San Giuliano, appealed directly to his counterpart, Secretary of State P.C. Knox.

In their various approaches, the Italian authorities belatedly acknowledged the epidemic of Asiatic cholera, but they urged the United States to conceal the fact from the public. In exchange for collusion with its own policy of secrecy, Italy would agree to full cooperation in allaying all reasonable American anxieties about the disease. On condition of confidentiality, the Italian Department of Public Health would furnish the American embassy with full details of its comprehensive programme of anti-cholera measures designed to eliminate the disease from Italian territory, and it undertook to provide daily health bulletins of cases and deaths. In addition, the Italians agreed to open a quarantine station (*asilo degli emigranti*) at both Naples and Palermo, the two ports of departure for sailings to New York. Representatives of the USPH&MHS would have full rights of access to these stations, and all sanitary procedures – the disinfection of personal effects, the confiscation of suspect produce, the bacteriological examination of faeces – would be carried out under their supervision. In addition, the Italian Government promised to assign a Royal Navy doctor designated a

'Sanitary Commissioner' to accompany every transatlantic crossing. Unlike the average ship's doctor, the navy physicians would have specialist training in the laboratory diagnosis of cholera and in the sanitary procedures to be taken aboard ship in the event that a case broke out at sea.

Finally, the Commissariat of Emigration agreed to provide an inspector at Ellis Island in the person of Dr M. Serrati, a naval physician. Serrati's mission was to assist the American authorities in the maintenance of public order on Hoffman and Ellis Islands, the two quarantine stations where arriving Italian steerage passengers were held for observation. Held by a foreign government for purposes that were often unclear and uncertain of their ultimate fate, the detainees were, in the words of the Commissariat, 'excited to the point of threatening serious disturbances'. In these circumstances, Serrati's mission was to 'comfort and often to discipline the masses of our emigrants'.[84]

Serrati also served the diplomatic function of soothing the tempers of the doctors attached to the USPH&MHS in New York Harbor. Appalled at the numbers of arriving Italians they were compelled to isolate and examine, and at the frequency with which cholera broke out among the immigrants, the American doctors urged the government to close the borders to passengers from Italy. The Italian doctor assumed the tasks of reassuring his Ellis Island colleagues of Italian good faith and of assisting the US immigration officials in the performance of their duties.[85] As the Commissariat described what rapidly became his *modus operandi*,

> As soon as a steamer carrying Italian emigrants docked, the Inspector took care to write to the Royal Commissioner aboard describing the most convenient hours for meals, the best timing and location for the medical examinations (women at one end of the ship, men at the other), and so on. Before the American bacteriologists boarded the ship, the Inspector arrived to speak with the emigrants in order to convince them of the necessity of medical examinations. Nor did he leave the vessel until all samples had been taken. Thus over 30,000 emigrants were examined in little more than four months; and only one refused to submit to the procedure.[86]

The Italian argument was that the combination of such measures constituted 'virtual compliance' with the Paris Convention. The spirit of the treaty would be honoured by means of a free flow of information between the two governments and the erection of an effective sanitary shield to protect the United States. Only the letter of the Convention with reference to informing the press, the public and the international community would be violated. In exchange, the interests of the United States would be fully protected and friendly relations between the two countries would persist.

From Rome, John Leishman, the American Ambassador, provided his government with unequivocal advice in favour of accepting the Italian proposal. His argument was that the State Department should take into account the economic dependence of Italy upon foreign tourists and the export of perishable foodstuffs. In addition, he pressed Washington to give due consideration to the patriotic significance of the celebrations marking the fiftieth anniversary of national unification. Any power taking the initiative in forcing quarantine and destroying the festivities would generate enormous 'antagonistic feeling among the people' and the 'consequent odium' of the Italian government. It would be unfortunate for a non-European power to take the first step, especially when the Italian central government was making 'herculean efforts' to stamp out the infection.[87] To Leishman's exhortations, San Giuliano added a sombre warning that to reveal the real state of public health would create an immediate danger to law and order, and the result could be to spread the disease still further. The conservative administration of President William Howard Taft chose not to embarrass the Italian government on the very issue of the vulnerability of the nation to cholera that had been so successfully exploited in 1910 by syndicalists, socialists and republicans. The Republican President did not wish to give credibility to the campaign of subversives and revolutionaries; nor did he wish lightly to deprive American employers of a major supply of cheap labour.

Under the pressure of these considerations, the American government agreed on 21 June to accede to the Italian request that secrecy be preserved. Secretary of State Knox instructed Ambassador Leishman by telegram that,

> In response to representations of the Italian Government as to the danger of disorder growing out of the existence of cholera in Italy and pending the measures being taken by that Government to deal with that cause of apprehension, the Government of the United States will be glad to take especial care to discourage any exaggerated and alarmist reports in this country on this subject … The Government of the United States of course cannot relax in any particular its measures of precaution both at ports of departure and at ports of arrival which are enjoined by its laws. Bills of health must therefore be filled out as usual, but the Treasury Department informs this Department that it will be immaterial if such bills of health be forwarded by the consuls under seal to the officers for whom they are intended. You may instruct the proper consuls as to the situation and in defense of the present telegram, and I trust the response this instruction will enable you to make to the Minister of Foreign Affairs will be recognized as entirely considerate of every proper wish on the part of the Government of Italy.
>
> You may inform the Minister of Foreign Affairs that this Government is happy to accede to his request that, for the present, no unnecessary publicity will be given as to the existence of cholera in Italy.
>
> You will also notify consuls that bills of health, after completion, shall be given to the Master of the vessel, sealed, and knowledge of contents to be known only to the consul and the medical officer; not even the Master is to know the contents.[88]

From the third week of June until the final outburst of cholera in Sardinia in 1912, therefore, the United States colluded in two respects with the Italian policy of concealment. First of all, during this sensitive period no American official made public reference to the epidemic prevailing in Italy. Secondly, in its subsequent reports relating to cholera, the United States Government knowingly published the 'laundered' figures provided by the Italian authorities in their public health bulletins – figures that were known to be misleading. In 1912, the Surgeon-General's *Annual Report* shed the following retrospective and false light on the Italian experience of cholera, 1910–12:

Italy was invaded by cholera in August, 1910. The disease was epidemic from August 17, 1910 to January 30, 1911, during which period there were 1,840 cases with 804 deaths. The disease broke out again in June, 1911, and from June 8 to December 31, 1911, there were 15,985 cases with 6,022 deaths. During the present year cholera was not reported until August 14, when cases appeared in Cagliari, in Sardinia. In Cagliari there were 30 cases with 8 deaths reported between August 14 and September 10, 1912.[89]

It was perhaps a gesture of diplomatic courtesy that the Surgeon-General marginally reduced the number of deaths listed by the Italians themselves: their secret bulletins recorded not 6,022 but 6,146 deaths from cholera in 1911.[90] Such a small discrepancy, however, is unimportant. The substantial reason that the Surgeon-General's figures were false is that they validated the systematic manipulation of statistics on which the Italian bulletins of health were based and against which officials like Henry Geddings had so vigorously protested. Against the informed judgment of its own officers in the field, the Surgeon-General's office published an official United States account of the sixth pandemic that coincided with the version of events that the Italian government published a year later, in 1913. Nowhere in the report of either government is there any suggestion that the city of Naples suffered a major outbreak.[91]

Despite such dutiful cooperation first in the subversion of the Paris Convention and later in the suppression of unpleasant truths, the United States Public Health Service rapidly became aware that the Italian Government was not content with breaking the international treaty. It also violated the secret accord with the Americans by providing them with information that had no relationship with medical reality. For Secretary of State Knox, the regular bulletins of health compiled by the Department of Public Health and secretly delivered to the American Embassy were the basis for his willingness to accede to the Italian request for secrecy. Timely and full disclosure, he argued, were the spirit, if not the letter, of the Convention. As long as the Public Health Service received accurate and prompt information, it could take appropriate measures to protect the interests of the United States.[92] 'Virtual compliance' with the Convention was sufficient for pragmatic purposes. For Giolitti's government, however, the purpose of the bulletins was not to inform the Americans but to mislead them. From the Italian perspective, their only purpose was to persuade the United States that Rome had the situation firmly in control.

From the outset, the officials of the USPH&MHS stationed in Italy complained bitterly that the covert agreement between the two countries was not being honoured. At Palermo, Dr Di Bartolo, the Acting Surgeon attached to the United States Consulate, warned Washington that the very first bulletin was blatantly false. According to the offending document, which covered the four days from 19 to 22 June, there were only ten deaths in the city. Hernando de Soto, the Consul, commented that, 'From private information and upon careful investigation made by Dr Di Bartolo, ... there is no doubt that since June 18 there have been at least 25 to 30 deaths from cholera per day, although the Foreign Office ... only reports 29 cases and 10 deaths in Palermo from June 19th to June 22nd.'[93]

A systematic attempt to deceive rather than inform – an attempt that was all too apparent from the outset – was integral to Giolitti's public health strategy. At Genoa, La Spezia, Catania and Livorno, the American Consuls complained that the disease raged in all four cities while the Italian authorities continued to present them with bulletins declaring the ports free from infection. When challenged, the Prefects vehemently denied any possibility that cholera was present.[94]

From Naples, Geddings reported that his service during the time of cholera was a bitter and painful experience. Because of its strategic position as the port of departure for emigration to North America, Naples was the most sensitive centre of all for Italian officials and the one where they were most committed to maintaining the fiction of total immunity to cholera. In his highly delicate posting, therefore, Geddings was inevitably confronted with determined and unexpected attempts at concealment practised by the Italians even to the disadvantage of their putative partners in conspiracy. 'I charge', he wrote in frustration,

> that the Italian authorities, by their accepted policy of delay, deception and evasion of all the requirements of the provisions of the Convention of Paris, are responsible for the introduction of cholera into the United States, and the trouble, anxiety and expense incident thereto. This is the second year in which opportunity has been afforded to observe the operations of the said Convention, and as one of the signatories thereto I am reluctantly compelled to record my belief that it operates to the advantage of the knave and to the detriment of the honest man.[95]

The United States Public Health Service, Geddings elaborated, was promised bulletins at frequent and regular intervals. In practice, however, the information arrived unpredictably and with such delay that it was virtually worthless. The consulate at Naples was compelled to base decisions on reports that were from one to two weeks out of date. After repeated protests, the Department of Public Health promised daily reports, but in practice nothing ever changed with regard to either regularity or accuracy. Furthermore, the sanitary bulletins were both unclear and unreliable. Geddings explained that,

> The promised reports ... are so incomplete and in such a form as to be practically valueless, as they never mention when a suspected place has been confirmed or released from suspicion, nor do they give information of value as to the relative positions of the places in their respective provinces, and the ease of communication between them, nor what precautions have been taken. Nor do I believe that the information, such as it is, is of any real value, inasmuch as it is incomplete, and I believe designedly so.[96]

Against the protests of Geddings and the other officials of the USPH&MHS stationed in Italy, American policy was to maintain secrecy as long as the Italian authorities cooperated with the practical sanitary procedures thought necessary to prevent cholera from reaching the American mainland. At the highest levels, therefore, it was determined not to allow a certain persistent duplicity to escalate into a diplomatic incident and a domestic crisis for a friendly government engaged in combat with left-wing subversion.

How far official statistics for the epidemic departed from the reality of the epidemic as both American and Italian public health officials understood it in secret cannot be quantified with precision because no comprehensive and reliable records survive. On the other hand, the files of the Department of Public Health provide firm proof that bulletins that were deceptively compiled by the Italian Department of Public Health, begrudgingly delivered to the Americans, and belatedly published were a sheer invention. The bills of health were the end result of a three-stage filtering process. At the first stage, the communes in every province affected by the disease collated the reports of confirmed cases within their territory and provided the Prefect with the total. Here was a first opportunity for concerned local officials to protect their image. At the second stage, the Prefect edited the various municipal responses in the province of his jurisdiction and forwarded them to the Department of Public Health. At the third stage, the Department in Rome again manipulated the numbers by allowing only 'bacteriologically confirmed' cases and deaths to be recorded. Three times cleansed by officials with clear instructions to minimize the extent of the emergency as far as was consistent with plausibility, the figures that emerged at the end of the process bore only a tenuous relationship to truth.

As evidence of the early stages of the process of statistical editing, a run of municipal and prefectoral reports assessing the magnitude of the epidemic survives in the archives of the Department of Public Health. Unfortunately, these documents are neither comprehensive nor extensive: records are available for only a limited number of provinces and they shed only a very partial light on medical events within the administrative boundaries to which they refer. In those provinces for which reports are extant, however, two conclusions emerge with great clarity – first, the presence of the epidemic in defiance of all official pronouncements; and, second, the considerable discrepancy between the information the state received from prefects and municipal officials on the one hand and the official statistics that it delivered to the Americans and ultimately published on the other. Naples, where Italian officials persistently asserted that no epidemic at all took place, provides the most extreme and important example. It is salutary, however, to consider several other instances before turning to Naples because they unmistakably suggest that the deception perpetrated by the state was systematic and all-pervasive. Cagliari, Venice and Palermo are useful illustrations.

In the province of Cagliari, where the epidemic claimed its last victims in the summer of 1912, the Italian Department of Statistics and the United States Surgeon-General published accounts suggesting that only 30 cases and 8 deaths occurred. The Prefect of Cagliari, however, had informed his superiors in the Ministry of the Interior of an outbreak with a very different order of magnitude.

According to the Prefect, 83 cases, 54 deaths and 96 asymptomatic carriers had been confirmed by laboratory testing. Furthermore, the official stationed in Sardinia clearly indicated that the figures he furnished were significantly understated. His orders, he slyly reminded his readers, were to act with the 'maximum prudence', and he explicitly stated that large numbers of additional cases had not been reported to his office.[97]

Venice provides a second example. The bulletin received by the American authorities in 1911 and the published Italian statistics of 1913 assert that in the province of Venice 116 people died of cholera in 1911.[98] The information received by the Department of Public Health, however, was significantly at variance with this figure. Professor Giordano, the Provincial Officer of Health, compiled a lengthy report on the epidemic of 1911 within his jurisdiction between the first cases on 22 May and the last on 2 November.[99] He stated that the province had suffered 778 reported cases of cholera, of which 605 had been bacteriologically confirmed, and 262 deaths – more than double the 'official' total. Other provinces present the same pattern. At Aquila, 60 deaths from cholera were listed in the state mortality tables, but the provincial officer of health recorded 271 cases and 159 deaths.[100] At Forlí, the government registered 18 deaths instead of the 60 reported by the provincial officer of health.[101] And in Massa Carrara the conflicting mortality figures were 45 and 77.[102]

Apart from Naples, the province that played the most significant role in the epidemic of 1911 was Palermo. There the official figure for the whole province was 873 deaths from cholera.[103] The information available to the state was very different. According to the detailed account written by Dr Barile, an Inspector of the Department of Public Health assigned to investigate conditions in the Sicilian capital, the commune of Palermo alone experienced 2,461 cases of cholera and 1,542 deaths.[104]

Naples, however, provides the most significant illustration of the way in which statistics were fabricated. Fortuitously, since important sanitary documents received by the Department of Public Health have been preserved, it is possible to follow the laundering of the cholera statistics at each level until the final myth – that no epidemic at all took place – was produced. Although, as we have seen, the southern metropolis has vanished from all discussion of the sixth pandemic, the secret and already carefully 'laundered' health bulletins compiled by the Department and furnished to the American Embassy indicate that in fact Naples was the most severely afflicted city in Italy. Of the 6,146 official deaths in Italy from Asiatic cholera during the course of the year, more victims were listed in the confidential bulletins as having died in the province of Naples (873) and in the region of Campania (2,162) than in any others.[105] Because the purpose of the bulletins was not to illuminate but to reassure, they maintain an artful discretion by providing statistics for the province of Naples and the region of Campania, but not for the city itself. Although not impossible, it was improbable that cholera would cause thousands of deaths in the surrounding region without affecting the capital.

By good fortune, this conclusion can be confirmed. The health bulletins represent the end product of the process of statistical refinement that Giolitti's government initiated. In the case of Naples, not only the health bulletin but also the confidential municipal table of cholera deaths on which the bulletin was based, have survived. The original local assessment can therefore be compared with the bulletin, with public statements and with the published official statistics. The municipal table provides evidence at variance with all other accounts of the medical events of 1911. The Palazzo San Giacomo and the Italian state pubicly claimed that the disease had been successfully eradicated in 1910, and that the city remained permanently cholera-free throughout 1911. According to the secret municipal table, however, an epidemic of Asiatic cholera began in the city of Naples on 3 May 1911 and lasted until mid-September, causing a total of 1,340 deaths and 2,231 cases.[106] Although there are grounds to suspect that these municipal figures had themselves been edited and should be regarded as understated, they are important in establishing a number of important considerations. First of all, the local report demonstrates both that (1) Naples was indeed at the centre of the sixth pandemic as Geddings and his subordinates had argued throughout and that (2) the pandemic itself was of a severity radically different from the benign and strictly limited outburst suggested by official accounts. According to the Town Hall, the city of Naples alone had far more victims than the state in its health bulletin for American consumption attributed to the entire province.

Furthermore, the distribution of deaths by borough confirms the apprehensions felt by the critics of the local administration and its conduct of urban renewal. Once again cholera remorselessly exposed the fact that, despite the claims of the Mayor, Alderman Giulio Rodinò and Orazio Caro, Naples was far from being medically unified in a state of general and equitable salubrity. The epidemic laid bare the enduring sanitary inequalities of the metropolis. Although there is good reason not to take even the confidential figures of the Neapolitan City Hall at face value, there is no reason to doubt the relative share of the general misfortune borne by each *sezione*. The governors of the city had no interest in magnifying the evidence of major disparities in sanitary provision. According to the confidential municipal documents, which contain a small discrepancy by recording a total of 1,332 victims in the borough figures rather than the 1,339 victims indicated elsewhere, the cholera deaths in the city were distributed as indicated in Table 7.3.

A striking feature of the Neapolitan outburst of 1911 was that its geography was strongly influenced by the pattern of the achievements and limitations of *risanamento*. The *sezioni* of Porto and Pendino, which had been among the most severely decimated boroughs in the city in every cholera visitation of the nineteenth century, no longer contributed disproportionately to the bills of mortality. Porto and Pendino had been successfully 'thinned out', and their worst slums had been demolished. As we have seen, however, the refugees from the slum clearances in these boroughs had found accommodation in neighbouring Vicaria and, to a lesser extent, Mercato. It was to Vicaria above all that the social

Table 7.3. *Cholera deaths in Naples, 1911*

Sezione	May	June	July	August	September
S. Ferdinando	7	35	17	4	1
Chiaia	10	44	35	19	3
S. Giuseppe	0	4	11	1	2
Montecalvario	11	32	23	14	1
Avvocata	4	33	26	10	1
Stella	6	34	26	15	3
S. Carlo all'Arena	4	55	19	7	0
Vicaria	28	158	87	45	0
S. Lorenzo	3	37	15	11	0
Mercato	22	79	47	31	3
Pendino	3	24	10	4	0
Porto	1	31	17	5	1
Vomero	1	3	7	5	2
Posillipo	0	2	3	2	0
Fuorigrotta	11	49	8	5	1
Miano	3	21	3	0	0
Pisariola	2	18	12	1	0
Harbour	0	0	3	1	0
Total	116	659	369	180	18

problems of the Lower City had been exported, and it was here that the cholera raged most severely during the summer of 1911, killing 318 (24 per cent) of the cholera victims reported by City Hall to the Department of Public Health.

Although these municipal figures prove that a substantial epidemic of Asiatic cholera did in fact ravage Naples despite both contemporary and subsequent denials, there are two telling indications that the statistics furnished by a reluctant city council substantially underestimated the real extent of the misfortune – probably by a factor of approximately 100 per cent. The first indication arises from the aggregate mortality figures for the summer of 1911 in comparison with the 'normal' summers of 1908, 1909 and 1910 when the city was not affected by cholera. Naples was afflicted in the months from May to September 1911 with a 'mortality bulge' well in excess of the cholera mortality acknowledged by City Hall in its table. The contrast between 1911 and the three preceding years is demonstrated in Table 7.4.[107]

During the months that Asiatic cholera prevailed in Naples in 1911, there was therefore an 'excess mortality' of approximately ten people a day in May and August, and of approximately thirty-five deaths a day during the months of June and July. On the basis of these figures, it is possible, as a rough approximation, to hazard the guess that it would be far closer to reality and more consistent with the evidence to believe that 2,600 people perished of cholera in Naples in 1911

Table 7.4. *Summer mortality in Naples, 1908–11*

Month	Deaths	Daily average of deaths	Deaths per 1,000 inhabitants
1908: population 597,178 (on 1 January)			
May	1,219	39	2.04
June	1,239	41	2.07
July	1,111	36	1.86
August	994	32	1.66
1909: population 604,299			
May	1,098	35	1.82
June	1,147	38	1.90
July	1,201	39	1.99
August	1,109	36	1.83
1910: population 612,191			
May	1,153	37	1.88
June	1,101	37	1.80
July	1,169	38	1.91
August	1,013	33	1.65
1911: population 625,891			
May	1,474	48	2.35
June	2,471	82	3.95
July	2,142	69	3.42
August	1,495	48	2.39

than to agree with the figure of 1,300 people provided by City Hall. By the contemporary standards of western Europe, in the wake of the bacteriological breakthroughs of Robert Koch, and in the context of a city specifically designed to be immune to epidemics of infectious disease, a cholera epidemic of such a magnitude was a major medical calamity.

The existence of the 'mortality bulge' is incontrovertible. There is, however, the possibility of an alternative medical explanation – namely, that the 'excess deaths' were due to the outbreak of another disease rather than Asiatic cholera. Apart from the implausibility of the supposition that Naples was swept contemporaneously by two separate epidemic diseases, there is is no suggestion in the contemporary medical literature of the passage of such an epidemic.

Indirect evidence that the real explanation can only be Asiatic cholera comes from the most unlikely and most unintentional source of all – a report by Orazio Caro, the foremost opponent of all suggestions that Naples could possibly experience a return of the pestilence from Bengal.[108] Writing to Dr Alessandro Messea, an Inspector-General of the Department of Public Health, Caro did not, of course, admit the existence of cholera. He did, however, accept the existence of the 'elevated mortality' of the summer of 1911, when the rate of death in the city doubled.

Caro's unconvincing attempt to explain the problem away unwittingly lends weight to the theory of cholera. According to Caro, years of high mortality are not always in need of a specific explanation. On the contrary, they need to be seen in a longer time perspective in which years of significantly raised mortality recur in a regular cyclical pattern. Therefore, 1911 should be understood as a simple recurrence of a 'normal' cycle of raised mortality, which had last taken place in Naples in 1896. As the mechanism involved, Caro pointed to an immediate local climactic factor in order to avoid invoking cholera. In 1911, he argued, Naples experienced a prolonged heat wave, with the temperature rising to an average of 27.8 degrees Centigrade in the final ten days of July. Such conditions, he argued, had accentuated the mortality from common endemic illnesses and especially from gastro-enteritis. The extra deaths of the summer of 1911, therefore, were 'in large part of intestinal origin', but they were not due to Asiatic cholera.[109] Given Caro's history of using the diagnosis of gastro-enteritis and given the vested interests that he was known to defend, his clumsy account creates suspicion and does nothing to weaken the alternative explanation that Henry Geddings offered – that Naples was swept by a major epidemic of Asiatic cholera.

Having estimated the extent of the epidemic in the city, one is also in a position to offer a revisionist appraisal of the magnitude of the mortality from cholera in the nation as a whole. Here it is necessary to recall the explanation given by Giovanni Raineri for his major innovation of 1910 in the way that the state reported deaths from the disease. In order to minimize the importance of the medical crisis facing the nation, the Department of Statistics at Raineri's direction recorded only those deaths that had been 'bacteriologically confirmed'. Scholars such as Forti Messina who have discounted the numerical significance of the Italian experience of the sixth pandemic in comparison with the vastly more deadly epidemics of the nineteenth century have made an important methodological error in their evaluation of the statistical evidence. Unaware of Raineri's new procedure, they have committed the mistake of failing to compare like with like.

It is a methodological error to use official statistics concerning the epidemic of 1910–12 for the purpose of making comparisons with any earlier outbreaks of the disease. In 1910–12 the state entirely altered the basis on which it made its calculations of mortality. In all previous epidemics of Asiatic cholera in Italy, deaths were recorded on the basis of the diagnoses provided by attending physicians or coroners. Beginning in 1910, the state elected instead to record only deaths certified as authentic Asiatic cholera by laboratory agglutination tests. By the new statistical procedure, which was devised solely to deceive, the Italian state recorded 805 deaths in 1910 and 6,145 in 1911. The difference between these figures and the real number of cholera victims was enormous. As Raineri explained with regard to the outbreak of 1910, the difference between the number of 'bacteriologically confirmed' deaths and the number of actual human beings who died of cholera was of the order of 225 per cent (i.e., 1,811 deaths as opposed to 805).

The proportions given by Raineri with respect to 1910 can be applied to the official statistics of 1911, which were compiled on the basis of the same criteria. That such a procedure yields plausible results is confirmed by a 'control' group – the six provinces already noted of Aquila, Cagliari, Forlí, Massa Carrara, Palermo and Venice. In these localities two sets of figures survive – the number of 'bacteriologically confirmed' deaths and the number of human victims reported by local authorities. Furthermore, they are randomly selected on the basis of the accidental fact that parallel sets of records are available to measure their mortality from cholera (see Appendix, Table A7). Taken together, these six provinces in 1911 suffered 1,120 'bacteriologically confirmed' deaths and 2,154 reported deaths, and the latter figure was 192 per cent greater than the former. The ratio involved, therefore, is approximately in line with the discrepancy suggested by the Minister responsible for state statistics. Furthermore, since these provinces provide samples taken from North, South and Centre, and since they account for a significant fraction – approximately one-sixth – of all of the official deaths from cholera in Italy in 1911, it seems reasonable to assume that roughly similar proportions would prevail everywhere in the nation. Raineri's suggestion of 225 per cent, therefore, is likely to yield results that are useful, provided that we remember that they are no more than an approximation and that precision is impossible.

On this assumption, one can convert the statistics of 'bacteriologically confirmed' cholera deaths into an estimate of the number of people who perished by the simple procedure of multiplying the published figure of 6,145 deaths by 225 per cent and expressing the product in round figures. The result of this calculation is the conclusion that, in 1911, nearly 14,000 deaths from cholera occurred in Italy excluding Naples, which was officially free of the disease and for which there are therefore no official published statistics. With regard to Naples, however, we have already arrived at the suggestion that 2,500 people died of Asiatic cholera in the city during the summer of 1911. For Italy as a whole, therefore, a rough estimate made on the basis of the best available evidence is that over 16,000 Italians died of cholera in 1911 and approximately 18,000 for the whole course of the outbreak of 1910–12.

Even this estimate is conservative. It is an attempt only to quantify the number of cholera deaths known to the authorities. The reports in the files of the Department of Public Health, however, frequently state that there were large but necessarily unspecifiable numbers of fatalities from the epidemic that were diagnosed as due to other causes. Such misdiagnoses were sometimes deliberate, as the authorities at Torre Annunziata observed. In many instances physicians colluded with patients who were terrified of being taken against their will to hospital isolation wards. When the reputation of so many hospitals as places of cure was negative, some physicians believed that they were increasing the chances of survival of their patients by not reporting them to the authorities. Most importantly, however, as the Prefect of Cagliari noted, misdiagnosis was the direct result of the state campaign of secrecy. To suppress all discussion of cholera and to deny its presence in Italy was to disarm the medical profession in its contest with an exotic tropical disease of which few doctors had any experience. Ignorance deprived patients of appropriate treatment and the public health authorities of essential information. The Italian military noted in alarm that its own channels of information uncovered 'absolutely certain reports' of cholera in localities of which the civilian authorities were unaware.[110] The 18,000 deaths of which the state was aware must therefore be supplemented with significant but unknowable numbers of victims whose real cause of death was not recognized or not reported. A more audacious attempt to quantify the Italian disaster was made by an American journalist stationed in Rome. In the freer climate that prevailed in Italy after the easing of the censorship in September, the correspondent of the *New York Times* reported that the epidemic of 1911 had already claimed in excess of 32,000 lives in Italy, and that the infection persisted in extensive areas of the peninsula.[111]

Expressed in these various terms ranging from a minimum of 18,000 fatalities to perhaps as many as 32,000, the sixth pandemic looms far larger as a national misfortune than has previously been recognized. This fact is important to understand the events that occurred in Naples itself. Unless it is appreciated that the Italian state confronted a substantial medical crisis, it is impossible to understand why the government devoted such energy to suppressing all knowledge of the occurrence. The larger estimate is important because it provides a vital missing clue necessary for an explanation of the conspiracy that took place. Precisely because the threat that they faced was so serious, the authorities were determined that no-one should ever know.

ENFORCING THE BAN

Against international leaks

The Italian and Neapolitan events of 1911 constitute a unique moment in the European history of Asiatic cholera. Italy in 1911 is the only known example in which a western nation succeeded both in concealing a substantial and widespread epidemic of the disease from its population during its course and in subsequently misleading posterity with regard to its magnitude and significance. While this process was unfolding at the national level, the city of Naples became the sole documented instance in which a major cholera epidemic was entirely expunged from all public records. There are adequate sources, as we have seen, to establish the fact that such a process took place in the summer of 1911. Having determined, therefore, the course of the events that occurred, we can confront the further question of how the national and local authorities, from Giovanni Giolitti to Mayor Francesco Del Carretto, enforced their ban on medical knowledge. It is important to explain their ability to carry out so ambitious a conspiracy of silence.

Success in such an enterprise depended on the capacity to forestall both international and domestic leaks. Internationally, it was essential to prevent foreign powers, which had independent sources of information about conditions in Italy, from exposing the truth about medical conditions in the peninsula and the Italian violation of the Convention of Paris. The greatest concern was for those nations that were likely to exercise the greatest vigilance because of their extensive intercourse with Italy or their geographical proximity. The United States and France posed particular threats to Giolitti's policy of concealment. It was impossible indefinitely to prevent all knowledge of the disease from reaching the authorities in these two countries as they received large numbers of Italian immigrants and maintained active consular and public health services in Italy. It could prove feasible, however, to delay their awareness and to prevent them from making what they learned public.

In dealing with foreign governments, the Italian strategy was, first, to promote delay by a systematic campaign of misinformation and denial. When total obfuscation was no longer possible, the Department of Public Health minimized the extent of the crisis and attempted to demonstrate that it had the situation in control. At the same time the Foreign Office skilfully argued (1) that public knowledge of the disease could prove medically counter-productive and economically ruinous, creating a crisis of public order in which the epidemic could thrive but trade would collapse; (2) that subversives and revolutionaries would benefit from the issue of public health in Italy; and (3) that secret accommodations could be reached to protect the vital interests concerned. The Foreign Office also threatened diplomatic complications and commercial reprisals if foreign nations attempted to invoke the full rigour of the Convention of Paris.

How well such a mixture of manipulation, argument and menace could work was demonstrated in the case of the United States. Despite serious reservations by the Public Health and Marine Hospital Service, the American Government followed what appeared to be the course of least resistance: it agreed to collude with the strategy of secrecy and subsequently even to publish information furnished by the Italians that it knew to be false.

Fortified by this success in their dealings with Washington, Italian officials then devoted special attention to the very delicate issue of the American Consulate in Naples. Naples presented a thorny problem for several reasons. It was the centre where the disease raged most fiercely, where Italian interest in avoiding damaging revelations was most acute, and where the state-sponsored deceit was most comprehensive. Unfortunately for the purposes of deception, Naples was also the city in Italy that represented the greatest sanitary threat to the United States. Because of emigration, it should be reiterated, the United States kept careful watch on medical conditions in the city through the representatives of its Public Health Service under the direction of Henry Geddings. From the Italian perspective, therefore, there was a constant danger that the energetic and well-informed doctor would present alarming news to Washington – news that would destroy the credibility of Italian claims to be in control of the emergency and would lead the US Government to limit immigration, to insist on the full application of the provisions of the Convention of Paris, and to make a very public disclosure.

Limiting the damage that Geddings and his assistants W. King and Buonocore could cause to Giolitti's conspiracy therefore became a major priority. The campaign to staunch this dangerous potential leak involved a series of initiatives. A first ruse was to attempt to undermine Geddings's influence and credibility by defaming his character. Beginning in the early weeks of 1911, therefore, Neapolitan officials and the press publicly claimed that the unhappy American official was a drunken and incompetent dandy with an inflated salary – 3,000 lire a month, according to the industrialist and municipal councillor Gennaro De Luca.[112] His sole interest, they claimed, was to exaggerate every medical rumour in order to justify his excessive wages in the eyes of his employers. It would, therefore, be in the best interest of harmonious relations between the two countries for the Department of State to recall its unreliable official or for the Italian Foreign Office to deport him.

The initiative in the attempt to undermine Geddings was not just local, however. The Foreign Office under San Giuliano suggested to the American government that its Neapolitan health official had overstayed his welcome, and the Italian Ambassador to Washington officially registered the disapproval of his government.[113] This stratagem was not entirely successful because Geddings was kept in post, but it did lead Surgeon-General Wyman to order an official investigation into his subordinate's behaviour and to instruct him to, 'Be conciliatory and guarded in language'.[114] Geddings himself believed that he was about to be dismissed, and a bitter rift did indeed develop between Geddings and the American Consul at Naples, William H. Handley. The Consul possessed no medical training or prior experience of cholera, but he thought that the doctor was an alarmist who recklessly alienated his host country. Geddings was shunned by Neapolitan polite society, but the Consul was lionized as much more *simpatico*. One must assume that during this important period Geddings's influence was much diminished, as the instigators of the campaign had intended.[115]

Not content to discredit Geddings, the Italians also attempted to destroy his usefulness and that of his colleagues to the United States as sources of information. One tactic employed by Italian officials was systematically to deny the Consulate at Naples all information. The most sinister and violent technique, however, was the attempt to silence Geddings, King and Buonocore with the threat to murder them if they did not keep silent. On 20 July 1911 Buonocore received a signed letter from the Camorra referring to the recent assassination of the New York policeman Giuseppe Petrosino, the scourge of the criminal underworld in his native city, by a team of mafia hit men. The letter stated,

> Unless you relieve our city of its misery within two days' time, the same will happen to you as happened to Giuseppe Petrosino. The American doctor [i.e. Geddings] will also be killed.
> Consider the fact that your sister will share your fate.[116]

Particularly alarming to the three American public health officials serving in Naples was the blatant connivance of the police with the Camorra attempt to intimidate them. Although the death-threat had been ostentatiously signed, the police never succeeded in making any arrests, and the authorities even denied the existence of the 'black hand' in Naples. Only the personal intervention of the American Ambassador with the Ministry of the Interior in Rome persuaded them to provide Geddings and his two associates with armed police protection.[117] Again, one can only suppose that, in the dangerous and hostile atmosphere created around them, the officials' effectiveness as gatherers of intelligence was limited, and that their ardour to seek out victims of cholera somewhat diminished. The leak of information from Naples by means of American public health officials was not stopped, but it was slowed.

A final possible threat of discovery posed by American officials was unintentional. The measures upon which the State Department and the Surgeon-General insisted in their agreement with Italy were impossible to conceal. Five days of floating quarantine for shiploads of steerage passengers in Naples harbour were highly visible, and certain to lead to conjecture and rumour about their purpose. Unwelcome publicity was all the more inevitable because the isolation of the emigrants from the city had enormous economic ramifications for the entire population of Naples as Luzzatti's tormentors had made abundantly clear in the early months of the year. With regard to the quarantine, the Italians had no room for manoeuvre because the United States was adamant on this point. The challenge for the state, therefore, was to invent a plausible explanation that both justified the sanitary procedures supervised by Geddings and at the same time denied that they were the result of infection in the city.

The official explanation was prominently published in the Italian press in mid-July.[118] At the very moment that over thirty people a day were dying of Asiatic cholera in the city, the authorities insisted that it was impossible for the disease to have returned to Naples. Renewal had provided Naples with the insurmountable barriers of the Serino aqueduct and the new sewer system. The Serino water was 'the most pure in existence', and the Neapolitan sewers formed 'one of the most complete and hygienic networks in the world'. No city in the civilized world was better defended against the threat of cholera than Naples. Therefore, the possibility that the quarantine measures affecting emigrants were due to the presence of epidemic disease could be discounted *a priori*.

According to this reasoning, the real purpose of such measures was not medical, but political. Frequently the steamships calling at Naples for the embarkation of emigrants had already called at ports in Dalmatia or the eastern Mediterranean, where cholera was raging. There was, therefore, always the danger that the disease would break out during the North Atlantic crossing, when it would be impossible to prove to the American authorities that Naples was not the source of the illness. The rigorous terms of the Convention of Paris would then be invoked to the detriment of Italy and its leading seaport. During the prevalence of cholera in the Middle East and the Balkans, therefore, it was a sound defence of Italian economic interests to ensure that the peninsula remained above suspicion by isolating passengers before embarkation.[119]

Among European powers, the most important nation to be silenced was France. Like the United States, France was certain eventually to become aware of the epidemic disease prevailing in Italy. Because of the extensive commercial and population exchanges between the two nations, the French Embassy also kept a vigilant watch on public health in Liberal Italy. The French Consul at Florence, for instance, was aware that cholera had broken out; he sent anxious reports to Paris; and he pressed the Prefects for accurate and detailed information.[120] Similar news did not arrive from Venice, the Italian Prefect boasted, only because he had successfully corrupted the foreign consuls stationed in the city and had persuaded them not to report what they saw concerning public health to their respective governments.[121]

Even the correspondent of the Parisian newspaper *Le Matin* observed the mysterious departure of whole families from the neighbourhood surrounding the French Embassy at the Piazza Farnese in Rome. The victims were transported to hospital in secret at night and their homes were subsequently disinfected although no public announcement concerning the state of public health in the capital was made. Not so easily deceived, the journalist reported that cholera had broken out in the city.[122] Furthermore, because of the temporary migration of labourers to southern France, the disease was likely to be exported to Provence, reversing the direction followed by the infection in the summer of 1884. And in fact Asiatic cholera broke out at Marseilles in August and September, causing 120 unreported deaths in the city in August alone and perhaps an equal number in September.[123]

In dealing with the medical anxieties felt in Paris, the Italians used the same combination of initial denials followed by reassurances, misinformation, appeals and threats that they had already used so effectively with Washington. French consular officials also met a wall of obstruction and falsehood in their attempts to elicit accurate information. The Consul at Florence, for instance, sought in August 1911 to investigate reports he had received of cholera in various localities in Tuscany. In framing his reply, the Prefect of Arezzo hesitated between outright lying and transparent stonewalling. Reporting his uncertainty as to which alternative would be more effective, he informed his superior at the Ministry of the Interior that, 'I could answer that all such reports are false and that in this province the conditions of public health are absolutely ideal. Or else I could reply ... that for the moment the press of duties prevents me from employing sanitary personnel for researches of a statistical nature.'[124]

In addition, it was Giolitti's good fortune that the French authorities possessed their own reasons for wishing to keep the outbreak of cholera confidential. Fearing popular alarm and disruption to trade if Marseilles were publicly declared an infected port, the French government, like the American, agreed to keep the matter secret. The French Government contented itself with imposing a ban on Italian pilgrims – a measure that it thought would prevent the entry into

France of some of the poorest class of Italian travellers while causing the least possible economic disturbance.[125] Indeed, M. Grégoire, the Prefect of the Department of Bouches-du-Rhone, joined the Italians in requesting that the American authorities not insist on the letter of the Convention of Paris. In a letter to A. Gaulin, the American Consul-General at Marseilles, he argued that, 'There have been a few cases of cholera nostras, which could not be held to justify the issuance of foul bills of health to vessels sailing from our port.'[126]

The final important foreign threat to the conspiracy of silence came from Argentina. In the Italian determination to conceal the presence of cholera, the South American Republic was an important factor because it was, after the United States, the major destination for emigrants from the Mezzogiorno. In 1910, for example, the number of Italian emigrants who departed for the various countries of North and South America was divided as shown in Table 7.5.[127]

In the new century the majority of those who made the journey to Argentina, an overwhelmingly agricultural country, were temporary migrants – farm labourers nicknamed the *golondrinas* ('swallows') – who departed via Genoa and, to a much smaller extent, Naples in the early autumn. Authentic nomads of two worlds, they left Italy after harvesting wheat in the Northern Hemisphere in order to repeat the agricultural cycle on the Argentinean frontier in the Southern. After disembarking in Argentina, they began work in the fields of the north of the country and moved steadily south, following the ripening of the corn. Finally, when spring returned to Italy, the swallows made the journey home again in time for another agricultural year. (The opposite seasonal patterns that distinguished emigration via Naples for North America from emigration via Genoa for South America are clearly demonstrated by Table A8 in the Appendix.) At the height of the Giolittian period, there was also a substantial demand for Italian navvies to lay the railroad lines necessary to complete the settlement of the country. With this volume of migration in constant movement, there was a clear danger that cases of cholera originating in Italy would break out either during the twenty-day crossing or after arrival at La Plata and then spread throughout the country.[128]

Argentina was steadfastly determined to avoid the importation of epidemic disease to South America, and its resolve was reinforced by the severe national problem of underpopulation relative to the vast expanse of its national territory. Argentina was too thinly settled to contemplate a demographic disaster.[129] The determination of the Republic was reinforced by the memory of the great epidemic of 1886–88 when a moment's lapse in vigilance had led to disaster. Argentina's response to the ravages of the fifth pandemic in Europe had been drastic: the Republic had closed its ports to all vessels from the infected continent. Unhappily, however, an exception had been made for the steamship *Perseo*, which carried Italian immigrants from Genoa, where cholera prevailed. The health authorities at the river port of Rosario had been impressed by the presence on board of the returning Minister Plenipotentiary to Italy, and by the mendacious assurances of the ship's captain that the health of the passengers and crew was perfect. With the disembarkation of the Italians on the shores of

Table 7.5. *Italian emigration to North and South America, 1910*

Country of destination	No. of emigrants
United States	262,554
Argentina	104,718
Brazil	19,331
Canada	10,209
Uruguay and Paraguay	2,072
Peru, Bolivia, Chile	661
Columbia, Venezuela, Equador, Guyana	602
Mexico	499
Guatemala, Salvador, Honduras, Nicaragua, Costa Rica	206
Total	400,852

the River Paraná on 12 October, the misfortunes of Argentina began. Despite draconian attempts to contain the infection with military cordons that severed all lines of communication in the country, the contagion spread remorselessly throughout all fourteen provinces of the Confederation.[130] In the alarming report of the American Consul at Buenos Aires as early as December 1886,

> In Mendoza the development of the disease has been most remarkable, and the population of that city of 20,000 has been almost decimated; and in the country districts the disease was equally fatal. In Tecuman the number of cases has on some days been as high as 500, of which about one-half proved fatal ... In nearly all the other interior cities the disease has been very virulent and fatal, but not confining itself to centers of population, it has ravaged entire provinces, and farmers [*estancieros*] and camp men have in great numbers succumbed to it.[131]

An awareness of the public health dangers posed by immigration in a time of cholera and the resolve to avoid a repetition of the laxity of 1886 deeply affected the public health policies of the Argentinean Government. In pursuit of this objective, the Republic not only signed the Paris Convention of 1903 but also reinforced it by negotiating a supplementary South American sanitary convention in 1904 with Brazil, Paraguay and Uruguay. Because of the scale of Italian immigration to its shores, Argentina anxiously followed sanitary news from Italy. During the Italian outbreak of 1910 it had established a precedent by invoking the two international sanitary conventions with respect to Italian shipping. Under their terms, all steamships arriving in South America from Italian ports were obliged to call first at Rio de Janeiro, where an Argentinean doctor boarded the vessel for the final leg of the journey to Buenos Aires. Officially designated a 'Sanitary Commissioner', the doctor was responsible for carrying out a thorough inspection of the passengers and crew. If there was no cause for alarm and more stringent measures, the first- and second-class passengers were allowed to disembark upon arrival at the Argentinean seaport, but steeragers were required to undergo five days of quarantine at the infamous lazaretto on the island of Martin Garcia. To monitor Italian medical conditions more closely, Argentina also assigned a health inspector to the two ports of Genoa and Naples.

At the end of March 1911, the emergency sanitary provisions of the previous autumn had been allowed to lapse. The administration of President Roque Saens Peña remained alert, however, to the danger of importing cholera in the event of a recrudescence of the disease in Italy. It also grew increasingly suspicious with regard to conditions in the Italian peninsula. Argentina lacked the resources to deploy a permanent service abroad comparable to the USPH&MHS, and its two sanitary inspectors had been recalled in the spring. But the Republic instructed its consuls to remain watchful and it carefully monitored all reports regarding sanitary conditions in Europe. In mid-July the Italian export of cholera cases to New York and Marseilles had given rise to scattered press notices both in Europe and in North America. These reports were widely published in newspapers in Buenos Aires.[132] The public agitation of the Association for the Defence of the Interests of the Twelfth Electoral District in Naples against the measures imposed by the United States in the harbour at Naples further attracted enormous interest in South America, and confirmed the Argentinean National Department of Hygiene that the impending large-scale arrival of Italian immigrants for the agricultural season posed a serious medical threat.[133]

On 20 July the authorities at Buenos Aires decided to act to defend the health of their people by again applying the measures that had worked successfully the previous year – sanitary commissioners and quarantine at Martin Garcia. Because these procedures were based on precedents that the Italian authorities had accepted for the entire period from September 1910 until March 1911, the Argentineans did not anticipate the eruption of a diplomatic incident. In the very different political conditions prevailing in Italy under the Giolitti ministry, however, the unilateral and public announcement that Italian ports were infected was unacceptable. On 21 July, in response to the Argentinean initiative, the Commissariat of Emigration cabled the Italian Consul at Rio de Janeiro, instructing him to inform all captains of vessels flying the Italian flag that Argentinean doctors should not be allowed aboard in any official capacity but only as ordinary first-class passengers.[134] Concurrently, on the occasion of the docking of the steamer *Re Vittorio* at La Plata, the National Department of Hygiene ordered the Italians aboard to be taken into quarantine, provoking – in the account of the Buenos Aires daily *La Prensa* – an 'uprising' among the passengers that was contained only with the intervention of the Argentinean navy.[135]

Here was a major crisis for the policy of concealment that the Foreign Office under San Giuliano immediately and adroitly deflected. The Italian countermeasure was timed to coincide with the next docking of an Italian steamship at Buenos Aires – that of the *Savoia* at the end of July. When the Department of Hygiene again attempted to assert its authority over the thousand immigrants aboard the emigrant steamer, the Italian government announced that the precedent of 1910 had no validity and that the terms of the Convention of Paris were inoperative. The reason was that in the summer of 1911 no Italian port had been declared infected. Argentina was not motivated, the Italians asserted, by considerations of public health at all. The real purpose of the Argentinean quarantine, according to the Italian government, was to enable the Republic to make a show of strength at Italian expense.

According to the same logic, the timing of the gesture was finely calculated to please the ardent clericalists in both Argentina and in Italy by embarrassing the Italian Liberal state in the midst of its patriotic celebrations. The Vatican had responded to the jubilee by proclaiming 1911 a 'year of mourning' as the 'fiftieth anniversary of the spoliation of the Church'. In accordance with this intransigent position, Pope Pius X attempted to sabotage the national festivities. He issued what was popularly termed the 'anti-tourist bull', urging Catholics abroad to refrain from visiting Italy during the year; he threatened to close the Vatican Museums during the Expositions; and he ordered that no Consistory would be held and that papal audiences would be severely curtailed. *Osservatore romano*, the papal newspaper, described the Exhibition at Rome as a 'colossal organization for the exploitation of foreigners'.[136] Finally, with the Pope's encouragement, priests fomented labour disputes among the Catholic workers engaged in the construction projects associated with the festivities, causing stoppages and delays in the completion of many phases of the preparations.[137] In this tense atmosphere, it was easy for Giolitti to exploit anti-clerical sentiment for his own purpose by charging that Catholic Argentina in its public health policies was simply colluding with the Church and the enemies of the nation. This religiously motivated outrage was not to be tolerated, and it was unthinkable that Argentinean physicians would ever be allowed to violate Italian sovereignty by claiming authority aboard ships flying the Italian flag. The lurid conditions at the lazaretto at Martin Garcia, which was reported to be flooded when the Italian 'swallows' were confined there, further provoked Italian fury.[138]

In reply to the alleged Argentinian provocation, Giolitti on 30 July 1911 instructed the Ministry of Foreign Affairs to announce a ban on all Italian emigration to Argentina – a measure presented to the nation as a defence of Italian national interests and an effective economic reprisal against a nation dependent on Italian labour.[139] On 5 August this decree was followed by another suspending emigration to Uruguay, which had resolved to honour the 1904 South American Sanitary Convention by supporting Argentina's demands.[140] The Commissariat of Emigration gave instructions to the police to reject all applications for passports to the two offending nations filed by manual labourers and to exercise rigorous surveillance at all ports and border crossings in order to prevent attempts to circumvent the decrees.

To avoid revealing the real conditions that had led the Argentineans to their decision regarding quarantine, Giolitti's government was prepared to create a full-scale international incident. Furthermore, it succeeded because the xenophobic feeling it unleashed obscured the public health considerations that had originally motivated Buenos Aires. The press and members of parliament were vociferous and unanimous in their praise of Giolitti's apparently resolute and defiant decision. Public discussion was effectively deflected from considerations of health to such matters as national pride; the chauvinism of a 'young Republic' that needed to be taught a lesson by a European power; the brutal treatment of Italian nationals by South American employers; the poor training and corruption of the Argentinean doctors who sought to be paid while they travelled first class on Italian ships; and the calculated insult of a nation that had declined to send a delegation to honour the Italian kingdom on the fiftieth anniversary of its founding. The isolated voice of the Vatican newspaper *Osservatore romano*, which took Argentina's part in the dispute, only strengthened Giolitti's case.[141] Cholera was not discussed, and even the tens of thousands of Italian peasants who were financially ruined by the ban on emigration were soon forgotten. After investing everything they owned in the purchase of passage overseas, they suddenly and unexpectedly discovered that they were unemployed.[142] Since the ban was revoked only on 24 August 1912, their plight is apparent in the deep trough in the numbers of Italian emigrants to Argentina in 1911 and in the still abnormally low figures for 1912, as demonstrated in Table 7.6.[143] According to the calculations of the Commissariat, approximately 100,000 potential emigrants were prevented from departing during the year that the ban was in force, and the profits of Argentinean farmers were decimated.[144]

The most important factor of all in Giolitti's success in preventing the Argentinean crisis from exposing the medical reality was the popularity of his decision with the Socialist Party and the trade-union movement. The Italian Left had long argued that the conditions experienced by Italian migrant labourers in Argentina were brutally exploitative. They received low pay and harsh treatment at the hands of South American farmers, and any attempts to protest or to organize made them liable to violent police measures, arbitrary arrest and sudden deportation.[145] Argentinean employers, however, were vulnerable to pressure in the labour market because the country was chronically short of labour, and the gap was only filled by the immigrants from Italy. The most effective means to improve conditions, Italian socialists and union leaders argued, was to make use of the weapon of the boycott, which they also employed as a means of wringing concessions from landlords at home in the Po Valley. Alceste De Ambris, the northern farm workers' leader who had spent years in South America, had long advocated the idea that the boycott was the weapon of choice in both situations. His view, furthermore, had been officially adopted by the Argentinean Socialist Party and trade union confederation, which appealed to their comrades in the Second International to prevent labourers from migrating from Europe until wage concessions had been made and civil liberties guaranteed in the Republic.[146]

In order to defend Italian emigrants in this manner, however, De Ambris and other socialists concerned with Italians overseas needed support from the Italian authorities. Such support, however had never been forthcoming, and Italian diplomats in Argentina were notorious for their indifference to the lot of their

Table 7.6. *Italian emigration to Argentina, 1910–13*

Year	Total emigration	Emigrants to Argentina
1910	651,475	104,718
1911	533,844	32,719
1912	711,446	72,154
1913	872,598	111,500

compatriots. For this reason, Giolitti's sudden decision to ban emigration to La Plata as the demand for labour approached its annual peak was viewed by the Left in Italy as the long awaited boycott that would induce farmers in Argentina to make concessions to their workforce. Far from alienating the Italian labour movement, therefore, Giolitti found himself hailed as the champion of defenceless workers against feudal oppression in Buenos Aires. *Avanti!*, the socialist paper, greeted the Prime Minister's decision with rapture and eagerly took up the task of justifying the measure to the nation.[147]

Furthermore, with the support of the Italian Left, Giolitti was able to outflank and undermine his dangerous opponent in Naples – the Association for the Defence of the Interests of the Twelfth Electoral District. Before the eruption of the conflict with Argentina, the Association had launched a campaign reminiscent of the effort that had proved so successful against Luzzatti. Under the leadership of the Deputy Monfredini, the movement noisily demanded that the health regulations in Naples be revoked and threatened strikes and lockouts if he failed to act. With the explosion of the diplomatic rupture with Argentina, however, Giolitti, now supported by the Socialist Party and the unions, was able to argue that it was the senseless agitation of the Association that had given Argentina the pretext of cholera to strike its blow at Italian dignity and national interests. It was the Association which was to blame for slow activity in the Naples harbour and for the hopes of the tens of thousands of workers who could no longer depart. In the end of July, the Association lost the vital mass support of the Borsa del Lavoro, and it collapsed as a major political force in the city. Political discussion in Naples moved from the issues of hygiene and disease to questions far more congenial to Giolitti, such as national honour and workers' rights. Instead of being exposed by Argentina's action and dangerously pressed by the Association, Giolitti emerged from the incident stronger and more popular. And he had gained additional time for his silent battle against disease.[148]

In this manner the Italian state preserved its medical secret. In so doing, however, Giolitti, together with the American and French Governments that agreed to cooperate with his policy, assumed a heavy responsibility. By failing to provide public notification of the presence of Asiatic cholera as required by international treaty, these authorities took the risk of spreading the disease abroad. Particularly in this era of mass emigration, there was a clear and immediate danger that people travelling from infected localities would carry the bacillus with them to their destinations. Foreign nations that were not apprised of the danger at all or that, like the United States, were misled as to its scope and prevalence were medically disarmed, and their citizens were placed at risk. How real the danger could be was demonstrated by the fact that immigrants arriving from Italy in the summer of 1911 repeatedly succumbed to cholera in New York Harbor. As we have seen, cholera even reached the American mainland on three separate instances. Italians were also the cause of limited outbreaks at Marseilles, in France, and in the villages near Tarragona in Spain.[149] In each case the infection was successfully contained, but such good fortune owed nothing to the Italian Department of Public Health, which was prepared to take the gamble of enabling the sixth pandemic to spread through its inaction.

Another serious responsibility was the danger to which foreign travellers to Italy were exposed without their knowledge. Failure publicly to alert the international community of the prevalence of cholera exposed legions of tourists, pilgrims and visitors to the great patriotic festivals at Turin and Rome to the risk of contracting cholera. The Italian government not only provided no warning, but it also actively encouraged foreigners to come and positively denied that there was any reason for alarm concerning their health. By remaining silent, the American Surgeon-General and the French public health service, both of whom belatedly and partially learned of the truth, provided no better protection to their own nationals. In secret correspondence with anxious and well-informed citizens who remembered the one official warning that the United States government published in January at the instigation of Henry Geddings, Surgeon-General Walter Wyman advised that they cancel their plans to visit the Italian peninsula. In mid-July, for instance, Wyman agreed that young Durr Friedley, who was planning a European Grand Tour after graduation from Harvard, should rethink his plans. Friedley was fortunate in enjoying privileged access to medical information because his father was a personal friend of leading health officials.[150]

Although the American Surgeon-General took such a forbidding stance in private, in public Wyman honoured the agreement struck between Secretary of State Knox and the Italian Foreign Office. His conduct in this regard was not without censure. Harrison Morris, the Commissioner-General of the American delegation to the International Exposition at Rome, protested vehemently to Wyman about Italian concealment and American complicity. Having discovered the reality of cholera through direct observation, he wrote in these terms:

> Simply as a citizen who travels, may I ask whether it is considered adequate to publish only the very unreliable records given out by Italy? There has been, we know, an absolute conspiracy of suppression. No paper in Italy has been allowed to print the word cholera. This naturally leads some people to travel thither who may be infected; and it seems to me a great lapse in international service not to correct it.[151]

Since there are no records of the health of foreign visitors in 1911, it is impossible to know whether, and to what extent, travellers to Italy suffered the consequences of their lack of information. At the very least, however, one must conclude that they were not given the opportunity of choice in the matter of their own health.

Against domestic leaks

Freed from the anxiety that the United States, France or Argentina would expose the real nature of the medical emergency they confronted, Italian officials concentrated on preventing the truth from seeping out at home while the epidemic prevailed. Their success depended in large measure on the fact that they had powerful allies in the political and economic interests for whom notification of Italy as an infected nation would have been ruinous. The outcry in Naples between the announcement of the presence of cholera in September 1910 and the revocation in March 1911 of the last sanitary measures affecting the port fully demonstrated how unpopular open admission could become. Giolitti's chosen course of policy enjoyed a measure of ardent and aroused support. Concealment was not simply an authoritarian diktat imposed from Rome.

The dilemma facing the organizers of medical orthodoxy was that there were also strategically placed people – doctors, journalists, officials at every level – who had access to troubling information about sanitary conditions and who believed in full public disclosure for a variety of reasons. Many physicians and public officials advocated full notification as the only effective method of organizing an effective programme of public health. Some opponents either of Giolittian rule at the national level or of the ruling faction in local government saw in cholera and the sanitary conditions it exposed a possible means of attacking the regime or those who wielded power under it. The 'popular bloc' had taken this line in Naples in 1910, and the left-wing newspapers *Roma* and *La Propaganda* fitfully and intermittently returned to the issue in 1911. Other advocates of disclosure rejected Giolitti's approach for pragmatic reasons, like Sidney Sonnino. The conservative former Prime Minister argued that the strategy of secrecy was self-defeating because it led the state into a morass of unending contradictions and confusion. He wrote in August that, 'It seems to me that one could reproach the authorities for having surrounded cholera in so much mystery. The system of telling lies has the disadvantage that one never knows how to begin telling the truth again.'[152]

A clear irony of the summer of 1911 was that, as the nation celebrated its freedom and its constitution, Giovanni Giolitti, who frequently intervened personally to ensure compliance with the policy of concealment, demonstrated a decidedly illiberal ambition to achieve the total control of information concerning public health. The means the Prime Minister and his allies employed were both legal and illegal. They were directed at those people most likely to be aware of the epidemic and most able to expose what they knew to the public at large – officials, journalists and the medical profession.

One means to exert such control was ideological exhortation. During the jubilee celebrations marking the fiftieth anniversary of Italian unification, the country was swept by gusts of patriotic fervour and nationalism. Exhibitions at Turin and Rome were at the heart of the festivities. At Turin a new stadium said to rival the Coliseum was built in time to accommodate grand displays held on two successive days at the start of May. On the first day the crowd paid homage to the past achievements of the Italian race and on the second to its future glories. These events, the *Corriere della sera* boasted, took place before crowds that were larger than those that attended the Olympics or even the Harvard–Yale football game in America. After the opening festivals of patriotic pride, where, according to *The Times*, the enthusiasm of the crowds 'surpassed ordinary limits',[153] the momentum of the fervour was maintained throughout the following summer. At frequent intervals new grand pavilions on the banks of the Po River opened. Each pavilion was intended to demonstrate an aspect of the power of Italian agriculture, industry and military force, or the artistic and technological accomplishments of other nations from around the world. Italian civilization was thus celebrated by enormous daily throngs of visitors from all parts of Italy and by multitudes of tourists and dignitaries from abroad,[154] bearing what the daily paper *La Tribuna* termed the 'universal homage of the civilized world'.[155]

Rome provided the other major forum for the outpouring of national feeling with its own concurrent Exhibition, where the various Italian regions sponsored pavilions celebrating the diversity of the nation; the state organized exhibits of Italian ethnography, archaeology, music and fine arts; and the city arranged both informal evenings of food, drink and entertainment at the Piazza d'Armi and gala receptions on the Capitoline Hill. The capital also hosted parades, festivities and oratory. The events of the Roman Exhibition then culminated in the inauguration of a series of grandiose public buildings – the National Stadium, the Palace of Justice, Parliament and, on 4 June, the Monument to Victor Emmanuel II. This colossal marble folly dedicated to the 'liberator king' performed no utilitarian purpose. Rising symbolically above the buildings of previous eras, it served only to proclaim the glory of the new Italy. The elaborately decorated Monument, whose first stone had been ceremonially laid in 1885, had cost the nation 40 million lire to build – approximately a third of the cost for the renewal of Naples.[156]

Finally, the national celebration was marked outside the two historic capital cities of Turin and Rome. There were smaller occasions – flower festivals, Risorgimento fetes and holidays in honour of the Italian constitution, all designed to carry the patriotic message of the power and promise of the 'Third Italy' to provincial centres and small towns.[157]

Giolitti was frequently the keynote speaker in the midst of this perambulating celebration of *italianità*. It was expedient for him to make use of the fanfare to divert attention from his medical problem. Retrospectively surveying the events of the summer, the journal of the Royal Hygiene Society noted in September that nationalist fervour had provided a significant distraction from the medical emergency. 'Fortunately for us, for the Exhibitions, and for the Right Honourable Giolitti,' it commented, the sanitary conditions of the country are good. There was a moment of fear on account of the disease that could not be named, but the storm was followed by a clear sky. Perhaps the only people who regret this tranquillity are speculators, the enemies of the nation, the purveyors of specific remedies, and those who advertise their wares every time our unhappy country experiences a calamity....

Now, I repeat, the moment of fear is over, and almost no one is still thinking of cholera. A wave of patriotism is absorbing everyone's attention, and it hides the reality of things – the reality of many of our miseries.'[158]

More menacingly, Giolitti also exploited the outburst of nationalist sentiment – the 'apotheosis of Italian unity', in the words of the *Corriere della sera*[159] – in the interest of imposing an authoritarian orthodoxy in the field of public health. In parliament, in city halls like the Palazzo San Giacomo and in the press, defenders of Giolitti's medical mythology were not content merely to assert that Italy was cholera-free. They also injected a disturbing new element into the discussion of the issue of health. In order to mobilize opinion against the doubters and questioners, the proponents of the new orthodoxy asserted that to entertain the notion that Italy could again be visited by cholera was illegitimate. The notion was 'anti-national', 'anti-patriotic', treasonous, and even an instance of what was now termed 'sanitary defeatism'. In Naples the month of July was marked by noisy street demonstrations against American quarantine measures and in favour of the view that the city, by renewal, had been forever immunized against the cholera. The discussion of medical issues was invested with the symbolism and rhetoric of military conflict, and the advocates of scientific measures against epidemic disease were regarded as dangerously un-Italian. Public opinion was a powerful force protecting the ban on the use of the word 'cholera'.

The new criminalization of medical dissent was intended to intimidate and suppress, and it was accompanied by police measures of persuasion and repression. With respect to persuasion, one of Giolitti's constant political preoccupations was the attempt to mould public opinion by cultivating the press. The failure to understand the influence of the media in an era of mass politics was, in his view, one of the great errors that had undermined the premiership of his conservative opponent Sidney Sonnino. To avoid repeating Sonnino's error, Giolitti attempted to preserve good relations with 'friendly' papers and correspondents with the clear intention that his own version of events would always find a sympathetic and ready forum. To that end, the Ministry of the Interior, under Giolitti's direction, secretly paid substantial sums to papers and their writers. Correspondents from a long list of papers received secret monthly retainers varying from 50 lire to 150 lire a month to guarantee that a helpful gloss would be put on political events in their articles. As an anonymous collaborator explained,

If they are paid and properly advised, we can generally obtain the useful result that they will sound a favourable note in the presentation of events. In particular, we can then rest assured that they will not transmit news items exaggerated by our opponents, or that they will transmit them in a muffled manner, or that they will follow the reports with some appropriate comments concerning their reliability.[160]

In 1911, therefore, Giolitti was well placed to call in outstanding debts by demanding of his network of 'friendly' journalists and subsidized papers that potentially embarrassing accounts of Asiatic cholera not be transmitted.

If his interlocutors proved less pliant, Giolitti and the Prefects under his command made use of more forceful means. A fully documented case is that of the medical profession in Venice, where two cases of Asiatic cholera were 'bacteriologically confirmed' by Koch's laboratory tests at the end of May. Alarmed by the event and the silence in which it was enveloped, the Medical Association of the City and Province of Venice met on 31 May to protest against the official policy of secrecy and to call instead for a public campaign of information and health education as an essential component of a rational and scientific campaign against cholera. The Association also registered its dissatisfaction with the unaccustomed position in which the profession found itself, ignored by the state and 'kept in the dark by the general directives of maximum secrecy imposed by the government'. Its assembly then voted a strongly worded resolution, 'deploring the stupidity [*insipienza*] of the national and local government authorities who have concealed the real sanitary condition of the city ..., thereby hindering the legitimate work of the medical professions'.[161] The resolution demanded 'means of hygienic propaganda and preventive medicine'. Acting on its convictions, the Association also printed 2,000 copies of a pamphlet intended for the general public outlining the danger of Asiatic cholera and the measures that the residents of the city could take to protect themselves.

In the repressive climate of the summer of 1911 such defiance of the strategy of secrecy was intolerable. Prefect Nasalli responded by ordering the police to conduct night-time raids of the premises of the printers used by the Association and to conduct searches at the central post office and the central railroad station. Their orders were to intercept and confiscate all copies of the pamphlet before it became public knowledge. Belatedly and retroactively, the Prefect also sought authorization from the public prosecutor to 'render the confiscation definitive'. At the same time Giolitti's representative intervened with the local press to forestall any mention of the occurrence.[162]

Carefully following such threats to his plans, Giolitti was not satisfied that these precautions would guarantee the full obedience that he demanded. He therefore telegrammed careful instructions to Nasalli. His wire stated that, 'I deeply deplore the rash and *criminal* agitation of the hospital doctors. Summon the leaders of the movement immediately and inform them of the responsibilities they will face if they persist in an agitation that is an actual crime against their city and their country.'[163] The persuasive means available to prefects in their encounters with recalcitrant physicians were explained in the course of a parliamentary interrogation by Casolini, the Deputy from Catanzaro. For publicly expressing alarmist views on medical matters, doctors could be arrested and charged under the Penal Code for criminal incitement.[164]

Thus instructed by his master, Nasalli did not rest after the general disciplinary measures he had already taken. Now he turned his attention to the leadership of the Association and to the press, which might share their views. On 2 June, as directed, he summoned the President of the Medical Association, Dr Giordano, who was known to be an indignant and outspoken critic of the Giolittian conspiracy, and the other leading physicians in the city. The Prefect confided his thoughts to Rocco Santoliquido, the Director-General of Public Health. Nasalli cabled that,

> I shall call him [Giordano] again, and I shall meet individually with the other most influential physicians, who are all perfectly aware of the true situation as they themselves carried out the bacteriological examinations of the two cases that were brought to the hospital. The most important newspapers continue to keep silent ... Two of the others deal with the matter of public health, but only to print denials and to calm anxieties. Nevertheless, I shall call upon them to shut up completely because that is even more calming.[165]

The government was still not entirely reassured. There was still the problem that the diplomatic representatives of foreign governments in the city of Venice and elsewhere might hear rumours and seek clarification regarding the situation. Giolitti therefore wrote to San Giuliano instructing him on how Italian officials should respond to all inquiries. It was important, he wrote, to remind them of the success of the anti-cholera campaign of the autumn of 1910 and of the watchfulness of the Italian authorities, who would promptly report any suspicious cases that occurred. Regarding any disturbing accounts of illness that they had already heard, Nasalli and other officials placed in such a situation should adopt their own form of the following words: 'Naturally reports of gastro-intestinal infections are occurring on a daily basis, because such infections are common both in Italy and elsewhere.'

Any more serious reports were only 'baseless suppositions' by an 'ignorant population'. It could also prove useful, the Prime Minister continued, to quote Dr Vivante, the Director of the municipal Office of Hygiene. Vivante, 'who is one of the most eminent bacteriologists in Italy', had concluded that the 'sanitary conditions of Venice are excellent'. Meanwhile, the Italian diplomatic service could combat 'tendentious rumours spread to our detriment'.[166]

By 8 June, according to the report of Inspector-General Alessandro Messea of the Department of Public Health, conditions in Venice had been settled to Giolitti's satisfaction. As a highly placed functionary, Dr Messea's loyalties were not to his fellow physicians in the Medical Association but to the Ministry of the Interior to which he owed his appointment. He reported that the 'unspeakable publication' printed by his profession had been unanimously condemned by all of the economic interests of the city, which were directly affected. Furthermore, 'the Venetian press has learned the ways of silence', and the only source of concern was that the scare had caused 'the most exaggerated reports' to appear in foreign newspapers. The local tourist industry had been seriously injured as a result. Fortunately, however, the most serious mishap – the necessity of notifying the international community that the Adriatic seaport was an infected city – had been avoided. That was a signal cause of relief because to have broken the silence by listing Venice as the first infected locality would have placed the whole of the nation under intense medical scrutiny. The result would have been an unstopp- able chain reaction by which it became necessary to notify center after center until even the strategic city of Naples was listed as contaminated, with untold harm to Italian interests.[167]

The repression in Venice was no aberration, but the logical application of a consistent national policy. Everywhere in Italy subversive ideas on the issue of Asiatic cholera were subject to police intervention. Officials were ordered to deny information to the press and the public, and the Ministry of the Interior exercised careful surveillance over newspapers and forbade all use of the cholera word. In the matter of public health, the police also attempted to sever communications between journalists and the papers for which they wrote, whether in Italy or abroad. To this end, the state censored all telegrams and interrupted telephone services.[168] The province of Milan illustrates the ways in which this strategy operated. There the Prefect assured Giolitti that there was no danger of un- welcome leaks in his territory. In a cable to his employer, he announced that, 'I have given formal and severe instructions that all telegrams containing infor- mation regarding cholera must always be presented to me.'[169]

The diligent official expressed anxiety that not all of his colleagues were equally alert. Specifically, he worried that a telegram with details of public health in Campania had been allowed to be sent from Caserta to a certain signor De Negri in Como. Fortunately, he had intercepted the offending wire and had prevented it from being delivered. But the implications of such a rent in the curtain of silence surrounding the disease were vexing. As he expressed it,

> I must add that it seems to me highly deplorable that the responsible authorities in Caserta have allowed telegrams reporting such serious facts to be despatched ... And what is worse is that the telegrams in question travel half the length of the Kingdom, needlessly causing alarm wherever they pass and causing harm in this city.'[170]

Alarmed that leaks of such a nature were possible from the very region where silence was most desired, Giolitti responded by intervening personally to repri- mand the Prefect of Caserta and to prevent a recurrence. In the words of the Prime Minister's instructions, 'I invite you to give me an explanation in this matter and to assure me with regard to the orders you have given to make certain that this grievous incident not be repeated.'[171] The leak from Caserta, however, was the exception. Elsewhere the police scrupulously carried out their assign- ment, and successfully stopped communications about cholera sent by correspon- dents from reaching such papers as *La Nazione, Messaggero* and *Giornale d'Italia*.[172]

In the highly sensitive city of Naples, private citizens as well as newspapermen could find that their communications had become the object of police censorship. The lawyer Alberto Aliberti, for example, discovered that the telephone at his residence was tapped, that the line was interrupted, and that the texts of his calls were transcribed and filed at the Ministry of the Interior. He became an object of state attention because he was known as a 'defeatist' during the 1911 epidemic. On 15 June, for instance, he phoned his contacts in Milan and informed them that Naples was experiencing at least forty cases of cholera a day.[173]

Where exhortation and censorship were insufficient, the Prefecture and City Hall at Naples employed more rigorous methods of the kind used against Henry Geddings and his associates. Officials and health personnel thought to be unreliable with regard to the medical orthodoxy were threatened with dismissal on the authority of the Prefect. Geddings noted that a serious obstacle in the way of obtaining accurate intelligence was that his informants were afraid of being not only sacked but also imprisoned if they were discovered.[174] John Leishman, the American Ambassador, further informed the Secretary of State that dissenting officials were menaced with physical violence, although he did not speculate on how or by whom such campaigns of intimidation were organized.[175]

All of the ingenuity employed by the state to maintain the veil of secrecy would have been unavailing if the progress of the disease through major cities like Naples and Palermo had been accompanied by riot and the collapse of public order. An abortive day of action in Naples in July had helped to alert the government of Argentina. Violent fracas in the streets, assaults on doctors, vigilantism and revolt – the range of popular responses that played so prominent a part in the events of 1884 – would have alerted both the nation and the international community to the medical emergency. An essential component of Giolitti's strategy, therefore, was the ability to devise an anti-cholera campaign that effectively combated the disease without giving rise to large-scale social tensions. A major sanitary offensive had to be reconciled with the imperatives of silence and discretion.

In sanitary terms, the 1911 offensive against cholera in Naples was unsurprising. Although implemented under the direction of the national Department of Public Health rather than the local Office of Hygiene as in 1910, the main directions of the operation were the same. Just as in 1910, the authorities sought to identify and remedy the major public sources of contamination liable to spread the disease with epidemic force – the water supply, the trade in second-hand garments, the fruit and vegetable markets, and the waters of the harbour and the Sebeto River. As if following a well-established tradition, the Department ordered the closing of wells and cisterns; sealed all cesspits; cleared, cleansed and disinfected the sewer mains; swept the streets; banned swimming and the harvesting of shellfish in the harbour; prohibited sewage farming in the market gardens to the east of the city; proscribed the rag trade; and inspected markets, restaurants and taverns. The sale of edible goods directly in the streets, where sanitary regulations were impossible to enforce, was forbidden. Throughout the summer huxters disappeared from the streets of the city.

The real novelty of the campaign of the Department of Public Health was its stress on silence. To carry out its objective, the Department divided the Lower City, which was most at risk, into thirteen zones, each of which was provided with a sanitation team under the direction of a doctor. The task of each team was to inspect every house and street where a case of cholera was reported; to remedy all causes of insalubrity; to search the neighbourhood for further undiscovered cases; and to discover and destroy all of the personal clothing and linen belonging to patients. Most importantly, each team was instructed to win the trust of the populace of its zone, to break down the remaining barriers of suspicion between the people and the medical profession, between the political authorities and the populace.

To ensure that there was no repetition of the stormy scenes of the past, the squads avoided all appearance of exercising a police function. Their orders were not to operate by force or intimidation but only by reason and persuasion. Furthermore, the physicians in command were chosen among the public health doctors who knew the areas; the teams made no sudden, lightning raids; they avoided theatrical displays of their power; and they went about their tasks unarmed and without an escort of municipal guards. To eliminate animosities based on class differences and the suspicion of outsiders, the squads were composed of working men from the districts in which they operated – builders, street sweepers and artisans who knew the neighbourhood and its residents intimately.

Reporting that in the matter of discretion the teams exceeded all expectations, Inspector-General Mauro Jatta described their operating methods as follows:

> The people of Naples are filled with prejudices and distrust. But if one takes the trouble to overcome their initial suspicion, they are easily convinced by reason. In general, Neapolitans are mild in their manners, but they refuse to tolerate authoritarian methods and any lack of respect. They are unable to resist anyone who goes in their midst with a smile, polite manners and no thought of gain, ... and who respects their deeply held beliefs, especially in the matter of religion. ...
>
> All of the physicians, disinfectant personnel and workers employed in the public health service were instructed to use courtesy and never to resort to force, but only to persuasion.[176]

Adopting these methods, Jatta continued, the squads were greeted with some hostility at the outset, but they were rapidly accepted and soon even welcomed as friends of the people. Most important to Giolitti, the teams were soon 'allowed to carry out their tasks without anyone taking any notice.'[177]

Just as in 1884, so in 1911 the Italian government clearly demonstrated the educative role of the state in its strategies of defence against epidemic disease. The policy pursued by the authorities is one of the most important variables in determining the popular response to invasions of cholera. In 1884 a coercive policy of prophylaxis spread terror by conveying the lesson that outsiders were dangerous and that they should be repulsed by military force. In 1911, by contrast, the decision to place the principal emphasis on gaining public trust sent the very different message that there was no reason to panic or to resort to violent self-defence because the state had the situation firmly in control. The lowered sense of alarm that resulted was an important factor in Giolitti's largely successful strategy of concealment.

CONSEQUENCES

The Giolittian strategy of public health achieved the purposes for which it was intended. By preserving secrecy, the Prime Minister avoided the political conflict between Rome and Naples that played so prominent a part in the downfall of Luigi Luzzatti. In the summer of 1911 there were no embarrassing interpellations in the Chamber of Deputies; there was no threat of anarchy or rebellion in Naples itself; and the parliamentary delegation from the city presented no threat of mass resignations.

By the same means the Liberal Prime Minister preserved the patriotic festivities at Rome and Turin; he avoided publicly tarnishing the reputation of the regime for modernity by allowing a display of severe and widespread hygienic deficiencies; he forestalled disruption to trade, tourism and emigration to North America; and he minimized the social disturbances that had so frequently accompanied epidemic cholera in the past.

Thus the positive accomplishments of secrecy were evident primarily in the realms of politics and economics. In medical terms, the legacy of Giolitti's anti-cholera strategy is more negative. Concealment was achieved at a high cost in life and suffering borne by his fellow countrymen. One important reason was that the determination to preserve silence extended to the willingness to deny Italian physicians the most recent information concerning developments in the treatment of the disease. Most dramatic and significant in this regard was the rejection, on grounds of expediency, of the application by Leonard Rogers, the English cholera expert practising at the Calcutta Medical College, to visit Naples in order to explain his recent therapeutic breakthrough to the Italian medical community. On the Calcutta cholera ward between 1906 and 1909, Rogers perfected the technique of rehydration therapy. At the urging of eminent Italian physicians, he applied in the summer of 1911 to the Italian Ministry of the Interior for permission to demonstrate his methods at the Cotugno Hospital. The refusal was especially surprising because, as the *British Medical Journal* observed, the Italian authorities normally placed no restrictions on British physicians wishing to practise in Italy. Normally, it was sufficient for a British doctor to have his name on the *Register* kept by the General Medical Council in order to be cleared to exercise his profession in Italy.[178]

As we have seen, the idea of replacing the bodily fluids lost by cholera patients through purging and vomiting was one of the earliest and most persistent therapeutic notions relating to cholera. The concept of rehydration was adopted during the first pandemic, and it was renewed during the course of every invasion of the disease. Attempts persisted because rehydration provided a means of countering the most characteristic and devastating clinical sign of cholera. As Rogers explained, in normal blood the ratio of corpuscles to serum is 45 per cent corpuscles and 55 per cent serum. Even in mild cases of Asiatic cholera this proportion was altered disastrously to at least 71 per cent corpuscles and 29 per cent serum, representing a loss of one-third of the liquid portion of the blood. In severe cases, this loss could double to two-thirds of the fluid of the serum. Similar proportions of the saline content of the blood were lost to circulation.[179]

Experimental rehydration procedures yielded dramatic but ephemeral results throughout the nineteenth century. Copious saline injections restored warmth, colour and animation to the bodies of patients; and relieved the most painful symptoms, such as cramps and asphyxia. Unfortunately, the improvement was only fleeting, and patients invariably relapsed within hours; and heroically repeated injections ended only in a succession of disappointments. In the early decades of the nineteenth century failure ensued for a range of different reasons such as embolism until hypodermic technology had been improved; from septicaemia until the germ theory taught that the water used had to be sterile; and from a lack of understanding of the quantities of solution to be used. Still more intractable was the conceptual problem that researchers replaced the lost blood fluids with isotonic saline solutions – solutions, that is, of salt concentrations identical to that of blood in an effort to replace like with like. Isotonic saline solutions are not retained, so that the injected fluid and the patient were lost.

Rogers made the decisive refinements in 1908.[180] With modern techniques of measuring the specific gravity of blood and blood pressure, he was able precisely to calibrate the quantity of fluid to be injected. He also discovered that hypertonic solutions – much more saline than blood itself – promote retention, thereby preventing the lethal choleraic discharge of fluid into the intestine. Given time, the patient's bodily defences would destroy the cholera germ; the problem until Rogers's innovation was that, in the majority of cases of the disease, death resulted from acute shock and its complications beforehand. At the Calcutta Medical Hospital, the English doctor and his precisely calculated hypertonic solutions reduced mortality in cases of acute cholera to less than 20 per cent. In addition to rehydration, Rogers administered solutions of permanganate orally as a means of neutralizing the cholera toxin in the digestive tract. His results were published in the *Proceedings of the Royal Society* in 1909.

In his memoirs *Happy Toil: Thirty-Five Years of Tropical Medicine*, the English physician discussed the reaction of the Italian Ministry of the Interior to his efforts to disseminate his findings for the benefit of Italian doctors and their patients. Having returned to England on home leave in 1911, Rogers learned through private contacts with physicians in Rome of the Italian epidemic of Asiatic cholera. Already an international authority in the field of tropical diseases and the correspondent in India of the *British Medical Journal*, he was anxious to demonstrate the effectiveness of his rehydration methods in a European context. He therefore made official enquiries regarding the possibility of doing so at Naples or Venice. Naples was especially appropriate because of its unhappy primacy in matters of cholera and because of its prominence as a medical centre. In reply, he recalled,

> I received information that ... an English doctor would not be welcomed –
> apparently because the disease had not been declared, as it ought to have been in
> accordance with the terms of the Venice [*sic*] Cholera Convention. The reason for the
> failure to notify the disease was the fear of upsetting the tourist traffic.[181]

Undeterred, Rogers travelled in mid-July to Rome, where he was refused permission by the Ministry of the Interior to enter Italian hospitals in an official capacity – despite the urgent advocacy by leading Italian authorities on cholera.

After further intense medical pressure, most strenuously applied by members of the medical faculty at Palermo, who had previously arranged for a translation of his paper of 1909, the Ministry arranged a limited compromise. A visit by Rogers to a major medical centre on the mainland was ruled out because it would attract unwelcome publicity and would constitute too flagrant an admission of the presence of cholera in Italy. Rogers was therefore refused permission to enter the cholera wards at Naples or Venice. He was allowed instead to take his rehydration apparatus to Sicily, where his presence would be less visible, and where any resulting publicity would be less damaging because it could be plausibly stated that the outbreak was confined to the island. There was also to be a strict time limit. Initially, his permission extended for a period of only two days, which were ultimately renewed for a total of three weeks.

Rogers referred to these weeks spent in July at the Lazzaretto della Guadagna at Palermo as 'the most remarkable experience of my varied life'.[182] One reason for the salience of this period in his memory was his amazement at the sheer number of cholera cases in the hospital – 'more than I had ever seen at one time in India'.[183] Sicily was in the midst of a substantial epidemic. Other reasons also abounded – the difficulties posed by the lack of a common language in which to communicate to the medical staff consisting of Professor Vincenzo Romano and five medical students under his direction; the enormous success of the trial that he made of his new methods; and the enthusiasm of Professor Romano, the Medical Director of the cholera ward, who described the therapeutic procedures introduced by Rogers as 'nothing short of the miraculous'.[184] Romano wrote a letter of gratitude and tribute in which he termed Rogers 'the first doctor in the world' and the 'star of medical science'.[185] The final explanation for the indelible impression of this Palermitan experience, Rogers noted, was his bitter encounter with the indifference of the Italian state to the welfare of its people. The Ministry of the Interior denied Rogers any extension of his stay beyond three weeks; it made no effort to inform the profession at large of the life-saving capabilities of rehydration therapeutics; and it never sent Rogers an acknowledgment of his efforts, a contribution to cover his expenses, or any communication at all.[186] In the priorities of the Department of Public Health, the maintenance of a prudent silence outweighed the interest of Italian citizens in the first effective means of dramatically reducing mortality from Asiatic cholera. Despite the clear demonstration of the effectiveness of Rogers's procedures, the state refused to publicize his visit and its significance. Secrecy thus took a heavy toll in human suffering. Thousands perished while an effective treatment was confined to an obscure ward in Palermo.

The consequences of state-sponsored ignorance were most apparent at Naples, the epicentre of the epidemic. In Naples, the treatment of Asiatic cholera had not altered substantially since 1884, apart from the abandonment of Cantani's lethal acidic irrigation of the gut. At the Cotugno Hospital the prevailing theory of the disease was the view advocated during the last great epidemic of the nineteenth century by Mariano Semmola – that cholera was an intoxication of the central nervous system. As Montefusco wrote with reference to the classic symptoms of *cholera gravis*,

It is necessary to conclude that at least the major portion of those symptoms beyond the digestive apparatus are related to nervous disorders caused by the choleraic toxins. Indeed Semmola admitted that diarrhoea itself, in the early stages of the disease, was not the result of local irritation by the *Vibrio cholerae* but should be regarded instead as the first effect of the poisoning of the nerve centres and of the abdominal sympathetic nerve, as these undoubtedly influence circulation and the digestive functions of the intestine.'[187]

Just as the paradigm of the disease adopted on the Cotugno cholera ward was reminiscent of the era of Semmola and Cantani, so the principal therapeutic procedures employed under Montefusco's direction echoed measures desperately attempted during the catastrophe of 1884. Some of these procedures were intended to facilitate the elimination of the cholera toxin, such as the exhibition of calomel, which was employed as a diuretic, and hot baths, which were regarded as a means to stimulate perspiration. As in every previous epidemic, however, so in 1911 repeated failures with the ascendant theory led to the desperate recourse to a wide variety of alternative approaches. In addition to eliminant therapy, therefore, stimulants were administered – caffeine, camphor, strychnine and alcohol; oxygen was inhaled to combat asphyxia; tincture of iodine was adopted to suppress excessive vomiting; and efforts were made to support the system by means of hypodermoclysis and subcutaneous injections of what were termed 'physiological' or isotonic saline solutions.

In addition, a highly experimental and limited trial was made of what was termed 'etiological therapeutics' – the effort to neutralize the cholera toxins directly in the body. For Montefusco, an encouraging recent idea in cholera management was the development of anti-cholera serum by injecting animals with the *Vibrio cholerae* in the hope that the antibodies they produced could be utilized to treat human sufferers. The first trials on human beings were conducted at St Petersburg, where the results were profoundly discouraging, producing a mortality rate of 75 per cent.[188] Undeterred by failures in Russia, the Cotugno experimented with the administration of serum to forty-one patients during the early weeks of the 1911 epidemic. The results, however, were as discouraging as in Russia: only eleven patients recovered, so that the rate of mortality using the 'etiological therapy' was 73.2 per cent, and Montefusco concluded that it was clinically worthless.[189]

At the very moment when Leonard Rogers was demonstrating his therapeutic breakthrough at Palermo, the incomplete statistics for the Cotugno in 1911 suggest that the Naples hospital for infectious diseases achieved a mortality rate of approximately 50 per cent among the cholera patients it treated – a rate roughly in accord with the norm in every outbreak of cholera since 1830 and more than triple the rate simultaneously but secretly recorded by Rogers and his

Table 7.7. *Patient statistics: Cotugno Lazaretto,*
3 May to 31 August 1911

Admitted	1,395
Discharged	773
In care	42
Dead on arrival	44
Deaths within two hours of admission	68
Deaths two or more hours after admission	468

colleagues at Palermo. On Professor Romano's cholera ward the recovery rate reached 85 per cent, and Rogers explained that a full recovery should be the normal expectation of a normally healthy person who received proper treatment at an early stage of the disease.[190] By contrast, incomplete and confidential municipal figures for the Cotugno cholera ward, called the 'lazaretto', were those shown in Table 7.6.[191] Thus the policy of secrecy had the immediate effect of denying cholera patients on the Italian mainland the benefit of the only effective therapy available.

In addition to promoting an unnecessarily high rate of mortality among the victims of the disease, secrecy almost certainly prolonged the epidemic itself. The epidemic first flared up at Naples in May, and the last known deaths in the city occurred in September, while elsewhere in Italy sufferers continued to perish until November. Such a lengthy outburst, which contrasts strikingly with the experience of all other industrial nations in the West during the final cholera pandemic, suggests such a conclusion. As the Venetian medical profession had protested, concealment disarmed the nation's physicians and it prevented an educational campaign among the general public. Secrecy prevented the armed forces from taking adequate precautions concerning the movement of troops because there was no official means of knowing which provinces were infected. For the same reason, it was impossible for education authorities to know whether schools should be shut and examinations cancelled or postponed. Because of the resulting administrative confusion and delay, the progress of the disease was facilitated and, once established, it was correspondingly more difficult to diagnose, isolate and eradicate. State policy therefore bears a significant share of the responsibility for the extent of the Italian misfortune in 1911, and this fact itself in turn supplied the authorities with yet another reason to preserve the silence.

The negative consequences of Giolitti's policy were not, however, solely medical. Democratic principles were among the most notable casualties. Having unilaterally taken the decision to mislead parliament, the press and the Italian public, the ministry pursued a course of policy for which there could be no public accountability. The executive denied the Chamber its constitutional right of oversight. There was no discussion of the medical emergency in parliament either during the outbreak or subsequently. In stark contrast to the precedents set by Depretis in the 1880s and of Luzzatti in 1910, Giolitti never presented a retrospective account to the Chamber, allowing it to criticize the administration and compel its officials to explain their conduct.

The only parliamentary consideration of the disaster of 1911 took place in March 1912 in the inauspicious context of a consideration of the budget of the Ministry of the Interior. On that occasion the deputy Murri expressed a considerable anxiety about the health of democracy in Italy. Overwhelmed by the enthusiasm and unanimity of the Libyan War, the Chamber, he complained, had not discussed the normal affairs of state with the requisite attention. There had been a serious lack of debate, passion and conflict in parliament, which had contented itself with meekly acquiescing in the decisions of the executive. 'But the Chamber', he reasoned, 'must not be unanimously for the Government. On our own behalf we must represent something in the play of national affairs . . .'[192]

The administration made certain, however, that the cholera epidemic would not provide the opportunity for such a re-assertion of parliamentary authority. Through its control of the legislative time-table, the government presented public health not as a topic to be considered on its own, but as part of an overall discussion of the budget of the most important Italian ministry. The time available for consideration of the epidemic was shared by such other urgent matters as law and order, emigration, socialism and taxation. The entire matter was concluded on two days – 8 and 9 March 1912.

On 8 March, Undersecretary of State Falcioni opened the debate in a manner that gave little indication of a willingness of the cabinet to submit itself to democratic scrutiny. Referring to infectious diseases generally and without ever mentioning cholera by name, he stated the position of the ministry, which was that,

> The Department of Public Health is very well organized; it has done and is doing all that is necessary to prevent the spread of any disease of an epidemic character.
>
> And then, if you will allow me, . . . one of the best means of preventing the spread of epidemic diseases is to discuss them as little as possible. And the reason for this emerges clearly from the facts, and is not just an impression. Unfortunately, there is a foreign press that delights in embroidering a fantasy out of alleged infectious diseases that we in Italy generally do not have, but that other nations do.
>
> The great advantage foreigners possess is that, unlike us, they preserve a prudent silence in these matters – which is exactly the opposite of how we behave![193]

In pursuit of this line of reasoning, Falcioni called on the press to pay no heed to the discussion and to avoid reporting the 'inaccurate information' presented by ordinary deputies.[194]

During the debate that ensued several deputies raised the issue of epidemic cholera – 'the disease we aren't allowed to mention'[195] – and called upon Giolitti to explain the causes for so great a misfortune. With regard to 'interrogations', however, it was the minister's prerogative to respond to all of the questions raised *en bloc* rather than considering them one by one. The results were that

Giolitti's response was brief and inconclusive, that he successfully avoided any acknowledgement of the epidemic, and that he never uttered the forbidden word 'cholera'. Mysteriously, too, despite the enormous anti-cholera campaign of the summer and autumn, the budget for the Ministry of the Interior did not include any sums specifically allocated to cover the costs of the disaster that had swept the nation. Cholera disappeared once more – this time from the national budget.[196]

Such political procedures were dangerous, and they formed part of a larger process by which the Liberal state slowly succumbed to a terminal illness that ended with Mussolini's March on Rome in 1922. The political ramifications of epidemic cholera for the Italian state are the subject of the Conclusion.

Conclusion: Neapolitan cholera and Italian politics

Neapolitan experience between 1884 and 1911 vindicates Asa Briggs and Louis Chevalier in their early insight that Asiatic cholera was a major transformative experience in the societies it affected, linking the history of medicine to the broader concerns of political, social, cultural and urban history. The ravages of the city of Naples in this period constitute an ideal test case for such a perspective because they occur so late. The fifth and sixth pandemics that mark the boundaries of this study were unlike the dramatic events of the 1830s that have most attracted historians. By the time the infection broke out in the boroughs of Porto and Mercato in the summer of 1884, it was an all too familiar visitor; its aetiology was largely understood; the mortality it caused had greatly diminished; and the medical and political authorities of the day understood the preventive measures that needed to be taken to prevent further epidemics. In 1910 and 1911 cholera could even be described as a disease whose time had passed because highly effective means existed to prevent, contain and treat it.

Even in such circumstances, cholera had a major impact on the history of the city. A major reason in 1884 is what might be termed its moral chronology. Morally, the epidemic of that year was the first for which the new Liberal regime could be held responsible. United Italy had already been devastated by a major epidemic of cholera in the 1860s. At that early date, however, the overthrow of the *ancien régime* was too recent and the new order too precariously established for it to be held accountable for the conditions that promoted Asiatic cholera. By 1884, however, the Liberal state had been in place for nearly a quarter of a century, and the close link between cholera on the one hand and poverty, filth and the urban environment on the other hand were well established. The authorities in every nation in Europe were aware of measures that could be taken in order substantially to reduce their citizens' risk of contagion.

Politically, therefore, the outbreak of 1884 was the first cholera epidemic of Liberal Italy – the first in which the claims of the Risorgimento to embody progress and social improvement were brought under close scrutiny and found wanting. Outlining his vision of the social consequences of national independence and free institutions, Cavour had declared in 1847:

> Let us act in such a manner that all of our fellow citizens, but the poor more than the rich, share in the benefits of an advance in civilisation and of an increase in wealth. In this way we shall find a peaceful and Christian solution to the great social question – the question that others wish to resolve with dreadful subversion and fearful tumult.[1]

It was a 'binding duty', he announced, to 'improve both the material and the moral conditons of the lower classes'.[2]

By 1884 there were no indications in Naples that the new regime had even begun to address such promises of social change. The return of cholera dramatically raised the issue of the achievements of the Liberal revolution. Cholera had enormous potential locally as a catalyst for political disaffection because epidemic disease was already at the centre of municipal debate. All currents of opinion were in agreement that cholera was a social disease in that its ravages were clear indications of sanitary neglect, economic hardship and dietary deficiency. The work of John Snow, Max von Pettenkofer and Robert Koch left no doubt that the weight of contemporary scientific opinion supported such a conclusion. Locally, this general indictment was powerfully reinforced by the fact that the city council under the leadership of mayors San Donato, Giusso and Amore – variously representing the Historical Left, the Catholics and the Historical Right – had commissioned official studies of the sanitary conditions of its population in relation to epidemic disease, had identified the leading risk factors, and had drawn up extensive plans for their correction. The reports by the physician and sanitary reformer Marino Turchi in particular were widely read and influential. It was accepted by all informed opinion that the sources of epidemic disease in the city were eradicable, but that the magnitude of the hygienic crisis required the commitment and support of the national political leadership.

Geography powerfully underlined the issue of responsibility for the medical disaster. The fact that in 1884 the disease devastated Naples almost solely made the details of the sanitary arrangements and economic misery of the city issues of national concern. Furthermore, as the former capital of the Kingdom of the Two Sicilies, Naples was regarded as the touchstone by which the issue of the treatment of the South by the new regime could be measured. Cholera, in other words, was not regarded as a misfortune, but – much more explosively – it was considered an injustice. The disease became a metaphor for all of the discontents of southerners under a political order dominated by Piedmont. The epidemic of 1884 formed a powerful catalyst for the crystallization of the twin issues of the 'Question of Naples' and the 'Southern Question' as two of the most important issues in Italian national life.

In the case of Naples, therefore, the anxiety of Pelling and Rosenberg that the importance of cholera has been overestimated by historians is almost certainly misplaced. Far from being an exotic import that created a moment of high drama and then departed without involving the long-term ills of the society, cholera became the vehicle through which Neapolitans gave expression to their discontents and their demands for change. For this reason, the disease is an essential moment for the historian wishing to examine the social and political structures of the city, and the attitudes of contemporaries towards them. But it needs to be stressed that cholera in Naples is far more than just a useful tool for historical investigation and a rich source of documentation regarding social conditions and *mentalités*. More fundamentally, it was for Neapolitans themselves a foremost means for the articulation of their grievances at their status as an internal colony condemned by the Italian state to the distress of economic decline, poverty and unregulated urbanization. It also follows that, having been taken up as a metaphor for the whole of the 'Problem of Naples', cholera became the standard against which progress was measured and the commitment of the regime to the welfare of the city was judged.

From the standpoint of the national political leadership, cholera therefore posed a most unwelcome political as well as a medical challenge. Already by 1884 the governors of Italy were preoccupied with the problems posed by the 'passive revolution' of the Risorgimento in which the legitimacy of the new regime was never firmly established in the Mezzogiorno. In the 1860s the precariousness of Liberal authority had been revealed by the split between the Catholic Church and the Liberal state as well as by the prolonged civil war in the southern provinces euphemistically termed 'Brigandage'. Hardly had the new order been established by force of arms than the regime experienced the shock of the elections of 1874, when the 'Historical Left', representing above all the discontents of southerners, gained a stunning success in the Mezzogiorno and powerfully contributed to the formation of the Depretis government in 1876. In the middle of the same decade, the protests of southerners were then officially legitimated by the drastic conclusions of the great investigation by Leopoldo Franchetti and Sidney Sonnino into the conditions of the island of Sicily.[3] In this already charged atmosphere the devastations of cholera in the Lower City of Naples provided the occasion for the concentration of the attention of the whole nation on the squalid misery and insalubrity of the Neapolitan poor – themes that were to provide an enduring cultural legacy in the works of such writers as Axel Munthe, Jessie White Mario, Pasquale Villari, Matilde Serao, Francesco Saverio Nitti and Arturo Labriola.

Only by appreciating the multiple depths of the crisis presented by the outburst of cholera in 1884 is it possible to explain the response of the state. An epidemic in Naples was not only a threat to the health of the nation; it was also a challenge to the legitimacy of Liberal rule. Catholic enemies of the regime immediately established the connection, arguing that the onset of the fifth pandemic in Italy demonstrated the hollow nature of the promises of the Risorgimento and exposed the sordid reality of Liberal misgovernment. Furthermore, the events of September 1884 dramatically confirmed the alienation of

Neapolitans from the political institutions of the regime. As the emergency reached its height, the writ of City Hall ceased to run in the boroughs of the Lower City.

In this threatening context, the royal visit and the unprecedented and rapid passage of the 'special law' to finance urban renewal by parliament were more than gestures of humanitarian solidarity with the sufferings of the great southern seaport. They were also intended to prevent intransigent Catholics on the right and socialist activists on the left from fishing in the troubled waters of social misery and from transforming despair into an active and dangerous sense of injustice. Along with the overt sanitary purpose of combating contagion, *risanamento* carried the powerful subliminal message that Liberal Italy was at last fully committed to answering the grievances of the Mezzogiorno.

Risanamento, therefore, was of far more than local importance. It served as a symbol, and it established a precedent for state intervention in the South through large-scale public works. Indeed, the long-term Liberal strategy for overcoming the economic underdevelopment of the South was by means of further 'special laws' authorizing the investment of capital in massive state programmes. Since the rebuilding of the Lower City was the prototype, it offers an instructive lesson. There is a close correspondence between the problem of public health and the contemporary economic issue of the development of the South. Liberal spokesmen for the 'Southern Question' – Giustino Fortunato, Pasquale Villari, F.S. Nitti – believed that the redemption of the Mezzogiorno was essentially a matter of massive capital investment. Nitti was the most coherent and influential advocate of this approach. North and South, in his conception, occupied different positions on a common path leading to modernity. The relative backwardness of the Mezzogiorno was merely a result of its systematic starvation of capital by a state dominated by northern interests. Taxation, tariffs and public spending north of Rome drained the South of resources, undermined its industry, and imprisoned it in a condition of permanent disadvantage. The remedy was a series of 'special laws' that would encourage northern entrepreneurs to invest in the region through tax incentives, subsidized power and favourable contracts. Such measures would enable the South to 'take off' into sustained economic growth.

The difficulty with this approach was that its effect in practice has never been to close the gap. The investment of northern capital alone has served only to reinforce underdevelopment, to reproduce the southern position of semi-colonial dependence, and to dissipate resources in the channels of patronage and clientele politics. The needs of the South were not essentially quantitative, but qualitative: what was required was not so much more capital but rather a programme of fundamental structural reforms. The effect of a strategy to develop the Mezzogiorno through imitation of the North and through the action of northern investors has been to confirm northern domination.

The issue of public health is not utterly dissimilar. In the late nineteenth and early twentieth centuries the South suffered from enormous medical and hygienic as well as economic backwardness. A major reason was the administrative framework within which public health policies were applied. Italian sanitary legislation, which was modelled on the example of Piedmont, devolved the major responsibility and expense of public health upon the commune without regard to regional disparities. This approach, which penalized the inhabitants of impoverished communities, guaranteed sanitary dualism. Naples was not a uniquely unhappy exception but a representative example of a general pattern. Municipalities throughout the Mezzogiorno were similarly indebted, maladministered and unable to defend the public welfare. To delegate public health to the commune in the economically backward provinces of the Mezzogiorno was to institutionalize the lack of provision. The conditions prevailing in Naples were not due to the neglect of the Palazzo San Giacomo alone; they were also the result of a systematic and permanent regional inequality.

Policy reinforced the deficiencies created by inappropriate administrative structures. Public health strategies in the Mezzogiorno imitated the experience of the very different societies of northern Italy and northern Europe. The defence of Naples against cholera through *risanamento* depended on transplanted procedures that had little purchase in their new context. To invest medical and economic capital in a city where the Camorra held sway was as unlikely, in the absence of prior reform of its social and political infrastructures, to produce health as to invest economic capital without structural reform was to generate industrial development. Renewal and rebuilding were doomed because the funds upon which they depended were inevitably dissipated in the established channels of patronage and corruption. *Risanamento* was the prototype of a pattern of spending on public works in the South that, instead of yielding health and development, led only to private enrichment.

Within the confines of a single city, the Neapolitan medical crisis of 1910 and 1911 bore a definite resemblance to the larger events of the crisis of the Liberal state after the First World War. Previous history ensured that the outbreak of cholera in 1910 presented more than just a sanitary emergency. It symbolized the breakdown of political trust. For cholera to return to a city that had been so expensively renewed and so ostentatiously proclaimed to be invulnerable was to reveal the full extent of local maladministration and the depths of the cynicism of the ruling elites in matters affecting public welfare. To Neapolitans at the height of the Giolittian era, therefore, cholera signified betrayal as well as disease. It was this consciousness that fuelled the semi-revolutionary ambitions of the Popular Bloc to sweep the ruling political classes from power on the strength of a campaign based on the issue of public health.

Giolitti's response to the medical and political challenge illustrates certain prominent features of Italian Liberal rule. From the time of his assumption of power at the turn of the century, the Piedmontese Prime Minister had followed a consistent strategy of attempting to solve the chronic Italian problem of governability by broadening the bases of the state. He feared that to employ repressive means alone to confront subversion in the manner of Crispi, Di Rudiní and Pelloux in the 1890s would prove counter-productive, extending and radicalizing political opposition. Giolitti sought instead to de-fuse tensions by adopting a substantial programme of social and political reforms – the legalization of the right to strike, the neutrality of the state in industrial disputes, support for a policy of wage increases, the reform of local taxation, and above all the broad extension of the suffrage. The intention behind these liberal concessions was conservative – to use liberal means to reinforce the power of the state.

As a far-sighted and astute conservative, Giolitti attached two essential limits to his willingness to contemplate reform. One was that the opponents he was prepared to bring into the political arena be moderate reformists rather than revolutionaries. The toleration extended to strikes launched for traditional trade-union and economic objectives did not extend to movements led by anarcho-syndicalists and revolutionary socialists. Against the latter he was prepared to use violent and merciless repression. The second vital qualification was that his liberalization applied to the North but not to the South of the peninsula. Here was a careful calculation of the means necessary to preserve political power. His majority in parliament would remain impregnable even if political opponents made substantial inroads among the deputies elected from the northern provinces provided the other half of the members elected from the Mezzogiorno voted with near unanimity for the government of the day.

Janus-headed, Giolitti's political system could be described as liberal in the North and authoritarian in the South. In a famous protest at Giolitti's policies in the Mezzogiorno, the reformist socialist leader from Apulia, Gaetano Salvemini, described the premier's rule as 'the minister of the underworld'.[4] In Sicily, Campania and Apulia, Giolitti closed both eyes during election campaigns while his faithful supporters unleashed reigns of terror by the Mafia, the Camorra and the notorious Apulian *mazzieri*. Far from democratic, the electoral process throughout the Giolittian era in the South was marked by every manner of fraud, corruption and illegality. Similarly, the history of the workers' movement in Apulia – the only region in the South where Giolitti faced a powerful and well-organized revolutionary opposition – was marked by persistent police inti-midation and marked by recurring incidents of savagery when the police opened fire on strikers and demonstrators. In Salvemini's telling phrase, Giolitti viewed his strategy south of Rome as a market transaction in which he bought the Deputy and sold the Prefect.[5]

Seen against this background, the highly illiberal conduct first of Luzzatti and then of Giolitti during the cholera epidemic of 1910–11 forms part of a consistent, long-term *modus operandi*. When the disease first broke out in Apulia, the thinking of the Luzzatti ministry was one of violent military repression. The language of official documents is that of war. The country was on a 'war footing'; prophylaxis was a 'campaign' and a 'battle' waged with 'weapons', 'outposts' and 'sentinels'; and the outbreak of the disease was an 'attack'. Such a military paradigm for disease rationalized the massive intervention of central govern-ment.[6] It also eased the decision to rely on the army and the police, and justified the use of violence, coercion and a calculated campaign of xenophobia. The danger to civil liberties in Bari and Foggia provinces was all the greater because, from the perspective of the national medical planners, the inhabitants of Apulia were not really fellow-citizens, but colonials towards whom the troops behaved like an army of occupation. The summer of 1910 thus posed the 'Southern Question' in its starkest terms, exposing the depth of the abyss that separated the Mezzogiorno from the rest of Italy, and revealing the violent potential of the Liberal state towards the 'dangerous classes' of the South.

When the disease broke out in Naples in September, Luzzatti's reaction was marked by a moment of indecision. On the one hand, it was impossible to contemplate a military anti-cholera operation of the Apulian sort in the great metropolis. Such a highly visible and illegal use of violence would have created a vast backlash of outrage and condemnation that the ministry could not have survived. On the other hand, the evolution of events in the city took a particularly menacing political direction that placed it well beyond the outer parameters that Giolitti had established for toleration. In Naples, the campaign to overthrow the ruling majority on the municipal council was led by syndicalist, republican and socialist subversives; and the initiative they took directly challenged the legitimacy of the regime and its policies in the South. While Luzzatti prevaricated, the sanitary issue exploded into a national crisis that helped to precipitate Luzzatti's final political demise.

Upon returning to power, Giolitti confronted the new and more serious epidemic of 1911 with resolute rigour. The policy he applied was the logical extension to public health of the system with which he had dominated the nation since the turn of the century. When confronted with a challenge that touched the bases of legitimacy of the regime, Giolitti had always been prepared to jettison constitutional niceties and the legal rights of citizens in the interest of *raison d'état*. In 1911 the epidemic centred in the South – at Naples and Sicily – threatened to undermine Liberal hegemony. International treaties, the well-being of nations to which Italians travelled and of visitors to Italy, the right of parliament to oversee the executive and of the press to report events, and the right of victims of the disease to the best available treatment – all of these were subordinated to the demands of maintaining power while the Prime Minister sanctioned the use of repressive means to impose a veil of silence. The events of 1911 were no novel departure in Giolittian rule but the medical facet of his southern strategy.[7]

Unfortunately for the regime, there was an insoluble moral contradiction that eroded the authority of Liberal rule and helped to prepare the political terrain for its overthrow. The ethical claim to authority of the Liberal order was based on such fundamental political principles as parliamentary sovereignty, the rule of law and civil liberties. Giolitti's commitment to such values, however, was not absolute but conditional upon their value in preserving the dominance of his party. Inevitably, the frequent exhibition of electoral fraud and violence in Apulia and Sicily bred cynicism, distrust and sullen resentment. Similarly, his display of power in setting aside truth, the interests of the ill, and parliamentary prerogatives during the cholera months in 1911 eroded the moral foundations of Liberal statecraft. Furthermore, Giolitti's selective willingness to set aside legality itself conveyed a dangerous message to the personnel who manned the state bureaucracy – a message from which they were ultimately to draw their own conclusions when Liberal Italy faced still greater challenges. And the process of moral erosion, once established, proved irreversible. The cholera epidemic of 1911 was one more instance of the way in which the disregard for the law and the constitution created an atmosphere of suspicion and disrespect surrounding the state, and the vigorous response of the state to the crisis suggests not that the regime was strong but that it was vulnerable to challenge because its authority was precarious.

Appendix

Appendix

Table A1. *Male deaths from cholera classified by occupational group: Italy, 1884*

Occupation	I	II
Labourers	285	17.0
Soldiers	182	9.0
Clerks and scribes	162	8.0
Carpenters, cabinet-makers, clog-makers	156	8.8
Farm workers, day labourers	126	9.3
Farmers, gardeners	123	1.0
Waiters	118	8.6
Shopkeepers, tradesmen	110	5.9
Cobblers	97	5.5
Blacksmiths, gunsmiths	94	9.1
Bricklayers	84	5.4
Boatmen, seamen	72	8.0
Porters	70	5.9
Itinerant trades	68	20.7
Policemen, municipal guards, customs guards	58	17.5
Coachmen, cabmen	53	8.7
Cooks, food friers	51	9.4
Prisoners	50	5.1
Tailors	50	5.7
Landlords, affluent men	49	1.5
Pensioners	45	2.8
Tavern-keepers, wine-sellers, innkeepers	40	7.4
Shop assistants	39	11.7
Barmen	36	9.9
Engravers, painters, sculptors	34	9.6
Hairdressers	32	16.2
Priests	32	3.0
Carters	30	4.5
Bakers	25	14.7

Appendix

Table A1. (*contd*)

Occupation	I	II
Typographers	25	8.3
Students, pupils	24	5.4
Officers	23	15.6
Coppersmiths, tinsmiths, brassworkers	22	8.6
Founders	21	29.6
Butchers	20	7.1
Teachers	20	6.2
Beggars	20	2.9
Bakers	18	5.0
Ragpickers	17	21.5
Lawyers, notaries	17	4.9
Tobacco vendors	14	6.8
Dyers and varnishers	14	6.2
Shepherds	14	3.8
Charcoalburners	14	12.5
Pork-butchers and sausage vendors	13	7.6
Doctors	13	5.2
Weavers and spinners	11	2.6
Messengers	9	11.7
Confectioners and pastry chefs	9	8.8
Stone-cutters, pavers, stone-masons	9	3.2
Mattress-makers	8	5.0
Nurses	7	8.3
Pharmacists	7	5.6
House-painters	5	7.2
Farriers	5	7.1
Quarriers and miners	5	3.1
Boatsmen and sailors on rivers and lakes	0	0
Other professions	403	5.6
Total	3,158	3403

Note: Column I: Absolute numbers of deaths
Column II: Percentage of all deaths of members of the group caused by Asiatic cholera

Table A2. *Deaths from cholera by province: Italy, 1884*

Region	Province	No. of communes affected	No. of deaths
Piedmont	Alessandria	25	72
	Cuneo	82	1,655
	Novara	23	100
	Turin	54	404
	Total	184	2,231
Liguria	Genoa	57	1,438
	Porto Maurizio	6	48
	Total	63	1,486
Lombardy	Bergamo	131	531
	Brescia	43	108
	Como	3	2
	Cremona	58	207
	Mantua	7	13
	Milan	23	48
	Pavia	30	97
	Sondrio	1	5
	Total	296	1,011
Veneto	Belluno	0	0
	Padua	1	1
	Rovigo	18	87
	Treviso	0	0
	Udine	0	0
	Venice	3	7
	Verona	0	0
	Vicenza	0	0
	Total	22	95
Emilia	Bologna	13	48
	Ferra	6	55
	Forlí	0	0
	Modena	16	93
	Parma	16	196
	Piacenza	2	2
	Ravenna	1	0
	Reggio nell'Emilia	17	141
	Total	71	535
Tuscany	Arezzo	0	0
	Florence	0	0
	Grosseto	0	0
	Livorno	1	5
	Lucca	8	11
	Massa and Carrara	14	232
	Pisa	8	7
	Siena	0	0
	Total	31	255

Table A2. (*contd*)

Region	Province	No. of communes affected	No. of deaths
Marches	Ancona	0	0
	Ascoli Piceno	1	1
	Macerata	0	0
	Pesaro and Urbino	1	6
	Total	2	7
Umbria	Perugia	1	1
Lazio	Rome	2	6
Abruzzi and Molise	Aquila	7	126
	Campobasso	12	81
	Chieti	5	33
	Teramo	0	0
	Total	24	240
Campania	Avellino	13	23
	Benevento	11	7
	Caserta	51	253
	Naples	54	7,994
	Salerno	28	147
	Total	157	8,424
Apulia	Bari	0	0
	Foggia	2	2
	Lecce	1	0
	Total	3	2
Basilicata	Potenza	1	15
Calabria	Catanzaro	0	0
	Cosenza	1	5
	Reggio	0	0
	Total	1	5
Sicily	Caltanissetta	0	0
	Catania	0	0
	Girgenti	0	0
	Messina	0	0
	Palermo	0	0
	Siracusa	0	0
	Trapani	0	0
	Total	0	0
Sardinia	Cagliari	0	0
	Sassari	0	0
	Total	0	0
Grand total		858	14,299

Table A3. *Deaths from gastro-enteritis in Naples, 1911*

Month	Population under 5 years of age	Population over 5 years of age
January	36	10
February	27	9
March	47	9
April	25	16
May	72	11
June	134	16
July	144	19
August	68	17
September	34	126
October	8	27
November	16	11
December	18	15

Source: Archivio Centrale dello Stato, Direzione Generale della Sanità, 1882–1915, b. 177 bis, fasc. Colera; dati statistici. 'Morti per gastro-enterite ed enterite acuta nei singoli mesi dell'anno 1910'.

Table A4. *Daily wages of farm workers in Italy, 1905*

Month	Wages in US dollars
January	$0.26
February	$0.27
March	$0.31
April	$0.34
May	$0.37
June	$0.44
July	$0.45
August	$0.38
September	$0.33
October	$0.32
November	$0.31
December	$0.29
Minimum	$0.26
Maximum	$0.45
Mean	$0.34*

Note: * The pay of $0.34 differs from the mean of $0.40 to $0.50 mentioned on page 267 because the latter figures include allowances of food and drink that were the norm in most of the Italian countryside. The Commission was at special pains to stress that these meagre Italian rural wages were not compensated by the low cost of the necessities of life. Indeed, the Commission found no substantial difference in the cost of living between Italy and the United States.
Source: Direzione Generale della Statistica e del Lavoro, *Annuario statistico italiano*, second series, 1(1911) (Rome, 1912), p. 156.

Table A5. *Steerage fares from Naples to New York, 1905–11*

Year	Highest fares (lire)	Lowest fares (lire)
1905	190	130
1906	180	125
1907	187	123
1908	200	138
1909	210	170
1910	210	175
1911	210	175
1912	210	175

Source: Commissariato Generale dell'Emigrazione, *L'emigrazione italiana dal 1910 al 1923* (Rome, 1926), vol. I, p.431.

Table A6. *Deaths from cholera in Italy in 1911*

Province	Deaths
Alessandria	33
Ancona	2
Aquila	60
Arezzo	0
Ascoli Piceno	0
Avellino	91
Bari	105
Belluno	0
Bergamo	14
Bologna	7
Brescia	0
Cagliari	66
Caltanissetta	166
Campobasso	307
Caserta	740
Catania	364
Catanzaro	82
Chieti	61
Como	0
Cosenza	56
Cremona	0
Cuneo	0
Ferrara	28
Florence	1
Foggia	116
Forlí	18
Genoa	266
Girgenti	278
Grosseto	0
Lecce	36
Livorno	370
Lucca	3
Macerata	0
Mantua	0
Massa Carrara	45
Messina	88
Milan	8
Modena	0
Naples	873
Novara	3
Padua	4
Palermo	830
Parma	0
Pavia	0
Perugia	0

Appendix

Table A6. (*contd*)

Province	Deaths
Pesaro-Urbino	47
Piacenza	0
Pisa	8
Porto Maurizio	0
Potenza	13
Ravenna	0
Reggio Calabria	2
Reggio Emilia	9
Rome	131
Rovigo	16
Salerno	432
Sassari	6
Siena	6
Siracusa	62
Sondrio	0
Teramo	7
Turin	0
Trapani	150
Treviso	0
Udine	0
Venice	116
Verona	0
Vicenza	0
Total	6,146

Table A7. *Reported deaths and bacteriologically*
confirmed deaths, Italy 1911

Province	Bacteriologically confirmed deaths	Reported deaths
Cagliari	8	54
Venice	116	252
Aquila	60	159
Forlí	18	60
Massa e Carrara	45	77
Palermo	873	1,542
Total	1,120	2,154

Note: For these samples the reported deaths were 192% greater
than the bacteriologically confirmed deaths

Table A8. *Monthly departures of emigrants from Naples*
and Genoa, 1909

Month	Port of departure	
	Genoa	Naples
January	6,820	13,703
February	5,344	20,991
March	8,846	39,971
April	9,283	32,278
May	6,129	25,049
June	4,894	12,337
July	3,076	7,908
August	7,162	6,356
September	11,288	11,311
October	22,737	10,029
November	21,041	7,920
December	10,126	5,791
Total	116,746	193,644

Notes

INTRODUCTION

1 My early work on the epidemic of 1910 was incorporated in my article, 'Cholera in Barletta', *Past and Present*, no. 132 (August 1991), pp. 67–103.

2 Asa Briggs, 'Cholera and Society in the Nineteenth Century', *Past and Present*, no. 19 (October 1961), pp. 76–96. Chevalier's pioneering work in the social history of cholera is Louis Chevalier, ed., *Le choléra: la première épidémie du XIXs siècle* (La Roche-sur-Yon, 1958).

3 Charles E. Rosenberg, 'Cholera in Nineteenth-Century Europe: A Tool for Social and Economic Analysis', *Comparative Studies in Society and History* 8 (1966), pp. 452–463.

4 Margaret Pelling, *Cholera, Fever and English Medicine, 1825–1865* (Oxford, 1978).

5 *Ibid.*, pp. 3–4.

CHAPTER 1: A CITY AT RISK

1 The official figure for the population of Naples in 1881 was 494,000. Municipio di Napoli, *Relazione sul V Censimento Generale della Popolazione e sul I Censimento Industriale* (Naples, 1912), p. 32. For figures relative to the population and the area of the city, see also Rocco De Zerbi, 'Relazione della commissione sul disegno di legge presentato dal presidente del consiglio ministro dell'interno (Depretis): Disposizione per provvedere alla pubblica igiene della città di Napoli', seduta del 15 dicembre 1884, *Camera dei deputati, Legislatura XV-Sessione 1882–86, Raccolta degli atti stampati per ordine della camera*, vol. XXII, n. 261–A, pp. 1–2.

2 Speech of Salvatore Trinchese, 22 July 1890, *Atti del consiglio comunale di Napoli*, 1890, p. 642. The eminent Bavarian hygienist Max von Pettenkofer refused to stay longer than three days in the city, and he drank only beer during his sojourn. Speech by Teodosio De Bonis, 22 February 1882, *Atti del consiglio comunale di Napoli*, 1882, p. 153.

3 Speech of 31 December 1873, *Atti del consiglio comunale di Napoli*, 1874, p. 12.

4 On the geography of the Old City, see Municipio di Napoli, *Progetto per lo*

ampliamento della città e risanamento delle zone insalubri: relazione (Naples, 1884), pp. 16–19.

For a compelling recent description of the contrast between the Upper and Lower Cities, see Paolo Macry, 'Borghesie, città e Stato. Appunti e impressioni su Napoli, 1860–1880', *Quaderni storici*, 19 (1984), pp. 339–383. Naturally, as Macry notes, it is important to make qualifications and distinctions. Within the Upper City there were gradations of wealth between San Giuseppe, the wealthiest of the twelve *sezioni* at one extreme and the fringes of San Carlo and San Lorenzo, where there were neighbourhoods whose conditions approximated those of nearby Vicaria and Pendino. The privileged borough of San Ferdinando contained the fishermen's quarter of Santa Lucia, one of the most impoverished of all. Similarly, in the Lower City Vicaria was the least disadvantaged of the four boroughs while Mercato had the unhappy distinction of being the poorest of all. Furthermore, the plebeian sea of the Lower City contained scattered islands of genteel respectability such as the grand Via Toledo. Even after all refinements, however, Macry still finds it useful to invoke the Disraelian analogy of 'two nations' to describe the social abyss between the Upper City and the Lower.

5 Mortality statistics were provided by the Alderman responsible for public health, Dr. Teodosio De Bonis. Speech of 22 June 1884, *Atti del consiglio comunale di Napoli*, 1884, pp. 522–527.

6 On the anxiety in the Third Republic about population and degeneration, see Eugen Weber, *France, Fin de Siècle* (Cambridge, Mass. and London, 1986), pp. 9–26.

7 Francesco Saverio Nitti, *Napoli e la questione meridionale* (Naples, 1903). pp. 57–58.

8 Speech of 22 July 1890, *Atti del consiglio comunale di Napoli*, 1890, p. 642.

9 Nitti, *Napoli*, p.1.

10 Speech by Faraone, 16 May 1874, *Atti del consiglio comunale di Napoli*, 1874, pp. 458–460.

11 Rocco De Zerbi, *Colera del 1884: Croce Bianca e Croce Rossa* (Naples, 1884), p. 3.

12 Speech by Michele Foucault, 30 August 1881, *Atti del consiglio comunale di Napoli*, 1881, p. 557; and speech by Teodosio De Bonis, 22 February 1882, *Atti del consiglio comunale di Napoli*, 1882, p. 153. See also speech by De Bonis, 23 December 1882, *Atti del consiglio comunale di Napoli*, 1882, p. 1028. Although retrospective diagnosis is inevitably suspect, it is possible to speculate that the disease was Malta fever.

13 Proposal by councillor Errico Spasiano, 21 October 1876, *Atti del consiglio comunale*, 1876, p. 400.

14 Speech of Nicola Trudi and interruption of the mayor, 17 October 1876, *Atti del consiglio comunale di Napoli*, 1876, p. 379.

15 Speech by Nicola Amore, 19 January 1885, *Atti del consiglio comunale di Napoli*, 1885, p. 15

16 *Innocents Abroad* (Hartford, Conn., 1869), p.315.

17 *La epidemia colerica e le condizioni sanitarie di Napoli* (Naples, 1884), p.6.

18 Speech by alderman T. De Bonis, 25 June 1884, *Atti del consiglio comunale di Napoli*, 1884, pp. 522–527.

19 Official figures provided by the U.S. government are in Edward O. Shakespeare, *Report on Cholera in Europe and India* (Washington, 1890), p. 141. Slightly different figures are in Alexandrine Tkatcheff, 'Un mois à Naples pendant l'épidémie cholérique de 1884', *Gazette hebdomadaire des sciences médicales de Montpellier*, 7 (1885), p. 69.

20 Rocco De Zerbi, 'Relazione della commissione sul disegno di legge presentato dal presidente del consiglio ministro dell'interno (Depretis): Disposizione per provvedere alla pubblica igiene della città di Napoli', seduta del 15 dicembre 1884, in Camera dei deputati, Legislatura XV-Sessione 1882–86, *Raccolta degli atti stampati per ordine della Camera*, vol. XXII, n. 261–A, pp. 2–3.

21 *Il ventre di Napoli* (Naples, 1973).

22 Direzione Generale della Statistica, *Statistica delle cause di morte nei comuni capoluoghi di provincia o di circondario e delle morti violente avvenute in tutto il regno, anno 1884* (Rome, 1885), p. xxvii.

23 The Via Fico is described in detail in the article 'La cronaca: il problema della salute pubblica', *Il Mattino* 28–29 September 1910.

24 *Innocents Abroad*, p. 316.

25 'Special Correspondence: Letters From Italy', *British Medical Journal*, 5 April 1884, pp. 693–694.

26 Marcellin Pellet, *Napoli Contemporanea, 1888–1892*, trans. Francesco D'Ascoli (Naples, 1989), pp. 19–20.

27 Marino Turchi, *Sulla igiene pubblica della città di Napoli: osservazioni e proposte* (Naples, 1862), p. 7.

28 Municipio di Napoli, *Progetto per lo ampliamento della città e risanamento delle zone insalubri: relazione* (Napoli, 1884), p. 21. On overcrowding in the Lower City, see also Giustino Fortunato, 'La città e la plebe', in *Scritti politici*, ed. F. Barbagallo (Bari, 1981), pp. 29–33.

29 Twain, *Innocents Abroad*, p. 316.

30 Ameury Duval, *Tableaux de Naples et de ses Environs*, in Gregoire Orloff, *Mémoires Historiques, Politiques et Littéraires sur le Royaume de Naples* (Paris, 1821), vol. V, pp. 267 and 289–290.

31 Eugenio Fazio, 'Il colera del 1884 in Napoli', *Giornale della Reale Società Italiana d'Igiene*, 7 (1885), p. 467; and Alexandrine Tkatcheff, 'Un mois à Naples pendant l'épidémie cholérique de 1884', *Gazette hebdomadaire des sciences médicales de Montpellier*, 7 (1885), p. 57 and p. 57, n.1.

32 Pellet, *Napoli*.

33 'La cronaca: il problema della salute pubblica', *Il Mattino* 28–29 September 1910.

34 Speech of 10 November 1884. *Atti del consiglio comunale di Napoli*, 1884, p. 704.

35 'Il grave problema della salute pubblica', *Il Mattino*, 2–3 October 1910.

36 This is a line from the poem ''O Funneco', in Alberto Consiglio, ed., *Antologia dei poeti napoletani* (Milan, 1978), p. 125.

37 'La cronaca: il problema della salute pubblica', *Il Mattino*, 28–29 September 1910.

38 Turchi, *Sulla igiene*.

39 *Letters from a Mourning City*, trans. Maude Valerie White (London, 1887).

40 The original description, published in the *Fanfulla*, appeared in translation in the article 'The Sanitary Condition of Naples', *Times*, 27 September 1884.

41 Speech by Achille Nardi, September 1886. *Atti del consiglio comunale di Napoli*, 1886, pp. 842–843.
42 Pellet, *Napoli*, p. 19.
43 National Archives. Record Group 84: Records of Foreign Service Posts. Consular Reports: Naples, Italy, volume 012. Despatch of Frank G. Haughwout to Hon. John Davis, Assistant Secretary of State, 22 December 1884, no. 50, pp. 229–230.
44 *Ibid.*, p. 236.
45 Archivio di Stato di Napoli, Prefettura, b. 3625, fasc. Condizioni igieniche delle case al largo S. Erasmo ai Granili. Letter of sixteen tenants to Sig. Prefetto della Provincia, 16 September 1885, n. 25148.
46 A helpful discussion of the living conditions of Neapolitan bricklayers is Alfredo Minozzi, 'L'operaio muratore di Napoli', *Riforma sociale*, 3:5 (1896), pp. 777–808.
47 *Ibid.*, pp. 784–785, 794–796.
48 In 1884 the American consul at Naples conducted an extensive investigation into wages and the conditions of labour in Naples. See National Archives. Record Group 84: Records of Foreign Service Posts. Consular Posts: Naples, Italy, volume 012. Despatch of Frank G. Haughwout to Hon. John Davis, Assistant Secretary of State, 22 December 1884, n. 50, pp. 228–250.
49 Minozzi, 'L'operaio', p. 803.
50 On the building trade and its intimate relationship with the boarding-houses of the borough of Porto, see Francesco P. Rispoli, *La Provincia e la città di Napoli* (Naples, 1902), pp. 69 and 94–96.
51 John Snow, 'On the Mode of Communication of Cholera', reprinted in *Snow on Cholera* (New York, 1936; 1st edn, 1855), p. 18.
52 Michael Durey, *The Return of the Plague: British Society and the Cholera, 1831–1832* (London, 1979), pp. 33–35.
53 Snow, *Snow on Cholera*, p. 18.
54 Luigi Romanelli, *Clinica delle malattie da infezione acute ovvero rendiconto statistico, etiologico, clinico e terapeutico degl'infermi spediti e curati nell'Ospedale della Conocchia nel 1881* (Naples, 1885), p. 86.
55 *Il colera e la carità: cenno storico dell'epidemia di Napoli del 1884* (Naples, 1884), p. 24. For a description of the *locande* in the city, see also Minozzi, 'L'operaio', pp. 785–787.
56 For discussions of the distinction between 'sporadic' and 'epidemic' cholera in the *Lancet*, see for example: Bendshye, 'On the Origin and Treatment of Sporadic Cholera', *Lancet* (1830–1, vol. 2), pp. 258–261; 'Westminster Medical Society: The Cholera, Its Nature and Treatment', *Lancet* (1831–2, vol. 1), pp. 340–346; 'Paris', *Lancet* (1873, vol. 2), pp. 435–436; 'Medical Societies. Royal Medical and Chirurgical Society', *Lancet* (1885, vol. 1), p. 564; and 'Cholera: Current Notes, Comments and Criticism', *Lancet* (1892, vol. 2), 790–792.
57 Snow, *Snow on Cholera*, p. 17.
58 Archivio di Stato di Napoli, Prefettura, b. 3625, fasc. Reclamo Viscussi Giuseppe sulle vacche e capre in città. Letter of Giuseppe Viscussi to Sig. Conte Sanseverino and Signori della Commissione igienica della città di Napoli, 5 March 1885.
59 Speech by Giuseppe Crotonei, 27 May 1888, *Atti del consiglio comunale di Napoli*, 1888, p. 295.

60 On the hazards posed by laundresses, see Archivio Centrale dello Stato. Ministero dell'Interno, Direzione Generale della Sanità, 1882–1915, b. 249 bis, fasc. Napoli: cholera. Mauro Jatta, 'Profilassi per il colera di Napoli: 1911', pp. 6–7.

61 For documents regarding the brass foundries in Lower City, see Archivio di Stato di Napoli, Prefettura, b. 3621, fasc. Fonderie di metalli nella sezione di Pendino in Napoli.

62 Archivio di Stato di Napoli, Prefettura, b. 3621, fasc. Fonderie di metalli nella sezione di Pendino. Letter of residents of the Vico Strettola agli Orefici to Signore Prefetto della Provincia di Napoli, 26 October 1881.

63 Archivio di Stato di Napoli, Prefettura, b. 3621, fasc. Fonderie di metalli nella sezione Pendino in Napoli. Letter of Minister of the Interior to Prefetto di Napoli, 27 October 1883, n. 30169. On the trade in coffins, clothing and bodies for dissection from the cemetery, see the speech of Councillor Camillo Agrelli, 7 February, 1874, *Atti del consiglio comunale di Napoli*, 1874, vol. 2, pp. 195–196.

64 On the street-sweeping practices of the city, see the discussion by Salvatore Trinchese, speech of 22 July 1890, *Atti del consiglio comunale di Napoli*, 1890, pp. 641–643.

65 On the cesspits (*pozzi neri*) of the city, see Nicola Amore, speech of 6 February 1885, *Atti del consiglio comunale di Napoli*, 1885, p.18; and speech by Councillor Florenzano, 11 February 1885, pp. 36–37.

66 For a detailed discussion of street-sweeping and waste removal, see the speech of Councillor Lucci, 13 November 1903, *Atti del consiglio comunale di Napoli*, 1903, vol. 2, pp. 560–673.

67 Speech by Lucci, 13 November 1903, *Atti del consiglio comunale di Napoli*, 1903, vol. 2, pp. 558–569.

68 On the microbial link established between the city and the *padulani*, see Orazio Caro, *L'evoluzione igienica di Napoli* (Naples, 1914), p. 213. The practice of sewage farming was not eliminated in the nineteenth century, however, but was still a major source of risk in 1911. See Archivio Centrale dello Stato. Ministero dell-'Interno, Direzione Generale della Sanità, 1882–1915, b. 249 bis, fasc. Napoli: cholera. Mauro Jatta, 'Profilassi per il colera di Napoli: 1911', pp. 11–13.

69 On the wells in use in 1884, see Nicola Amore, Report on the Sanitary Service during the Cholera Epidemic, 30 October 1884, *Atti del consiglio comunale di Napoli*, 1884, vol. 2, esp. pp. 681–682.

70 A recent study of the Carmignano aqueduct is Giuseppe Fiengo, *L'acquedotto di Carmignano e lo sviluppo di Napoli in età barocca* (Florence, 1990).

71 The classic discussion of the Neapolitan water supply is Marino Turchi, *Sulle acque e sulle cloache della città di Napoli* (Naples, 1865). The discussion here is also based on Salvatore De Renzi, *Osservazioni sulla topografia medica del Regno di Napoli*, 3 vols. (Naples, 1828–30), esp. vol. I, pp. 50–55; Caro, *L'evoluzione igienica*; Edward O. Shakespeare, *Report on Cholera in Europe and India* (Washington, 1890), esp. pp. 120–123; and discussions in the city council such as the speech by T. De Bonis, *Atti del consiglio comunale di Napoli*, 1884, pp. 522–527. Also useful is Giuseppe Saredo, *Relazione della R. Commissione d'inchiesta per Napoli sulla amministrazione comunale* (Rome, 1901), vol. II, pp. 58–141.

72 The number of cisterns was discussed by Nicola Amore, Report on the Sanitary

Service during the Cholera Epidemic, 30 October 1884, *Atti del consiglio comunale di Napoli*, 1884, vol. 2, pp. 681–682.

73 Alexandrine Tkatcheff, 'Un mois à Naples pendant l'épidémie cholérique de 1884', *Gazette hebdomadaire des sciences médicales de Montpellier*, 7 (1885), pp. 68–69.

74 Shakespeare, *Report on Cholera*, pp. 121–122.

75 Federico Sirignano, *Relazione igienico-sanitaria circa l'epidemia cholerica del 1884 nella sezione Pendino* (Naples, 1885), p. 13.

76 Robert Koch, *Professor Koch on the Bacteriological Diagnosis of Cholera, Water-Filtration and Cholera, and the Cholera in Germany during the Winter of 1892–93*, trans. George Duncan (Edinburgh, 1894), p. 61.

77 National Archives. Record Group 84: Records of Foreign Service Posts. Consular Posts, Naples, Italy, volume 012. Despatch of Frank G. Haughwout to Hon. John Davis, Assistant Secretary of State, 22 December 1884, n. 50, p. 237.

78 For recent discussions of the role of seafood in the spread of cholera, see Eric D. Mintz, Tanja Popovic, and Paul A. Blake, 'Transmission of *Vibrio cholerae* 01', in I. Kaye Wachsmuth, Paul A. Blake, and Ørjan Olsvik, *Vibrio cholerae and Cholera: Molecular to Global Perspectives* (Washington, DC, 1994), pp. 349–351; William B. Baine, Mirella Mazzotti, Donato Greco, Egidio Izzo, Alfredo Zampieri, Giusseppe Angioni, Mario Di Gioia, Eugene J. Gangarosa, Francesco Pocchiari, 'Epidemiology of Cholera in Italy in 1973', *Lancet* (1974, vol. 2), pp. 1370–1374; Paul A. Blake, Mark L. Rosenberg, Jose Bandeira Costa, Pedro Soares Ferreira, Cesar Levy Guimaraes, and Eugene J. Gangarosa, 'Cholera in Portugal, 1974', *American Journal of Epidemiology*, 105 (1977), pp. 337–343; and Robert Tauxe, Luis Seminario, Roberto Tapia, and Mario Libel, 'The Latin American Epidemic', in Wachsmuth, *et al.*, eds., *Vibrio cholerae*, pp. 337–339.

79 Speech of Councillor Camerlingo, 4 July 1903, *Atti del consiglio comunale di Napoli*, 1903, vol. 2, p. 8.

80 Report on the budget of 1881, 14 July 1881, *Atti del consiglio comunale di Napoli*, 1881, pp. 360–376.

81 *Ibid.*, p. 371.

82 Unites States House of Representatives, 48th Congress, 2nd Session, Ex. Doc. 54, Part 1, *United States Consular Reports. Labor in Europe. Reports from the Consuls of the United States in the Several Countries of Europe on the Rates of Wages, Cost of Living to the Laboring Classes, Past and Present Wages, &c., in Their Several Districts, in Response to a Circular from the Department of State Requesting Information on These Subjects* (Washington, 1885). Hereafter this report will be referred to as *United States Consular Reports. Labor in Europe.*

83 For the letter of explanation provided by the Secretary of State, see *ibid.*, pp. 1–7. In the words of the Secretary of State, 'an intelligent understanding of the conditions of the existing relations of labor and wages to capital and enterprise in other countries is indispensable to a correct judgment upon problems affecting the laboring and employing classes in our own country.'

84 National Archives. Record Group 84: Records of Foreign Service Posts. Consular Posts: Naples, Italy, volume 012. Despatch of Frank G. Haughwout to Hon. John Davis, Assistant Secretary of State, 22 December 1884, n. 50, p. 228

85 *Ibid.*, pp. 231–232.

86 *Ibid.*, pp. 229–230.
87 *Ibid.*, p. 243.
88 *Ibid.*, p. 229.
89 *Ibid.*, p. 239.
90 *Ibid.*, p. 235.
91 *Ibid.*, pp. 234–235.
92 *Ibid.*, pp. 241–242.
93 The comparative conclusions of the Department of State with regard to wages in Europe and the United States are to be found in *United States Consular Reports. Labor in Europe*, pp. 178–193. The statistics furnished here are drawn from figures for the general trades, p. 181.
94 On the Neapolitan fishing industry, see Rispoli, *La Provincia*, pp. 18–26; and 'I Pescatori di Napoli', *Il Piccolo*, 11 October 1884. On the reputation of S. Lucia as one of the neighbourhoods most in need of renewal, see Archivio Comunale di Napoli. Gennaro Sambiase Duca di San Donato, 'Discorso-programma del sindaco', 5 October 1876, *Atti del consiglio comunale di Napoli*, 1876, p. 296.
95 Councillor Folinea, speech of 5 May 1887, *Atti del consiglio comunale di Napoli*, 1887, p. 311.
96 National Archives. Records of the US Department of State, Re: Internal Affairs of Italy, 1910–1929, Publication no. M527, category 865.12, Microfilm Roll 25. Report of Ernest E. Evans, American Vice-Consul at Naples, 'Burial Customs and Costs in Naples, Italy', to Homer M. Byington, American Consul-General, 4 August 1927, p. 4.
97 Speech of 19 April 1902, *Atti del consiglio comunale di Napoli*, 1902, vol. 1, p. 427. Nitti a year later suggested a figure of 150,000 unemployed in Naples. *Napoli*, p. 60.
98 Municipio di Napoli, *Progetto per lo ampliamento della città e risanamento delle zone insalubri: relazione* (Napoli, 1884), p. 21.
99 Speech by Baron Savarese, 15 January 1874, *Atti del consiglio comunale di Napoli*, 1874, pp. 111–112.
100 Saredo, *Relazione della R. Commissione*, pp. 45–46.
101 For a discussion of the economic condition of Naples, see the speech by Vincenzo Pizzuti, 31 December 1873, *Atti del consiglio comunale di Napoli*, 1874, pp. 7–34; and the speech by Baron Savarese, 15 January 1874, *ibid.*, pp. 109–113.
102 Speech of Baron Savarese, 15 January 1874, *Atti del consiglio comunale di Napoli*, 1874, p. 112. A study of the growth of poverty in Naples in the two decades following unification is Rocco De Zerbi, 'La miseria di Napoli', *Nuova antologia* 48 (1879), pp. 737–758.
103 Speech by Vincenzo Pizzuti, 31 December 1873, *Atti del consiglio comunale di Napoli*, 1874, p. 22.
104 Report by Vincenzo Pizzuti, 6 March 1876, *Atti del consiglio comunale di Napoli*, 1876, p. 129.
105 *Ibid.*, p. 136.
106 Speech of 23 December 1873, *Atti del consiglio comunale di Napoli*, 1874, pp. 6–34 and esp. p. 7.
107 Report by Vincenzo Pizzuti, 6 March 1876, *Atti del consiglio comunale di Napoli*, 1876, p. 136.

108 On the defects of the taxation policies pursued by the Neapolitan town council between 1861 and 1901, Saredo, *Relazione della R. Commissione*, vol. I, esp. pp. 274–319.

109 Speech by Angelo Incagnoli, 13 January 1865, *Atti del consiglio comunale di Napoli*, 1865, p. 44.

110 Rispoli, *La Provincia*, p. 96.

111 *Ibid.*, p. 105.

112 On the populism of the Camorra, see Marcella Marmo, 'La Camorra e lo stato liberale', in Francesco Barbagallo, ed., *Camorra e criminalità organizzata in Campania* (Naples, 1988), esp. pp. 24–25. On the customs of the Camorra, see Ferdinando Russo and Ernesto Serao, *La camorra: origini, usi, costumi e riti dell'annorata soggietà* (Naples, 1970). Cf. also Cesare Lombroso, *L'homme criminel* (Paris, 1895), vol. II, pp. 539–558.

For 'social banditry' the classic works are Eric J. Hobsbawm, *Bandits* (London, 1969), esp. pp. 13–23, 34–60, and 94–115; and *Primitive Rebels: Studies in Archaic Forms of Social Movement in the 19th and 20th Centuries* (New York, 1969), esp. pp. 13–56. More sombre assessments of the Mafia include Pino Arlacchi, *Mafia, Peasants and Great Estates: Society in Traditional Calabria* (Cambridge, 1983); Anton Blok, *The Mafia of a Sicilian Village, 1860–1969: A Study of Violent Peasant Entrepreneurs* (New York, 1975); and Jane and Peter Schneider, *Culture and Political Economy in Western Sicily* (New York, 1976).

113 Fabbroni's testimony is printed in 'Il processo Cuocolo', *Il Mattino* 12 July 1911.

114 Saredo, *Relazione della R. Commissione*, vol. 1, p. 70.

115 The organizational structure of the Camorra was discussed in detail by the Camorra leader Gennaro Abbatemaggio during the Cuocolo trial in 1911, when he turned witness for the prosecution in exchange for immunity. See esp. 'La confessione di Abbatemaggio', *Il Mattino* 30–31 January 1911.

116 'Il processo Cuocolo', *Il Mattino* 9–10 June 1911,

117 Quoted in Luigi Miscilli Migliorini, 'Povertà e criminalità a Napoli dopo l'unificazione: il questionario sulla camorra del 1875', *Archivio storico per le province napoletane* 98 (1980), pp. 567–615. The classic discussion of the collusion of Ferdinand II and the camorra is Marc Monnier, *La Camorra* (Paris, 1863), ch. 5, pp. 145–172.

118 On the collusion between the Liberals and the Camorra, see Monnier, *La Camorra*, ch. 7, pp. 173–200.

119 On this point see Marcella Marmo, 'Tra le carceri e i mercati. Spazzi e modelli storici del fenomeno camorrista', in Paolo Macry and Pasquale Villani, ed., *Storia d'Italia. Le regioni dall'Unità a oggi: La Campania* (Turin, 1990), pp. 689–730. On the collusion between the Bourbons and then the Liberals and the Camorra, see Giuseppe Alongi, *La camorra: studio di sociologia criminale* (Turin, 1890), pp. 24–25, 34–36, 106, 117–119.

120 Monnier, *La Camorra*, p. 160.

121 For a discussion of the Neapolitan abattoir, see Saredo, *Relazione della R. Commissione*, vol. II, pp. 486–536.

122 *Ibid.*, vol. II, p. 488.

123 Report of 22 January and 14 February 1874, *Atti del consiglio comunale di Napoli*, 1874, pp. 149–151; and pp. 214–216.

124 On this point, see Paolo Frascani, 'Mercato e commercio a Napoli dopo l'Unità', in Macry and Villani, ed., *La Campania*, esp. pp. 198–199.

125 Saredo, *Relazione della R. Commissione*, vol. II, p. 150. On the activity of the Camorra, see Alongi, *La Camorra*, esp. ch. 5, pp. 95–113; and Monnier, *La Camorra*, ch. 4, pp. 95–123.

126 The text of the reply is in Migliorini, 'Povertà e criminaltà', p. 592.

127 On this point see *Ibid.*

128 Speech of 31 March 1909, *Atti del consiglio comunale di Napoli*, 1909, pp. 580–588.

129 De Renzi, *Osservazioni*, vol. II, pp. 21–22.

130 Speech of 22 February 1874, *Atti del consiglio comunale di Napoli*, 1874, p. 274.

131 Interpellation of 29 May 1883, *Atti del consiglio comunale di Napoli*, 1883, pp. 540–541.

132 Nitti, *Napoli*, p. 1.

133 The idea of a mild form of cholera, variously termed 'choleraic diarrhoea' or 'premonitory diarrhoea', that precedes the attack of proper 'malignant cholera' was widespread in the medical literature of the century. Some representative examples are: 'Statistical Results of the Treatment of Cholera and Diarrhoea', *Lancet* (1855, vol. 1), pp. 438–439; 'The Treatment of Cholera', *Lancet* (1866, vol. 2), pp. 153–154; 'Tannic Acid Injections in Cholera', *Lancet* (1885, vol. 1), pp.352–353. See also A.J. Wall, *Asiatic Cholera: Its History, Pathology and Modern Treatment* (London, 1893), ch. 5, esp. pp.98–101.

   For a discussion of 'premonitory diarrhoea' by the mayor of Naples after the epidemic of 1884, see the speech by Nicola Amore, 12 November 1884, *Atti del consiglio comunale di Napoli*, 1884, p. 729.

134 Pellet, *Napoli*, p. 165. Matilde Serao reported that in 1884 Naples contributed 16 million lire to the total of 60 million lire generated by the national lottery. *Il paese di Cuccagna* (Milan, 1891), p. 372.

135 Serao, *Il paese di Cuccagna*.

136 *Ibid.*, p. 156.

137 Pellet, *Napoli*, pp. 176–177. On the importance of the lottery to the poor of Naples, see also Serao, *Il paese di Cuccagna*, pp. 39–46.

138 On the camorra and the underground lottery, see Monnier, *La Camorra*, pp. 109–110.

139 For Gramsci's concept of 'passive revolution', see *Selections from the Prison Notebooks of Antonio Gramsci*, ed. and trans. Quintin Hoare and Geoffrey Nowell Smith (London, 1971), esp. pp. 105–120.

140 For a review of the sanitary practices of the Liberal government between 1848 and the advent of cholera in 1884, see Carlo Zucchi, 'Della competenza scientifica e giuridica del medico nell'esercizio dell'amministrazione sanitaria', *Giornale della Reale Società Italiana d'Igiene*, 8 (1886), pp. 17–59.

141 *Ibid.*, p. 24.

142 Christopher Seton-Watson, *Italy from Liberalism to Fascism, 1870–1925* (London, 1967), p. 50, n. 6.

143 Vincenzo Pizzuti, 'Sul bilancio del Municipio di Napoli: Relazione al Consiglio Comunale presentata dall'Assessore V. Pizzuti nella tornata del 6 marzo 1876', *Atti del consiglio comunale di Napoli*, 1876, pp. 108–111.

144 On the revelations made during the Casale trial, see below, Chapter 6.

145 Speech by Faraone, 16 May 1874, *Atti del consiglio comunale di Napoli*, 1874, pp. 459–460.

146 Rocco De Zerbi, *Colera del 1884: Croce bianca e croce rossa* (Napoli, 1884), p. 16.

147 Speech of 7 October 1865, *Atti del consiglio comunale di Napoli*, 1865, p. 559.

148 Speech of 16 May 1874, *Atti del consiglio comunale di Napoli*, 1874, p. 459–460.

149 'Il problema del risanamento di Napoli', *Corriere della sera*, 14–15 September 1884.

150 Saredo, *Relazione della R. Commissione*, vol. II, pp. 710–711.

151 *Ibid.*, p. 712.

152 Speech of 5 October 1876, *Atti del consiglio comunale di Napoli*, 1876, p. 294.

153 *Ibid.*

154 Giulio Melisurgo, 'Le morie di Napoli (II)', *Il Piccolo*, 8 October 1884.

155 Raffaele Parisi, ' A Napoli: le impressioni della Croce Bianca', *Corriere della sera* 17–18 September 1884.

156 Raffaele Parisi, 'Le impressioni d'un volontario della Croce Bianca a Napoli', *Corriere della sera*, 4–5 October 1884.

157 Alfonso Scirocco, *Politica e amministrazione a Napoli nella vita unitaria* (Naples, 1972), p. 82.

158 On the cultural background to the demand for the free circulation of ideas in Italy by the Liberal movement, see Kent Roberts Greenfield, *Economics and Liberalism in the Risorgimento: A Study of Nationalism in Lombardy, 1814–1848* (Baltimore, 1965).

159 'The Italian Medical Association', *Lancet* (1876, vol. 1), p. 185.

160 On the growing unity of the Italian medical profession under the Liberal regime, see 'Medical Congress at Turin', *Lancet* (1876, vol. 2), pp. 236; and 625–626.
    The history of the Italian medical profession in the modern period has still to be written, but see Paolo Frascani, 'Il medico nell'Ottocento', *Studi storici*, xxiii (1982), pp. 617–637; and Paolo Fracasini, 'Ospedali, malati e medici dal Risorgimento all'età giolittiana', in F. Della Peruta, ed., *Storia d'Italia' Annali, 7: Malattia e medicina* (Turin, 1984), p. 297–331.

161 For a listing of the members of the Faculty of Medicine and Surgery, see *Annuario della R. Università degli Studi di Napoli. Anno scolastico 1883–84* (Naples, 1884), pp. 19–23. For the distribution by faculty of the 5,368 students enrolled for the academic year 1896–7, see *Regia Università degli Studi di Napoli, Annuario Scolastico 1896–97* (Naples, 1897), p. 300.

162 *Il gattopardo* (Milan, 1958), ch. 7.

163 Direzione Generale della Statistica, *Annuario statistico italiano. Anno 1886* (Rome, 1887), Table III, p. 109.

164 The gender reference here is intentional because the medical profession was still closed to women.

165 Saredo, *Relazione della R. Commissione*, vol. I, p. 428.

166 *Ibid.*

167 *Ibid.*, p. 429.

168 *Ibid.*, p. 430. The problem of the cost of medicine and dietary prescriptions for the poor was raised as a serious impediment to proper medical care by Giuseppe

Buonomo in 1874 during the course of municipal discussion of public health. Speech of 16 May 1874, *Atti del consiglio comunale di Napoli*, 1874, vol. 2, pp. 461–462.

169 The civilian hospitals, excluding the special infirmary for syphilis, were the following: Gesù e Maria, Loreto, Pellegrini, Pace, Pacella, Incurabili, S. Maria della Vita and S. Eligio. For a brief outline of the specialisms of the various hospitals in the city, see *Bollettino ebdomadario dell'ufficio di statistica della città di Napoli*, 1875, no. 1 (1–7 January 1875).

170 Direzione Generale della Statistica, *Annuario statistico italiano. Anno 1886* (Rome, 1887), p. 251.

CHAPTER 2: FROM PROVENCE TO THE BAY OF NAPLES

1 Edward O. Shakespeare, *Report on Cholera in Europe and India* (Washington, 1980), p. 5.

2 National Archives, Washington, D.C. Record Group 84: Records of Foreign Service Posts. Consular Posts: Naples, Italy, Volume 012. Despatch of U.S. Consul B.D. Duncan to John Davis, Assistant Secretary of State, 30 June 1883, n. 36.

3 On the outburst of 1883 at Marseilles, see Comité Médical des Bouches-du-Rhône. Commission Scientifique, 'Séances extraordinaires, 4 juillet–8 août: Le choléra', *Marseille médical*, 21 (1884), p. 485. The deaths from cholera at Marseilles in the summer of 1883 were also reported as 'unquestionable' by the American consul. See Frank H. Mason, 'Progress of the Epidemic in Marseilles', August 19, 1884, in United States Bureau of Foreign Commerce, *Cholera in Europe in 1884. Reports from Consuls of the United States* (Washington, DC, 1885), pp. 15–16.

4 Consul Benjamin F. Peixotto, United States Consulate, Lyons, 'Cholera in France and throughout Europe', United States Bureau of Foreign Commerce, *Cholera in Europe*, p. 28.

5 A report that discusses the suspicions surrounding the *Sarthe*, if only to reject them, is F. Gendron, *Notes et observations sur l'épidémie cholérique à Toulon en 1884* (Paris, 1885).

6 The movements of the *Sarthe* from 1 April 1884 were described by M. Brouardel, *Bulletin de l'Académie de Médecine*, 2nd series, 13:2 (July–December) (1884), pp. 839–843. The result of the investigation was the conclusion that the *Sarthe* was not responsible for the epidemic.

7 'Le Choléra à Toulon', *Le Temps* 25 June 1884.

8 The naval regulations concerning the repatriation of the personal effects of French military personnel are discussed by Sirus Pirondi, 'Du choléra sur les côtes de la Méditerranée', *Marseille médical* 21 (1884), pp. 449–451.

9 Consul Frank H. Mason, 'Origin and Character of the Cholera Now Prevailing in Marseilles and Toulon', July 7, 1884, in United States Bureau of Foreign Commerce, *Cholera in Europe*, p. 5.

10 The French policy of secrecy was noted by the Italian Government. Giovanni Battista Morana, *Il colera in Italia negli anni 1884 e 1885: Relazione a S.E. il Cav. Avv. Agostino Depretis* (Rome, 1885), p. 3.

11 'The Cholera in Toulon', *Times*, 24 June 1884.

12 *Ibid.*

13 For a discussion of the sanitary conditions prevailing at Toulon and Marseilles, see 'Report of the Lancet Special Sanitary Commission on Marseilles and Toulon', *Lancet* (1885, vol. 1), pp. 1142–1143 and 1179–1180. Useful observations on the state of hygiene in the two cities are also made by the American consul Frank Mason, 'Preventive and Curative Methods', July 17, 1884, in United States Bureau of Foreign Commerce, *Cholera in Europe*, pp. 6–9.

14 Consul Benjamin F. Peixotto, United States Consulate, Lyons, 'Cholera in France and throughout Europe', July 17, 1884. United States Bureau of Foreign Commerce, *Cholera in Europe*, p. 28.

15 On the outbreak of cholera at Marseilles, see 'Le Choléra', *Le Temps,* 26 June 1884.

16 See, for example, 'Il cholera a Tolone e a Marsiglia', *Corriere della sera,* 28–29 June 1884.

17 *Atti del consiglio comunale di Napoli,* 1884, pp. 521–528.

18 R. Zampa, 'Storia del colera del 1884 in Italia', *Gazzetta di medicina pubblica: organo ufficiale per gli atti del consiglio di sanità di Napoli,* 16 (1885), pp. 112–113.

19 For the replies of the mayors to the questionnaire, see Ministero di Agricoltura Industria e Commercio. Direzione Generale della Statistica, *Statistica della emigrazione italiana negli anni 1884 e 1885* (Rome, 1886), pp. 7–143.

20 *Ibid.,* pp. 14–15.

21 *Ibid.,* pp. 8–9.

22 Ministero di Agricoltura Industria e Commercio. Direzione Generale della Statistica, *Statistica della emigrazione italiana per gli anni 1884 e 1885* (Rome, 1886).

23 In 1883 91.8 per cent of seasonal and 78.6 per cent of long-term emigrants were male. Ministero di Agricoltura, Industria e Commercio. Direzione Generale della Statistica, *Statistica della emigrazione italiana. Anno 1883* (Rome, 1884), Table 3, p. x. Of the temporary emigrants in 1883, 54.52 per cent departed in the three months of February, March, and April. *Ibid.,* p. xv.

24 For a description of the employment opportunities Italian immigrants found in southern France, see Erminio Albonico, *Saggio di una prima inchiesta sulla emigrazione italiana in Europa* (Milan, 1921), pp. 11–13.

25 Ministero di Agricoltura Industria e Commercio. Direzione Generale della Statistica, *Statistica della emigrazione italiana per gli anni 1884 e 1885* (Rome, 1886), p. 218.

26 On the incident at Aigues-mortes and the tensions that led up to it, see Teodosio Vertone, 'Antécédents et causes des évènements d'Aigues-mortes', in Jean-Baptiste Duroselle and Enrico Serra, ed., *L'emigrazione italiana in Francia prima del 1914* (Milan, 1978), pp. 107–138. On the hostility towards Italians at this period in the Third Republic, see Eugen Weber, *France, Fin de Siècle* (Cambridge, Mass. and London, 1986), pp. 133–141.

27 For the monthly health bulletin for October 1884, see *Marseille médical,* 21 (1884), pp. 691–701.

28 'Cholera in New Fields', *New York Times,* 7 September 1884.

29 'Southern Italy', *The Times,* 9 July 1884.

30 'Cronaca', *Il Piccolo,* 24 June 1884.

31 'Il cholera', *Il Piccolo,* 25 June 1884.

32 The classic statement of the opposition between the two medical philosophies of cholera is Erwin H. Ackerckneckt, 'Anticontagionism between 1821 and 1867', *Bulletin of the History of Medicine*, 22 (1948), pp. 562–593.

The revisionist position that the opposition between the two sides has been all too frequently exaggerated was formulated by Margaret Pelling, *Cholera, Fever and English Medicine, 1825–1865* (Oxford, 1978).

33 Pettenkofer's views were extensively discussed by the *Lancet*, and articles penned by him frequently appeared in its pages. Among the discussions of Pettenkofer's theories, see 'Epidemiological Society', *Lancet* (1866, vol. 1), p. 10; 'Professor Pettenkofer on Cholera', *Lancet* (1869, vol. 1), p. 133; 'Pettenkofer's Views on the Origin of Cholera', *Lancet* (1869, vol. 2), p. 345; 'Pettenkofer on Cholera', *Lancet* (1883, vol. 2), p. 155; and 'Bacteriology and Epidemiology', *Lancet* (1886, vol. 1), pp. 310–312. The text of an interview with Pettenkofer is 'Scientific Investigation into the Causes of Cholera. A Report of Interviews with Prof. Max von Pettenkofer at Munich, Nov. 1868', *Lancet* (1869, vol. 1), pp. 3–4. For articles by Pettenkofer, see Max von Pettenkofer, 'Cholera', *Lancet* (1884), pp. 769–771, 816–819, 861–864, 904–905, 992–994, 1042–1043, 1086–1088.

34 Max von Pettenkofer, 'Cholera', *Lancet* (1884, vol. 2), p. 769.

35 Max von Pettenkofer, *Cholera: How to Prevent and Resist It*, trans. Thomas Whiteside Hime (London, 1875), pp. 39–40.

36 *Ibid.*, p. 40.

37 'Il cholera a Tolone e a Marsiglia', *Corriere della sera*, 28–29 June 1884; and 'Le Choléra', *Le Temps*, 30 June 1884.

38 'Le Choléra à Toulon', *Le Temps*, 24 June 1884.

39 'Il Cholera', *Corriere della sera*, 28–29 June 1884.

40 'The Cholera', *Times*, 19 July 1884.

41 Consul Frank H. Mason, 'Situation at Marseilles and Toulon', 31 July 1884, in United States Bureau of Foreign Commerce, *Cholera in Europe*, pp. 10–11.

42 'Le Choléra', *Le Temps*, 30 June 1884.

43 Statistics for the troops present at Toulon were: soldiers – 1,830; marines – 3,313; sailors – 5,099; total – 10,242. See speech by M. Le Roy de Méricourt, 1 July 1884, *Bulletin de l'Académie de Médecine*, 2nd series, 13:2 (July–December) (1884), p. 838.

44 'The Cholera', *Times*, 4 July 1884.

45 'The Cholera', *Times*, 1 July 1884.

46 The higher estimate for Toulon is that of the *New York Times*. 'The Cholera in Europe', *New York Times*, 6 July 1884. For an estimate of the numbers who fled Marseilles, see 'Down among the Dead Men', *New York Times*, 27 July 1884.

47 *Bulletin de l'Académie de Médecine*, 2nd series, 13:2 (1884), pp. 913–914.

48 'The Cholera', *Times*, 1 July 1884.

49 'Il Cholera', *Corriere della sera*, 7–8 July 1884; and 'The Cholera', *Times*, 5 July 1884.

50 'Il Cholera', *Corriere della sera*, 7–8 July 1884.

51 'The Dreaded Cholera', *New York Times*, 1 July 1884. A slightly different account of Belot's fate was reported by the Parisian paper *Le Radical*. According to this account, Belot took his life when he was overcome by grief after his wife had succumbed to the disease. 'Le Choléra', *Le Radical*, 1 July 1884.

52 'Le Choléra', *Le Radical*, 14 July 1884.
53 'The Cholera in Europe', *New York Times*, 6 July 1884.
54 'The Cholera', *Times*, 30 June 1884.
55 'Il Cholera', *Corriere della sera*, 29–30 June 1884.
56 'The Cholera', *Times*, 1 July 1884.
57 Statistics for the 1865 epidemic are found in 'Le Choléra', *Le Temps*, 30 June 1884. On the plague of insects, see 'Il Cholera', *Corriere della sera*, 29–30 June 1884.
58 Lev. 18.5: 'You shall observe my institutions and my laws: the man who keeps them shall have life through them.' Similarly the Fifth Commandment promised: 'Honour your father and your mother, that you may live long in the land which the Lord your God is giving you.' Exod. 20:12.
59 On this point, see Nancy G. Siraisi, *Medieval and Early Renaissance Medicine: An Introduction to Knowledge and Practice* (Chicago and London, 1990), pp. 7–9.
60 Acts 12:23.
61 St. John 9:3.
62 Num. 12:9–12.
63 2 Kgs. 5:26–27.
64 2 Chr. 26:16–26.
65 1 Sam. 5:6–12.
66 'The Cholera', *Times*, 1 July 1884.
67 'The Cholera', *Times*, 26 July 1884.
68 2 Kgs. 20. On the views of the Archbishop of Paris, see 'Le Choléra et l'Archevêque de Paris', *Le Petit Var*, 29 July 1884.
69 'Cholera Still Spreads', *New York Times*, 17 August 1884. See also 'The King and the Cholera', *New York Times*, 5 October 1884, which described the cholera epidemic as a 'political factor' in both Italy and France.
70 Giuseppe Ferrigno, *Il colera in Palermo nel 1885* (Palermo, 1886).
71 *Ibid.*, pp. 13–14.
72 *Ibid.*, p. 23.
73 'Una nuova lettera del Card. Arc. di Napoli', *L'Osservatore romano*, 31 August 1884.
74 'Una pastorale del Card. Celesia', *L'Osservatore romano*, 25 November 1885.
75 'La morale dei casi di Sicilia', *Civiltà cattolica*, 26:4 (1885), iv, pp. 129–138. The reference was to Massimo D'Azeglio, *Degli ultimi casi di Romagna* (1846).
76 A clear exposition of the Jesuits' view of the epidemic of 1884 is 'Il colera: flagello e maestro', 7 October 1884, *Civiltà cattolica*, 8 (1884). pp. 129–142.
77 'Cronaca contemporanea: il *cholera-morbus* ad Ancona', *Civiltà cattolica*, 16:3 (1865), pp. 486–487.
78 *Ibid.*, p. 489.
79 'Cose italiane: il colera nelle Puglie', *Civiltà cattolica*, 61:2 (1910), pp. 624–625.
80 'Cholera and Politics', *New York Times*, 19 August 1884.
81 'Cholera in New Fields', *New York Times*, 7 September 1884.
82 *Ibid.*
83 'Il Cholera', *Corriere della sera*, 29–30 June 1884.
84 For the text of Dr. Brouardel's report to the Academy of Medicine on 1 July, see *Bulletin de l'Académie de Médecine*, 2nd series, 13:2 (1884), pp. 839–852.

85 The text of Herisson's speech is printed in 'Le Choléra', *Le Temps*, 28 June 1884.
86 *Ibid.*, p. 854.
87 Speech of Louis Pasteur, 1 July 1884, *Bulletin de l'Académie de Médecine*, 2nd series, 13:2 (1884), pp. 856–857.
88 See the speeches by Dr. Marey and Dr. Brouardel, 19 August 1884, *Bulletin de l'Académie de Médecine*, 2nd series, 13:2 (1884), pp. 1059–1154.
89 On Koch's interview, see 'The Cholera', *Times*, 7 and 10 July 1884.
90 'Course of the Pestilence', *New York Times*, 27 July 1884.
91 'The Trip to Marseilles', *New York Times*, 10 August 1884.
92 On the early confusion at the Pharo and the improvement that had taken place by late July see 'The Cholera', *Times*, 2 August 1884.
93 The systems of therapy adopted by the Pharo Hospital are briefly considered in 'Cholera News Bad Again', *New York Times*, 3 August 1884.
94 'Down among the Dead Men', *New York Times*, 27 July 1884.
95 'Cholera News Bad Again', *New York Times*, 3 August 1884.
96 'Cholera in Europe', *New York Times*, 1 August 1884.
97 Epicarmo Corbino, *Annali dell'economia Italiana* (Naples, n.d.), vol. III, esp. pp. 1–3, 102, 116, 173, 183.
98 Archivio di Stato di Napoli, Prefettura, b. 3525, fasc. Nappa Salvatore.
99 The following discussion of the administrative means devised to combat plague in Europe between the seventeenth century and the nineteenth is based primarily on Daniel Panzac, *Quarantaines et lazarets: L'Europe et la peste d'Orient (XVIIe–XXe siècles)* (Aix-en-Provence, 1986) and *La peste dans l'Empire ottoman, 1700–1850* (Leuven, 1985); and Jean-Noël Biraben, *Les hommes et la peste en France et dans les pays européens et méditerranéens*, 2 vols. (Paris, 1975–6).

   On the measures adopted by the Kingdom of the Two Sicilies, see Gino Leonardo Di Mitri, *Regolamenti di sanità marittima nel Regno delle Due Sicilie (1820 e 1853)* (Gallatina, 1992).
100 Useful descriptions of the measures taken to safeguard Languedoc from infection from neighbouring Provence are provided by Paul Gaffarel and Marquis de Duranty, *La Peste de 1720 à Marseille et en France* (Paris, 1911), pp. 553–586; and C. Carrière, M. Courdurie and F. Rebuffat, *Marseille ville morte: La Peste de 1720* (Marseilles, 1968), pp. 127–155.
101 The coercive experiment in Russia is well discussed by Roderick E. McGrew, *Russia and the Cholera, 1823–1832* (Madison, Wis. and Milwaukee, 1965).
102 R.J. Morris, *Cholera, 1832: The Social Response to an Epidemic* (London, 1976), p. 31.
103 'History of the Rise, Progress, Ravages, etc. of the Blue Cholera of India', *Lancet* (1831–2, vol. 1), pp. 241–284 and esp. 280–283.
104 Auguste Gerardin and Paul Gaimard, *Du choléra-morbus en Russie, en Prusse et en Autriche, pendant les années 1831 et 1832* (Paris, 1833, 3rd edn; 1st edn. 1832), pp. 6–7.
105 *Ibid.*, pp. 12–14.
106 'The Progress of Cholera', *Lancet* (1865, vol. 2), 189–190.
107 'The Progress of Cholera', *Lancet* (1883, vol. 2), p. 159. See also 'The Cholera', *Lancet* (1883, vol. 2), pp. 207–208.

108 The objections of the majority of European cholera authorities to the idea of sanitary cordons and land-based quarantines are discussed, for example, by M. Brouardel, 'Rapport de la Commission sur le choléra prise dans le sein du Comité consultatif sur les mesures de préservation du choléra', *Bulletin de l'Académie de Médecine*, 2nd series, 13:2 (1884), pp. 913–936. See also the many articles on quarantine published in the *Lancet*, such as 'The Cholera', *Lancet* (1883, vol. 2), pp. 207–208; and 'Epidemiological Society of London', *Lancet* (1886), vol. 2, pp. 1077–1078.

109 On the work of the International Sanitary Conference of 1874, see *Lancet* (1874, vol. 2), pp. 20–21, 104–105, 175–176. The history of quarantine in the nineteenth century is surveyed, with particular reference to Britain, by J.C. McDonald, 'The History of Quarantine in Britain during the 19th Century', *Bulletin of the History of Medicine*, 25 (1951), pp. 22–44.

110 E. De Renzi, 'Sul cholera di Napoli (1884)', *Rivista clinica e terapeutica*, 7 (1885), p. 70.

111 R. Zampa, 'Storia del colera del 1884 in Italia', *Gazzetta di medicina pubblica: organo ufficiale per gli atti del consiglio di sanità di Napoli*, 16 (1885), p. 177.

112 *Ibid.*, p. 171.

113 Zampa, 'Storia del colera', p. 191. Comparative statistics for the two epidemics are also provided by Morana, *Il colera in Italia*, pp. 72–74.

114 Morana, *Il colera in Italia*, pp. 75–76.

115 *Ibid.*, p. 88.

116 The most exhaustive accounts of the Italian sanitary system of 1884 are the discussion by Morana, *Il colera in Italia*; and Shakespeare, *Report on Cholera*.

117 Morana, *Il colera in Italia*, pp. 100–105.

118 'Un mois à Naples pendant l'épidémie cholérique de 1884', *Gazette Hebdomadaire des Sciences Médicales de Montpellier*, 7 (1885), p. 125.

119 'Guarding against Cholera', 25 July 1884, in United States Bureau of Foreign Commerce, *Cholera in Europe*, p. 63.

120 Morana, *Il colera in Italia*, pp. 6–10.

121 *Ibid.*, pp. 14–18.

122 *Gazzetta di medicina pubblica*, 16 (1885), p. 130.

123 For a description of the lazaretto at Pian di Latte, see Dr. Gimbert, 'Etudes des lazarets du Pian de Latte et de Nice pendant l'épidémie du choléra de 1884', *Nice médical*, 10 (1886), pp. 177–188.

124 Consul Frank G. Haughwout, 'Outbreak and Course of the Cholera in Naples', 22 September 1884, in United States Department of Foreign Commerce, *Cholera in Europe*, pp. 45–47.

125 Zampa, 'Storia del colera', pp. 113–114.

126 *Ibid.*, p. 114.

127 Francesco Pierotti, *Relazione del colera a Spezia* (Spezia, 1884), p. 3.

128 *Ibid.*, p. 19.

129 Zampa, 'Storia del colera', p. 117.

130 *Ibid.*, p. 138.

131 'Le Choléra', *Le Temps*, 19 August 1884.

132 Morana, *Il colera in Italia*, p. 20.

133 Direzione Generale della Statistica, *Annuario statistico italiano. Anno 1886* (Rome, 1887), Tav. XII bis, p. 145.

134 *Times*, 31 July 1884.

135 Morana, *Il colera in Italia*, p.27.

136 The following account of events at La Spezia is based primarily on the following: Pierotti, *Relazione*; F. Fiorani, 'Il colera di Spezia', *Giornale medico del R. esercito e della R. marina*, 23 (1885), pp. 230–242; and Stefano Oldoini, 'Storia delle epidemie di cholera avvenute nel Comune di Spezia durante gli anni 1884–85–86', *Annali universali di medicina e chirurgia*, 63 (1887), pp. 337–383.

137 F. Fiorani, 'Il colera di Spezia', p. 241. Statistics for the population and for the numbers of victims of cholera at La Spezia are provided by Morana, *Il colera in Italia*, pp. 72–74.

138 Pierotti, *Relazione*, p. 16.

139 Oldoini, 'Storia delle epidemia', p. 343.

140 For vivid accounts of the sufferings of La Spezia, see Pierotti, *Relazione*; and Zampa, 'Storia del colera', pp. 112–113, esp. pp. 188–190.

141 On the disorders of Calabria, see Morana, *Il colera in Italia*, pp. 22–31.

142 On the outbreak at Isernia, see Arnaldo Cantani and V.A. Margotta, 'Il Colera nel Circondario d'Isernia: Relazione della Commissione delegata dal Ministero a provvedere ai mezzi per arrestarne la diffusione', *Gazzetta di medicina pubblica*, 16 (1885), pp.39–45.

143 Report of 30 October 1884, *Atti del consiglio comunale di Napoli*, 1884, pp. 664–665. For another prominent advocate of the Isernia theory, see De Renzi, 'Sul colera di Napoli (1884)', p. 58.

144 'Cholera in New Fields', *New York Times*, 7 September 1884.

145 *Ibid.*

146 G. Somma, *Relazione sanitaria sui casi di colera avvenuti in sezione Porto durante la epidemia dell'anno 1884* (Naples, 1885), p. 3.

147 Morana, *Il colera in Italia*, pp. 67–69.

148 National Archives. Record Group 84: Records of Foreign Service Posts. Consular Posts: Naples, Italy. Despatch of B.D. Duncan to John Davis, Assistant Secretary of State, 30 June 1883, n. 36.

149 For details of the demonstration, see 'Dimostrazioni a Napoli', *Corriere della sera*, 11–12 July 1884.

150 Agostino Depretis, *Discorsi parlamentari* (Rome, 1892), vol. VIII p. 496.

151 'Il colera di Napoli: I lazzaretti ed i provvedimenti di preservazione delle isole', *Giornale medico del R. esercito e della R. marina*, 23 (1885), pp. 735–748.

152 *Ibid.*, p. 736.

153 See in particular Stefano Oldoini, 'Storia delle epidemie', pp. 337–383; and Pierotti, *Relazione*.

154 Pierotti, *Relazione*, p. 3.

155 'Cholera in the Province of Genoa', 30 August 1884, in United States Bureau of Foreign Commerce, *Cholera in Europe*, p. 36.

156 The account of Varignano above is based above all on Pierotti, *Relazione*.

157 Pierotti, *Relazione*, pp. 10–11.

158 For statistics on the numbers of deaths from cholera at La Spezia, see Stefano Oldoini, 'Storia delle epidemie', pp. 351–352.

159 Somma, *Relazione*, p. 3; Eugenio Fazio,' Il colera del 1884 in Napoli', *Giornale della Reale Società Italiana d'Igiene*, 7 (1885), p. 464.
160 Cimitero dei Colerosi, Naples. Registro: 17 August to 15 November 1884.
161 Archivio di Stato di Napoli, Prefettura, b. 3626, fasc. 'Notizie richieste dal Ministero circa i legni approdati al lazzaretto di Nisida nell'anno 1884.' Telegram of the Prefect of Naples to Ministero dell'Interno, 9 September 1885, n. 234.
162 Archivio di Stato di Napoli, Prefettura, b. 3626, fasc. 'Tariffa viveri al lazzaretto di Nisida.' Letter of Capitano Comandante il Distaccamento, 6o Reggimento Bersaglieri to Prefetto della Provincia di Napoli, 27 June 1884, n. 18286.
163 On the measures to isolate Nisida by land and see, see Archivio di Stato di Napoli, Prefettura, b. 3626, fasc. 'Cordone sanitario alla spiaggia di Coroglio'.
164 Archivio di Stato di Napoli, Prefettura, b. 3626, fasc.'Tariffa viveri al lazzaretto di Nisida'. Letter of Capitano Comandante il Distaccamento, 6o Reggimento Bersaglieri to Prefetto della Provincia di Napoli, 27 June, 1884, n. 18286.
165 Archivio di Stato di Napoli, Prefettura, b. 3626, fasc. 'Caputo Luigi: Chiede di essere nominato guardia avventizia al lazzaretto di Nisida'. Letter of Direttore del Lazzaretto di Nisida A. di Martino to Prefetto della Provincia di Napoli, 7 October 1885, n.27352.
166 On the administrative comparison of lazarettos with prisons rather than hospitals, see Di Mitri, *Regolamenti di sanità*, p. 29.
167 Archivio di Stato di Napoli, Prefettura, b. 3626, fasc. 'Tariffa viveri al lazzaretto di Nisida'. Letter of Capitano Comandante il Distaccamento, 6o Reggimento Bersaglieri to Prefetto della Provincia di Napoli, 27 June 1884, n. 18286.
168 Archivio di Stato di Napoli, Prefettura, b. 3626, fasc. 'Tariffa viveri al lazzaretto di Nisida.' Letter of Capitano Comandante il Distaccamento, 6o Reggimento Bersaglieri to Prefetto di Napoli, 27 June 1884, n. 18286.
169 'Il cholera a Napoli', *Osservatore romano*, 6 September 1884.
170 'Atti della Reale Società Italiana d'Igiene', 1 March 1885, *Giornale della Reale Società Italiana d'Igiene*, 7 (1885), p. 410.
171 See, for example, 'Cronaca', *Roma*, 6 and 7 August 1884.
172 *Ibid.*
173 The American report on the epidemic of 1884–7 also regarded the maritime route as the most likely source of the contamination of both La Spezia and Naples. Shakespeare, *Report on Cholera*, pp. 9–10.
174 *Ibid.*, p. 9.

CHAPTER 3: DEATH IN NAPLES

1 For the official municipal figures for the epidemic, see Municipio di Napoli, *Statistica Generale del Colera dalla mezzanotte del 17 agosto a quella del 4 novembre 1884* (Naples, 1884).
2 For a discussion of the Sunday celebrations, see 'The Cholera in Naples', *The Sanitarian*, 13 (1884), p. 503.
3 On the incident at the primary school and the subsequent lottery, see 'The Cholera', *Times*, 12 September 1884; and 'Cronaca', *Roma*, 27 August 1884.
4 'Cholera in New Fields', *New York Times*, 7 September 1884.
5 Robert Koch, 'Lecture at the First Conference for Discussion of the Cholera

Question (1884)', in *Essays of Robert Koch*, trans. K. Codell Carter (New York, Westport and London, 1987), p. 162. On the pernicious effect of alcohol, see also Cesare Lombroso, *Crime: Its Causes and Remedies*, trans. Henry P. Horton (Boston, 1911), p. 88.

6 For the text of the speech by De Bonis, see *Atti del consiglio comunale di Napoli*, 1884, pp. 522–527.

7 *Ibid.*, p. 526.

8 Speech of 8 November 1884, *Atti del consiglio comunale di Napoli*, 1884, p. 701.

9 On 30 October mayor Nicola Amore reported on the manner in which the executive committee had used its emergency powers. See *Atti del consiglio comunale di Napoli*, 1884, pp. 662–672. The following account of the health initiatives of the Amore administration is largely based on that report. See also Federico Sirignano, *Relazione igienico-sanataria circa l'epidemia colerica del 1884 nella sezione Pendino* (Naples, 1884).

10 Sirignano, *Relazione*, pp. 1–10.

11 National Archives. Record Group 84: Records of Foreign Service Posts. Consular Posts: Naples, Italy, volume 012. Report of Frank G. Haughwout, 'Outbreak and Course of the Cholera Epidemic in Naples', to Hon. William Hunter, Second Assistant Secretary of State, 23 September 1884, n. 43, pp. 202–203.

12 Vincenzo Muro, *Sulla epidemia cholerica napoletana del 1884: considerazioni etiologiche, cliniche e terapeutiche* (Naples, 1885), pp. 29–30.

13 Eugenio Fazio, *La epidemia colerica e le condizioni sanitarie di Napoli* (Naples, 1884), p. 7.

14 'Un mois à Naples pendant l'épidémie cholérique de 1884', *Gazette hebdomadaire des sciences médicales de Montpellier*, 7 (1885), p. 125.

15 On the advice for individual prophylaxis, see Arnaldo Cantani, *Istruzioni popolari concernenti il cholera asiatico* (Naples, 1884), esp. pp. 18–25. See also E. De Renzi, 'Sul colera di Napoli (1884)', *Rivista clinica e terapeutica*, 7 (1885), p. 69.

16 Cimitero della Pietà, Naples: Cholerosi, 17 August to 15 November 1884.

17 Eugenio Fazio, 'Il colera del 1884 in Napoli', *Giornale della Reale Società Italiana d'Igiene*, 7 (1885), p. 461.

18 Direzione Generale della Statistica, *Statistica delle cause di morte nei comuni capoluoghi di provincia o di circondario e delle morti violente avvenute in tutto il regno, anno 1884* (Rome, 1885), p. xxvii.

19 Direzione Generale della Statistica, *Statistica delle cause di morte nei comuni capoluoghi di provincia o di circondario e delle morti violente avvenute in tutto il regno, anno 1884* (Rome, 1885), Table F, p. xxviii.

20 Consul Frank G. Haughwout, 'Outbreak and Course of the cholera in Naples', 22 September 1884; and 'Progress of the Cholera in Naples', Naples, 2 October 1884, United States Bureau of Foreign Commerce, *Cholera in Europe in 1884. Reports from Consuls of the United States* (Washington, 1885), pp. 45 and 49. On the underreporting of cases, see also De Zerbi, *Colera del 1884: Croce Bianca e Croce Rossa* (Naples, 1884), p. 61.

It is revealing that in 1887, well after the end of the epidemic, Councillor Arlotta makes use of the figure of 9,000 victims from the epidemic. Speech of 22 May 1887, *Atti del consiglio comunale di Napoli*, 1887, p. 163.

21 'The Cholera', *Times*, 27 September 1884. For another newspaper report of the mendacity of official figures, see 'Cholera in New Fields', *New York Times*, 7 September 1884.
22 Municipio di Napoli, *Statistica Generale del Colera dalla mezzanotte del 17 agosto a quella del 4 novembre 1884* (Naples, 1884).
23 Frank G. Haughwout, 'Progress of the Cholera in Naples', Naples, October 2, 1884, United States Bureau of Foreign Commerce, *Cholera in Europe*, p. 49.
24 Eugenio Fazio, 'Il colera del 1884', p. 465.
25 'The Cholera in Naples', *The Sanitarian*, 13 (1884), pp. 502–505.
26 This point was stressed by Alexandrine Tkatcheff, 'Un mois à Naples pendant l'épidémie cholérique de 1884', *Gazzette hebdomadaire des sciences médicales de Montpellier*, 7 (1885), p. 69.
27 E. De Renzi, 'Sul colera di Napoli (1884)', p. 71.
28 Speech of 19 December 1884, in *Atti del parlamento italiano: Camera dei deputati, Sessione 1882–83–84 (1a della XV Legislatura), Discussioni*, X, pp. 10375.
29 'The Cholera', *Times*, 27 September 1884. Unfortunately, persistent efforts to locate letters, diaries and memoirs written by the cholera fugitives have proved fruitless.
30 Vincenzo Pagano, *Il cholera e la carità: cenno storico dell'epidemia di Napoli del 1884* (Naples, 1884), p. 55.
31 Fazio, *La epidemia colerica*, pp. 50–51.
32 G. Ciaramelli, *Sul cholera del 1884: relazione al sindaco di Napoli* (Naples, 1884), p.27.
33 Fazio, *La epidemia colerica*, p. 11.
34 Frank G. Haughwout, 'Outbreak and Course of the Cholera in Naples', 22 September 1884, in United States Bureau of Foreign Commerce, *Cholera in Europe*, pp. 43–44.
35 Rocco De Zerbi, 'Relazione della commissione sul disegno di legge presentato dal presidente del consiglio ministro dell'interno (Depretis): Disposizione per provvedere alla pubblica igiene della città di Napoli', seduta del 15 dicembre 1884; in Camera dei deputati, Legislatura XV-Sessione 1882–86, *Raccolta degli atti stampati per ordine della Camera*, XXII, n.261–A, pp. 2–3.
36 Pagano, *Il cholera e la carità*, p. 8.
37 'Il Cholera', *Osservatore romano*, 28 September 1884.
38 'Plague scenes in Naples', *New York Times*, 14 September 1884.
39 'Cronaca', *Roma*, 8 September 1884.
40 'Plague scenes in Naples', *New York Times*, 14 September 1884.
41 'The Cholera', *Times*, 12 September 1884. Another account of these events is 'The Cholera in Naples', *New York Times*, 10 Sept. 1884.
42 'Il Cholera a Napoli', *Osservatore romano*, 16 September 1884.
43 For a discussion of the religious processions and their exploitation by criminal elements in the city, see Pagano, *Il cholera e la carità*, p. 16. See also, 'Il Colera a Napoli', *Corriere della sera*, 13–14 Sept. 1884.
44 A description of the scenes that took place outside the municipal premises is provided by Pagano, *Il cholera e la carità*, p. 15.
45 *Ibid.*, p. 121.

46 Eugenio Fazio, 'Il colera del 1884 in Napoli', *Giornale della Reale Società Italiana d'Igiene*, 7 (1885), pp. 466–467. Contemporary accounts often record the 'cure' rate. Since, with retrospective wisdom, it is apparent that no 'cure' was available in 1884, I have substituted the more neutral term 'discharge' rate.

47 'Il cholera a Napoli', *Osservatore romano*, 11 October 1884.

48 'The Cholera in Naples', *New York Times*, 10 Sept. 1884.

49 For a description of the disorganization prevailing at the Conocchia Hospital in the early days of the epidemic, see Alexandrine Tkatcheff, 'Un mois à Naples', p. 56.

50 See in particular *The Magic Mountain*, trans. H. T. Lowe-Porter, 2 vols. (London, 1927). For an interesting discussion of attitudes to tuberculosis, see Susan Sontag, *Illness as Metaphor* (London, 1977). The discussion here owes much also to René and Jean Dubos, *The White Plague: Tuberculosis, Man and Society* (London, 1953) and to Claude Quetel, *The History of Syphilis* (Baltimore, 1990). On plague literature, see David Steel, 'Plague Writing: From Boccaccio to Camus', *Journal of European Studies*, 11 (1981), pp. 88–110.

51 Thomas Mann, *Death in Venice*, trans. H. T. Lowe-Porter (London, 1928).

52 Giovanni Verga, *Mastro-Don Gesualdo* (Milan, 1979).

53 'Proposal for Improving the Treatment of Cholera by the Aid of a Travelling Commission', *Lancet* (1831–2, vol. 2), pp. 731–732.

54 A classic account of the disease is by the French physiologist F. Magendie, *Lezioni sul cholera-morbus* (Milan, 1832). Other useful accounts are Nathaniel F. Pierce and Arabino Mondal, 'Clinical Features of Cholera', in Dhiman Barua and William Burrows (eds.), *Cholera* (Philadelphia, 1974), pp. 209–220; A. J. Wall, *Asiatic Cholera: Its History, Pathology, and Modern Treatment* (London, 1893), pp. 30–63; R. Pollitzer, *Cholera* (Geneva, 1959), pp. 683–735; Giuseppe Spada, *Memoria statistica e clinica degl'infermi di cholera-morbus trattati nell'ospedale di S.a M.a di Loreto nell'estate di 1854* (Naples, 1854), pp. 22–26; and Leonard Rogers, *Cholera and Its Treatment* (London, 1911), pp. 89–137.

Since each pandemic has distinctive qualities of its own, it is important to consult specific discussions of the pathology of the Neapolitan outbreak in 1884. A well-informed report for the *sezione* Pendino is Sirignano, *Relazione*, esp. pp. 10–30.

55 James Alderson, 'Lectures on Clinical Medicine', *Lancet* (1867, vol. 1), p. 35.

56 'History of the Progress of the Malignant Cholera in England and Scotland', *Lancet* (1831–2, vol. 1), pp. 669–684.

57 On the occurrence of 'dry cholera' in Naples in 1884, see G. Somma, *Relazione sanitaria sui casi di colera avvenuti in sezione Porto durante la epidemia dell'anno 1884* (Naples, 1885), p. 9.

58 The full range of cholera cases was discovered by Robert Koch as a result of bacteriological examinations performed during the after-epidemic at Hamburg in 1893. Cf. Robert Koch, *Professor Koch on the Bacteriological Diagnosis of Cholera, Water-Filtration and Cholera, and the Cholera in Germany during the Winter of 1892–93*, trans. George Duncan (Edinburgh, 1894), pp. 77–79.

59 Wall, *Asiatic Cholera*, p. 39.

60 *Ibid.*, p. 41.

61 *Ibid.*, pp. 42–43.

62 For a discussion of the reaction stage, see Rogers, *Cholera and Its Treatment*, pp. 100–103.

63 Roderick E. McGrew, *Russia and the Cholera, 1823–1832* (Madison and Milwauke, 1965); quoted in Richard J. Evans, *Death in Hamburg: Society and Politics in the Cholera Years, 1830–1910* (Oxford, 1987), p. 448.

64 Patrice Bourdelais and Jean-Yves Raulot, *Une peur bleue: Histoire du choléra en France, 1832–1854* (Paris, 1987), pp. 114–115.

65 E. De Renzi, 'Sul colera di Napoli (1884)', p. 64.

66 Evans, *Death in Hamburg*, esp. pp. 445–450.

67 Ibid., p. 449.

68 Direzione Generale della Statistica, *Statistica delle cause di morte nei comuni capoluoghi di provincia o circondario e delle morti violente avvenute in tutto il regno, anno 1884* (Rome, 1885), Table H, p. xxxi.

69 Evans, *Death in Hamburg*, pp. 199–200.

70 Ann-Mari Svennerholm, Gunhild Jonson, and Jan Holmgren, 'Immunity to *vibrio cholerae* Infection', in I. Kaye Wachsmuth, Paul A. Blake, and Ørjan Olsvik, eds., *Vibrio cholerae and Cholera: Molecular to Global Perspectives* (Washington, D.C., 1994), pp. 267–268; and Michael L. Bennish, 'Cholera: Pathophysiology, Clinical Features, and Treatment', *Ibid.*, p. 248.

71 Roger I. Glass, Ann-Mari Svennerholm, Barbara J. Stoll, M.R. Khan, K.M. Belayet Hossain, M. Imdadul Huq, and Jan Holmgren, 'Protection against Cholera in Breast-fed Children by Antibodies in Breast Milk', *New England Journal of Medicine*, 308 (1983), p. 1389.

72 Shousun C. Szu, Rajesh Gupta, and John B. Robbins, 'Induction of Serum Vibriocidal Antibodies by O-Specific Polysaccharide-Protein Conjugate Vaccines for Prevention of Cholera', in Wachsmuth, Blake, and Olsvik, *Vibrio cholerae*, p. 383.

73 'Westminster Medical Society', *Lancet* (1849, vol. 2), p. 459.

74 For discussion of the terror spread by post-mortem muscular convulsions in cholera, see 'National Westminster Medical Society', *Lancet* (1849, vol. 2), pp. 459–460; 'Medical Societies: Royal Medical and Chirurgical Society', *Lancet* (1850, vol. 1), p. 156; and Wall, *Asiatic Cholera*, p. 54.

75 Arnaldo Cantani, *La cura del cholera mediante l'ipodermoclisi e l'enteroclisi* (Naples, 1884), p. 14.

76 The precautions taken at the Cholera Cemetery are described in the article 'Il Cimitero dei colerosi a Napoli', *Corriere della sera*, 14–15 Sept. 1884.

77 See, for example, Torquato Oliveti, *Della morte apparente nei cholerosi, del modo di farli risorgere e della sola cura giovevole nel cholera asiatico* (Naples, 1886); and Francesco Oliveti, *Brevi cenni sul colera asiatico e nuovo mezzo curativo* (Naples, 1884), esp. p. 16.

78 'Il cholera a Napoli', *Osservatore romano*, 26 September 1884.

79 An excellent overview of the evolution of therapeutics in the nineteenth century is John Harley Warner, *The Therapeutic Perspective: Medical Practice, Knowledge, and Identity in America, 1820–1885* (Cambridge, Mass., 1986). Warner's subject is the American experience, but since medicine was the most cosmopolitan of professions and since American physicians closely followed European medical fashions, the main lines of development were similar.

There is, unfortunately, no work of similar quality devoted to therapeutics in Europe or, more particularly, Italy. With regard to the treatment of cholera, a first attempt was made by Norman Howard-Jones, 'Cholera Therapy in the Nineteenth Century', *Journal of the History of Medicine*, 17 (1972), pp. 373–395. The discussion of cholera therapy here is based above all on a reading of all of the articles on cholera in *The Lancet* between 1829 and 1911.

80 The theory of cholera as a poisoning of the nervous system persisted throughout the century. An early formulation was that of George Hamilton Bell, who was regarded by the *Lancet* as having provided the most plausible account of the disease. He explained the etiology of cholera on the basis of three principles:

1. The great ganglionic or sympathetic system of nerves, is possessed of a power wholly unconnected with cerebral influence, which it may retain after the brain and spinal marrow are removed, and which may exist while these retain the full exercise of their functions.

2. To this system belong the circulation and distribution of blood; and it consequently has a most important share in regulating secretion, and in carrying on the involuntary functions. And,

3. To the suspension of this power of the system, is to be ascribed the disease which has obtained the name of Cholera Asphyxia.

    Quoted in 'History of the Rise, Progress, Ravages, &c. of the Blue Cholera of India', *Lancet* (1831–32, vo. 1), p. 257.

81 This view was explained by the physician Edward Smith in his paper 'On the Primary or Essential Seat of Cholera' delivered to the Royal Medical and Chirurgical Society in 1855. Cf. 'Medical Societies', *Lancet* (1855, vol. 1), pp. 262–263.

    For an illustration of the persistence in the 1860s of the interpretation of the symptoms of cholera as caused by a general paralysis of the sympathetic or ganglionic nervous system, see Review of William Sedgwick, *On the Nature of Cholera as a Guide to Treatment*, in *Lancet* (1866, vol. 2), pp. 548–549.

82 For Dr. Johnsons's representative analysis of cholera as an intoxication of the nervous system, see 'Westminster Medical Society: The Cholera. Its Nature and Treatment', *Lancet*, 1831–2, i, pp. 340–342.

83 J.L. Gray, 'Observations on the Treatment of Tropical Diseases', *Lancet* (1869, vol. 1), p. 600.

84 For an example of a physician who advocated opening the jugular vein, see the comments of Dr Whiting to the Westminster Medical Society. 'Westminster Medical Society: The Cholera. Its Nature and Treatment', *Lancet* (1831–32, vol. 1), p. 346.

85 Quoted in 'History of the Rise, Progress, Ravages, etc. of the Blue Cholera of India', *Lancet* (1831–32, vol. 1) , p. 276.

86 On the use of ipecacuanha in Naples, see M. Thibault, 'Cholera Morbus of Naples', *Lancet* (1837–38, vol. 1), pp. 167–168,

87 'It appears', wrote William Henry of Hull in support of a depletive course of sulphate of zinc, 'that the spontaneous vomiting of incipient cholera does not disgorge that which is needful to be thrown off, and that an irritant calls into action such auxiliary powers, exceeding in effect all that can be possibly induced spontaneously, howsoever protracted the efforts.' 'The Treatment of Cholera by Calomel', *Lancet* (1849, vol. 2), pp. 409–410.

88 'Analyses of Communications Relating to the Pathology, Causes, and Treatment of Cholera', *Lancet* (1849, vol. 2), pp. 149–150.

89 For a description and illustration of such a device, cf. Joseph Rogers, 'A Convenient Form of Hot-Air Bath for an Invalid in Bed', *Lancet* (1867, vol. 2), pp. 624–625; and esp. 'Description of a Portable Hot-air and Vapour Bath', *Lancet* (1868, vol. 2), pp. 309–310.

90 Francis Anstie, 'On the Popular Idea of Counter-Irritation', *Lancet* (1869, vol. 1), pp. 290–291.

91 Sir William Gull, 'Address on Clinical Medicine. Delivered before the Clinical Society', *Lancet* (1872, vol. 1), pp. 139–140.

92 On the symbolic importance of venesection, see Warner, *The Therapeutic Perspective*, pp. 208–211.

93 'Statistical Results of the Treatment of Cholera and Diarrhoea', *Lancet* (1855, vol. 1), p. 438. For an additional report condemning the eliminative system, see 'The Results of Different Methods of Treating Cholera', *Lancet* (1855, vol. 1), p. 412.

94 See, for example, J.T. Gray, 'Observations on the Treatment of Tropical Diseases', *Lancet* (1869, vol. 1), pp. 599–600. A representative response to the use of emetics as part of a depletive strategy was the reaction of T.M. Greenhow, who wrote ('On the Treatment of Cholera', *Lancet* (1849, vol. 2), p. 91), that emetics were,

> at one time considered so essential and important. But we cannot commend their use, except in cases where the stomach is supposed to retain undigested food in considerable quantity. The intention with which they have been prescribe, of rousing the system, and re-exciting the action of the heart and arteries, is, we feel assured, fallacious. The circulation is depressed because the vessels are half emptied of their proper contents; and what remains is too viscid to be propelled by the muscular energy of the heart and arteries. It is not the stimulus of emetics by which this state of things can be corrected; and the exertion attendant on this operation can only increase the degree of general exhaustion.

95 'The Use of Purgatives', *Lancet* (1870, vol. 2), pp. 474–476. In a telling editorial against the therapeutics of depletion, *The Lancet* argued that elimination was,

> an integral part of a system of biology and pathology that was as purely imaginary as an Arabian Night's tale. Disease was supposed to be a definite something which invaded the organism from without, or else was concocted from some 'humour' natural to the organism, but accidentally present in morbid excess. In either case it was a positive and objective existence, which ought to be, and which could be, *eliminated*, or expelled from the body; a work which was always attempted by the *vis medicatrix naturae*, a mysterious power residing within the body, and constantly inspired by an almost personal animosity towards the hostile entities known as diseases. Unfortunately it appeared that the *vis medicatrix* was very often unequal to the completion of the task, and it was therefore the duty of the physician to assist by the employment of various *evacuant* remedies. The *vis medicatrix* was supposed to cast out the enemy in a haemorrhage, a sweat, a diarrhoea, or a diuresis, and so the physician was encouraged to imitate these processes in the full faith that he, too, might chase the lurking evil out of the body by such means. It was like a

rat-hunt in a barn with the barn-doors all left open. 'Therapeutic Traditions', *Lancet* (1872, vol. 1), pp. 49–50.

96 One of the most influential advocates of calomel in the treatment of cholera was Joseph Ayre. Early accounts of his therapeutic approach are his articles 'Efficiency of Calomel in the Treatment of Malignant Cholera', *Lancet*, (1831–2, vol. 2), pp. 271–274; and 'On the Remedial Powers of Calomel in Small and Frequent Doses in the Treatment of Malignant Cholera', *Lancet* (1833–4, vol. 2), pp. 889–892.

Undeterred by repeated failures at the bedside, Ayre was just as enthusiastic about mercury in the second pandemic as he had been in the first. See Joseph Ayre, 'Treatment of Cholera by Small and Repeated Doses of Calomel', *Lancet* (1849, vol. 2)i, pp. 327–328; 'On the Successful Treatment of Asiatic Cholera by Small and Frequently Repeated Doses of Calomel', *ibid.*, pp. 145–147; and 'The Cholera', *Lancet* (1854, vol. 1), pp. 536–538, 563–566, and 591–593.

97 C. Morehead, 'Notes on the Prevention and Treatment of Cholera', *Lancet* (1866, vol. 1), p. 62.

98 For a cautionary article on the employment of prussic acid in cholera therapy, see Richard Laming, 'On Medicinal Prussic or Hydrocyanic Acid', *Lancet* (1832–3, vol. 2), pp. 623–624.

99 For the use of phosphorus, see W. Batten, 'Malignant Cholera. Treatment of Its Advanced Stages with Phosphurs. – Preparation of a Phosphorus Pill', *Lancet* (1832–3, vol. 2), pp. 694–696.

100 'The Cholera', *Lancet* (1867, vol. 2), p. 114. In 1848 the *Lancet* enumerated fifty specifics commonly deployed as remedies for Asiatic cholera. Cf. Joshua Waddington, 'Remarks on the State of Pathological Science Illustrated by an Enumeration of Cholera Specifics!', *Lancet* (1848, vol. 2), p. 703.

Even sugar had its advocates as a sovereign remedy for the disease. Cf. J. Innis Mackintosh, 'Treatment of Cholera with Sugar', *Lancet* (1854, vol. 1), pp. 384–385.

101 S. Dickson, 'Memoranda on the Epidemic Cholera of India', *Lancet* (1829–30, vol. 2), pp. 238–239. Counter-irritation continued as a strategy of physicians in the course of the second pandemic. Cf. 'Analyses of Communications Relating to the Pathology, Causes, and Treatment of Cholera', *Lancet* (1849, voll 2), pp. 149–15; Francis E. Antsie, 'On the Popular Idea of Counter-irritation', *Lancet* (1869, vol. 1), pp. 290–291; and John G. French, 'On the Philosophy of Counter-irritation as Applied in Practice', *Lancet* (1869, vol. 1), pp. 359–360.

With regard to arsenic in particular, the case was made that its curative powers were based on its ability to produce the 'reflected portrait' of the pathology of cholera. Cf. William Hitchman, 'Arsenic in Cholera', *Lancet* (1857, vol. 2), p. 534.

102 For an instance of the antiphlogistic approach, see *Lancet* (1831–2, vol. 1), p. 277. Creosote also persisted as the sedative of choice for many physicians. Cf. Review of E.A. Parkes, *Researches into the Pathology and Treatment of the Asiatic or Algid Cholera* (London, 1847), in *Lancet* (1848, vol. 1), pp. 13–14.

103 On the methods of François Broussais, see Bourdelais and Raulot, *Une peur bleue*, pp. 127–140.

104 George W. Balfour, 'On the Treatment of Cholera by Strychnine', *Lancet* (1867, vol. 1), pp. 8–9.

105 For a brief overview of the early attempts at rehydration during the first pandemic, see McGrew, *Russia and the Cholera*, pp. 143–152.

106 Charles Clark, 'On Cholera, Its Nature and Treatment', *Lancet* (1846, vol. 1), p. 652.

107 See for example 'Physiological Society of London', *Lancet* (1855, vol. 1), p. 611.

108 For a discussion of the experiments in Britain by Latta and O'Shaughnessy with saline solutions, and of the transfusion of human and animal blood by François Magendie and others on the Continent, see 'The Cases of Cholera Successfully Treated by Large Aqueous Injections', *Lancet* (1831–2, vol. 2), pp. 184–286.

For an account of Professor Dieffenbach's experiments with blood transfusion during the first pandemic at Berlin, see 'The Transfusion of Blood in Malignant Cholera', *Lancet* (1832–3, vol. 1), pp. 202–203. On transfusion in London during the second pandemic, see C.H.F. Routh, 'Report of a Case of Cholera Treated by Transfusion', *Lancet* (1849, vol. 2), pp. 71–73.

109 'The Cases of Cholera Successfully Treated by Large Aqueous Injections', *Lancet* (1831–2, vol. 2) p. 284.

110 For a letter by Thomas Latta describing his briefly encouraging therapeutic results and then their ultimate failure, see Letter of Thomas Latta, 23 May 1832, *Lancet* (1831–2, vol. 2), pp. 274–276. For a further account of the fleetingly beneficial effects of saline injections, see W.C. Anderson, 'Effects of Saline Venous Injection in Cholera', *Lancet* (1832–3, vol. 2), p. 111.

For the much later period of the 1860s, see Hermann Beigel, 'Treatment of Cholera by Hypodermic Injections of Warm Water', *Lancet* (1866,vol. 2), pp. 352–353.

111 For discussions of galvanism as a means to combat the want of energy in the nervous system in cholera, see Charles F. Favell, 'On the Employment of Galvanism in Cases of Malignant Cholera', *Lancet* (1832–3, vol. 1), pp. 710–713; and 'Galvanism in Cholera', *Lancet* (1859, vol. 2), p. 571.

112 On the inhalation of chloroform, see James Hill, 'Treatment of the Cholera by Chloroform &c. in Peckham House (Poor) Asylum', *Lancet* (1848, vol. 2), p. 514.

113 Deputy Inspector-General Maclean, 'Lecture on the Treatment of Cholera', *Lancet* (1866, vol. 2), p. 114; and (1866, vol. 2), pp. 165–166.

114 John Gason, 'Cholera: Its Nature and Treatment', *Lancet* (1865, vol. 2), pp. 697–698.

115 See 'Analysis of Pamphlets on Cholera', *Lancet* (1849, vol. 2), pp. 16–17, where the technique for restoring animation to the patient was described as follows:

> The manner of applying it in the hospital of Berlin was as follows: – As soon as the patient was stripped of his clothes he was placed in the wooden bath before mentioned; one assistant-nurse supported him in an upright sitting position, whilst another assistant dished a bucket of cold water on his head and back; he then took another bucket of cold water, and poured it equally quick on his face, thorax and abdomen. The patient was then partially wiped dry, and lifted into bed, when sometimes he was wiped drier, and hot jars applied to his feet. As soon as this was done, a large sheet, saturated in cold

water, and folded up, was placed on his abdomen as a cold fomentation; another similar piece of wet linen was placed on his head. This process was repeated three times in the twenty-four hours.

116 T.G. Tebay, 'Remarks on Cholera Treatment and the Eliminative Theory', *Lancet* (1866, vol. 2), pp. 203–204.
117 T. Senise, 'Terapia del colera', *Rivista clinica e terapeutica*, 7 (1985), esp. pp. 475–476.
118 *The Therapeutic Perspective*, pp. 235ff.
119 *Lancet* (1833–4, vol. 1), p. 110.
120 See Koch, *Professor Koch*, pp. 1–23 for a detailed description of the technical improvements in cultivation that were made before a fully reliable test for the vibrio cholerae was available.
121 'Koch's Theory Assailed', *New York Times*, 5 October 1884.
122 Emanuel E. Klein, *The Bacteria in Asiatic Cholera* (London and New York, 1889).
123 See Koch, *Professor Koch*, pp. 64–150.
124 G. Manfredonia, *Sul cholera morbus infierito in Napoli nel 1884: osservazioni patologiche cliniche* (Naples, 1885), p. 16.
125 A clear statement of the physiological position is Mariano Semmola, 'New Therapeutic Researches upon the Asiatic Cholera', in United States Bureau of Foreign Commerce, *Cholera in Europe*, pp. 52–55.
126 *Ibid.*, p. 53.
127 See Manfredonia, *Sul cholera morbus*; and Giuseppe Amalfi, *Gli oppiacei nel colera ed un'ipotesi (epidemia di Napoli del 1884)* (Naples, 1885).
128 *Ibid.*, p. 53.
129 Ciaramelli, *Sul cholera del 1884*, pp. 7–10, 14–18.
130 Cantani's classic discussion of his procedure is *La cura del colera*. For a briefer expression of the main lines of his therapeutic thought, see also Arnaldo Cantani, *Il colera* (Naples, 1884).
    The attempt to attack the cholera bacillus directly by irrigating the small intestine with disinfectants was attempted as late as the outbreak in Hamburg in 1892. Cf. Evans, *Death in Hamburg*, pp. 336–338. A weak point in this important work, however, is the discussion of therapeutics. His brief outline of enteroclysis is presented confusingly as a return to the therapeutics of purging.
131 For a description of the procedure employed for hypodermoclysis, see Luigi Stefanoni, 'Come si curano i colerosi a Napoli', *Corriere della sera*, 18–19 September 1884.
132 Cantani, *La cura del colera*, p. 27.
    The attempt to treat cholera by acid was not, however, entirely new. Between 1849 and 1853 a previous 'acid treatment' had undergone widespread trials in the Habsburg Empire, and had been recommended by some English physicians as well. In the earlier version, however, the acid had been drunk instead of being administered in the form of an enema; and no link had been made with the idea of destroying the still unknown cholera bacillus. W. Reeves, 'The Treatment of Cholera by Acids', *Lancet* (1853, vol. 2), p. 354.
133 'Tannic Acid Injections in Cholera', *Lancet* (1885, vol. 1), pp. 352–353. By the 1890s Cantani himself abandoned carbolic acid in favour of tannic, and regarded

the former as lethally corrosive. Cf. 'Professor Cantani on the Treatment of Cholera', *Lancet* (1892, vol. 2), pp. 681–682.

134 For a description of Cantani's methods, see also 'Treatment of Cholera by Hypodermoclysis and Enteroclysis', *Lancet* (1885, vol. 2), p. 637.

135 Cantani, *La cura del colera*, pp. 24–25.

136 *Ibid.*, pp. 25–26.

137 Semmola, 'New Therapeutic Researches', p. 52.

138 Gaetano Rummo, 'Sulla cura del colera', *La Medicina contemporanea*, 1 (1884), pp. 473–476 and 543–548.

139 A. Cantani and F. De Simone, 'L'acido tannico contro l'avvelenamento ptomain-ico del cholera', *Giornale internazionale delle scienze mediche*, 10 (1888), pp. 257–259.

140 'Cronaca', *Roma*, 3 and 5 September 1884.

141 Orazio Caro, *L'evoluzione igienica di Napoli (Cenni storici – osservazioni e pro-poste – dati statistici)* (Naples, 1914), p. 169.

142 *Ibid.*, p. 169.

143 Alfonso Montefusco, *Clinica e terapia delle malattie acute* (Naples, 1912), p. 36.

144 *Ibid.*, p. 49.

145 For another negative assessment of hypodermoclysis and enteroclysis by a municipal doctor who employed them, see Somma, *Relazione*, pp. 15–21.

146 The electric bath was discussed in mid-September at the Naples Academy of Medicine. See 'Adunanza ordinaria del 14 settembre 1884', *Resoconto delle adunanze e dei lavori della R. Accademia Medico-chirurgica di Napoli*, 38:1 (January–March 1884), pp. 259–260.

147 Pietro Smurra, 'L'enteroclisi e l'ipodermoclisi nella cura del colera', *Gazzetta di Medicina pubblica*, 16 (1885), pp. 65–83.

148 *The Great Fear: Rural Panic in Revolutionary France* (Paris, 1932, trans. 1982).

149 Fazio, *La epidemia colerica*, pp. 51–52.

150 Professor E. Albanesi, a leading figure in the anti-cholera campaign in Palermo, closely observed the fear of poisoning. Attempting to explain the phenomenon, he wrote:

> For such a belief in poisoning one can find a plausible pretext in the very febrile activity into which the proverbial municipal indolence converts itself. It is a fact that municipalities which had never paid much attention to their administration suddenly rushed into all sorts of regulations, and immedi-ately ordered abundant disinfections as soon as they saw a great calamity approaching. In order to protect public health they often exceeded the limits of assiduity; and the people, who are generally neglected and frequently ill-treated, suddenly perceiving that they were the subject of most assiduous care, observing that their misfortune increased with the multiplication of public services, and terrified by the general calamity, were unable to discriminate between good and evil, suspected something must be wrong, refused assist-ance, shut themselves up, barricaded the doors of their houses, and when one offered them any aid, replied, 'Let me die in peace.' Quoted in Edward O. Shakespeare, *Report on Cholera in Europe and India* (Washington, 1890), p. 137.

151 'Un mois à Naples pendant l'épidémie cholérique de 1884', *Gazette hebdomadaire des sciences médicales de Montpellier*, 7 (1885).
152 'Il Cholera a Napoli', *Osservatore romano*, 13 September 1884.
153 'Da Napoli', *Osservatore romano*, 30 August 1884.
154 'Cronaca', *Roma*, 27 August 1884.
155 Direzione Generale della Statistica, *Annuario statistico italiano. Anno 1886.* (Rome, 1887), p. LVI.
156 *Ibid.*, table IV, pp. 116–123.
157 *Ibid.*, p. LVI.
158 Direzione Generale della Statistica, *Statistica delle cause di morte nei comuni capoluoghi di provincia e di circondario e delle morti violente avvenute in tutto il Regno, anno 1884* (Rome, 1885), pp. xv–xvi.
159 Direzione Generale della Statistica, *Annuario statistico italiano. Anno 1886.* (Rome, 1887), p. 159.
160 *Ibid.*
161 Direzione Generale della Statistica, *Statistica delle cause di morte nei comuni capoluoghi di provincia o di circondario e delle morti violente avvenute in tutto il regno, anno 1884* (Rome, 1885), Table L, pp. xlii –xlv.
162 *Ibid.*, Table V, pp. 58–59.
163 Direzione Generale della Statistica, *Statistica delle cause di morte nei comuni capoluoghi di provincia o di circondario e delle morti violente avvenute in tutto il regno, anno 1884* (Rome, 1885), Table M, pp. xlvi –xlvii.
164 'Plague Scenes in Naples', *New York Times*, 14 September 1884.
165 Somma, *Relazione*, p.4.
166 For press reports of the fruit demonstrations, see 'The Cholera', *Times*, 12 September 1884; and 'Il cholera a Napoli', *Osservatore romano*, 10 September 1884.
167 'A l'Etranger', *Le Petit Var*, 19 September 1884; and 'A Naples', *Le Petit Var*, 28 September 1884.
168 On the observation of traditional fetes during the epidemic of 1884, and their effects on the course of the disease, see Shakespeare, *Report on Cholera*, p. 123.
169 Fazio, 'Il colera del 1884', pp. 461–452.
170 'A Napoli', *Corriere della sera*, 6–7 September 1884.
171 See for example 'Il Cholera', *Corriere della sera*, 2–3 September 1884; and 'Il Cholera', *Il Piccolo*, 1 September 1884.
172 An example is Fazio, *La epidemia colerica*, p. 51. The Deputy Rocco De Zerbi used such terms in a speech. See 'La riunione della Croce Bianca a Napoli', *Corriere della sera*, 6–7 October 1884.
173 'Da Napoli', *Osservatore romano*, 30 August 1884.
174 The events in the Borgo Loreto are described by the articles 'Brutte scene a Napoli', *Corriere della sera*, 30–1 August 1884; and 'Cronaca', *Roma*, 27 August 1884.
175 'Cronaca', *Roma*, 26 August 1884.
176 'Il Cholera', *Corriere della sera*, 28–29 August 1884. See also 'Cronaca', *Roma*, 26 August 1884.
177 Archivio di Stato di Napoli, Prefettura di Napoli, b. 3540, fasc. Giannattasio

Luigi, Lancellotti Ernesto, Ferraro Guglielmo – Arrestati per disordine nell-'ospedale della Conocchia. Letter of Direzione delle Carceri Giudiziarie to Sig. Prefetto della Provincia di Napoli, 27 August 1884; and Letter of il Procuratore del Re Reggente la Questura to Ill.mo Signor prefetto della Provincia di Napoli, 27 August 1884, n. 45045.

178 For a description of the Chiaia riot, see 'A Napoli', *Corriere della sera*, 9–10 September 1884; and 'The Cholera', *Times*, 10 September 1884.

179 'Il Cholera a Napoli', *Corriere della sera*, 14–15 September 1884.

180 'Cronaca', *Roma*, 12 January 1885.

181 On the new penal regime in Naples, see Archivio di Stato di Napoli, Prefettura, b. 3540. Letter of Direttore Generale, Direzione Generale delle Carceri, Ministero dell'Interno to Sigori Prefetti del Regno, 4 September 1884, n. 25479; and Letter of Direttore della Casa di Pena S. M. Apparente, to Ill.mo Sig. Prefetto della Provincia, 2 Sept. 1884, n. 25116.

182 Archivio di Stato di Napoli, Prefettura, b. 3556. Letter of Direttore Generale, Direzione Generale delle Carceri, Ministero dell'Interno, 2 December 1884, n. 33686.

183 The events at the prisons are described by 'Il Cholera a Napoli', *Corriere della sera*, 11–12 September 1884; 'Napoli', *Osservatore romano*, 12 September 1884; and 'Il Cholera a Napoli', *Osservatore romano*, 13 September 1884.

184 'Southern Italy', *Times*, 4 September 1884.

185 On the poisoning hysteria during the bubonic plague, see Jean-Noël Biraben, *Les hommes et la peste en France et dans les pays européens et méditerranéens*, 2 vols. (Paris, 1975–6), esp. vol. I, pp. 57–67; vol.II, pp. 22–23; and, for Italy in particular, Paolo Preto, *Epidemia, paura e politica nell'Italia moderna* (Bari, 1987), pp. 5–117. See also Philip Ziegler, *The Black Death* (London, 1969), esp. ch. 5, pp. 84–109.

186 On the Milan epidemic of 1630 and the *colonna infame*, see Preto, *Epidemia, paura e politica*, pp. 35–76, and 104–117. Manzoni's work on the witchhunt is *Storia della colonna infame* (Naples, Genoa, Città di Castello, 1928; 1st edn 1842).

187 Manzoni, *Storia della colonna infame*, p. 48.

188 'The Indian Cholera', *Lancet* (1830–1, vol. 2), p. 422.

189 McGrew, *Russia and the Cholera*, pp. 106–107.

Summarizing the frenzied social reaction that accompanied the first pandemic, Richard Evans has recently written that, 'The progress of the disease across Europe in the early 1830s was marked by a string of riots and disturbances in almost every country it affected. Popular opinion did not accept that cholera was a hitherto unknown disease, but considered instead that an attempt was being made to reduce the numbers of the poor by poisoning them. Riots, massacres and the destruction of property took place across Russia, swept through the Habsburg empire, broke out in Königsberg, Stettin and Memel in 1831 and spread to Britain the next year, affecting cities as far apart as Exeter and Glasgow, London, Manchester and Liverpool.' (Richard J. Evans, 'Epidemics and Revolutions: Cholera in Nineteenth-century Europe', *Past and Present*, no. 120 (August 1988), pp. 131–132).

190 In 1887 Albanesi published an article, 'Cholera, and the Duties of Governments

and Countries during Epidemics', which was published in English translation by the American government in Shakespeare, *Report on Cholera*, pp. 128–141.

191 *Ibid.*, p. 137n.

192 Michael Durey, *The Return of the Plague: British Society and the Cholera, 1831–2* (London, 1979); Norman Longmate, *King Cholera: The Biography of a Disease* (London, 1966); and R.J. Morris, *Cholera 1832: The Social Response to an Epidemic* London, 1976).

193 Durey, *Return of the Plague*, p. 157.

194 Louis Chevalier, *Le choléra: la première épidémie du XIXe siècle* (La Roche-sur-Yon, 1958), p. xv.

195 'The Cholera in Paris', *Lancet* (1831 –2, vol. 2), p. 62.

196 *Ibid.*, pp. 21–24. See also René Baehrel, 'Epidémie et terreur. Histoire de sociologie', *Archives Historiques de la Révolution Française*, 23 (1951), esp. pp. 113–122; and François Delaporte, *The Cholera in Paris, 1832* (Cambridge, Mass., 1986), esp. pp. 6–10, and 47–72.

In the United States native-born Americans frequently attributed the ravages of the first pandemic to the sinfulness and filth of Irish Catholic immigrants. Cf. Alan M. Kraut, *Silent Travelers: Germs, Genes, and the 'Immigrant Menace'* (New York, 1994), ch. 2, pp. 31–49.

197 Keith Thomas, *Religion and the Decline of Magic* (London, 1971).

198 See above, Chapter 2.

199 The four epidemic waves in Britain ending in 1866 are surveyed by Longmate, *King Cholera*.

200 Evans, *Death in Hamburg*, pp. 292–293, 295.

201 *Ibid.*, p. 367.

CHAPTER 4: SURVIVAL AND RECOVERY

1 Municipio di Napoli, *Statistica Generale del Colera dalla mezzanotte del 17 agosto a quella del 4 novembre 1884* (Naples, 1884).

2 There was an outbreak in Paris in November, but it was of limited severity, producing a total of some 900 fatalities. The Parisian epidemic did not create a crisis commensurate with the experience of Provence and Naples earlier in the year, and it failed to attract international attention in the same manner. For brief accounts, see 'The Annus Medicus 1884', *Lancet* (1884, vol. 2), pp. 1151–1161; and H. Tomkins, 'Some Brief Notes on the Late Outbreak of Cholera in Paris', *Lancet* (1885, vol. 1), pp. 511–512.

3 'The Cholera', *Times*, 13 September 1884.

4 'Notizie del cholera', *La Nazione*, 25 September and 16 October 1884.

5 For a report on the initiative of the Società Operaia, see 'Cronaca', *Roma*, 31 August 1884.

6 On the origins of the Società Operaia, see Alfonso Scirocco, *Democrazia e socialismo a Napoli dopo l'unità (1860–1878)* (Naples, 1973), pp. 62–74.

7 'Il Cholera', *Osservatore romano*, 18 September 1884.

8 R. De Zerbi, *Cholera del 1884: Croce Bianca e Croce Rossa* (Naples, 1884), pp. 6–7. For a report on the volunteers, see also 'Cronaca', *Roma*, 18 September 1884.

9 'La riunione della Croce Bianca a Napoli', *Corriere della sera*, 6–7 October 1884.

10 Felice Cavallotti, *Lettere, 1860–1898*, ed. Cristina Vernizzi (Milan, 1979), p. 210.

11 De Zerbi, *Cholera del 1884*, pp. 59–60.

12 *Ibid.*, pp. 59–60.

13 *Ibid.*, p. 29.

14 *Ibid.*, p. 64.

15 Vincenzo Pagano, *Il Cholera e la carità: cenno storico dell'epidemia di Napoli del 1884* (Naples, 1884), pp. 37–38.

16 De Zerbi, *Cholera del 1884*, pp. 61–62.

17 'The Cholera', *Times*, 3 October 1884.

18 There is an excellent description of the miracle of the blood and of its significance for Neapolitans in Serao, *Il paese di Cuccagna* (Naples, 1902), ch. 10, pp. 184–208.

19 'Il Cholera', *Il Piccolo*, 10 September 1884.

20 'The Cholera at Naples', *Times*, 30 September 1884.

21 'Cronaca', *Il Piccolo*, 19–20 September 1884.

22 *Ibid.*

23 For brief accounts of the King's visit to Busca, see 'Il Re fra i colerosi', *Corriere della sera*, 27–28 August 1884; and 'Il Cholera a Busca', *Osservatore romano*, 29 August 1884.

24 For a recent assessment of King Umberto, see Denis Mack Smith, *Italy and its Monarchy* (New Haven and London, 1989), pp. 71–143.

25 'Italy', *Lancet* (1884, vol. 2), p. 437.

26 'Le choléra', *Le Temps*, 13 September 1884.

27 'Plague Scenes in Naples', *New York Times*, 14 September 1884.

28 'Deaths Due to Cholera', *New York Times*, 28 September 1884.

29 'The Cholera', *Times*, 16 September 1884.

30 'Le choléra', *Le Temps*, 19 September 1884.

31 An assessment of the visit of the King to Naples is, 'The King and the Cholera', *New York Times*, 5 October 1884. See also 'The Cholera Epidemic in Southern Europe', *Lancet* (1884, vol. 2), pp. 499–500.

32 'Una nuova lettera del Card. Arc. di Napoli', *Osservatore romano*, 31 August 1884.

33 The actions of Cardinal Archbishop San Felice are reported on an almost daily basis throughout the months of September and October 1884 in the column 'Il Cholera a Napoli' in the papal newspaper *Osservatore romano*. The discussion here is based primarily on these reports.

34 'The Cholera', *Times*, 4 September 1884.

35 For the views of the paper *Roma*, see the column 'Cronaca' during the last week of August and throughout September 1884. See also 'The King and the Cholera', *New York Times*, 5 October 1884.

36 For a clear exposition of the intransigent Catholic position in Sicily, see 'La morale dei casi di Sicilia', *Civiltà cattolica*, XXXVI (1885), iv, pp. 129–138.

37 'Il Cholera a Napoli', *Osservatore romano*, 16 September 1884.

38 Pagano, *Il cholera e la carità*, pp. 40–41.

39 For an account of the financial interventions of the Bank of Naples during the cholera epidemic, see the report of 7 December 1884, *Atti del Consiglio Generale del Banco di Napoli (1884)*, pp. 44–46.

40 'Relazione del Consiglio di amministrazione al Consiglio generale per lo esercizio 1883', *Atti del Consiglio Generale del Banco di Napoli (1884)*, Allegato A, p. 5.
41 Archivio del Banco di Napoli. Verbali del Consiglio di Amministrazione del Banco di Napoli, 1884, 'Situazione del Banco di Napoli al 31 del mese di dicembre 1883', 19 January 1884, n. 14.
42 Speech of 13 January 1888, *Atti del consiglio comunale di Napoli*, 1888, pp. 22 –23.
43 Municipio di Napoli, *Statistica Generale*.
44 *Atti del consiglio comunale di Napoli*, 1884, vol. 2, p. 665.
45 Nicola Amore summarized the initiatives undertaken by the city during the epidemic on 30 October 1884. See *Atti del consiglio comunale di Napoli*, 1884, vol. 2, pp. 662–672.
46 Ciaramelli, *Sul cholera del 1884*, pp. 37–38.
47 Marino Turchi, G. Albini, Francesco Viziola, 'Rapporto sul lavoro del dott. Francesco d'Agostino, dal titolo La Meteorologia ed il Cholera', in Reale Accademia Medico-chirurgica di Napoli, *Resoconto delle adunanze e dei lavori*, 39:2 (April–December, 1885), pp. 82–83.
48 Patrice Bourdelais and Jean-Yeves Raulot, *Une peur bleue: Histoire du choléra en France, 1832–1854* (Paris, 1987), pp. 161–162.
49 For a report on the rains in the second week of October, see 'The Cholera', *Times*, 11 October 1884.
50 Consul Frank G. Haughwout, 'Outbreak and Course of the cholera in Naples', in United States Bureau of Foreign Commerce, *Cholera in Europe in 1884. Reports from Consuls of the United States* (Washington, 1885), p. 44.
51 Stanislao D'Alessandro, *Studi sul cholera dal punto di vista etiologico generale e speciale relativamente all'epidemia in Napoli del 1884 nella Sezione S. Lorenzo* (Naples, 1885), p. 24. See also Eugenio Fazio, *La epidemia colerica e le condizioni sanitarie di Napoli* (Naples, 1884), p. 56.
52 National Archives. Record Group 84: Records of Foreign Service Posts. Consular Posts: Naples, Italy, volume 012. Despatch of Frank G. Haughwout to Hon. William Hunter, Second Assistant Secretary of State, 'Outbreak and Course of the Cholera Epidemic in Naples", 23 September 1884, n. 43, p. 206.
53 *Ibid*.
54 Fazio, *La epidemia colerica*, p. 54.
55 On the relation between the Nunziatella celebrations and the epidemic surge, see Dottor G. Paoletti, 'Il colera di Napoli e le misure di difesa individuale e collettiva', *Rivista internazionale di clinica e terapia* 5 (1910), p. 282.

A description of the *ottobrate* and their medical consequences is in National Archives. Record Group 84: Records of Foreign Service Posts. Consular Posts: Naples, Italy, volume 012. Despatch of Frank G. Haughwout to William Hunter, Second Assistant Secretary of State, 13 October 1884, n. 48, pp. 223–224.
56 Robert Koch, *Professor Koch on the Bacteriological Diagnosis of Cholera, Water-Filtration and Cholera, and the Cholera in Germany during the Winter of 1892–93*, trans. George Duncan (Edinburgh, 1894), pp. 72–73.
57 Orazio Caro, *L'evoluzione igienica di Napoli (Cenni storici – osservazioni e proposte – dati statistici)* (Naples, 1914), p. 298.
58 Michael Durey, *The Return of the Plague: British Society and the Cholera, 1831–2* (London, 1979).

59 Charles E. Rosenberg, 'Cholera in Nineteenth-Century Europe: A Tool for Social and Economic Analysis', *Comparative Studies in Society and History*, 8 (1966), p. 452, emphasis added.

60 See Durey, *The Return of the Plague*; Norman Longmate, *King Cholera: The Biography of a Disease* London, 1966); R.J. Morris, *Cholera 1832: The Social Response to an Epidemic* (London, 1976); Bourdelais and Raulot, *Une peur bleue*; Louis Chevalier, *Le choléra: la première épidémie du XIXe siècle* (La Roche-sur-Yon); François Delaporte, *The Cholera in Paris, 1832* (Cambridge, Mass., 1986); Ange-Pierre Leca, *Et le choléra s'abattit sur Paris, 1832* (Paris, 1982); and Roderick E. McGrew, *Russia and the Cholera, 1823–1832* (Madison and Milwaukee, 1965).

61 Charles E. Rosenberg, *The Cholera Years: The United States in 1832, 1849 and 1866* (Chicago, 1962); and Geoffrey Bilson, *A Darkened House: Cholera in Nineteenth-Century Canada* (Toronto, 1980).

62 Richard Evans, *Death in Hamburg: Society and Politics in the Cholera Years, 1830–1910* (Oxford, 1987).

63 Anna Lucia Forti Messina, *Società ed epidemia: il colera a Napoli nel 1836* (Milan, 1979).

64 'L'Italia dell'Ottocento di fronte al colera', *Storia d'Italia, Annali 7: Malattia e Medicina*, ed. F. Della Peruta, (Turin, 1984), pp. 469–470.

65 For statistics for the earlier outbreaks of cholera in Naples, see above, Chapter 1.

CHAPTER 5: REBUILDING: MEDICINE AND POLITICS

1 On the 'mortality revolution', see Philip D. Curtin, *Death by Migration: Europe's Encounter with the Tropical World in the Nineteenth Century* (Cambridge, 1989), esp. chs 1 and 2, pp. 1–61.

2 A brief overview of renewal in nineteenth-century Italy is Alberto Mioni and Michela Barzi, 'Sventrare la città: il risanamento urbano, 1870–1920', in Franco Della Peruta, ed., *Vita civile degli italiani: società, economia, cultura materiale. Città, fabbriche e nuove culture alle soglie della società di massa, 1850–1920* (Milan, 1990), pp. 50–69.

3 Speech of 25 April 1887, *Atti del consiglio comunale di Napoli*, 1887, vol. 1, p. 190.

4 For a brief discussion of the models considered by the Neapolitan planners, see Giuseppe Russo, *Napoli come città* (Naples, 1966), esp. Chapter 11, pp. 303–333.

    The discussion here of the rebuilding of Paris is based primarily on the following: Louis Girard, *La Politique des Travaux Public du Second Empire* (Paris, 1952); David Pinkney, *Napoleon III and the Rebuilding of Paris* (Princeton, 1958); and Georges Haussmann, *Mémoires du baron Haussmann*, 3 vols. (Paris, 1890–3).

5 Alberto Marghieri, *Intorno al problema edilizio della città di Napoli* (Naples, 1911), p. 16.

6 Speech of 10 January 1885, *Atti del parlamento italiano. Camera dei senatori. Legislature XV, Sessione 1882–86. Discussioni*, p. 3023.

7 For discussions by Max von Pettenkofer of his views on the etiology of Asiatic cholera, there was extended coverage in *The Lancet*. See 'Scientific Investigation into the Causes of Cholera. A Report of Interviews with Prof. Max von Pettenkofer at Munich, Nov. 1868. By Dr. D. Douglas Cunningham and Dr. Timothy Lewis',

Lancet (1869, vol. 1), pp. 3–4; 'Pettenkofer's Views on the Origin of Cholera', *Lancet* (1869, vol. 2), p. 345; 'Review of Max von Pettenkofer, *Cholera: How to Prevent and Resist It*, trans. by Thomas Witeside Hime (London, 1875)", *Lancet* (1875, vol. 2), pp. 760–761; 'Pettenkofer on Cholera', *Lancet* (1883, vol. 2), p. 155; Max Von Pettenkofer, 'Cholera', *Lancet* (1884, vol. 2), pp. 769–771, 816–819, 861–864, 904–905, 992–994, 1042–1043, 1086–1088; 'Cholera Conference at Berlin', *Lancet* (1885, vol. 1), pp. 911–913, 961–962; 'Bacteriology and Epidemiology', *Lancet* (1886, vol. 1), pp. 310–312; 'Cholera Forecasts', *Lancet* (1887, vol. 1), p. 1246; 'Von Pettenkofer's Latest Views on Cholera', *Lancet* (1887, vol. 2), pp. 339–340; 386–387; 'Cholera: Current Notes, Comments and Criticism', *Lancet* (1892, vol. 2), pp. 790–792.

See also Max von Pettenkofer, *Cholera: How to Prevent and Resist It*, trans. Thomas Whiteside Hime (London, 1875); and *Outbreak of Cholera among Convicts* (London, 1876).

8 Municipio di Napoli, *Proposte e documenti per la esecuzione del progetto di risanamento delle sezioni Porto, Pendino, Mercato, Vicaria* (Naples, 1887), p. 27.

9 *Ibid.*, p. 59.

10 'Sul cholera di Napoli (1884)', *Rivista clinica e terapeutica*, 7 (1885), pp. 63–65.

11 Adolfo Giambarba, *Relazione tecnica sul progetto di risanamento delle sezioni Porto, Pendino, Mercato, Vicaria*, in Municipio di Napoli, *Proposte e documenti*, p. 60.

12 Rocco De Zerbi, 'Relazione della commissione sul disegno di legge presentato dal presidente del consiglio ministro dell'interno (Depretis): Disposizione per provvedere alla pubblica igiene della città di Napoli', in Camera dei deputati, Legislatura XV-Sessione 1882–86, *Raccolta degli atti stampati per ordine della Camera*, vol. XXII, seduta del 15 dicembre 1884, n.261–A, p. 7.

13 Marghieri, *Intorno al problema edilizio*, p. 24.

14 Marghieri, *Intorno al problema edizio*, pp. 24–25.

15 Max von Pettenkofer, 'Cholera', *Lancet* (1884, vol. 2), p. 770.

16 Pettenkofer, *Cholera*, pp. 37–38.

17 Speech of 11 February 1885. *Atti del consiglio comunale di Napoli*, 1885, p. 39.

18 For the text of the sanitary code, see 'Proposta di regolamento d'igiene pubblica e di polizia sanitaria', *Atti del consiglio comunale di Napoli*, 1886, tornata del 26 gennaio 1886, pp. 55–66; and tornata del 28 gennaio 1886, pp. 68–84.

19 A short outline of the main features of the new sewer network is provided by the Alderman De Rosenheim in a speech of 20 February 1885. *Atti del consiglio comunale di Napoli*, 1885, p. 698. The official municipal plan for the sewers of Naples prepared by G. Bruno is Comune di Napoli: Consiglio Superiore dei Lavori Pubblici, *Fognatura della città di Napoli: ultimi studi e proposte definitive* (Naples, 1885).

20 Max von Pettenkofer, 'Cholera', *Lancet* (1884, vol. 2), pp. 770–771.

21 A concise history of the Serino aqueduct is provided by Orazio Caro, *L'evoluzione igienica di Napoli (Cenni storici – osservazioni e proposte – dati statistici* (Naples, 1914), pp. 76–99.

22 Giuseppe Saredo, *Relazione della R. commissario straordinario al consiglio comunale di Napoli* (Naples, 1891), vol. I, p. 65.

23 For an instance of Pettenkofer's critique of the English for their obsession with water in the propagation of cholera, see Max von Pettenkofer, 'Cholera', *Lancet* (1884, vol. 2), pp. 863 and 904. See also Pettenkofer, *Outbreak of Cholera* (London, 1876), p. 74.

24 Saredo, *Relazione della R. commissione*, vol. I, p. 913.

25 Teodosio De Bonis, speech of 20 February 1885, *Atti del consiglio comunale di Napoli*, 1885, pp. 53–55; and speech of 19 December 1885, pp. 869–871.

26 For the speech of Agostino Depretis on 27 November 1884 presenting the bill to finance the renewal of Naples, see Camera dei deputati, Legislatura XV-Sessione 1882–86, *Raccolta degli atti stampati per ordine della Camera*, vol. XXII, n. 261, pp. 1–6.

27 Speech of 19 December 1884, *Atti del parlamento italiano: Camera dei deputati*, Sessione 1882–83–84 (1a della XV Legislatura), Discussioni, Vol. X, pp. 10370–10372.

28 Speech of 17 November 1884, Camera dei deputati, Legislatura X-Sessione 1882–86, *Raccolta degli atti stampati per ordine della Camera*, vol. XXII, n. 261, p. 1.

29 On the results of the elections of 1874, see Giuliano Procacci, *Le elezioni del 1874 e l'opposizione meridionale* (Milan, 1956), esp. 9–16.

30 On the relations between San Donato and Depretis, see Cesare Magni, *Vita parlamentare del duca di San Donato patriota e difensore di Napoli* (Padua, 1968), esp. pp. 111–124.

31 Pasquale Villari noted the term by which the bill was known in a speech to the Senate on 10 January 1885. *Atti del parlamento italiano. Camera dei senatori Legislatura XV, Sessione 1882–86. Discussioni*, p. 3018.

32 Haussmann, *Mémoires*, vol. II, pp. 35–36.

33 This argument is used, for example, by Cavour in his budget speech before the Chamber of Deputies on 11 April 1854. Cf. Camillo di Cavour, *Discorsi parlamentari*, vol. VIII (Florence, 1869), esp. pp. 160–161. Cavour used the same principle in a speech to the Senate on 19 December 1854. Cf. Camillo di Cavour, *Discorsi parlamentari*, vol. IX (Florence, 1870), pp. 174–175.

34 See 'Tornata di venerdì 19 dicembre 1884', in *Atti del parlamento italiano: Camera dei deputati, Sessione 1882–83–84 (1a della XV Legislatura), Discussioni*, Vol. X, p. 10440.

35 Alberto Marghieri, Speech of 25 and 27 April 1887, *Atti del consiglio comunale di Napoli*, 1887, pp. 174–199 and 202–215.

36 *Ibid.*, p. 197.

37 *Ibid.*, p. 212.

38 *Ibid.*

39 *Ibid.*, p. 213.

40 Marghieri, *Intorno al problema edilizio*, p. 16.

41 Speech of 27 April 1887, *Atti del consiglio comunale di Napoli*, 1887, p. 213.

42 Nardi, speech of 3 May 1887, *Atti del consiglio comunale di Napoli*, 1887, p. 303. Nardi's camorra associations were revealed during the famous lawsuit of Alberto Casale against the socialist newspaper *La Propaganda*, in which the Alderman appeared as a witness on Casale's behalf. Cf. 'Processo Casale – giornale *Propa-*

ganda', Avanti!, 24 October 1900; and 'Gesta dell'affarismo e violenze del governo', *Avanti!*, 21 December 1900.

43 Speech of Nicola Amore, 5 May 1887, *Atti del consiglio comunale di Napoli*, 1887, p. 352.

44 *Ibid.*, p. 214.

45 Speech of 24 February 1888, *Atti del consiglio comunale di Napoli*, 1888, p. 173.

46 Nardi, speech of 3 May 1887, *Atti del consiglio comunale di Napoli*, 1887, p. 303.

47 Speech of 30 April 1887, *Atti del consiglio comunale di Napoli*, 1887, pp. 237–260.

48 See councillor Folinea, speech of 5 May 1887, *Atti del consiglio comunale di Napoli*, 1887, p. 311.

49 *Atti del consiglio comunale di Napoli*, 1887, pp. 202–213. The landlords are the subject of pages 202–212, and the poor of pages 212–214. Marghieri repeated in 1888 his estimate that 87,000 people would be evicted by the renewal programme. Speech of 30 January 1888, *Atti del consiglio comunale di Napoli*, 1888, p. 172.

50 Municipio di Napoli, *Proposte e documenti*, p. 31.

51 *Ibid.*, pp. 31–43.

52 For the text of Article 6 of the contract, see *Atti del consiglio comunale di Napoli*, 1888, p. 234.

53 Leopoldo Di Maio, Campodisola, and Alberto Marghieri, speeches of 24 February 1888, *Atti del consiglio comunale di Napoli*, 1888, pp. 170–175.

54 Speech of 24 February 1888, *Atti del consiglio comunale di Napoli*, 1888, p. 173.

55 'Lo sventramento affaristico', *Osservatore romano*, 24 October 1884.

56 *Ibid.*, p. 174.

57 For Giusso's explanation of the artificiality of the compensation extended by the city to the proprietors, see his speech of 30 April 1887, *Atti del consiglio comunale di Napoli*, 1887, esp. pp. 247ff.

58 *Ibid.*, p. 248. The official version of the expenses of expropriation is Municipio di Napoli, *Proposte e documenti*, pp. 13 and 16–20.

59 *Ibid.*, pp. 249–250.

60 G. Giusso, speech of 30 April 1887, *Atti del consiglio comunale di Napoli*, 1887, p. 247.

61 Speech of 24 February 1888, *Atti del consiglio comunale di Napoli*, 1888, p. 169.

62 Procacci, *Le elezioni del 1874*, p. 47. The comment by Franchetti and Sonnino was in *La Sicilia* (Florence, 1926), vol. II, p. 344, n.1.

63 On the issue of privatization, see Alberto Marghieri, speech of 25 April 1887, *Atti del consiglio comunale di Napoli*, 1887, pp. 174–199, and Speech of 27 April 1887, *ibid.*, pp. 202–215.

64 Nicola Amore, speech of 7 May 1887, *Atti del consiglio comunale di Napoli*, 1887, p. 351.

65 Councillor Menichili, speech of 3 May 1887, *Atti del consiglio comunale di Napoli*, 1887, p. 291.

66 Municipio di Napoli, *Proposte e documenti*, pp. 21–22.

67 Parlati, Speech of 10 March 1894, *Atti del consiglio comunale di Napoli*, 1894, pp. 144–145.

68 *Ibid.*, p. 145.

69 For a discussion of the municipal anxiety over this point, see *ibid.*, pp. 145–148.

70 For the estimate of costs for demolition and roadwork, see Alberto Marghieri, speech of 25 April 1887, *Atti del consiglio comunale di Napoli*, 1887, pp. 175–190.

71 Alberto Marghieri, speech of 25 April 1887, *Atti del consiglio comunale di Napoli*, 1887, p. 193. The arguments in favour of private enterprise were summarized by councillor Menichili, speech of 3 May 1887, *Atti del consiglio comunale di Napoli*, 1887, pp. 292–293; and by mayor Nicola Amore, speech of 5 May 1887, *Atti del consiglio di Napoli*, 1887, esp. pp. 358–362.

72 On the issue of the *lotto unico*, see Alberto Marghieri, speech of 25 April 1887, *Atti del consiglio comunale di Napoli*, 1887, pp. 193ff.

73 Parlati, speech of 28 April 1887, *Atti del consiglio comunale di Napoli*, 1887, p. 223; and G. Giusso, speech of 30 April 1887, *Atti del consiglio comunale di Napoli*, 1887, p. 237–260.

74 *Ibid.*, p. 224.

75 *Ibid.*, p. 223.

76 The reasons for the adoption of a single contractor for the whole of the project are explained in Municipio di Napoli, *Proposte e documenti*, pp. 24–28. Cf. also councillor de Rosenheim, speech of 6 May 1887, *Atti del consiglio comunale di Napoli*, 1887, p. 322.

77 Marghieri's arguments in favour of a single contractor are contained in his speech of 25 April 1887, *Atti del consiglio comunale di Napoli*, 1887, pp. 193–196.

78 Alberto Marghieri, speech of 25 April 1887, *Atti del consiglio comunale di Napoli*, 1887, p. 198.

79 Municipio di Napoli, *Proposte e documenti*, p. 28.

80 For Marghieri's position regarding subcontracting, see speech of 25 April 1887, *Atti del consiglio comunale di Napoli*, 1887, p. 199. Arlotta reached identical conclusions. See speech of 2 May 1887, *Atti del consiglio comunale di Napoli*, 1887, pp. 264–265.

81 Speech of 25 April 1887, *Atti del consiglio comunale di Napoli*, 1887, p. 198.

82 Arlotta, speech of 2 May 1887, *Atti del consiglio comunale di Napoli*, 1887, pp. 264–265.

83 Saredo, *Relazione della R. commissione*, vol. I, pp. 678–685.

84 Nardi, speech of 24 August 1888, *Atti del consiglio comunale di Napoli*, 1888, pp. 989–990.

85 Imbriani, speech of 2 October 1890, *Atti del consiglio comunale di Napoli*, 1890, p. 723. On the fraudulent stock transaction, see also Achille Nardi, speech of 10–11 October 1903, *Atti del consiglio comunale di Napoli*, 1903, vol. 2, pp. 225–226.

86 Speech of 24 August 1888, *Atti del consiglio comunale di Napoli*, 1888, pp. 1020–1021.

87 On this point see Salvatore Fusco, speech of 10 February 1890, *Atti del consiglio comunale di Napoli*, 1890, pp. 100–101.

88 Archivio di Stato di Napoli, Prefettura, b. 4279, Letter of mayor of Naples to Prefect of the Province of Naples, 21 April 1890, n. 12963.

89 'Il colmo', *Il Piccolo*, 8–9 November 1889.

90 'Napoli', *Il Piccolo*, 7–8 November 1889.

91 'Napoli', *Il Piccolo*, 10–11 November 1889.

92 'Napoli: Dove abiteremo?' *Il Piccolo*, 10–11 December 1889.

93 'Napoli: autosventramento', *Il Piccolo*, 25–6 September 1889.
94 See, for example, 'Napoli: Perché cadono le case?', *Il Piccolo*, 22–3 March 1890; 'Napoli: Perché le case rovinano', *Il Piccolo*, 26–7 March 1890; 'Napoli che sprofonda', *Il Piccolo*, 30–1 May 1890; and 'Soliti disastri', *Il Piccolo*, 3–4 July 1890.
95 Interpellation of 4 December 1889, *Atti del consiglio comunale di Napoli*, 1889, pp. 1340–1341.
96 Speech of 10 February 1890, *Atti del consiglio comunale di Napoli*, 1890, pp. 94–97.
97 'Napoli: per gli infortuni sul lavoro', *Il Piccolo*, 11–12 October 1890.
98 Salvatore Fusco, speech of 10 February 1890, *Atti del consiglio comunale di Napoli*, 1890, pp. 98–101.
99 *Ibid.*
100 *Ibid.*, p. 725.
101 Speech of 2 October 1890, *Atti del consiglio comunale di Napoli*, 1890, pp. 723–724.
102 Quoted in Archivio di Stato di Napoli, Prefettura, busta 4279, fascio Napoli: opere di risanamento. Vigilanza disposta per evitare disastri, Letter of the mayor of Naples to the prefect of Naples, 1 May 1890,n. 29694.
103 Archivio di Stato di Napoli, Prefettura, busta 4279, fascio Napoli: opere di risanamento. Vigilanza disposta per evitare disastri, Letter of Pagliani, Ministero dell'Interno, Direzione della Sanità Pubblica to Prefect of Naples, 6 May 1890, n. 20940B.
104 Saredo, *Relazione della R. commissione*, p. 440.
105 *Ibid.*, vol. I, p. 437.
106 *Ibid.*, p. 237.
107 Archivio di Stato di Napoli, Prefettura, busta 4279, fascio Napoli: opere di risanamento. Vigilanza disposta per evitare disastri, Petition to Prefect of the City [*sic*], 11 April 1890.
108 Archivio di Stato di Napoli, Prefettura, busta 4279, fascio Napoli: opere di risanamento. Vigilanza disposta per evitare disastri, Unsigned letter to Prefect of the Province of Naples, 14 January 1890.
109 Saredo, *Relazione della R. commissisone*, vol. I, pp. 437–438.
110 *Ibid.*, vol. I, p. 436.
111 *Ibid.*, pp. 437–438.
112 Arlotta, speech of 20 March 1894, *Atti del consiglio comunale di Napoli*, 1894, p. 224.
113 Speech of 18 February 1901, *Atti del consiglio comunale di Napoli*, 1902, p. 153.
114 Speech of 19 April 1902, *Atti del consiglio comunale di Napoli*, 1902, p. 427.
115 Speech by Leone, 19 April 1902, *Atti del consiglio comunale di Napoli*, 1902, p. 427.
116 Speech by Councillor De Pezzo, 29 April 1902, *Atti del consiglio comunale di Napoli*, 1902, p. 508.
117 The issue of timing was dealt with by Salvatore Fusco, speech of 17 March 1894, *Atti del consiglio comunale di Napoli*, 1894, pp. 190–191.
118 The difficulties of the Company for the Renewal of Naples were explained to the

city council by Parlati, speech of 10 March 1894, *Atti del consiglio comunale di Napoli*, 1894, pp. 145–147.

119 Salvatore Fusco, speech of 17 March 1894, *Atti del consiglio comunale di Napoli*, 1894, p. 200.

120 Parlati, speech of 10 March 1894, *Atti del consiglio comunale di Napoli*, 1894, p. 147.

121 For the text of Nicola Amore's speech of 21 March 1894, see *Atti del consiglio comunale di Napoli*, 1894, pp. 234–241.

122 Amore, speech of 21 March 1894, *Atti del consiglio comunale di Napoli*, 1894, p. 235.

123 *Ibid.*

124 Salvatore Fusco, speech of 17 March 1894, *Atti del consiglio comunale di Napoli*, 1894, p. 195.

125 Speech of 20 March 1894, *Atti del consiglio comunale di Napoli*, 1894, pp. 217–219.

126 Saredo, *Relazione della R. commissione*, vol. I, pp. 624–625.

127 Marghieri, *Intorno al problema edilizio*, p. 31.

128 Municipio di Napoli, *Relazione sul V censimento generale della popolazione e sul I censimento industriale* (Naples, 1912).

129 Marghieri's gloomy appraisal of the results of renewal is *Intorno al problema edilizio*.

130 *Ibid.*, pp. 9–10.

131 Serao, *Il ventre di Napoli* (Naples, 1973), pp. 99–101.

132 Municipio di Napoli, *Relazione sul V censimento*, p. 32.

133 *Ibid.*, p. 33.

134 The survival of the *fondaci* is reported in Comune di Napoli, *Riordinamento della numerazione civica e della nomenclatura stradale* (Naples, 1906), p. 18.

135 Municipio di Napoli, *Relazione sul V censimento*, p. 33.

136 *Ibid.*, p. 33, n.1.

137 'Il grave problema della salute pubblica', *Il Mattino*, 30 September to 1 October 1910.

138 *Ibid.*

139 *Ibid.*

140 'La cronaca: il problema della salute pubblica', *Il Mattino*, 25–6 September 1910.

141 *Ibid.*

142 Comune di Napoli, *Annuario storico-statistico-topografico del comune di Napoli, anno 1909–1910* (Naples, 1912), pp. 70–71.

143 On trachoma in Giolittian Naples, see Antonio Mincione, 'Il tracoma ed il problema sociale della sua profilassi', *Gazzetta internazionale di medicina, chirurgia, igiene, interessi professionali*, 1909, pp. 147–151; 183–187; Ernesto Sgrosso, 'Sul tracoma: dati statistici desunti dall'Ambulatorio della Clinica oculistica della R. Università di Napoli (1 January 1902 to 30 June 1904). Nozioni riassuntive sul tracoma. Profilassi. Reparti ospedalieri ed ambulatorii per tracomatosi', *La Medicina italiana*, 5 (1907), pp. 565–569, 607–614; and Giulio Valenti, 'Distribuzione geografica del tracoma in Italia', *La Clinica oculista*, 3 (1902), pp. 1122–1126.

144 Prospero Guidone, 'La questione ospedaliera a Napoli', *Roma*, 30 July to 1 August 1910.

145 Speech of 20 February 1911, *Atti del consiglio comunale di Napoli*, 1911, vol. 1, pp. 378–379.

146 Caro, *L'evoluzione igienica*, p. 133.

147 'Una visita al Cotugno', *Roma*, 17–18 September 1910.

148 Alfonso Montefusco, *Resoconto dell'Ospedale Cotugno pel triennio 1902–1904* (Naples, 1905), p. 7.

149 Speech of 19 May 1911, *Atti del consiglio comunale di Napoli*, 1911, vol. 1, pp. 862–863. Two physicians who inspected the Cotugno and reported on its lamentable conditions to the city council in 1906 were Councillors Masullo and Semmola. Cf. speeches of 25 January 1906, *Atti del consiglio comunale di Napoli*, 1906, vol. 1, pp. 187–191. Neapolitan doctors, Masullo reported, often refused to diagnose infectious diseases accurately for fear that their patients would be taken to the Cotugno Hospital, where they were certain to die.

150 Archivio Storico del Comune di Napoli, Atti della Giunta Municipale di Napoli, Deliberazione presa nella tornata del 24 agosto 1910, n. 12.

151 For the report of the Vice-Chancellor of the University, Luigi Miraglia, on the renewal of the Medical Faculty, see R. Università degli Studi di Napoli, *Annuaro per l'anno scolastico, 1896–97* (Naples, 1897), pp. iii–xxiv.

152 Roger Cooter, 'Anticontagionism and History's Medical Record', in Peter Wright and Andrew Treacher, eds., *The Problem of Medical Knowledge: Examining the Social Construction of Medicine* (Edinburgh, 1982), pp. 94–95. Cooter finds that British anticontagionism early in the century was associated with political radicalism. The thesis advanced here is that the related doctrine of miasmo-contagionism in the 1880s provided support for the Neapolitan ruling elites instead.

The attempt to place medical theory in its social and political context owes much to the seminal essay of Erwin H. Ackerknecht, 'Anticontagionism between 1821 and 1867', *Bulletin of the History of Medicine*, 22 (1948), pp. 562–593.

153 Regia Università degli Studi di Napoli, *Annuario scolastico, 1896–1897* (Naples, 1897), p. xix.

154 The significance was not lost on the population of the city. The eviction of the nuns from their convent of the Sapienza provoked a heated debate in the city council and led to violent clashes in the street between Catholics and anticlericalists. Cf. 'Cronaca contemporanea: cose italiane', *Civiltà cattolica*, 37:4 (1886), pp. 242–244.

155 For a full description of the operation of the Office of Hygiene by its creator and first director, see Caro, *L'evoluzione igienica*, pp. 112–163.

156 *Ibid.*, p. 115.

157 *Ibid.*, pp. 122–123.

158 Speech of 16 May 1874, *Atti del consiglio comunale di Napoli*, 1874, vol. 2, pp. 460–462.

159 Ackerknecht, 'Anticontagionism', pp. 562–593.

160 See Margaret Pelling, *Cholera, Fever and English Medicine, 1825–1865* (Oxford, 1978); and Cooter, 'Anticontagionism'.

161 Richard Evans, *Death in Hamburg: Society and Politics in the Cholera Years, 1830–1910* (Oxford, 19870, pp. 270–275.

CHAPTER 6: THE RETURN OF CHOLERA: 1910

1 For detailed accounts of the epidemic, see Archivio Centrale dello Stato, Ministero dell'Interno, Direzione Generale della Sanità, b. 176, fasc. Colera: istruzioni per prevenire lo sviluppo del colera, 1901–1906, 'Ministero dell'Interno: appunto per il Signor Direttore Generale,' n.d. The assessment of the menace to Italy is Archivio Centrale dello Stato, Ministero dell'Interno, Direzione Generale della Sanità, b. 176, fasc. Colera: istruzioni per prevenire lo sviluppo del colera, 1901–1906, 'Programma delle misure preventive contro il pericolo di un'epidemia colerica in Italia: Relazione a S.E. il Ministro', 16 September 1905.

2 The lack of preparation along the Adriatic coast was discussed on 19 December by Senator Maragliano: *Atti parlamentari della camera dei senatori, legislatura XXIII, sessione 1909–1911, discussioni*, vol. VI, pp. 3870–3886.

3 *Annual Report of the Surgeon General of the Public Health Service of the United States for the Fiscal Year 1911* (Washington, DC, 1912), p. 98.

4 The report which identified fishermen as the probable importers of the cholera vibrio is Archivio Centrale dello Stato, Ministero dell'Interno, Direzione della Sanità, b. 181, fasc. Rapporti degli Ispettori sanitari sul colera, sottofasc. Episodi epidemici pugliesi, 'Documenti sugli episodi epidemici pugliesi, agosto-settembre 1910', pp. 10–12, 17–22.

5 *Ibid.*, p. 20.

6 There is a record of Rosa Quarto's burial on 17 August in Cimitero di Barletta, Registro (1910).

7 Archivio Centrale dello Stato, Ministero dell'Interno, Direzione Generale della Sanità, b. 225, fasc. Bari: affari generali e complessivi, sottofasc. Bari, no. 1392. Telegram, prefect Gasperini to Ministero dell'Interno, 20 September 1910.

8 Archivio Centrale dello Stato. Ministero dell'Interno, Direzione Generale della Sanità, 1882–1915, b. 225, fasc. Bari: affari generali e complessivi, sottofasc. Bari. Telegram of Prefect Gasperini to Ministry of the Interior, 20 September 1910, n. 1392.

9 In the period 1902–11 the average yearly number of emigrants from Bari province was 13,436. Istituto Nazionale di Economia Agraria, *Inchiesta sulla piccola proprietà coltivatrice formatasi nel dopoguerra* (Rome, 1935), vol. XV, p. 8.

10 Direzione Generale della Statistica e del Lavoro, *Annuario statistico italiano*, 2nd series, 1 (1911) (Rome, 1912), p. 24.

11 *Annual Report of the Surgeon General of the Public Health Service of the United States for the Fiscal Year 1912* (Washington, 1913).

12 The text of Calissano's speech is in *Il Giornale d'Italia*, 17 October 1910.

13 The desperate measures of the populace to escape detection are discussed by E. Rodingher, 'Una visita al lazzaretto di Trani', *Corriere della sera*, 23 August 1910.

14 *Corriere della sera*, 19 August 1910. On the obligation to report illness, see also Archivio Centrale dello Stato, Ministero dell'Interno, Direzione Generale della

Sanità, b. 234, fasc. Bari. Telegram, Del Bello to S.E. il Sottosegretario di Stato per gli Interni, 2 September 1910.

15 For informative articles on the sanitary vigilantes, see *Avanti!*, 6 September 1910 and *Corriere della sera*, 2 and 6 September 1910. For an official report, see Archivio Centrale dello Stato, Ministero dell'Interno, Direzione Generale della Sanità, b. 181, fasc. Rapporti degli ispettori sanitari sul colera, n. 29154. Telegram, Ispettore Generale Medico Ravicini to S.E. il Sottosegretario di Stato Int., 4 September 1910.

16 Quoted in Vito Lefemine, 'Colpe e responsabilità di uomini e di sistemi', *Avanti!*, 3 September 1910.

17 *Ibid.*

18 Archivio Centrale dello Stato, Ministero dell'Interno, Direzione Generale della Sanità, b. 181, fasc. Rapporti degli Ispettori sanitari sul colera, sottofasc. Episodi epidemici pugliesi, 'Documenti sugli episodi epidemici pugliesi, agosto-settembre 1910', p. 25.

19 Cesare Lombroso, *Crime: Its Causes and Remedies*, trans. Henry P. Norton (Boston, 1911), pp. 39–41.

20 Archivio Centrale dello Stato. Ministero dell'Interno, Direzione Generale della Sanità, b. 271, fasc. 'Vigilanza sugli zingari'. Telegram of Director-General of Public Security Pasquale Leonardi to Ministry of the Interior, 23 October 1910, n. 44557.

21 *Avanti!*, 22 August 1910.

22 *Il Messagero*, 25 August 1910.

23 E. Branzoli Zappi, 'Gli zingari', *Il Resto del carlino*, 5 September 1910.

24 Calissano's speech was on 17 December 1910. See *Atti del parlamento italiano: Camera dei deputati*, legislatura XXIII, sessione 1909–1910, discussioni, vol. IX, p. 10980.

25 The official version of events can be read in *Il Messagero*, 23 August 1910. The article contains an interview with Calissano.

26 R. Pollitzer, *Cholera* (Geneva, 1959), p. 43.

27 On the true state of the interned travellers, see the report by the sailing company that transported them, Archivio Centrale dello Stato, Ministero dell'Interno, Direzione Generale della Sanità, b. 271, fasc. 'Vigilanza sugli zingari', sottofasc. Bari, Società Nazionale di Servizi Marittimi, Venice, to Ill.mo Commendator Santoliquido, 20 August 1910.

28 Archivio Centrale dello Stato, Ministero dell'Interno, Direzione Generale della Sanità, b. 271, fasc. 'Vigilanza sugli zingari', sottofasc. Bari. Telegram of Gasperini to Ministero dell'Interno, Direzione Generale della Sanità, 5 September 1910, n. 29414.

29 E. Branzoli Zappi, 'Gli zingari', *Il Resto del carlino*, 5 September 1910.

30 Archivio Centrale dello Stato, Ministero dell'Interno, Direzione Generale della Sanità, 1882–1915, b. 271, fasc. 'Vigilanza sugli zingari'. Letter of Prefect of Piacenza to Mayors of the Province, 3 September 1910, n. 11748.

31 Archivio Centrale dello Stato. Ministero dell'Interno, Direzione Generale della Sanità, 1882–1915, b. 277, fasc. 'Specifici anticolerici'. Letter of Lorenzo Cortellino to S.E. on. Luigi Luzzatti, 23 August 1910.

32 'La fine del colera', *Il Messaggero*, 31 August 1910.
33 'Cronaca della città', *Il Resto del carlino*, 4 September 1910. On the misfortunes of gypsies during the cholera outbreak of 1910, see also A. Nappi, 'Zingari', *Il Giorno*, 28 August 1910.
34 On the exodus from Barletta, see Archivio Centrale dello Stato, Ministero dell-'Interno, Direzione Generale della Sanità, b. 234, fasc. Bari. Telegram of Gasperini to Ministero dell'Interno, 23 August 1910, n. 7921.
35 On the riot at Molfetta, see Gaetano Salvemini, 'I tumulti di Molfetta', *La Voce*, 2: 45 (20 October 1910), pp. 417–419.
36 Archivio Centrale dello Stato, Ministero dell'Interno, Direzione Generale della Sanità, 1882–1915, b. 181, fasc. Rapporti degli Ispettori sanitari sul colera', sottofasc. 'Episodi epidemici pugliesi', 'Documenti sugli episodi epidemici pugliesi, agosto–settembre 1910', pp. 27–28.
37 *Ibid.*, pp. 31–32.
38 Orazio Caro, *L'evoluzione igienica di Napoli (Cenni storici – osservazioni e proposte – dati statistici)* (Naples, 1914), pp. 273–274.
39 *Ibid.*, p. 164.
40 'Cose italiane: il colera nelle Puglie', *Civiltà cattolica*, 61:2 (1910), pp. 624–625.
41 'Cholera in Paris', *New York Times*, 15 November 1884.
42 *Ibid.* There are no modern studies of the final experience of Paris with cholera in 1884 and 1892–3, and the subject merits further attention. A preliminary reading of reports in *The Lancet, The Times, Le Temps*, the *New York Times* and *Le Petit Var* suggests that Paris was free of major social tensions during its final experiences of epidemic cholera.
43 'Spread of the Contagion in the French Capital', *New York Times*, 14 November 1884.
44 The course of the disease can be traced in the Parisian paper *Le Temps* between its outbreak in April and its end in November, especially in the months between July and October when there was a frequent column 'Le choléra'.
45 Asa Briggs, 'Cholera and Society in the Nineteenth Century', *Past and Present*, no. 19 (October 1961), p. 80.
46 Charles E. Rosenberg, 'Afterword', in *The Cholera Years: The United States in 1832, 1849 and 1866* (Chicago, 1962), p. 242.
47 For the works on Spain, see Vincent Bernard, 'Le choléra en Espagne au xixe siècle,' in Jean-Pierre Bardet, *et al., Peurs et terreurs face à la contagion: Choléra, tuberculose, syphilis aux xixe–xxe siècles* (Paris, 1988), pp. 43–55; Antonio Fernandez Garcia, *Epidemias y Sociedad en Madrid* (Madrid, 1985); and Esteban Rodriguez Ocana, *El colera de 1834 en Granda* (1983).
48 Richard Evans, 'Epidemics and Revolutions: Cholera in Nineteenth-Century Europe,' *Past and Present*, no. 120 (August, 1988), pp. 123–146.
49 'Epidemics and Revolution: The Rinderpest Epidemic in Late Nineteenth-Century Southern Africa', *Past and Present*, no. 138 (February 1993), pp. 112–143.
50 For a report on the course of the outbreak in Sardinia, see Archivio Centrale dello Stato, Ministero dell'Interno, Direzione Generale della Sanità, 1882–1915, b226, fasc. Cagliari, sottofasc. Relazione sull'epidemia colerica. Prefect of Cagliari, Epidemia colerica', 4 November 1912.

51 Evans, 'Epidemics and Revolutions', pp. 123–146.
52 Patrice Bourdelais and Jean-Yves Raulot, *Une peur bleue: Histoire du choléra en France, 1832–1854*, p. 37.
53 Giovanni Giolitti, *Memorie della mia vita* (Milan, 1922).
54 Major works on the Giolittian period in which the cholera epidemic is never mentioned include the documentary anthologies by Franco De Felice, *L'età giolittiana* (Turin, 1980), and Claudio Pavone, ed., *Dalle carte di Giovanni Giolitti: Quarant'anni di politica italiana*, vol. III *Dai prodromi della grande guerra al fascismo, 1910–1928* (Milan, 1962); the biography by Nino Valeri, *Giovanni Giolitti* (Turin, 1972); and the studies of the Giolittian era by Sergio Romano, *Giolitti: lo stile del potere* (Milan, 1989), Giampiero Carocci, *Giolitti e l'età giolittiana* (Turin, 1971), Giovanni Ansaldo, *Il ministro della buona vita* (Milan, 1949), and Alberto Aquarone, *L'Italia giolittiana* (Milan, 1988; 1st edn 1981).
    Influential recent monographs on modern Naples and Campania that ignore the cholera epidemic of 1910–11 are Giuseppe Galasso, *Napoli* (Bari, 1987); and Paolo Macry and Pasquale Villani, eds., *Storia d'Italia: Le regioni dall'Unità a oggi. La Campania* (Turin, 1990).
55 Alan M. Kraut, *Silent Travelers: Germs, Genes, and the 'Immigrant Menace'* (New York, 1994).
56 Anna Lucia Forti Messina, 'L'Italia dell'Ottocento di fronte al colera', in Franco Della Peruta, ed. *Storia d'Italia, Annali 7: Malattie e medicina* (Turin, 1984), pp. 469–470.
57 Pollitzer, *Cholera*, ch. 1, esp. pp. 41–45.
58 The term is used by Francesco de Miranda, 'Importante intervista col comm. Orazio Caro', *Il Giorno*, 12 October 1910.
59 See Caro, *L'evoluzione igienica*, esp. pp. 164–185; and 298–312.
60 *Ibid.*, pp. 302–303.
61 On the transformation of Vicaria, see *ibid.*, p. 307.
62 *Ibid.*, p. 165.
63 *Ibid.*, pp. 173–174.
64 *Ibid.*, p. 309.
65 See above, Chapter 3.
66 Archivio Centrale dello Stato, Ministero dell'Interno, Direzione Generale della Sanità, 1882–1915, b. 177 bis, fasc. Napoli e provincia: colera 1911, 'Casi e decessi di colera nell'anno 1910 in Napoli'.
67 Caro, *L'evoluzione igienica*, pp. 311–312.
68 *Ibid.*, p. 179.
69 Galasso, *Napoli* (Bari, 1987).
70 Ugo Fusco and Mario Soscia, 'Il colera in Italia ed a Napoli (Profilo storico)', *Aggiornamenti su Malattie Infettive ed Immunologia*, 19 (1973), pp. 1–10.
71 Giuseppe Russo, *Il risanamento e l'ampliamento della città di Napoli* (Naples, 1960).
72 *Ibid.*, p. 320.
73 *Ibid.*, p. 374.
74 A concise recent discussion of the crisis in Naples at the turn of the century is Alfonso Scirocco, *Politica e amministrazione a Napoli nella vita unitaria* (Naples,

1972), pp. 122–134. Cf. also Luigi Mascilli Migliorini, 'La vita amministrativa e politica,' in Galasso, ed., *Napoli*, pp. 176–194.

75 'Il comune di Napoli', *Avanti!*, 18 February 1910.

76 'Per le elezioni amministrative', *Roma*, 4 July 1910.

77 *Ibid.*

78 'Il comizio di ieri alla Borsa', *La Libertà*, 18 July 1910.

79 See, for example, 'Le elezioni amministrative', *Don Marzio*, 26–7 July 1910.

80 For the results of the provincial elections, see 'Le elezioni amministrative', *La Tribuna*, 26 July 1910.

81 'Cronaca: A Palazzo San Giacomo', *La Libertà*, 18 August 1910.

82 Christopher Seton-Watson, *Italy from Liberalism to Fascism* (London, 1967), pp. 262–264.

83 Giolitti's bill, as Seton-Watson explained, 'gave the vote to all male literates at the age of twenty-one, and to illiterates on completing their military service or on reaching the age of thirty'. *Italy from Liberalism to Fascism*, p. 282.

84 'Il colera alle porte di Napoli', *La Propaganda*, 20–21 August 1910.

85 Speech of 18 August 1910, *Atti del consiglio comunale di Napoli*, 1910, vol. 2, pp. 104–105.

86 'Cronaca: Napoli ed il colera', *La Libertà*, 18 September 1910.

87 'Cronaca: il colera ... che non c'è!', *La Libertà*, 17 September 1910.

88 Archivio Centrale dello Stato, Ministero dell'Interno, Direzione Generale della Sanità, 1881–1915, b. 274, fasc. affari vari, Bill of health of the steamship *Santana*, 20 September 1910.

89 National Archives. Record Group 90: Records of the Public Health Service. Central File, 1897–1923, box 057, category 397. Letter of H.D. Geddings to the Surgeon-General, 25 June 1912. For De Giaxa's official positions, see Regia Università degli Studi di Napoli, *Annuario per l'anno scolastico, 1896–97* (Naples, 1897), pp. 35–37. For evidence of De Giaxa's prominence as a cholera expert, see Alessandro Lustig, 'La recente epidemia colerica e l'evoluzione igienica dell'Italia,' *La Rassegna nazionale*, 177 (1911), p. 49.

90 National Archives. Record Group 90: Records of the Public Health Service. Central File, 1897–1923, box. 054, category 397. Letter of H. D. Geddings to the Surgeon-General, 7 September 1910.

91 On the nativism and xenophobia that formed one strand of American public health policy with regard to immigrants, see Kraut, *Silent Travelers*.

92 *Ibid.*

93 National Archives. Record Group 90: Records of the Public Health Service. Central File, 1897–1923, box 054, category 397. Despatch of Geddings to Surgeon-General, 26 September 1910.

Particularly revealing was the fact that the outburst of gastro-enteritis in September 1910 attacked a different age cohort from the diarrhoeal illness that regularly decimated the population of infants and toddlers during the hot months of the summer. The outburst was also suspiciously out of phase with the mortality of infants and small children. Municipal statistics illustrate these points, dividing the population into those under and those over 5 years of age (see Appendix, Table A3).

94 *Ibid.* On the conflict between Italian denials of cholera in Naples and the views of foreign consuls.
95 National Archives. Record Group 90: Records of the Public Health Service. Central File, 1897–1923, box 954, category 397, Letter of Geddings to Surgeon-General, 26 September 1910.
96 *Ibid.*
97 *Ibid.*
98 *Ibid.*
99 Archivio Centrale dello Stato, Direzione Generale della Sanità, 1882–1915, b. 225, fasc. Affari generali e complessivi, sottofasc. Lettera dell'assessore municipale di Roma, Prof. Rossi-Doria, to Direttore Generale della Sanità, 15 September 1910.
100 Session of 26 August 1910, *Atti del consiglio comunale di Napoli*, 1910, vol. 2, pp. 100–102.
101 Giuseppe Tropeano, 'Il pericolo di Napoli', *La Propaganda*, 17–18 September 1910.
102 'Un caso sospetto al vico Zite a Forcella', *Roma*, 26 August 1910.
103 See *Roma*, 10, 11, 12, 13, 14, 15 September 1910.
104 'Scenate selvaggie in sezione Mercato', *Roma*, 10 September 1910.
105 Archivio Centrale dello Stato, Ministero dell'Interno, Direzione Generale della Sanità, 1882–1915, b. 249bis, sottofasc. Napoli: cholera 1911, Mauro Jatta, 'Profilassi per il colera di Napoli: 1911', n.d.
106 Speech of 10 December 1910, *Atti del consiglio comunale di Napoli*, 1910, vol. 2, pp. 307–308.
107 Archivio Centrale dello Stato, Ministero dell'Interno, Direzione Generale della Sanità, 1882–1915, b. 227, fasc. Napoli, sottofasc. Prov. di Napoli: Recrudescenza del colera. Telegram of De Seta to Ministero dell'Interno, Direzione Generale della Sanità, 10 September 1910, n. 9075A.
108 Archivio Centrale dello Stato. Ministero dell'Interno, Direzione Generale della Sanità, 1882–1915, b. 273, fasc. Ministero Affari Esteri: Affari Generali. Telegram of San Giuliano to S.E. Luigi Luzzatti, 18 September 1910, n. 2184.
109 For the interview with Caro, see *Il Giorno*, 12 October 1910.
110 For the text of the official communiqué announcing the disease and the case of Ernesto Vigilante, see 'Un comunicato del Governo sulle condizioni sanitarie di Napoli', *Il Giorno*, 26 September 1910. On Vigilante's activities as a criminal, see 'Dal Cotugno a San Francesco', *Roma*, 1 November 1910.
111 National Archives. Record Group 90: Records of the Public Health Service. Central File, 1897–1923, box 054, category 397. Letter of Geddings to Surgeon-General, 26 September 1910.
112 'Naples Now Admits Cholera Is There', *New York Times*, 26 September 1910.
113 *New York Times*, 28 September 1910.
114 Archivio Centrale dello Stato, Ministero dell'Interno, Direzione Generale della Sanità, 1882–1915, b. 227, fasc. Napoli, sottofasc. Napoli: recrudescenza del colera. Telegram of De Seta to S.E. Calissano, 29 September 1910, emphasis added.
115 'La situazione sanitaria in Italia', *La Tribuna*, 29 September 1910.

116 'Le migliorate condizioni della salute a Napoli', *La Libertà*, 28 September 1910.
117 'Cronaca: il morbo decresce', *La Propaganda*, 1 October 1910.
118 'La salute pubblica a Napoli', *Don Marzio*, 22–3 August 1910.
119 'Il colera non c'è!' and 'Il colera a Napoli non c'è!', *Don Marzio*, 16–17 September 1910 and 17–18 September 1910.
120 'Per certe notizie allarmanti', *Don Marzio*, 14–15 September 1910.
121 'La salute pubblica a Napoli: L'epidemia decresce rapidamente' and 'La salute pubblica a Napoli', *Don Marzio*, 28–9 September and 2–3 October 1910.
122 'La salute pubblica a Napoli', *Don Marzio*, 2–3 October 1910.
123 'La giornata di ieri al Cotugno', *Roma*, 28 September 1910.
124 'La salute pubblica: pel risanamento igienico di Napoli', *Roma*, 1 October 1910.
125 'Cronaca', *Roma*, 5 October 1910. Ciccotti wrote an open letter calling for urban renewal as the major necessity of the city. See 'Lettera aperta dell'on. Ciccotti all'on. Francesco Girardi', *Roma*, 9 October 1910.
126 Giuseppe Tropeano, 'Il colera se ne va e il fango resta', *La Propaganda*, 1–2 October 1910.
127 National Archives. Record Group 84: Records of Foreign Services Posts. Consular Posts: Naples, Italy, volume 012. Despatch of B. Duncan to John Davis, Assistant Secretary of State, 10 July 1883, n. 40.
128 For a recent study concluding that poverty was the essential 'push' factor, see Francesco Paolo Cerase, *Sotto il dominio dei borghesi: sottosviluppo ed emigrazione nell'Italia meridionale, 1860–1910* (Assisi and Rome, 1975). Cerase rightly stresses, however, that poverty itself is not an explanation but a shorthand indicating underlying social and economic structures. A discussion of the poverty that led to the decision to emigrate, and of the causes underlying that poverty, is Ercole Sori, *L'emigrazione italiana dall'Unità alla seconda guerra mondiale* (Bologna, 1979), esp. pp. 69–118.
129 National Archives. Record Group 84: Records of Foreign Service Posts. Consular Posts: Naples, Italy, Volume 012. Despatch of Edward Camphausen to Hon. Assistant Secretary of State, 24 September 1888, n. 102, p. 485.
130 On the 'new immigration', see United States Senate, 51st Congress, 3d Session, Document no. 748, *Reports of the Immigration Commission. Emigration Conditions in Europe* (Washington, 1911), esp. pp. 12–39. Immigration from Italy is discussed in part II, pp. 137–239. For an overview of the 'new immigration' to the United States, see Alan M. Kraut, *The Huddled Masses: The Immigrant in American Society, 1880–1921* (Arlington Heights, Illinois, 1882).

For official analyses of the social composition of the mass movement, see Commissariato Generale dell'Emigrazione, *L'emigrazione italiana dal 1910 al 1923* (Rome, 1926), vol. II, Table X, pp. 28–29; and Direzione Generale della Statistica e del Lavoro, *Annuario statistico italiano*, 2nd series, 1 (1911) (Rome, 1912), p. 23.
131 *Ibid.*, p. 156. For the mean monthly wages, see Appendix, Table A4.
132 Poverty was suggested by the fact that southern Italians arrived in the United States with an average of $15.38 in 1908–9; $20.94 in 1910–11; and $26.30 in 1911–12. Commissariato Generale dell'Emigrazione, *L'emigrazione italiana dal*

1910 al 1923 (Rome, 1926), vol. II, p. 22. Even these sums were frequently only a ruse, consisting of funds lent to them to confound the immigration officers, who had instructions to deny admission to paupers.

133 See Francesco Saverio Nitti, *Scritti sulla questione meridionale*, vol. IV, *Inchiesta sulle condizioni dei contadini in Basilicata e in Calabria (1910)* (Bari, 1968), part I, esp. pp. 153–206. On the concept of 'rural democracy', see p. 34.

134 On the activities of Italian immigrants after their arrival in the United States there is a vast literature. For illuminating samples, see Kraut, *The Huddled Masses*; John W. Briggs, *An Italian Passage: Immigrants to Three American Cities, 1890–1930* (New Haven, Conn., 1978); and Michael Piore, *Birds of Passage: Migrant labour and Industrial Societies* (London, 1974).

135 An informative discussion of the demand for Italian immigrants in Argentina is Consul Baker of Buenos Aires, 'Agricultural Progress in the Argentine Republic,' in United States Department of State, *Consular Reports on Commerce, Manufacture, &c.*, no. 32 (August 1883), (Washington, DC, 1883), pp. 309–330.

136 On the 'prepaid' and contract labour systems, see 'Come viene promosso l'incitamento all'emigrazione secondo una scrittrice americana', in Commissariato Generale dell'Emigrazione, *Bollettino dell'emigrazione*, 1911, pp. 337–343. See also Sori, *L'emigrazione italiana*, pp. 295–298.

137 On the role of emigration agents, see Nicola Malnate, 'Gli agenti d'emigrazione,' *La Rassegna nazionale*, 180 (1911), pp. 484–510.

138 Sori, *L'emigrazione italiana*, p. 337.

139 Reproduced in Robert F. Foerster, *The Italian Emigration of Our Time* (New York, 1969, 1st edn 1924), p. 7.

140 Interpellation of On. Arlotta, 8 March 1911, *Atti della Camera dei deputati: Sessione 1909–1911, Legislatura XXIII, Discussioni*, vol. XI, p. 13063.

141 *Ibid.*, p. 13064.

142 On the role of emigration in the Neapolitan economy, see Francesco Saverio Nitti, 'Il porto di Napoli', in F.S. Nitti *Scritti sulla questione meridionale* (Bari, 1978), vol. III, pp. 187–226.

143 Commissariato Generale dell'Emigrazione, *L'emigrazione italiana dal 1910 al 1923* (Rome, 1926), vol. I, p. 13065.

144 'La cronaca: le locande degli emigranti', *Il Mattino*, 17–18 November 1910.

145 Speech of Luigi Luzzatti, *Atti della Camera dei deputati: Sessione 1909–1911, Legislatura XXIII, Discussioni*, p. 13162.

146 The first attempts to regulate the boarding-houses of Naples are discussed in 'Le locande degli emigranti', *Roma*, 6 November 1910.

147 Archivio Centrale dello Stato. Ministero dell'Interno, Direzione Generale della Sanità, 1882–1915, b. 287 bis, fasc. Napoli. Telegram of San Giuliano to S.E. on. Luigi Luzzatti, 6 September 1910, n. 2045.

148 Archivio Centrale dello Stato. Ministero dell'Interno, Direzione Generale della Sanità, 1882–1915, b. 287 bis, fasc. Napoli. Letter of President of the Cooperative of Locandieri, Giovanni Marino, to S.E. Ministro degli Esteri, October 1910.

149 Archivio Centrale dello Stato. Ministero dell'Interno, Direzione Generale della Sanità, 1882–1915, b. 287 bis, fasc. Napoli. Telegram of Lutrario to Prefect of Naples, 1 March 1911.

150 Archivio Centrale dello Stato. Ministero dell'Interno, Direzione Generale della Sanità, 1882–1915, b. 287 bis, fasc. Napoli. Telegram of Giolitti to Prefect of Naples, 25 May 1911, n. 14979.
151 'La cronaca: le locande degli emigranti', *Il Mattino*, 17–18 November 1910.
152 Archivio Centrale dello Stato. Ministero dell'Interno, Direzione Generale della Sanità, 1882–1915, b. 287, fasc. Emigrazione: Napoli e Palermo. Letter of Di Fatta to on. Min. Int. Dir. Gen. Sanità, 28 June 1911, n. 817R.
153 Session of 7 March 1911, *Atti della Camera dei deputati: Sessione 1909–1911, Legislatura XXIII, Discussioni*, vol. II, pp. 13024–13032.
154 *Ibid.*, p. 13027.
155 Interpellation of 7 March 1911, *Atti della Camera dei deputati, Sessione 1909–1911, Legislatura XXIII, Discussioni*, vol. II, p. 13020.
156 'Cronaca: le locande degli emigranti', *Il Mattino*, 17–18 November 1910.
157 'L'agitazione di Napoli contro la tutela degli emigranti', Avanti!, 25 February 1911.
158 'La riscossa della camorra', *Avanti!*, 6 March 1911.
159 'L'agitazione di Napoli contro la tutela degli emigranti', *Avanti!*, 25 February 1911.
160 'Immigrants Sent $275,000,000 Abroad in One Year', *New York Times*, 2 October 1910.
161 *Ibid.*
162 Giovanni Rapi figured prominently in the Cuocolo murder trial. On his activities, see, 'Criminal Band that Murdered Petrosino in Police Coils', *New York Times*, 11 September 1910.
163 National Archives. Record Group 90: Records of the Public Health Service. Central File, 1897–1923, box. 037, category 219, 'A Manual for the Mental Examination of Immigrants', prepared by Officers of the Public Health Service at Ellis Island, New York Harbor, n.d.
164 On the importance of trachoma, see National Archives. Record Group 90: Records of the Public Health Service. Central File, 1897–1923, box 036, category 397, Letter of J. W. Kerr, Assistant Surgeon-General, to Surgeon-General, 4 March 1910.
165 F. Hammond, the Acting Commissioner-General of the Bureau of Immigration in Washington, explained the significance of the classification of 'poor physique'. In his words,

> A certificate of this nature implies that the alien concerned is afflicted not only but illy adapted to the work necessary to earn his bread, but also but poorly able to withstand the onslaught of disease. It means that he is undersized, poorly developed, with feeble heart action, arteries below the standard size; that he is physically degenerate, and as such not only unlikely to become a desirable citizen, but also very likely to transmit his undesirable qualities to his offspring, should he, unfortunately for the country in which he is domiciled, have any.
>
> Of all causes for rejection outside of those for dangerous, contagious, or loathsome diseases, or for mental disease, that of 'poor physique' should

receive the most weight, for in admitting such aliens not only do we increase the number of public charges …, but we admit likewise progenitors to this country whose offspring will produce, often in an exaggerated degree, the physical degeneracy of their parents. National Archives, Record Group 90: Records of the Public Health Service. Central File, 1897–1923, Box. 036, category 219, Letter of F. Hammond to Walter Wyman, Surgeon-General, n.d., n. 48,462/3.

166 National Archives. Category 90: Records of the Public Health Service. Central File, 1897–1923, box 039, category 219, William Williams, Commissioner U.S. Immigration Service, 'Notice Concerning Detention and Deportation of Immigrants', 18 March 1911.

167 The admission process at Ellis Island and the danger of rejection are discussed in Kraut, *The Huddled Masses*, ch. 2, pp. 42–73. Kraut recognizes the fear of rejection, but underestimates the real danger, viewing the anxiety as chiefly psychological.

168 Archivio Centrale dello Stato, Direzione Generale della Sanità, 1882–1915, b. 287, fasc. Emigrazione: Napoli e Palermo. Letter of Di Fatta to Ministero dell'Interno, Direzione Generale dell'Emigrazione, 28 June 1911, n. 817R.

169 United States Senate, 53d Congress, 2d Session, Ex. Doc. No. 114, *Letter from the Secretary of the Treasury, in Response to the Senate Resolution of June 12, 1894, calling for facts in regard to the padrone system in connection with Italian immigration, transmitting a report from the Superintendent of Immigration and copies of a correspondence between the Italian ambassador at Washington, the Secretary of the Treasury, and a copy of instructions issued by the Treasury Department* (Washington, DC, 1894), p. 2.

170 'Relazione sulla gestione del 1910', *Atti del consiglio generale del Banco di Napoli*, 1911, pp. 11–17.

171 For a brief outline of Sacchi's visit, see 'Cose italiane', *Civiltà cattolica*, 61:2 (1910), p. 622.

172 As an example of Del Carretto's salesmanship, see Will J. Guard, 'Much-abused Naples Finds an Ardent Champion', *New York Times*, 21 August 1910.

173 *Ibid.*

174 'Cronaca: i nuovissimi barbari', *Roma*, 19 September 1910.

175 'La salute pubblica', *Roma*, 18 September 1910.

176 For the alarm in early 1910, see Archivio Centrale dello Stato, Ministero dell'Interno, Direzione Generale della Sanità, b. 181, fasc. Rapporti degli ispettori sanitari sul colera, sottofasc. Relazione circa l'andamento del colera in Italia, p. 5, 'L'andamento del colera in Italia', n.d.

On the measures taken in Milan and Novara respectively, see Archivio Centrale dello Stato, Ministero dell'Interno, Direzione Generale della Sanità, b. 227, fasc. Milano: Rapporto sulla profilassi del colera, Medico Provinciale di Milano, 'Sulla profilassi anticolerica', 30 September 1911; and b. 227 bis, fasc. Novara: affari generali, Medico Provinciale Alessandro Prati, 'La difesa sanitaria della provincia', 23 October 1911.

177 For the measures undertaken in August, see Caro, *L'evoluzione igienica*, pp.

165–166. See also Archivio Storico del Comune di Napoli, *Deliberazioni della giunta*, August and September 1910; and the interview with Rodinò originally published in *Il Mattino*, 1 November 1910. Giulio Rodinò outlined the measures that he had authorized in his speech of 17 August 1910, *Atti del consiglio comunale di Napoli*, 1910, vol. 2, pp. 104–105.

178 Speech of 18 August 1910, *Atti del consiglio comunale di Napoli*, 1910, vol. 2, p. 104.

179 'Le condizioni sanitarie in Italia', *La Tribuna*, 27 September 1910.

180 Caro, *L'evoluzione igienica*, p. 166.

181 On the measures undertaken by the Office of Hygiene in its anti-cholera campaign, see Caro, *L'evoluzione igienica*, pp. 166–170.

182 *Ibid.*, pp. 167–168.

183 On this measure, see 'Le condizioni sanitarie in Italia', *La Tribuna*, 1 October 1910.

184 Archivio Centrale dello Stato, Direzione Generale della Sanità, 1882–1915, b. 249 bis, fasc. Napoli, sottofasc. Segnalazione prefetti provincie marittime. Telegram of Ministero dell'Interno to Prefect of Naples, 25 September 1910.

185 Archivio Centrale dello Stato, Ministero dell'Interno, Direzione Generale della Sanità, 1882–1915, b. 274, fasc. affari vari, Letter of H. Geddings to representatives of the various shipping companies, 25 September 1910.

186 National Archives. Record Group 90: Records of the Public Health Service. Central File, 1897–1923, box 054, category 397. Despatch of Henry Bordewich, Consul-General, Norway, to Hon. Secretary of State, 10 December 1910.

187 National Archives. Record Group 90: Records of the Public Health Service. Central File, 1897–1923, box 054, category 397. Despatch of H. Geddings to Stuart J. Fuller, 30 December 1910.

188 The absence of the autumnal session is evident from the *Atti del consiglio comunale di Napoli*. On 10 December the opposition presented a motion protesting. *Ibid.*, 1910, vol. 2, p. 293.

189 See the speech of 20 February 1911 by Councillor Palomba, *Atti del consiglio comunale di Napoli*, 1911, vol. 1, p. 380.

190 'La salute pubblica: la recrudescenza del morbo', *Roma*, 24 September 1910. In the original, the word that I have translated as disease was 'snake' (*serpe*). The snake metaphor, however, fails completely in translation.

191 Archivio Centrale dello Stato, Ministero dell'Interno, Direzione Generale della Sanità, 1882–1915, b. 275, fasc. Ministero Guerra. Letter of Tenente Generale Medico Ispettore Capo, Ispettorato di Sanità Militare to Direzione Generale della Sanità Pubblica, 2 December 1910, n. 87/R.P.

192 On the desertion by the steamship companies, see 'Cholera is Keeping Liners from Naples', *New York Times*, 29 September 1910.

193 'Cronaca contemporanea: cose italiane', *Civiltà cattolica*, 62:3 (1911), pp. 374–375.

194 'Uno stato di cose intollerabile: l'agitazione dei locandieri', *Il Mattino*, 13–14 November 1911.

195 Edward Marshall, ' "Little Now in Cholera to Be Afraid of" Says Dr. Doty', *New York Times*, 16 October 1910.

196 'Le locande degli emigranti', *Roma*, 11 November 1910.

197 F.S. Nitti, speech of 9 March 1911, *Atti della camera dei deputati: Sessione 1909–1911, Legislatura XXIII, Discussioni*, vol. XI, p. 13102.

198 Speech of 10 March 1911, *Atti della camera dei deputati: Sessione 1909–1911, Legislatura XXIII, Discussioni*, vol. XI, p. 13160.

199 On Luzzatti's role as *rapporteur* for the emigration law of 1901, see 'Camera dei Deputati: Sull'emigrazione. Relazione della commissione sul disegno di legge presentato dal ministro degli affari esteri (Visconti-Venosta)', seduta del 3 luglio 1900. *Atti del parlamento italiano. Raccolta degli atti stampati per ordine della Camera. Legislatura XXI, Sessione 1900–1902*, II, n. 44 and 44 bis.

200 Commissariato Generale dell'Emigrazione, *L'emigrazione italiana dal 1910 al 1923* (Rome, 1926), vol. I, p. 660.

201 On the protest by the *locandieri*, see 'Cronaca: il comizio dei locandieri all'Umberto', *Roma*, 14 November 1910; 'Uno stato di cose intollerabile: l'agitazione dei locandieri', *Il Mattino*, 13–14 November 1910; and 'Cronaca: continua l'agitazione dei locandieri', *Il Mattino*, 14–15 November 1910.

202 On Striano's dubious background, see 'La riscossa della camorra', *Avanti!*, 6 March 1911.

203 'La cronaca: continua l'agitazione dei locandieri', *Il Mattino*, 14–15 November 1910.

204 Speech of 3 March 1911, *Atti del consiglio comunale di Napoli*, 1911, vol. 1, pp. 437–438.

205 On the bankruptcies in Naples in February, see 'Le condizioni sanitarie di Napoli e la diffamazione', *Osservatore romano*, 21 February 1911.

206 'Napoli contro i suoi diffamatori', *Il Mattino*, 16–17 February 1911.

207 'La campagna denigratoria contro la salute pubblica in Italia,' *Giornale d'Italia*, 10 March 1911. On the medical activities of Geddings, see Archivio Centrale dello Stato, Ministero dell'Interno, Direzione Generale della Sanità, 1882–1915, b. 273, fasc. Ministero Affari Esteri: affari generali, sottofasc. False notizie all'estero sullo stato sanitario. Letter of Prefect of Palermo to On. Ministero Interno, 1 February 1911, n. 4749.

208 'Italian Cholera Lingers', *New York Times*, 29 January 1911.

209 For a mention of the role of Orazio Caro in the Association, see 'Napoli gode la sua vittoria', *Osservatore romano*, 27 February 1911.

210 On the agitation in Naples, see 'Note di vita napoletana', *Avanti!*, 2 January 1911; 'Una grande agitazione a Napoli contro i padroni di casa', *Avanti!*, 11 January 1911; 'A Napoli', *Avanti!*, 21 January 1911; and 'Il problema delle pigioni a Napoli', *Avanti!*, 27 February 1911.

211 'Il comizio di iersera al Vasto', *Roma*, 22 January 1911.

212 On the position of Palomba, see 'La riscossa della camorra', *Avanti!*, 6 March 1911.

213 On Tropeano's views, see 'Il comizio di ieri contro il caro delle pigioni', *Roma*, 16 January 1911.

214 'La cronaca: per la vita e la salvezza del Porto', *Il Mattino*, 22–3 February 1911. See also 'Napoli proclama la serrata generale per protestare contro il Governo', *Giornale d'Italia*, 25 February 1911.

215 'Napoli si difende contro la morte', *Il Mattino*, 24–5 February 1911.

216 Quoted in 'La cronaca', *Il Mattino*, 24–5 February 1911. For Palomba's business associations, see 'La riscossa della camorra', *Avanti!*, 6 March 1911.

217 'La cronaca: il ricatto a Napoli', *Il Mattino*, 6–7 July 1911.

218 Archivio Centrale dello Stato, Direzione Generale della Sanità, 1882–1915, b. 287 bis, fasc. Napoli. Letter of Giovanni Marino to S.E. Ministro degli Esteri, October 1910.

219 'Il fenomeno Geddings al Consiglio Comunale e alla Camera di Commercio', *Il Mattino*, 18–19 February 1911.

220 Speech of 17 February 1911, *Atti del consiglio comunale di Napoli*, 1911, vol. 1, p. 344.

221 On the award to Geddings, see House of Representatives, 57th Congress, 1st Session, Report no. 174, *Dr. Eugene Wasdin and Dr. H. D. Geddings* (Washington, DC, 1902).

222 Archivio Centrale dello Stato, Ministero dell'Interno, Direzione Generale della Sanità, 1882–1915, b. 273, fasc. Ministero Affari Esteri: affari generali, sottofasc. False notizie all'estero sullo stato sanitario. Letter of February 1911.

223 'Il fenomeno Geddings al Consiglio Comunale e alla Camera di Commercio', *Il Mattino*, 18–19 February 1911.

224 'Come si svolge il grande e violento movimento', *Il Mattino*, 25–6 February 1911.

225 *Atti del consiglio comunale di Napoli*, 1911, vol. 1, pp. 386–387.

226 *Ibid.*, pp. 387–388.

227 See session of 24 February 1911, *Atti del consiglio comunale di Napoli*, 1911, vol. 1, pp. 386ff.

228 *Ibid.*, pp. 388–389.

229 On the events at Taranto, see 'Da Taranto', *Corriere della sera*, 31 December 1910; 'Un eccidio a Taranto', *Avanti!*, 1 January 1911, 'La verità sui fatti di Taranto', *Avanti!*, 4 January 1911; 'Gravi tumulti a Taranto', *Il Mattino*, 1–2 January 1911; 'Dopo i fatti di Taranto', *Il Mattino*, 5–6 January 1911; and 'Sanguinosi disordini a Taranto', *Corriere della sera*, 4 January 1911.

230 On the meeting in Rome, see 'Napoli si difende contro la morte', *Il Mattino*, 24–5 February 1911.

231 'Napoli ha vinto la sua battaglia', *Il Mattino*, 26–7 February 1911.

232 'La Camera con 173 voti di maggioranza rinnova la fiducia nel Gabinetto Luzzatti', *Corriere della sera*, 3 February 1911. The threat to the ministry was greater than the final tally of votes suggests.

233 'La riscossa della camorra', *Avanti!*, 6 March 1911.

234 For the parliamentary record of the discussion of emigration and public health, see sessions of 7 to 10 March 1911, *Atti della Camera dei deputati: Sessione 1909–1911, Legislatura XXIII, Discussioni*, vol. XI, pp. 13012–13170.

235 'L'emigrazione e il porto di Napoli alla Camera', *Corriere della sera*, 9 March 1911; and 'I discorsi di Luzzatti e Di San Giuliano alla Camera,' *Corriere della sera*, 11 March 1911.

236 For the text of Turati's intervention, see *Atti della Camera dei deputati: Sessione 1909–1911, Discussisoni*, vol. XI, pp. 13016–13023.

237 'La grande discussione per Napoli alla Camera', *Giornale d'Italia*, 8 March 1911.

238 'La questione degli emigranti trattata dall'on. Nitti alla Camera', *Corriere della sera*, 10 March 1911.

239 On the discussion in the Chamber on 10 March, see 'I discorsi di Luzzatti e Di San Giuliano all Camera', *Corriere della sera*, 11 March 1911.

CHAPTER 7: CONCEALMENT AND CRISIS: 1911

1 In February 1911 Geddings wrote to Wyman recalling his earlier confidential reports and protesting at the use that Wyman had made of them publicly. My account here is primarily based on this February despatch. See National Archives. Record Group 90: Records of the Public Health Service. Central File, 1897–1923, category 397, box 055. Despatch of H.D. Geddings to Surgeon-General Wyman, 14 February 1911. See also *Annual Report of the Surgeon General of the Public Health Service of the United States for the Fiscal Year 1911* (Washington, 1912), p. 98.

2 For an English-language version of Cusani's protest, see National Archives. Record Group 90: Records of the Public Health Service. Central File, 1897–1923, category 397, box 055. Letter of Ambassador Cusani to Hon. P.C. Knox, Secretary of State, 2 February 1911.

3 For the daily bulletins kept by the Department of Health with regard to all reported cases of Asiatic cholera and deaths for the whole of 1911, see Archivio Centrale dello Stato, Direzione Generale della Sanità, 1882–1915, b. 178 bis. The file is organized by bundles or 'fascicoli', one for each month.

4 From the safe distance of 1926, the Commissariat of Emigration confirmed the existence of Asiatic cholera in the spring of 1911. Commissariato Generale dell-'Emigrazione, *L'emigrazione italiana dal 1910 al 1923* (Rome, 1926), vol. I, p. 660.

5 Archivio Centrale dello Stato. Ministero dell'Interno, Direzione Generale della Sanità, 1882–1915, b. 250, fasc. Napoli, sottofasc. Torre Annunziata. Telegram of Lutrario to Prefect of Naples, 16 July 1911, n. 19741.

6 Archivio Centrale dello Stato. Ministero dell'Interno, Direzione Generale della Sanità, 1882–1915, b. 250, fasc. Napoli, sottofasc. Torre Annunziata. Telegram of Director-General of Public Health to Prefect of Naples, 16 July 1911.

7 Archivio Centrale dello Stato. Ministero dell'Interno, Direzione Generale della Sanità, 1882–1915, b. 226, fasc. Cagliari, sottofasc. Relazione sull'epidemia colerica. Report of prefect of Cagliari, 'Epidemia colerica', 4 November 1912, n. 1174.

8 Archivio Centrale dello Stato. Ministero dell'Interno, Direzione Generale della Sanità, 1882–1915, b. 275, fasc. Ministero Agricoltura, Industria e Commercio; Statistiche sul cholera, anni 1910 e 1911. Letter of Minister of Agriculture, Industry and Commerce to His Excellency the Minister of the Interior, 1 February 1912, n. 127.

9 Archivio Centrale dello Stato. Ministero dell'Interno, Direzione Generale della Sanità, 1882–1915, b. 275, fasc. Ministero Agricoltura, Industria e Commercio: Statistiche sul cholera, anni 1910 e 1911. Letter of Minister of Agriculture, Industry and Commerce to Director-General of Public Health, 8 January 1912, n. 21.

10 National Archive. Record Group 90: Records of the Public Health Service, Central

File, 1897–1923, category 397, box 056. Letter of H. Geddings to Surgeon-General, 30 October 1911.

11 Archivio Centrale dello Stato. Ministero dell'Interno, Direzione Generale della Sanità, 1882–1915, b. 250, fasc. Napoli, sottofasc. Pianura. Tel. of Ministero dell'Interno to Prefect of Naples, 6 May 1911.

12 *Annual Report of the Surgeon General of the Public Health and Marine Hospital Service of the United States for the Fiscal Year 1911* (Washington, 1912), esp. p. 97.

13 National Archive. Record Group 90: Records of the Public Health Service. Central File, 1897 to 1927, box 055. Despatch of W. W. King to Hon. John G.A. Leishman, Ambassador, 14 June 1911.

14 'La cronaca: il ricatto di Napoli', *Il Mattino*, 6–7 July 1911.

15 Archivio Centrale dello Stato. Ministero dell'Interno, Direzione Generale della Sanità, 1882–1915, b. 250, fasc. Napoli, sottofasc. Gragnano. Telegram of Prefect Ferri to Ministero dell'Interno, Direzione Generale della Sanità, 11 July 1911, n. 3654.

16 'La cronaca: il ricatto a Napoli', *Il Mattino*, 6–7 July 1911.

17 'Napoli protesta compatta contro lo strangolamento del suo porto', *Il Mattino*, 15–16 July 1911; 'L'Assemblea delle leghe portuali proclama la serrata generale del Porto', *Il Mattino*, 18–19 July 1911; 'La serrata generale è proclamata dalle leghe per venerdí mattina', *Il Mattino*, 20–1 July 1911; and 'La dignitosa e calma protesta di Napoli contro il governo', *Il Mattino*, 21–2 July 1911.

18 See National Archives. Record Group 90: Records of the Public Health Service. Central File, 1897–1923, box 055. Despatch of Ambassador John. G. Leishman to the Hon. the Secretary of State, 14 June 1911.

19 An English-language version of the text of the Convention was provided by H.D. Geddings to the American Government. See Henry Downes Geddings, 'Report of the International Sanitary Conference, Paris, 1903' (Unpublished MS, National Library of Medicine, History of Medicine Section, Washington, DC), p. 49.

20 *Ibid.*, p. 23.

21 *Ibid.*, pp. 49–50.

22 *Ibid.*, p. 24.

23 On the actual preventive measures taken at Naples under supervision by the United States Public Health and Marine Hospital Service from June 1911, see National Archives. Record Group 90: Records of the Public Health Service. Central File, 1897–1923, box 055. Letter of W. W. King to the Surgeon-General, 24 June 1911.

24 The duties imposed on the masters of ships by the U.S. Quarantine Regulations are outlined in *Annual Report of the Public Health and Marine Hospital Service of the United States for the Fiscal Year 1910* (Washington, 1911), pp. 89–90.

25 On employment restrictions affecting Italians in the United States in the summer of 1911, see National Archives. Record Group 90: Records of the Public Health Service. Central File, 1897–1923, box 055. Letter of Eugene P. King, Superintendent of Health, Providence, R.I., to Walter Wyman, 21 July 1921.

The immigrant destination cards are discussed by National Archives. Record Group 90: Records of the Public Health Service. Central File, 1897–1923, box 055.

Eugene H. Porter, Commissioner of Health, Albany, N.Y. to Walter Wyman, 19 July 1911.

26 For the American report on the Convention, see H. Geddings, MS.

27 On the role of central government in public health, see National Archives. Record Group 90: Records of the Public Health Service. Central File, 1897–1923, box 055. Letter of W.W. King to John G. Leishman, 14 June 1911.

This centralizing decision by the Italian prime minister represented one of the implications of the discrediting in the international medical community of Pettenkofer's localist theories since the decisive vindication of Koch's approach during the Hamburg–Altoona epidemic of 1892–1893. The Bavarian hygienist's approach to cholera had buttressed the authority of local officials in combating the disease because only they rather than central government possessed the detailed knowledge of the local subsoil ecology on which he insisted. Koch's methodology, in which the laboratory replaced local knowledge, provided the rationale for the Department of Public Health to replace City Hall as the directing centre of the campaign.

28 Archivio Centrale dello Stato. Ministero dell'Interno, Direzione Generale della Sanità, 1882–1915, b. 227, fasc. Napoli. Telegram of Giolitti to Prefect of Naples, 13 May 1911, n. 13816.

29 Archivio Centrale dello Stato. Ministero dell'Interno, Direzione Generale della Sanità, 1882–1915, b. 227, fasc. Napoli. Telegram of Giolitti to Prefect of Naples, 20 May 1911, n. 14343.

30 See, for example, 'Un ricatto a Napoli', *Osservatore romano*, 6 July 1911; and 'Polemiche sanitarie', *Osservatore romano*, 18 July 1911.

31 'Salus publica . . .', *Osservatore romano*, 20 August 1911.

32 See for instance 'Salus publica . . .', *Osservatore romano*, 20 August 1911; 'La salute pubblica a Livorno', *Osservatore romano*; and 'Le non liete condizioni sanitarie di alcune parti d'Italia', *Osservatore romano*, 22 August 1911; 'Cronaca italiana', *Osservatore romano*, 24 August 1911; 'L'epidemia colerica', *Osservatore romano*, 25 August 1911; and 'La salute pubblica in Italia', *Osservatore romano*, 26 August 1911.

33 'I delitti delle follie collettive', *Osservatore romano*, 29 August 1911.

34 For instances of the more militant position that began on 29 August, see 'I delitti delle follie collettive', *Osservatore romano*, 30 August 1911; 'La giornata rossa di Verbicaro', *Osservatore romano*, 30 August 1911; 'La salute pubblica e le responsabilità del Governo', *Osservatore romano*, 3 September 1911.

The Jesuit journal *Civiltà cattolica* also gave explicit attention to the cholera epidemic and the state policy of concealment. See, for example, 'Cronaca contemporanea', *Civiltà cattolica*, 62:3 (1911), pp. 234, and 374–375.

35 See 'Italy', *Lancet* (1911, vol. 1), p. 736; 'Italy: The Cholera Epidemic', *Lancet* (1911, vol. 2), p. 729; 'Cholera in Italy', *Lancet* (1911, vol. 2), p. 854; and 'Italy: The Cholera Epidemic in Italy', *Lancet* (1911, vol. 2), p. 861.

The *British Medical Journal* was tardier in its coverage of Italian events in 1911, publishing its first definite report of the epidemic in its issue of 16 September. See 'Cholera in Italy', *British Medical Journal* (1911, vol. 2), p. 631.

36 '*Annus Medicus*', *Lancet* (1911, vol. 2), p. 1856. According to this report, Italy suffered 15,459 cases and 5,757 deaths in forty-nine provinces.

37 On the 'yarns' in circulation, see 'Fifth Cholera Death from Liner Moltke', *New York Times*, 17 July 1911. On the cholera-scares at Auburn, Brooklyn and Staten Island, see 'Asiatic Cholera Startles Auburn', *New York Herald*, 2 July 1911; 'Federal Officials Confer on Cholera', *New York Herald*, 4 July 1911; and 'Asiatic Cholera Victim Dies at Hoffman Island', *New York Herald*, 16 July 1911.

38 For the early recognition that cholera was present in Italy, see 'Cholera Spreads to France', *New York Times*, 14 July 1911; 'Two More Die of Cholera', *New York Times*, 15 July 1911; 'Fifth Cholera Death from Liner Moltke', *New York Times*, 17 July 1911; 'Cholera Kills Boy; Eighth Death Here', *New York Times*, 18 July 1911; and 'Tenth Victim Dies of Cholera Here', *New York Times* 21 July 1911.

39 '2,300 Dead from Cholera', *New York Times*, 17 July 1911.

40 'Fifth Cholera Death from Liner Moltke', *New York Times*, 17 July 1911.

41 See, for example, the articles 'Cholera Has Killed over 30,000 in Italy', *New York Times*, 6 September 1911; 'Storm and Burn Cholera Hospitals', *New York Times*, 10 September 1911; and 'Frenzied Mob Frees Cholera Patients', *New York Times*, 17 October 1911.

42 For the letters suggesting cures for cholera, see Archivio Centrale dello Stato, Ministero dell'Interno, Direzione Generale della Sanità, 1882–1915, b. 277, fasc. Specifici anticolerici.

43 'I gravissimi fatti di Verbicaro pel colera', *Roma*, 29 August 1911.

44 *Ibid.*

45 *Ibid.*

46 Interpellation of Elefante, 17 July 1911, *Atti del consiglio comunale di Napoli*, 1911, vol. 2, p. 145.

47 Speech of 17 July 1911. *Atti del consiglio comunale di Napoli*, 1911, vol. 2, pp. 148–149.

48 For the record of the deliberations of the executive committee, see Archivio Storico del Comune di Napoli. Atti della Giunta Municipale, 1911.

49 See for example Archivio Storico del Comune di Napoli. Deliberazioni della Giunta Municipale, 1911. 'Estratto di deliberazione presa dalla Giunta Comunale nella tornata del 1 luglio 1911', n. 14.

50 Archivio Storico del Comune di Napoli. Deliberazioni della Giunta Municipale di Napoli, 1911. On the Maddalena barracks and the New Castle, see especially 'Deliberazione presa dalla Giunta Comunale nella tornata del dí 3 giugno 1911', n. 66.

51 Archivio Storico del Comune di Napoli. Deliberazioni della Giunta Municipale, 1911. 'Deliberazione presa dalla Giunta Comunale nella tornata del dí 3 giugno 1911', n. 66.

52 Archivio Storico del Comune di Napoli. Deliberazioni della Giunta Municipale, 1911, 'Deliberazione presa dalla Giunta comunale nella tornata del 6 giugno 1911', p. 2.

53 Archivio Storico del Comune di Napoli. Deliberazioni della Giunta Municipale di Napoli, 1911, 'Estratto di deliberazione presa dalla Giunta Comunale nella tornata de dí 6 giugno 1911', n. 18.

54 Archivio Storico del Comune di Napoli, Deliberazioni della Giunta Municipale, 1911, 'Estratto di deliberazione presa dalla Giunta Comunale nella tornata de dí 10 giugno 1911'.

55 Archivio Storico del Comune di Napoli. Deliberazioni della Giunta Municipale, 1911, 'Deliberazione presa dalla Giunta Comunale nella tornata de dí 17 giugno 1911', n. 37; and 'Estratto di deliberazione presa dalla Giunta Comunale nella tornata del 21 giugno', n. 57.

56 Archivio Storico del Comune di Napoli. Atti della Giunta Municipale di Napoli, Ottobre 1911, 'Deliberazione presa nella tornata del 17 ottobre 1911', n. 54. The word 'cholera' is used on a limited number of other occasions during the six months beginning in May 1911, but always with reference to 1910.

57 See Ospedale Domenico Cotugno. Cartelle mediche, 1910 and 1911.

58 Archivio Storico del Comune di Napoli. Deliberazioni della Giunta Municipale, 1911, 'Deliberazione presa dalla Giunta Comunale nella tornata de dí 21 giugno 1911, n. 48.

59 Archivio Storico del Comune di Napoli. Deliberazioni della Giunta Municipale, 1911. Report of Giulio Rodinò, 21 June 1911, n. 8432.

60 Archivio Storico del Comune di Napoli. Deliberazioni della Giunta Municipale, 1911. Report of Giulio Rodinò, 23 June 1911.

61 Archivio Storico del Comune di Napoli. Deliberazioni della Giunta Municipale, 1911. 'Estratto di deliberazione presa dalla Giunta Comunale nella tornata del 21 giugno', n. 57.

62 See above, Chapter 6.

63 Cimitero della Pietà, Naples. Registro, 1884: colerosi, 17 agosto a 15 novembre 1884.

64 Cimitero della Pietà, Naples. Registro, 1910 and 1911.

65 Alfonso Montefusco, *Clinica e terapia delle malattie acute* (Naples, 1912).

66 *Ibid.*, p. 55.

67 See 'Atti della Camera: sulla sistematica denigrazione sanitaria dell'Italia', *Giornale della Reale Società d'Igiene*, 33 (1911), pp. 126–127; and 'Cose d'attualità: le condizioni sanitarie del nostro paese', *ibid.*, pp. 410–411.

68 'Alcune osservazioni sulla recente epidemia colerica di Livorno (Luglio–Settembre 1911)', *Rivista critica di clinica medica*, 12 (1911), pp. 657–663.

69 As a medium of refrigeration, Neapolitans relied not on ice but rather on the purchase of packed snow. The American consul described the method by which the ice was acquired and transported to the city. 'During the coldest part of the winter,' he wrote, 'holes are dug on the mountains at an elevation of about 2500 or 3000 feet above the level of the sea. These holes are filled with snow, packed down as solid as possible and covered with the leaves of the chestnut tree to a sufficient height to protect the snow against rain etc. From these holes the snow is packed in straw mats or baskets, transported on mule or donkies [*sic*] to the nearest Railroad station and thence to the cities. The supply for Naples is brought from Monte S. Angelo about 16 miles from Naples' (National Archives. Record Group 84: Records of Foreign Service Posts. Consular Posts: Naples, Italy, volume 012. Despatch of Edward Camphausen to Hon. W.F. Wharton, Assistant Secretary of State, 21 January 1890, n. 139, p. 540).

70 National Archives. Record Group 90: Records of the Public Health Service. Central File, 1897–1923, box 057. Despatch of H.D. Geddings to Surgeon-General, 18 May 1912.

71 On the illnesses aboard the *SS Berlin*, see National Archive. Record Group 90: Records of the Public Health Service. Central File, 1897–1923, category 397, box 056. Despatch of H. Geddings to Surgeon-General, 8 August 1911.

72 On the cholera scare that followed the docking of the *Moltke*, see 'Fifth Cholera Death from Liner Moltke', and 'Tenth Victim Dies of Cholera Here', *New York Times*, 17 and 21 July 1911.

73 *Annual Report of the Surgeon General of the Public Health Service of the United States for the Fiscal Year 1912* (Washington, DC, 1913), pp. 189–190.

74 National Archives. Record Group 90: Records of the Public Health Service. Central File, 1897–1923, category 397, box 057. Despatch of George W. Stoner, 12 February 1912.

75 *Ibid.*

76 On the events surrounding the *Duca degli Abruzzi*, see National Archives. Record Group 90: Records of the Public Health Service. Central File, 1897–1923, box 055. Letter of John D. Anderson, Director, Office of Hygienic Laboratory, USPH&MHS to Surgeon-General, 29 July 1911 and letter of Edward Frances, Assistant Director, Office of Hygienic Laboratory, to Surgeon-General, 18 July 1911. On the outbreak at Auburn, see also 'To Watch Cholera Cases', *New York Times*, 3 July 1911.

77 Archivio Centrale Dello Stato. Ministero dell'Interno, Direzione Generale della Sanità, 1882–1915, b. 251, fasc. Palermo, sottofasc. Palermo: cholera. Telegram of Prefect Rovasenda to Min. Int. Sanità, 21 May 1911, n. 5804A; and Telegram of Prefect Rovasenda to Min. Int. Sanità, 23 May, n. 5952A.

78 'Come non si difese Palermo', *L'Ora*, 2–3 February 1912.

79 Archivio Centrale dello Stato. Ministero dell'Interno, Direzione Generale della Sanità, b. 181, fasc. Rapporti degli Ispettori sanitari sul colera, sottofasc. Palermo: Rapporto Ispettore Barile. Report of Ispettore di sanità Barile, 'Epidemia di colera: città e provincia di Palermo', 30 September 1911, p. 2.

80 National Archives. Record Group 90: Records of the Public Health Service. Central File, 1897–1923, box 055. Letter of Hernando de Soto to the Hon. Secretary of State, 26 June 1911.

81 The events at Palermo are discussed by an anonymous surgeon of the United States Public Health and Marine Hospital Service in an official report. See National Archives. Record Group 90: Reports of the Public Health Service. Central File, 1897–1923, box 055. 'Sanitary Conditions in Naples and Palermo, Italy', n.d.

82 National Archives. Record Group 90: Records of the Public Health Service. Central File, 1897–1923, box 055. Letter of Hernando de Soto to Hon. Secretary of State, 26 June 1911, n. 39.

83 On the date of the arrival of the *Berlin* as a turning point, see National Archives. Record Group 90: Records of the Public Health Service. Central File, 1897–1923, box 057. Report of H.D. Geddings to Surgeon-General, 29 May 1912.

84 Commissariato Generale dell'Emigrazione, *L'emigrazione italiana dal 1910 al 1923* (Rome, 1926), vol. I, p. 663.

85 *Ibid.*, pp. 663–664.

86 *Ibid.*, p. 664.

87 National Archives. Record Group 90: Records of the Public Health Service. Central

File, 1897–1923, box 055. Despatch of John G.A. Leishman to the Hon. Secretary of State, 14 June 1911.

88 National Archives. Record Group 90: Records of the Public Health Service. Central File, 1897 to 1923, box 055. Telegram to the American Ambassador, 21 June 1911.

89 *Annual Report of the Surgeon General of the Public Health Service of the United States for the Fiscal Year 1912* (Washington, DC, 1913), p. 190.

90 Archivio Centrale dello Stato. Ministero dell'Interno, Direzione Generale della Sanità, 1882–1915, b. 275, fasc. Ministero Agricoltura Industria e Commercio, sottofasc. Statistiche sul cholera anni 1910 e 1911, 'Numero di morti per colera nel 1911'.

91 For the published official Italian statistics concerning the 1911 epidemic, see Direzione Generale della Statistica e del Lavoro: Ufficio Centrale di Statistica, *Statistica delle cause di morte nell' anno 1911* (Rome, 1913), Table 1, pp. 2–31.

92 National Archives. Record Group 90: Records of the Public Health Service, Central File, 1897 to 1923, category 397, box 055. Letter of Secretary of State Knox to Secretary of the Treasury, 20 June 1911.

93 National Archives. Record Group 90: Records of the Public Health Service, Central File, 1897 to 1923, category 397, box 055. Letter of Hernando de Soto to the Hon. Secretary of State, 26 June 1911, n. 39.

94 National Archives. Record Group 90: Records of the Public Health Service, Central File, 1897–1923, category 397, box 056. Report of Consul-General James Smith, 'Sanitary Conditions at Genoa and Elsewhere in Italy', 19 July 1911.

95 National Archives. Record Group 90: Records of the Public Health Service, Central File, 1897–1923, category 397, box 056. Despatch of H. Geddings to Surgeon-General, 8 August 1911.

96 National Archives. Record Group 90: Records of the Public Health Service, Central File, 1897–1923, category 397, box 056. Report of H. Geddings to Surgeon-General, 2 August 1911.

97 Archivio Centrale dello Stato. Ministero dell'Interno, Direzione Generale della Sanità, 1882–1915, b. 226, fasc. Cagliari, sottofasc. Relazione sull'epidemia colerica. Report of Prefect of Cagliari, 'Epidemia colerica', 4 November 1912, n. 1174.

98 Archivio Centrale dello Stato. Ministero dell'Interno, Direzione Generale della Sanità, 1882–1915, b. 275, fasc. Ministero di Agricoltura Industria e Commercio, sottofasc. Statistiche sul colera anni 1910 e 1911. 'Numero di morti per colera nel 1911'.

99 Archivio Centrale dello Stato. Ministero dell'Interno, Direzione Generale della Sanità, 1882–1915, b. 228, fasc. Venezia. Professor Giordano, 'Il colera a Venezia nel 1911', December 1911.

100 Archivio Centrale dello Stato. Ministero dell'Interno, Direzione Generale della Sanità, 1882–1915, b. 225, fasc. Aquila: Rapporti del prefetto. Pietro Pellegrini, 'Relazione sulla epidemia di colera nella Provincia di Aquila', 14 November 1911.

101 Archivio Centrale dello Stato. Direzione Generale della Sanità, 1882–1915, b. 226, fasc. Forlí: Relazione sull'epidemia colerica del 1911. Leonardo Caravaggi, 'Il colera nella provincia di Forlí (estate-autunno 1911): relazione epidemiologica', 1912.

102 Archivio Centrale dello Stato. Ministero dell'Interno, Direzione Generale della Sanità, 1882–1915, b. 227, fasc. Massa e Carrara. Dr. Cucchia, 'Relazione sul colera, anno 1911', n.d.

103 Archivio Centrale dello Stato. Ministero dell'Interno, Direzione Generale della Sanità, 1882–1915, b. 275, fasc. Ministero Agricoltura Industria e Commercio, sottofasc. Statistiche sul colera anni 1910 e 1911. 'Numero di morti per colera nel 1911'.

104 Archivio Centrale dello Stato. Ministero dell'Interno, Direzione Generale della Sanità, 1882–1915, b. 181, fasc. Rapporti degli Ispettori sanitari sul colera, sottofasc. Rapporto Ispettore Barile. Inspector Barile, 'Epidemia di colera: città e provincia di Palermo', 30 September 1911.

105 Archivio Centrale dello Stato. Ministero dell'Interno, Direzione Generale della Sanità, 1882–1915, b. 275, fasc. Ministero Agricoltura Industria e Commercio, sottofasc. Statistiche sul colera anni 1910 e 1911, 'Numero di morti per colera nel 1911'.

The official number of deaths by province from Asiatic cholera in 1911 is presented in the Appendix (Table A6).

106 Archivio Centrale dello Stato. Ministero dell'Interno, Direzione Generale della Sanità, 1882–1915, b. 177 bis, fasc. Napoli e provincia: cholera 1911. Ufficiale sanitario, 'Casi e decessi di colera nell'anno 1911 a Napoli', 19 September 1911.

107 Archivio Centrale dello Stato. Ministero dell'Interno, Direzione Generale della Sanità, 1882–1915, b. 177 bis, fasc. Napoli e provincia: cholera 1911. 'Mortalità Generale del Comune di Napoli'.

108 Archivio Centrale dello Stato. Ministero dell'Interno, Direzione Generale della Sanità, 1882–1915, b. 177 bis, fasc. Napoli e provincia: cholera 1911. Letter of Orazio Caro to Comm. Messea, 20 August 1911.

109 *Ibid.*

110 Archivio Centrale dello Stato. Ministero dell'Interno, Direzione Generale della Sanità, 1881–1915, b. 275, fasc. Ministero Guerra. Letter of Tenente Generale Medico Ispettore Capo, Ispettorato di Sanità Militare to Direzione Generale della Sanità Pubblica, 2 December 1910, n. 87/R.P.

111 'Storm and Burn Cholera Hospitals', *New York Times*, 10 September 1911. See also the article 'Cholera Has Killed over 30,000 in Italy', *New York Times*, 6 September 1911.

112 Speech of 17 February 1911, *Atti del consiglio comunale di Napoli*, 1911, vol. 1, p. 344.

113 National Archives. Record Group 90: Records of the Public Health Service. Central file, 1898–1923, category 397, box 055. Letter of Frank MacNeal to Dr. Wyman, 11 February 1911.

114 National Archives. Record Group 90: Records of the Public Health Service. Central File, 1898–1923, category 397, box 055. Telegram of Wyman to Geddings, 6 February 1911.

115 National Archives. Record Group 90: Records of the Public Health Service, Central File, 1897–1923, category 397, box 056. Letter of H. Geddings to Surgeon-General, 30 October 1911.

116 For the text of the letter, see National Archives. Record Group 90: Records of the

Public Health Service, Central File, 1898–1923, category 397, box 056. Report of H. Geddings to Surgeon-General, 2 August 1911. For a report on the threat to Buonocore's life, see 'Dopo la vittoria di Napoli', *Osservatore romano*, 23 July 1911.

117 *Ibid.*

118 See, for example, 'Un tentativo di serrata e di sciopero generale a Napoli', *La Tribuna*, 22 July 1911.

119 *Ibid.*

120 Archivio Centrale dello Stato. Ministero dell'Interno, Direzione Generale della Sanità, 1882–1915, b. 273, fasc. Ministero Affari Esteri: vari, sottofasc. Francia. Telegram of Prefect of Arezzo to Ministero dell'Interno, 15 August 1911, n. 14889.

121 Archivio Centrale dello Stato. Ministero dell'Interno, Direzione Generale della Sanità, 1882–1915, b. 278, fasc. Condizioni sanitarie del regno. Telegram of Averna to Min. Int., Sanità, 5 June 1911, n. 6777.

122 Archivio Centrale dello Stato. Ministero dell'Interno, Direzione Generale della Sanità, 1882–1915, b. 273, fasc. Ministero Affari Esteri: vari, sottofasc. Francia. Telegram of Di Scalea to Min. Int. Dir. Gen. Sanità Pubblica, 13 August 1911, n. 1940.

123 National Archives. Record Group 90: Records of the Public Health Service, Central File, 1897–1923, category 397, box 055. Letter of Surgeon-General W. Wyman to Dr. C. O. Probst, 7 August 1911.

On cholera deaths in Marseilles in August, see National Archives. Record Group 90: Records of the Public Health Service, Central File, 1897–1923, category 397, box 056. Despatch of Consul-General A. Gaulin to Secretary of State, 14 September 1911. For the week ending 23 September 1911, the USPH&MHS received information that there were 41 cases and 26 deaths in Marseilles from Asiatic cholera. National Archives. Record Group 90: Records of the Public Health Service, Central File, 1897–1923, category 397, box 056. Despatch of Surgeon J.M. Eager to the Surgeon-General, 25 September 1911.

124 Archivio Centrale dello Stato, Direzione Generale della Sanità, 1882–1915, b. 273, fasc. Ministero Affari Esteri: vari, sottofasc. Francia. Telegram of Prefect of Arezzo to Ministry of the Interior, 15 August 1911, n. 14889.

125 Archivio Centrale dello Stato. Ministero dell'Interno, Direzione Generale della Sanità, 1882–1915, b. 273, fasc. Ministero Affari Esteri; Affari generali, sottofasc. Francia. Embassy of the French Republic, 'Note verbale', n.d.

126 National Archives. Record Group 90: Records of the Public Health Service, Central File, 1897–1923, category 397, box 056. Letter of Prefect Gregoire to Consul-General of the United States, n.d. The letter is preserved in English translation.

127 Direzione Generale della Statistica e del Lavoro, *Annuario statistico italiano*, 2nd series, 1 (1911) (Rome, 1912), p. 25.

128 On Italian emigration to Argentina, see 'L'emigrazione italiana per l'Argentina', in Commissariato dell'Emigrazione, *Bollettino dell'emigrazione*, 1909, pp. 877–888; 'Relazione sull'emigrazione italiana per l'estero nel 1909', in Commissariato dell'Emigrazione, *Bollettino dell'emigrazione*, 1910, esp. pp. 3288–3309;

and Commissariato Generale dell'Emigrazione, *L'emigrazione italiana dal 1910 al 1923* (Rome, 1926), vol.II, esp. pp. 207–271.
129 A.V. Vecchi, 'Il dissidio italo-argentino', *La Rassegna nazionale*, 181 (1911), pp. 14–18.
130 On the origins of the epidemic of 1886–1888 in Argentina, see Edward O. Shakespeare, *Report on Cholera in Europe and India* (Washington, 1890), pp. 350–361; Olga Bordi de Ragucci, *Colera e inmigracion, 1880–1900* (Buenos Aires, 1977), esp. ch. 3, pp. 47–74; and José M. Gabezon, 'El coléra en Buenos Aires,' *Revista Argentina de Ciencias Médicas*, 4 (1887), pp. 12–18.
131 Quoted in *ibid.*, p. 353.
132 See, for example, 'La epidemia de colera: la version norteamericana', *La Prensa*, 21 July 1911; and 'Medidas contra el colera', *La Prensa*, 22 July 1911.
133 For Argentinean coverage of the protests organized by the Association in Naples, see 'Las Protestas Popolares en Napoles', *La Prensa*, 22 July 1911.
134 'Salud Publica', *La Prensa*, 21 July 1911.
135 *Ibid.* For a retrospective Italian account of the sanitary dispute, see Commissariato Generale dell'Emigrazione, *L'emigrazione italiana dal 1910 al 1923* (Rome, 1926), vol. I, pp. 651–655. In this 1926 account, the Italian Government admitted that there was a cholera epidemic during the summer of 1911 'in some regions of Italy'. The Italian position remained, however, that the Argentinean response was unnecessary and unjustified.
136 'La cronaca di Roma', *Osservatore romano*, 26 May 1911.
137 On papal opposition to the Jubilee, see 'Pope May Spoil Italy's Fetes', *New York Times*, 5 March 1911 amd such articles in the *Osservatore romano* as '27 marzo 1861 – 27 marzo 1911', *Osservatore romano*, 28 March 1911 and 'La cronaca di Roma', *Osservatore romano*, 26 May 1911. Cf. also the comments by the socialist deputy Giuseppe Canepa in 'Atti della Camera: sulla sistematica denigrazione sanitaria dell'Italia', *Giornale della R. Società Italiana d'Igiene*, 33 (1911), p. 127.
138 For a description of Martin Garcia, see 'Il conflitto italo-argentino', *Osservatore romano*, 8 August 1911.
139 For the text of the decree suspending emigration to Argentina, see Commissariato Generale dell'Emigrazione, *Bollettino dell'emigrazione*, 1911, p. 670.
140 For an explanation of the crisis by an unnamed 'high official at the Foreign Office', see 'Il provvedimento del Governo contro l'Argentina', *Corriere della sera*, 1 August 1911. For the text of the decree suspending emigration to Uruguay, see Commissariato Generale dell'Emigrazione, *Bollettino dell'emigrazione*, 1911, p. 671.
141 See, for example, 'Un' ora grigia per la politica italiana', *Osservatore romano*, 1 August 1911. The Vatican attacked Giolitti's foreign policy for abruptly and unnecessarily destroying the 'idyllic relations' that existed between the two nations.
142 For examples of the manner in which the Italian action was defended in the press, see 'Il veto del Governo all'emigrazione in Argentina', *La Tribuna*, 1 August 1911; and 'La Repubblica Argentina ritirerà il provvedimento contro l'Italia', *La Tribuna*, 2 August 1911. For instances of the presentation of the issue by deputies as the defense of Italian dignity against Argentinean chauvinism, see

the interviews with Giovanni Camera and Castellino in 'L'Argentina partecipa ufficialmente alle feste pel Cinquantenario italiano', *La Tribuna*, 5 August 1911.

143 Commissariato Generale dell'Emigrazione, *Il movimento dell'emigrazione italiana negli anni dal 1910 al 1926* (Rome, 1927), p. 21.

144 Commissariato Generale dell'Emigrazione, *L'emigrazione italiana dal 1910 al 1923* (Rome, 1926), vol. I, pp. 654–655.

145 On the conditions of Italian labourers in Argentina, see Roberto Pallottino, 'Dall'Argentina al Brasile', *Avanti!*, 5 August 1911.

146 On the strategy to boycott Argentina, see 'Il pensiero di Alceste De Ambris sull'emigrazione in Argentina', *Avanti!*, 7 August 1911.

147 See, for example, Vincenzo Vacirca, 'L'Argentina e il proletariato italiano', *Avanti!*, 8 August 1911; and 'Un altro aspetto della questione Argentina', *Avanti!*, 10 August 1911.

148 For the socialist perspective on the Association and its responsibility for the crisis, see 'Lettere napoletane', *Avanti!*, 13 August 1911.

149 On the export of cholera to Spain, see National Archives. Record Group 90: Records of the Public Health Service. Central File, 1897–1923, category 397, box 056. Letter of Harry A. McBride, Vice and Deputy Consul-General, Barcelona, to the Hon. Secretary of State, 31 August 1911.

150 For the correspondence between Friedly and Wyman, see National Archives. Record Group 90: Records of the Public Health Service, Central File, 1898–1923, category 397, box 055. Letter of H.H. Friedly to Surgeon General, 21 July 1911 and telegram of Wyman to Friedly, 24 July 1911.

151 National Archive. Record Group 90: Records of the Public Health Service. Central File, 1898–1923, category 397, box 056. Letter of Harrison S. Morris to Dr. Walter Wyman, 19 September 1911.

152 Sidney Sonnino, *Carteggio, 1891–1913*, ed. Benjamin F. Brown and Pietro Pastorelli (Bari, 1981), p. 519.

153 'The Turin Exhibition', *Times*, 1 May 1911.

154 On the Exposition at Turin, see 'Cerimonie, feste e banchetti a Torino', *Corriere della sera*, 1–2 May 1911; 'Nuovi padiglioni e nuove mostre inaugurati a Torino', *Corriere della sera*, 3 May 1911; and 'All'esposizione di Torino', *Corriere della sera*, 4 May 1911.

155 'La stampa di tutto il mondo a Roma', *La Tribuna*, 2 May 1911.

156 On the Exposition at Rome, see 'Il monumento a Vittorio Emanuele II', *Corriere della sera*, 11 May 1911; 'I padiglioni regionali inaugurati ieri a Roma', *Corriere della sera*, 13 May 1911; 'Le feste giubilari', *Corriere della sera*, 14 May 1911; 'Le feste giubilari a Roma', *Corriere della sera*, 15 May 1911; 'Le feste cinquantenarie', *Corriere della sera*, 10 May 1911; 'Il monumento a Vittorio Emanuele', *Corriere della sera*, 3 June 1911; and 'Apoteosi dell'unità d'Italia', *Corriere della sera*, 5 June 1911. There are also extensive reports on the celebrations at Rome in *La Tribuna* for the period from 1 May until August 1911.

157 Cf., for example, 'L'inaugurazione della Mostra dei Fiori a Firenze', *Corriere della sera*, 8 May 1911; 'Le feste giubilari', *Corriere della sera*, 5 June 1911; and 'Catania nel cinquantenario: il monumento a Umberto I', *La Tribuna*, 31 May 1911.

158 'A.S.B.', 'Cose d'attualità: le condizioni sanitarie del nostro paese', *Giornale della Reale Società d'Igiene*, 38 (1911), pp. 410–411.

159 'L'apoteosi dell'Unità d'Italia', *Corriere della sera*, 5 June 1911.

160 Quoted in Nino Valeri, *Giovanni Giolitti* (Turin, 1972), p. 3.

161 Quoted in Archivio Centrale dello Stato. Ministero dell'Interno, Direzione Generale della Sanità, 1882–1915, b. 178 and 278, fasc. Condizioni sanitarie del Regno. Telegram of Prefect of Venice Nasalli to S.E. Min. Int., 1 June 1911, n. 1503.

162 *Ibid.*

163 Archivio Centrale dello Stato. Ministero dell'Interno, Direzione Generale della Sanità, 1882–1915, b. 178, fasc. Condizioni sanitarie del Regno. Telegram of Giolitti to Prefect of Venice, 1 June 1911, n. 15682. Emphasis added.

164 Interrogation of the Minister of the Interior, 8 March 1912, *Atti del parlamento italiano. Camera dei deputati. Legislature xxviii, Sessione 1909–11. Discussioni*, IV, p. 17756.

165 Archivio Centrale dello Stato. Ministero dell'Interno, Direzione Generale della Sanità, 1882–1915, b. 178, fasc. Condizioni sanitarie del Regno. Telegram of Nasalli to Min. Int. Sanità, 2 June 1911, n. 6535.

166 Archivio Centrale dello Stato. Ministero dell'Interno, Direzione Generale della Sanità, 1882–1915, b. 278, fasc. Condizioni sanitarie del Regno. Letter of Ministro dell'Interno to S.E. il Ministro degli Affari Esteri, 25 June 1911, n. 20300–1.

167 Archivio Centrale dello Stato. Ministero dell'Interno, Direzione Generale della Sanità, 1882–1915, b. 181, fasc. Rapporti degli inspettori sanitari sul colera, sottofasc. Venezia: Rapporto Ispettor Messea. Report of Inspector-General Alessandro Messea, 'Condizioni sanitarie di Venezia a tutto l'8 giugno 1911'.

168 The *New York Times* noted that, 'A strict censorship is maintained over telegraphic communications from Italy in regard to the cholera.' 'Cholera Spreads to France', *New York Times*, 14 July 1911.

169 Archivio Centrale dello Stato. Ministero dell'Interno, Direzione Generale della Sanità, b. 278, fasc. Affari riservati. Telegram of Prefect of Milan to Min. Int., 11 June 1911.

170 *Ibid.*

171 Archivio Centrale dello Stato. Ministero dell'Interno, Direzione Generale della Sanità, b. 278, fasc. Affari riservati. Telegram of Giolitti to Prefect of Caserta, 12 June 1911, n. 16712.

172 For examples, see Archivio Centrale dello Stato. Ministero dell'Interno, Direzione Generale della Sanità, b. 278, fasc. Affari riservati.

173 Archivio Centrale dello Stato. Ministero dell'Interno, Direzione Generale della Sanità, 1882–1915, b. 249 bis, fasc. Napoli, sottofasc. Napoli: colera. Fonogramma n. 1104, 15 June 1911, ore 9:30.

174 National Archives. Record Group 90: Records of the Public Health Service, Central File, 1897–1923, category 397, box 054. Letter of Henry Geddings to Surgeon-General, 26 September 1910.

175 National Archives. Record Group 90: Records of the Public Health Service, Central File, 1897–1923, category 397, box 055. Despatch of John G.A. Leishman to the Hon. Secretary of State, 14 June 1911.

176 Archivio Centrale dello Stato. Direzione Generale della Sanità, 1882–1915, b. 249

bis, fasc. Napoli: cholera. Mauro Jatta, 'Profilassi per il colera di Napoli: 1911', pp. 18–19.

177 *Ibid.*, pp. 19–20.

178 'Practice in Foreign Countries', *British Medical Journal* (1911, vol. 2), p. 586.

179 Leonard Rogers, *Cholera and Its Treatment* (London, 1911), p. 150.

180 On his techniques of rehydration, see Leonard Rogers, *Recent Advances in Tropical Medicine* (London, 1928), pp. 174–185; and especially *Cholera and Its Treatment* (London, 1911).

181 *Happy Toil: Fifty-five Years in Tropical Medicine* (London, 1950), p. 153.

182 *Happy Toil*, pp. 154–155.

183 *Ibid.*

184 For an article describing the rehydration therapy adopted by Rogers and the enthusiastic reception accorded it by Professor Romano, see 'New Cholera Cure Gives Good Results', *New York Times* 17 December 1911.

185 Romano's letter is printed in Rogers, *Happy Toil*, p. 156.

186 *Ibid.*, p. 157.

187 *Ibid.*, p. 35.

188 For the attempt at serum therapy at the Cotugno and its background, see Alfonso Montefusco, *Clinica e terapia delle malattie acute* (Naples, 1912), pp. 23–31.

189 *Ibid.*, pp. 28–31.

190 'New Cholera Cure Gives Good Results', *New York Times*, 17 December 1911.

191 Archivio Centrale dello Stato. Ministero dell'Interno, Direzione Generale della Sanità, 1882–1915, b. 177 bis, fasc. Napoli e provincia: cholera 1911. Municipio di Napoli, 'Statistica degli infermi ricoverati al Cotugno dal 3 maggio al 31 agosto 1911 nel lazzaretto'.

192 *Atti del parlamento italiano. Camera dei deputati. Legislatura XXIII, Sessione 1909–1912. Discussioni*, XV, p. 17750.

193 *Ibid.*, p. 17735.

194 *Ibid.*, p. 17737.

195 This was the description of the deputy Pasqualino-Vassallo, speech of 8 March 1912. *Ibid.*, p. 17755.

196 For Giolitti's speech on 8 March 1912, see *ibid.*, pp. 17815–24.

CONCLUSION: NEAPOLITAN CHOLERA AND ITALIAN POLITICS

1 Camillo Cavour, *Tutti gli scritti di Camillo Cavour*, ed. Carlo Pischedda and Giuseppe Talamo, vol. III (Turin, 1976), p. 1014.

2 *Ibid.*

3 L. Franchetti and S. Sonnino, *La Sicilia nel 1876*, ed. E. Cavalieri, 2 vols. (Florence, 1925).

4 *Opere*, vol. IV *Il ministro della malavita* (Milan, 1962) part I.

5 Gaetano Salvemini, 'Fu l'Italia prefascista una democrazia?', *Il Ponte*, 8 (1952), pp. 178–179.

6 The observations here owe much to Susan Sontag, *Illness as Metaphor* (London, 1977).

7 For a discussion of the limits of Giolitti's reforming impulses in the field of medicine with special reference to tuberculosis, see Tommaso Detti, 'La questione della tuberculosi nell'Italia giolittiana', *Passato e presente*, 1:2 (1982), pp. 27–60.

Select bibliography

ARCHIVAL SOURCES

Archivio del Banco di Napoli, Naples

Pandetta del Consiglio d'Amministrazione
Verbali del Consiglio d'Amministrazione

Archivio Centrale dello Stato, Rome

Ministero dell'Interno: Direzione Generale della Sanità, 1910–1920
Ministero dell'Interno: Direzione Generale della Sanità, 1881–1915

Archivio di Stato di Bari, Bari

Camera di Commercio
Prefettura: Sanità pubblica

Archivio di Stato di Barletta, Barletta

Deliberazioni del Consiglio Comunale (1910)
Deliberazioni della Giunta Municipale (1910)

Archivio di Stato di Napoli, Naples

Prefettura di Napoli

Archivio Storico del Comune di Napoli, Naples

Atti del Consiglio Comunale di Napoli
Atti della Giunta Municipale di Napoli

Archivio dell'Ospedale Domenico Cotugno, Naples

Cartelle mediche

Cimitero di Barletta, Barletta

Registro (1910)

Cimitero della Pietà, Naples

Colerosi, 17/8 1884–15/11 1884
Registro (1911)
Registro (1912)

National Archives, Washington, D.C.

Records of the Department of State, Re: Internal Affairs of Italy, 1910–29
US Department of State: Records of Foreign Service Posts

OFFICIAL PUBLICATIONS

Annual Report of the Supervising Surgeon-General of the Marine Health Service of the United States (Washington, D.C., 1901–1912)
Atti del consiglio comunale di Napoli
Atti del consiglio generale del Banco di Napoli
Atti del consiglio provinciale di Napoli
Atti del parlamento italiano
Ciaramelli, Gennaro, *Sul cholera del 1884: relazione al sindaco di Napoli* (Naples, 1884).
Commissariato Generale dell'Emigrazione, *Annuario statistico della emigrazione italiana dal 1876 al 1925* (Rome, 1926).
Commissariato Generale dell'Emigrazione, *Bollettino dell'emigrazione*
Commissariato Generale dell'Emigrazione, *L'emigrazione italiana dal 1910 al 1923*, 2 vols. (Rome, 1926).
Commissariato Generale dell'Emigrazione, *Il movimento dell'emigrazione italiana negli anni dal 1910 al 1926* (Rome, 1927).
Comune di Napoli, *Annuario storico-statistico-topografico del comune di Napoli, Anno 1909–1910* (Naples, 1912).
Riordinamento della numerazione civica e della nomenclatura stradale (Naples, 1906).
Comune di Napoli: Consiglio Superiore dei Lavori Pubblici, *Fognatura della Città di Napoli: ultimi studi e proposte definitive* (Naples, 1885).
Conti, Alfonso, *Relazione a S.E. il Presidente del Consiglio Ministro dell'Interno sull' amministrazione della provincia di Napoli* (Rome, 1889).
Convention Sanitaire Internationale de Paris (3 Décembre 1903) (Rome, 1910).
D'Alessandro, Stanislao, *Studii sul cholera dal punto di vista etiologico generale e speciale relativamente all'epidemia in Napoli del 1884 nella sezione S. Lorenzo* (Naples, 1885).
Depretis, Agostino, *Discorsi parlamentari*, vol. VIII (Rome, 1892).
Direzione Generale della Statistica e del Lavoro, *Annuario statistico italiano* (Rome, 1912).
Ermengem, Emile P. van, *Recherches sur le microbe du choléra asiatique: rapport présenté à M. le Ministre de l'Intérieur, le 3 novembre 1884* (Paris and Brussels, 1885).
Gerardin, Auguste and Gaimard, Paul, *Du choléra-morbus en Russie, en Prusse et en Autriche pendant les années 1831 et 1832* (Paris: 1833, 3rd edn).
Great Britain. Privy Council. Central Board of Health, *Rapporti relativi al morbo chiamato*

cholera-spasmodica nell'Indie e nella Russia compilati dalla Giunta di Sanità di Londra (Florence, 1831).

Ministero di Agricoltura, Industria e Commercio. Direzione Generale della Statistica, *Statistica della emigrazione italiana. Anno 1883.* (Rome, 1884).

Statistica della emigrazione italiana per gli anni 1884 e 1885 (Rome, 1886).

Ministero dell'Interno: Direzione Generale della Sanità, *Consigli popolari per la difesa individuale contro il colera* (Rome, 1907).

Istruzioni per i medici pratici per la difesa contro il colera (Rome, 1908).

Istruzioni per la diagnosi batteriologica del colera (Rome, 1907).

Istruzioni per le autorità sanitarie per la difesa contro il colera (Rome, 1907).

Istruzioni per le vaccinazioni anticoleriche (Rome, 1907).

Piano difensivo contro la diffusione del colera da applicarsi nei grandi centri e disposizioni relative alle località marittime (Rome, 1910).

Norme ed istruzioni per la difesa sanitaria alle frontiere terrestri e nell'interno del Regno contro la diffusione del colera e della peste (Rome, 1910).

Montefusco, Alfonso, *Resoconto dell'ospedale Cotugno pel triennio 1902–1904* (Naples, 1905).

Morana, Giovanni Battista, *Il colera in Italia negli anni 1884 e 1885: Relazione a S.E. il Cav. Avv. Agostino Depretis* (Rome, 1885).

Municipio di Napoli, *Progetto per lo ampliamento della città e risanamento delle zone insalubri: relazione* (Naples, 1884).

Proposte e documenti per la esecuzione del progetto di risanamento delle sezioni Porto, Pendino, Mercato, Vicaria (Naples, 1887).

Relazione sul V censimento generale della popolazione e sul I censimento industriale (Naples, 1912).

Statistica generale del colera dalla mezzanotte del 17 agosto a quella del 4 novembre 1884 (Naples, 1884).

Municipio di Napoli: Ufficio d'Igiene e di Sanità Pubblica, *Lo stato della salute pubblica in Napoli* (Naples, 1903).

Nespoli, Crescenzo, *Il colera di Napoli del 1884 riguardato dal punto di vista etiologico e clinico-terapico. Relazione all'Ill. Sindaco ed alla Commissione Sanitaria Municipale della Città* (Naples, 1884).

Office International d'Hygiène Publique, *Vingt-cinq ans d'activité, 1909–1933* (Paris, 1933).

Pierotti, Francesco, *Relazione del colera a Spezia* (Spezia, 1884).

Presutti, Errico, *Inchiesta parlamentare sulle condizioni dei contadini nelle provincie meridionali e nella Sicilia: Puglia* (Rome, 1910).

Raccolta ufficiale delle leggi e dei decreti del Regno d'Italia.

Saredo, Giuseppe, *Relazione della R. commissario straordinario al consiglio comunale di Napoli* (Naples, 1891) 2 vols.

Relazione della R. Commissione d'inchiesta per Napoli sulla amministrazione comunale (Rome, 1901).

Shakespeare, Edward O., *Report on Cholera in Europe and India* (Washington, DC, 1890).

Sirignano, Federico, *Relazione igienico-sanitaria circa l'epidemia colerica del 1884 nella sezione Pendino* (Naples, 1884).

Somma, Giuseppe, *Relazione sanitaria sui casi di colera avvenuti in sezione Porto durante la epidemia dell'anno 1884* (Naples, 1885).

Ufficio Centrale di Statistica, *Statistica delle cause di morte nell'anno 1911* (Rome, 1913).

United States Bureau of Foreign Commerce, Cholera in Europe in 1884. *Reports from Consuls of the United States* (Washington, DC, 1885).

United States Department of State, *Consular Reports on Commerce, Manufacture, & C.* (Washington, DC, 1833).

United States House of Representatives, 48th Congress, 2nd Session, Ex. Doc. 54, Part 1, *United States Consular Reports. Labor in Europe. Reports from the Consuls of the United States in the Several Countries of Europe on the Rates of Wages, Cost of Living to the Laboring Classes, Past and Present Wages, &., in Their Several Districts, in Response to a Circular from the Department of State Requesting Information on These Subjects* (Washington, DC, 1885).

United States House of Representatives, 57th Congress, 1st Session, Report no. 174, *Dr. Eugene Wasdin and Dr. H. D. Geddings* (Washington, 1902)

United States Senate, 53d Congress, 2d Session, Ex. Doc. No. 114, *Letter from the Secretary of the Treasury, in Response to the Senate Resolution of June 12, 1894, calling for facts in regard to the padrone system in connection with Italian immigration, transmitting a report from the Superintendent of Immigration and copies of a correspondence between the Italian ambassador at Washington, the Secretary of the Treasury, and a copy of instructions issued by the Treasury Department* (Washington, D.C., 1894)

United States Senate, 51st Congress, 3d Session, Document no. 748, *Reports of the Immigration Commission. Emigration Conditions in Europe* (Washington, DC, 1911).

R. Università degli Studi di Napoli, *Annuario per l'anno scolastico 1865–66* (Naples, 1865).

Annuario per l'anno scolastico 1883–84 (Naples, 1884).

Annuario per l'anno scolastico 1896–97 (Naples, 1897).

Annuario. Volume unico del 1909–10 e 1910–11 (Naples, 1911).

NEWSPAPERS

Avanti!, Rome
Il Buon senso, Barletta
Corriere della sera, Milan
Corriere delle Puglie, Bari
Don Marzio, Naples
Il Fieramosca, Barletta
Il Giornale d'Italia, Rome
Il Giorno, Naples
La Libertà, Naples
Il Mattino, Naples
Il Messaggero, Rome
The New York Herald, New York
The New York Times, New York
La Nazione, Florence
L'Osservatore romano, Rome
Le Petit Var, Toulon
Il Piccolo, Naples
La Prensa, Buenos Aires
La Propaganda, Naples

Il Pungolo, Naples
Le Radical, Paris
Il Resto del carlino, Bologna
Roma, Naples
Le Temps, Paris
The Times, London
La Tribuna, Rome

CONTEMPORARY JOURNALS

Annali universali di medicina e chirurgia, Milan
Bollettino ebdomadario dell'ufficio di statistica della città di Napoli, Naples
Boston Medical and Surgical Journal, Boston.
Bulletin de l'Académie de Médecine, Paris
Bulletin Général de Thérapeutique Médicale et Chirurgicale, Paris
The British Medical Journal, London
Civiltà cattolica, Florence
Clinica oculista, Palermo
Gazette Hebdomadaire des Sciences Médicales de Montpellier, Montpellier
Gazzetta internazionale di medicina, chirurgia, igiene, interessi professionali, Naples
Gazzetta medica di Torino, Turin
Gazzetta di medicina pubblica, Naples
Giornale di clinica, terapia e medicina pubblica, Naples
Giornale medico del R. esercito e della R. Marina, Rome
Giornale della Reale Società Italiana d'Igiene, Milan
Igiene moderna, Genoa.
Ingrassia: Giornale di medicina e chirurgia, Palermo.
The Lancet, London
Marseille Médical, Marseilles
Medical Record, New York
Medicina contemporanea, Naples
Nice-médical, Nice
Nuova antologia, Rome
The Practitioner, London
Raccoglitore medico, Forlí
Rassegna nazionale, Florence
Resoconto delle adunanze e dei lavori della Reale Accademia Medico-chirurgica di Napoli,
    Naples
Revista Argentina de Ciencias Médicas, Buenos Aires
Riforma sociale, Turin
Rivista d'igiene e sanità pubblica, Milan
Rivista internazionale di clinica e terapia, Naples
Rivista internazionale di medicina e chirurgia, Naples
Rivista clinica e terapeutica, Naples
Rivista di malattie infettive, Naples
Rivista di medicina pubblica, Naples
The Sanitarian, New York
La Voce, Florence

BOOKS AND ARTICLES

Note: Articles in journals from the period covered by the book are not listed. References to them appear only in the Notes.

Ackerknecht, Erwin H., 'Anticontagionism between 1821 and 1867', *Bulletin of the History of Medicine*, 22 (1948), pp. 562–593.

Agulhon, Maurice, ed., *Histoire de Toulon* (Toulouse, 1980).

Agulhon, Maurice, ed., *La Ville de l'Age Industriel: le Cycle Haussmannien* in *Histoire de la France urbaine*, vol. IV (Paris, 1983).

Albonico, Erminio, *Saggio di una prima inchiesta sulla emigrazione italiana in Europa* (Milan, 1921).

Aliberti, Giovanni, 'La 'Questione di Napoli" nell'età liberale (1861–1904)', in *Storia di Napoli*, vol. X (Naples, 1971), pp. 219–271.

Alisio, Giancarlo, *Napoli e il risanamento: recupero di una struttura urbana* (Naples, 1980).

Alongi, Giuseppe, *La camorra: studio di sociologia criminale* (Turin, 1890).

Amalfi, Giuseppe, *Gli oppiacei nel colera ed un'ipotesi (epidemia di Napoli del 1884)* (Naples, 1885).

Ansaldo, Giovanni, *Il ministro della buona vita* (Milan, 1949).

Aquarone, Alberto, *L'Italia giolittiana* (Milan, 1988; 1st edn 1981).

Ariès, Philippe, *The Hour of Our Death* (London, 1981).

   Images of Man and Death (Cambridge, Mass., 1985).

   Western Attitudes toward Death from the Middle Ages to the Present (London, 1976).

Arlacchi, Pino, *Mafia, Peasants and Great Estates: Society in Traditional Calabria* (Cambridge, 1983).

Baehrel, René, 'Épidémie et terreur. Histoire et sociologie', *Archives Historiques de la Révolution Française*, 23 (1951), pp. 113–146.

Baine, William D.; Mazzotti, Mirella; Greco, Donato; Iggo, Egidio; Zampieri, Alfredo; Angioni, Giuseppe; Di Gioia, Mario; Gangarosa, Eugene J.; and Pocchiari, Francesco, 'Epidemiology of Cholera in Italy in 1973', *Lancet* (1974, vol. 2), pp. 1370–1374.

Barbagallo, Francesco, ed., *Camorra e criminalità organizzata in Campania* (Naples, 1988).

   'Dal camorrista plebeo al criminale imprenditore: una modernizzazione riuscita', *Studi storici*, 29 (1988), pp. 549–555.

   Stato, parlamento e lotte politico-sociali nel mezzogiorno, 1900–1914 (Naples, 1976).

Bardet, Jean, *et al.*, *Peurs et terreurs face à la contagion: Choléra, tuberculose, syphilis xixe–xxe siècles* (Paris, 1988).

Barnet, Margaret C., 'The 1832 Cholera Epidemic in York', *Medical History*, 16 (1972), pp. 27–39.

Barracano, Gaetano, *Observations on the Cholera-Morbus* (Naples, 1853).

Bartrip, P.W.J., *Mirror of Medicine: A History of the BMJ* (Oxford, 1990).

Barua, Dhiman and Burrows, William, eds., *Cholera* (Philadelphia, 1974).

Bellew, Henry Walt, *The History Of Cholera in India from 1862 to 1881* (London, 1885).

Benyajatti, Chanyo and Keoplung, Muni, 'Metabolic Alkalosis, a Late Complication in Asiatic Cholera: A Case Study', *American Journal of Tropical Medicine and Hygiene*, 10 (1961), pp. 914–917.

Bilson, Geoffrey, *A Darkened House: Cholera in Nineteenth-Century Canada* (Toronto, 1980).

Biraben, Jean-Noël, *Les hommes et la peste en France et dans les pays européens et méditerranéens*, 2 vols. (Paris, 1975–6).

Black, George F., *A Gypsy Bibliography* (Edinburgh, 1909).

Blake, Paul A.; Rosenberg, Mark L.; Costa, Jose Bandeira; Ferreira, Pedro Soares; Guimaraes, Cesar Levy; and Gangarosa, Eugene J., 'Cholera in Portugal, 1974', *American Journal of Epidemiology*, 105 (1977), pp. 337–343.

Blok, Anton, *The Mafia of a Sicilian Village, 1860–1969: A Study of Violent Peasant Entrepreneurs* (New York, 1975).

Bardi de Ragucci, Olga, *Colera e immigracion, 1880–1900* (Buenos Aires, 1977).

Bourdelais, Patrice and Raulot, Jean-Yves, *Une peur bleue: Histoire du choléra en France, 1832–1854* (Paris, 1987).

Bousigue, Jean-Yves 'L'épidémie, objet de l'histoire: le choléra dans le canton des Cabannes (1854)', *Annales du Midi*, 97 (1985), pp. 411–426.

Bowring, John, *Observations on the Oriental Plague and on Quarantine, as a Means of Arresting its Progress* (Edinburgh, 1838).

Bowsky, William M., *The Black Death: A Turning Point in History?* (Huntington, N.Y., 1978).

Briggs, Asa, 'Cholera and Society in the Nineteenth Century', *Past and Present*, 19 (1961), pp. 76–96.

Briggs, John W., *An Italian Passage: Immigrants to Three American Cities, 1890–1930* (New Haven and London, 1978).

Brignoli, Marziano, *I lombardi della Sinistra storica (Da carteggi inediti di Agostino Depretis, Benedetto Cairoli, Cesare Corenti)* (Rome, 1985).

Brock, Thomas D., *Robert Koch: A Life in Medicine and Bacteriology* (Madison, Wisconsin, 1988).

Brunetti, Lodovico, *Fatti, considerazioni, conclusioni sul colera* (Padova, 1885).

Calvi, Giulia, *Histories of a Plague Year: The Social and the Imaginary in Baroque Florence*, trans. Dario Biocca and Bryant T. Ragan, Jr. (Berkeley, Los Angeles and Oxford, 1989).

Camus, Albert, *La peste* (Paris, 1947).

Cantani, Arnaldo, *Il colera* (Naples, 1884).
    La cura del cholera mediante l'ipodermoclisi e l'enteroclisi (Naples, 1884).
    Istruzioni popolari concernenti il cholera asiatico (Naples, 1884).

Caro, Orazio, *L'evoluzione igienica di Napoli (Cenni storici–osservazioni e proposte–dati statistici)* (Naples, 1914).
    La politica sanitaria del colera (Naples, 1911).

Carocci, Giampiero, *Giolitti e l'età giolittiana* (Turin, 1971).
    Agostino Depretis e la politica interna italiana (Turin, 1956).

Carrière, C., Courdurie, M. and Rebuffat, F. *Marseille ville morte: La Peste de 1720* (Marseille, 1968).

Cavallotti, Felice, *Lettere, 1860–1898*, ed. Cristina Vernizzi (Milan, 1979).

Cavour, Camillo, *Tutti gli scritti di Camillo Cavour*, ed. Carlo Pischedda and Giuseppe Talamo (Turin, 1976).

Cera, Vincenzo Leonardo, *Metodo curativo per la colera sviluppatasi in Napoli dallo scorcio di luglio 1854* (Naples, 1854).

Cerase, Francesco Paolo, *Sotto il dominio dei borghesi: Sottosviluppo ed emigrazione nell'Italia meridionale, 1860–1910* (Assisi and Rome, 1975).

Challice, John, *Should the Cholera Come, What Ought to Be Done?* (London, 1848).

Chevalier, Louis, ed., *Le choléra: la première épidémie du XIXe siècle* (La Roche-sur-Yon, 1958).

Christie, A.B., *Infectious Diseases: Epidemiology and Clinical Practice*, 2 vols (Edinburgh, London, Melbourne and New York, 1987).

Ciccotti, Ettore, *Sulla questione meridionale* (Milan, 1904).

Cipolla, Carlo M., *Cristofano and the Plague: A Study in the History of Public Health in the Age of Galileo* (London, 1973).

Fighting the Plague in Seventeenth-Century Italy (Madison, Wisc., 1981).

Clebert, Jean-Paul, *The Gypsies* (London, 1963).

Colapietra, Raffaele, *Giovanni Giolitti: Biografia politica e interpretazioni storiografiche* (Florence and Messina, 1973).

Consiglio, Alberto, ed., *Antologia dei poeti napoletani* (Milan, 1973).

Corbino, Epicarmo, *Annali dell'economia italiana*, 5 vols. (Naples, n.d.).

Cosmacini, Giorgio, *Storia della medicina e della sanità in Italia* (Bari, 1992; 1st edn 1987).

Countryman, Edward, *The American Revolution* (London, 1985).

Creighton, Charles, *A History of Epidemics in Britain*, 2 vols. (Cambridge, 1891–4).

Crombet, Paul, *Les Souvenirs d'Italie (1817–1826)* (Brussels and Rome, 1941).

Crosby, Alfred W., *America's Forgotten Pandemic: The Influenza of 1918* (Cambridge, 1989).

Curtin, Philip D., *Death by Migration: Europe's Encounter with the Tropical World in the Nineteenth Century* (Cambridge, 1989).

D'Ascoli, Francesco and D'Avino, Michele, *I sindaci di Napoli*, vol. 1 (Naples, 1974).

De Felice, Franco, *L'agricoltura in Terra di Bari* (Bari, 1971).

'L'età giolittiana', *Studi storici*, 10 (1969), pp. 114–190.

L'età giolittiana (Turin, 1980).

Defoe, Daniel, *A Journal of the Plague Year* (London, 1966).

Delaporte, François, *The Cholera in Paris, 1832* (Cambridge, Mass., 1986).

Della Peruta, Franco, ed., *Vita civile degli italiani: società, economia, cultura materiale. Città, fabbriche e nuove culture alle soglie della società di massa, 1850–1920* (Milan, 1990).

De Lorenzo, Ferruccio, *I giorni della grande paura* (Naples, 1980).

Demarco, Domenico, *Per una storia economica dell'emigrazione italiana* (Geneva, 1978).

Del Panta, Lorenzo, *Le epidemie nella storia demografica italiana (secoli XIV–XIX)* (Turin, 1980).

De Renzi, E., 'Sul colera di Napoli (1884)', *Rivista clinica e terapeutica*, 7 (1885), pp. 57–73.

De Renzi, Salvatore, *Osservazioni sulla topografia medica del Regno di Napoli*, 3 vols. (Naples, 1828–1830).

Detti, Tommaso, 'La questione della tuberculosi nell'Italia giolittiana', *Passato e presente*, 1: 2 (1982), pp. 27–60.

De Zerbi, Rocco, *Colera del 1884: Croce Bianca e Croce Rossa* (Naples, 1884).

Di Mitri, Gino Leonardo, *Regolamenti di sanità marittima nel Regno delle Due Sicilie (1820 e 1853)* (Gallatina, 1992).

Dols, Michael W., *The Black Death in the Middle East* (Princeton, 1977).

Dominique, A., *Le choléra à Toulon: étude historique statistique et comparative des épidémies de 1835, 1849, 1854, 1865 et 1884* (Toulon, 1885).

Dubos, René, *Pasteur and Modern Science* (Madison, Wisc., 1988).

Dubos, René and Dubos, Jean, *The White Plague: Tuberculosis, Man and Society* (London, 1953).

Durey, Michael, *The Return of the Plague: British Society and the Cholera, 1831–2* (London, 1979).

Duroselle, Jean-Baptiste and Serra, Enrico, ed., *L'emigrazione italiana in Francia prima del 1914* (Milan, 1978).

Duval, Amaury, *Tableaux de Naples et de ses Environs*, vol. 5 in Gregoire Orloff, *Mémoires Historiques, Politiques et Littéraires sur le Royaume de Naples* (Paris, 1821), pp. 251–465.

Esposito, Gennaro, ed., *Anche il colera: Gli untori di Napoli* (Milan, 1973).

Evans, Richard J., *Death in Hamburg: Society and Politics in the Cholera Years, 1830–1910* (Oxford, 1987).

'Epidemics and Revolutions: Cholera in Nineteenth-Century Europe', *Past and Present*, no. 120 (August 1988), pp. 123–146.

Eyler, John M., 'William Farr on the Cholera: The Sanitarian's Disease Theory and the Statistician's Method', *Journal of the History of Medicine*, 28 (1973), pp. 79–100.

Fazio, Eugenio, *La epidemia colerica e le condizioni sanitarie di Napoli* (Naples, 1884).

Fernandez Garcia, Antonio, *Epidemias y Sociedad en Madrid* (Madrid, 1985).

Ferrigno, Giuseppe, *Il colera in Palermo nel 1885* (Palermo, 1886).

Fiengo, Giuseppe, *L'acquedotto di Carmignano e lo sviluppo di Napoli in età barocca* (Florence, 1990).

Filipuzzi, Angelo, *Il dibattito sull'emigrazione: polemiche nazionali e stampa veneta (1861–1914)* (Florence, 1976).

Foerster, R.F., *The Italian Emigration of Our Times* (New York, 1969; 1st edn 1924).

Forti Messina, Anna Lucia, 'L'Italia dell'Ottocento di fronte al colera', in F. Della Peruta, ed., *Storia d'Italia, Annali 7: Malattia e Medicina* (Turin, 1984), pp.429–494.

Società ed epidemia: il colera a Napoli nel 1836 (Milan, 1979).

Fortunato, Giustino, *Carteggio, 1865–1911* (Bari, 1978).

Il mezzogiorno e lo stato italiano, 2 vols. (Florence, 1973).

Scritti politici, ed. F. Barbagallo (Bari, 1981).

Foucault, Michel, *The Birth of the Clinic* (London, 1989).

Fracasini, Paolo, 'Ospedali, malati e medici dal Risorgimento all'età giolittiana', in F. Della Peruta, ed., *Storia d'Italia, Annali 7: Malattia e medicina* (Turin, 1984), pp. 297–331.

Franchetti, L. and Sonnino, S., *La Sicilia* (Florence, 1926).

Frieden, Nancy M., 'The Russian Cholera Epidemic, 1892–93, and Medical Professionalization', *Journal of Social History*, 10 (1977), pp. 538–559.

Fucini, Renato, *Napoli a occhio nudo: lettere ad un amico* (Florence, 1878).

Fusco, Ugo and Soscia, Mario, 'Il colera in Italia ed a Napoli (Profilo storico)', *Aggiornamenti su Malattie Infettive ed Immunologia*, 19 (1973), pp. 1 –10.

Gaffarel, Paul and Duranty, Marquis of, *La Peste de 1720 à Marseille et en France* (Paris, 1911).

Galasso, Giuseppe, *Napoli* (Bari, 1987).

Galli, Tomaso, *Il colera* (Mantova, 1884).

Garcia, Fernandez, *Epidemias y Sociedad en Madrid* (Madrid, 1985).

Gendron, F., *Notes et observations sur l'épidémie cholérique à Toulon en 1884* (Paris, 1885).

Ghirelli, Antonio, *Napoli italiana: La storia della città dopo il 1860* (Turin, 1977).

Giolitti, Giovanni, *Memorie della mia vita* (Milan, 1922).

Girard, Louis, *La Politique des Travaux Publics du Second Empire* (Paris, 1952).

Glass, Robert I.; Svennerholm, Ann-Mari; Stoll, Barbara J.; Khan, M.R.; Belayet Hossain, K.M.; Huq, M. Imdadul; and Holmgren, Jan, 'Protection against Cholera in Breast-fed Children by Antibodies in Breast Milk', *New England Journal of Medicine*, 308:2 (1983), pp. 1389–1392.

Gottfried, Robert S., *The Black Death: Natural and Human Disaster in Medieval Europe* (New York and London, 1983).

Gramsci, Antonio, *Quaderni del carcere*, 4 vols. (Turin, 1977).

Greenfield, Kent Roberts, *Economics and Liberalism in the Risorgimento: A Study of Nationalism in Lombardy, 1814–1848* (Baltimore, 1965).

Grillandi, Massimo, *Francesco Crispi* (Turin, 1969).

Haussmann, Georges, *Mémoires du baron Haussmann*, 3 vols. (Paris, 1890–3).

Hay, Douglas, *et. al.*, *Albion's Fatal Tree: Crime and Society in Eighteenth-Century England* (London, 1975).

Heyningen, W. E. van and Seal, John R., *Cholera: The American Scientific Experience, 1947–1980* (Boulder, Col., 1983).

Hobsbawm, Eric J., *Bandits* (London, 1969).

　Primitive Rebels; Studies in Archaic Forms of Social Movement in the 19th and 20th Centuries (New York, 1959).

Hoffman, Elizabeth Newell, *The Sources of Mortality Changes in Italy since Unification* (New York, 1981).

Howard, John, *An Account of the Principal Lazarettos in Europe* (Warrington, 1789).

Howard-Jones, Norman, 'Cholera Therapy in the Nineteenth Century', *Journal of the History of Medicine*, 17 (1972), pp. 373–395.

Istituto Nazionale di Economia Agraria, *Inchiesta sulla piccola proprietà coltivatrice formatasi nel dopoguerra* (Rome, 1935).

Jeuland-Meynaud, Maryse, *La Ville de Naples après l'Annexation (1860–1915)*. (Paris, 1973).

Joslin, Benjamin F., *The Homoeopathic Treatment of Epidemic Cholera. Therapeutics and Repertory* (Philadelphia, 1885).

Kenrick, Donald and Puxon, Grattan, *The Destiny of Europe's Gypsies* (London, 1972).

Klein, Edward E., *The Bacteria in Asiatic Cholera* (London and New York, 1889).

Koch, Robert, *Essays of Robert Koch*, trans. K. Codell Carter (New York, Westport, London, 1987).

　Professor Koch on the Bacteriological Diagnosis of Cholera, Water-Filtration and Cholera, and the Cholera in Germany during the Winter of 1892–93, trans. George Duncan (Edinburgh, 1894).

Kraut, Alan M., *The Huddled Masses: The Immigrant in American Society, 1880–1921* (Arlington Heights, Illinois, 1982).

　Silent Travelers: Germs, Genes, and the 'Immigrant Menace' (New York, 1994).

Labriola, Arturo, *Il Segreto di Napoli e la leggenda della camorra* (Naples, 1914).

Lavedan, Pierre, *French Architecture* (London, 1979).

Leca, Ange-Pierre, *Et le choléra s'abattit sur Paris, 1832* (Paris, 1982).

Lecocq, Georges, *Le Choléra à Toulon en 1884: Notes d'un Étudiant* (Peronne, 1884).

Leonard, Charlene Marie, *Lyon Transformed: Public Works of the Second Empire, 1853–1864* (Berkeley and Los Angeles, 1961).

Lepidi-Chioti, Giulio, *Sulle acque potabili di Palermo* (Palermo, 1885).

Lewis, R.A., *Edwin Chadwick and the Public Health Movement, 1832–1854* (London, 1952).

Livon, Charles, *Recherches sur le Choléra* (Marseilles, 1884).

Lombroso, Cesare, *Crime: Its Causes and Remedies,* trans. Henry P. Horton (Boston, 1911). *L'homme criminel,* 2 vols. (Paris, 1895).

Longmate, Norman, *King Cholera: The Biography of a Disease* (London, 1966).

Lopriore, Salvatore, *Il colera: conferenza popolare d'igiene, tenuta in Capurso la sera del 3 ottobre 1910 nella sede del Circolo Operaio Indipendente* (Bari, 1910).

Luzzatti, Luigi, *La Libertà di coscienza e di scienza* (Milan, 1909). *Scienza e patria* (Florence, 1916).

McDonald, J.C., 'The History of Quarantine in Britain during the 19th Century', *Bulletin of the History of Medicine,* 25 (1951), pp. 22–44.

Macdowall, Cameron, *A Short Note on Peritoneoclysis, Hypodermoclysis and Vesicoclysis in Cholera* (London, 1886).

McGrew, Roderick E., *Russia and the Cholera, 1823–1832* (Madison and Milwaukee, 1965).

Mack Smith, Denis, *Italy: A Modern History* (Ann Arbor, 1959). 'The Latifundia in Modern Sicilian History', *Proceedings of the British Academy,* 51 (1965), pp. 87–93.

McManners, John, *Death and the Enlightenment* (Oxford, 1981).

Macnamara, N. C., *History of Asiatic Cholera from 1781 to July 1892* (London, 1892).

McNeill, William H., *Plagues and Peoples* (London, 1979; 1st edn 1976).

Macry, Paolo, 'Borghesie, città e Stato. Appunti e impressioni su Napoli, 1860 -1880', *Quaderni storici,* 19 (1984), pp. 339–383.

Macry, Paolo and Villani, Pasquale, eds., *Storia d'Italia: Le regioni dall'Unità a oggi. La Campania* (Turin, 1990).

Magendie, F., *Lezioni sul colera-morbus* (Milan, 1832).

Magni, Cesare, *Vita parlamentare del Duca di San Donato, patriota e difensore di Napoli* (Padua, 1968).

Manfredonia, Giuseppe, *Sul cholera morbus infierito in Napoli nel 1884: osservazioni patologiche cliniche* (Naples, 1885).

Mann, Thomas, *Death in Venice,* trans. H. T. Lowe-Porter (London, 1928). *The Magic Mountain,* trans. H. T. Lowe-Porter, 2 vols. (London, 1927).

Manzoni, Alessandro, *I promessi sposi* (Milan, 1903; 1st revised edn 1840–2). *Storia della colonna infame* (Naples,Genoa, Città di Castello, 1928; 1st edn 1842).

Marghieri, Alberto, *Intorno al problema edilizio della città di Napoli* (Naples, 1911).

Margotta, V. Antonio, *Relazione storico-medico-statistica sul colera del 1866 nella provincia di Napoli* (Naples, 1866).

Marmo, Marcella, *Il proletariato industriale a Napoli in età liberale, 1880–1914* (Naples, 1978).

Marquez, Gabriel Garcia, *Love in the Time of Cholera,* trans. Edith Grossman (London, 1989).

Matossian, Mary K., 'Death in London, 1750–1909', *Journal of Interdisciplinary History,* 16 (1985), pp. 183–197.

Mennuni, G., *L'Assistenza sanitaria in Barletta* (Barletta, 1906). *Statistica demografica e sanitaria del comune di Barletta nel quadrennia 1901–1904* (Barletta, 1905).

Migliorini, Luigi Mascilli, 'Povertà e criminalità a Napoli dopo l'unificazione: il questionario sulla camorra del 1875', *Archivio storico per le province napoletane,* 90 (1980), pp. 567–615.

Monnier, Marc, *La Camorra* (Paris, 1863).

Montefusco, Alfonso, *Clinica e terapia delle malattie acute* (Naples, 1912)

Morris, R. J., *Cholera 1832: The Social Response to an Epidemic* (London, 1976).

Muro, Vincenzo, *Sulla epidemia cholerica napoletana del 1884: considerazioni etiologiche, cliniche e terapeutiche* (Naples, 1885).

Nelli, Humbert S., *The Business of Crime: Italians and Syndicate Crime in the United States* (New York, 1976).

Neufeld, M.F., *Italy: School for Awakening Countries* (Ithaca, 1961).

The New English Bible (Oxford and Cambridge, 1970).

Nitti, Francesco Saverio, *Il mezzogiorno in una democrazia industriale: antologia degli scritti meridionalistici*, ed. Francesco Barbagallo (Bari, 1987).

  Napoli e la questione meridionale (Naples, 1903).

  Scritti sulla questione meridionale, 4 vols. (Bari, 1958–1978).

Noyes, John Humphrey, *Home-talks*, ed. Alfred Barron and George Noyes Miller (Oneida, 1875).

Oliveti, Francesco, *Brevi cenni sul colera asiatico e nuovo mezzo curativo* (Naples, 1884).

Oliveti, Torquato, *Della morte apparente nei cholerosi e del modo di farli risorgere e della sola cura giovevole nel cholera asiatico* (Naples, 1886).

Pacini, Filippo, *Della natura del colera asiatico* (Florence, 1866).

  Sulla causa specifica del colera asiatico (Florence, 1865).

Pagano, Vincenzo, *Il cholera e la carità: cenno storico dell'epidemia di Napoli del 1884* (Naples, 1884).

Paliotti, Vittorio, *La camorra. Storia, personaggi, riti della bella società napoletana dalle origini a oggi* (Milan, 1973).

Pankhurst, Richard, 'The History of Cholera in Ethiopia', *Medical History* XII (1968), pp. 262–269.

Panzac, Daniel, *La peste dans l'Empire ottoman, 1700–1850* (Leuven, 1985).

  Quarantaines et lazarets: L'Europe et la peste d'Orient (XVIIe–XXe siècles) (Aix-en-Provence, 1986).

Parkin, John, *On the Antidotal Treatment of Cholera* (London, 1846).

Pavone, Claudi, ed., *Dalle carte di Giovanni Giolitti: Quarant'anni di poitica italiana* (Milan, 1962).

Pellet, Marcellin, *Napoli Contemporanea, 1888–1892*, trans. Francesco D'Ascoli (Naples, 1989).

Pelling, Margaret, *Cholera, Fever and English Medicine, 1825–1865* (Oxford, 1978).

Petraccone, Claudia, *Napoli dal '500 all' '800: problemi di storia demografica e sociale* (Naples, 1974).

Pettenkofer, Max von, *Cholera: How to Prevent and Resist It*, trans. Thomas Whiteside Hine (London, 1875).

  Outbreak of Cholera among Convicts (London, 1876).

Petti, Giovanni, *Della epidemia colerica durata dal dì 25 luglio a mezzo settembre 1854* (Naples, 1854).

Phoofuto, Pule, 'Epidemics and Revolutions: The Rinderpest Epidemic in Late Nineteenth-Century Southern Africa', *Past and Present*, no. 138 (February 1993), pp. 112–143.

Pinkney, David, *Napoleon III and the Rebuilding of Paris* (Princeton, 1958).

Piore, Michael, *Birds of Passage: Migrant Labour and Industrial Societies* (Cambridge, 1974).

Pollitzer, R., *Cholera* (Geneva, 1959).

Porter, Roy and Dorothy, *In Sickness and in Health* (London, 1988).

Preto, Paolo, *Epidemia, paura e politica nell'Italia moderna* (Bari, 1987).

Procacci, Giuliano, *Le elezioni del 1874 e l'opposizione meridionale* (Milan, 1956).

Ramsey, Matthew, *Professional and Popular Medicine in France, 1770–1830: The Social World of Medical Practice* (Cambridge, 1988).

Reeves, William C., 'Can the War to Contain Infectious Diseases Be Lost?", *American Journal of Tropical Medicine and Hygiene*, 21 (1972), pp. 251–259.

Rehfisch, Farnham, ed., *Gypsies, Tinkers and Other Travellers* (London, 1975).

Richardson, Ruth, *Death, Dissection and the Destitute* (London, 1988).

Rispoli, Francesco P., *La Provincia e la città di Napoli* (Naples, 1902).

Rodriguez Ocana, Esteban, *El colera de 1834 en Granada* (1983).

Rogers, Leonard, *Cholera and Its Treatment* (London, 1911).

    Happy Toil: Fifty-five Years in Tropical Medicine (London, 1950).

    Recent Advances in Tropical Medicine (London, 1928).

Romanelli, Luigi, *Clinica delle malattie da infezione acuta ovvero rendiconto statistico, etiologico, clinico e terapeutico degl'infermi spediti e curati nell'Ospedale della Conocchia nel 1885* (Naples, 1885).

Romano, Ruggiero, *Napoli: dal Viceregno al Regno. Storia economica* (Turin, 1978).

Romano, Sergio, *Giolitti: lo stile del potere* (Milan, 1989).

Rose, R. B., 'Eighteenth Century Price Riots and Public Policy in England', *International Review of Social History*, 6 (1961), pp. 277–292.

Rosen, George, 'An Eighteenth Century Plan for a National Health Service', *Bulletin of the History of Medicine*, 16 (1944), pp. 429–436.

Rosenberg, Charles E., 'Cholera in Nineteenth-Century Europe: A Tool for Social and Economic Analysis', *Comparative Studies in Society and History*, 8 (1966), pp. 452–463.

    The Cholera Years: The United States in 1832, 1849 and 1866 (Chicago, 1962).

    Explaining Epidemics and Other Studies in the History of Medicine (Cambridge and New York, 1992).

Rudé, George, *The Crowd in History, 1730–1848* (London, 1981; 1st edn 1964).

Russo, Ferdinando and Serao, Ernesto, *La Camorra: origini, usi, costumi e riti dell' 'annorata soggietà'* (Naples, 1970).

Russo, Giuseppe, *Napoli come città* (Naples, 1966).

    Il Risanamento e l'ampliamento della città di Napoli (Naples, 1960).

Saccardo, Pietro, *Un rimedio sovrano contro il colera* (Venice, 1886).

Salvemini, Gaetano, *Opere*, 9 vols. (Milan, 1961–1978).

Scarano, Giovanni, 'Cenni sull'epidemia di colera del 1835 in Venezia e sugli esperimenti istituiti dal dott. Giacinto Namias', *Rivista di storia della medicina*, 11 (1967), pp. 78–89.

Schneider, Jane and Peter, *Culture and Political Economy in Western Sicily* (New York, 1976).

Scirocco, Alfonso, 'Dall'unità alla prima guerra mondiale', in *Storia di Napoli*, vol. X (Naples, 1971), pp. 1–124.

    Democrazia e socialismo a Napoli dopo l'unità (Naples, 1973).

    Politica e amministrazione a Napoli nella vita unitaria (Naples, 1972).

Serao, Matilde, *Il paese di Cuccagna* (Naples, 1902).

    Il ventre di Napoli (Naples, 1973).

Seton-Watson, Christopher I. W., *Italy from Liberalism to Fascism* (London, 1967).

Sfregola, Nicola, *Relazione storico-medica sulla epidemia colerosa di Barletta del 1865* (Bari, 1866).

Shearman, David J. C. and Finlayson, Niall D. C., *Diseases of the Gastrointestinal Tract and Liver* (Edinburgh, 1982).

Shryock, Richard Harrison, *The Development of Modern Medicine* (London, 1948).

Simon, John, *Public Health Reports*, ed. Edward Seaton, 2 vols. (London, 1887).

Siraisi, Nancy G., *Medieval and Early Renaissance Medicine: An Introduction to Knowledge and Practice* (Chicago and London, 1990).

Slack, Paul, *The Impact of Plague in Tudor and Stuart England* (London, 1985).

Snow, John, *On the Mode of Communication of Cholera*; reprinted in *Snow on Cholera* (New York, 1936), pp. 1–139.

Snowden, Frank M., 'Cholera in Barletta', *Past and Present*, no. 132 (August 1991), pp. 67–103.

   Violence and Great Estates in the South of Italy: Apulia,1900–1922 (Cambridge, 1986).

Sonnino, Sidney, *Carteggio, 1891–1913*, ed. Benjamin F. Brown and Pietro Pastorelli (Bari, 1981).

Sontag, Susan, *Illness as Metaphor* (London, 1977).

Sorcinelli, Paolo, *Nuove epidemie antiche paure: uomini e colera nell'ottocento* (Milan, 1986).

Sori, Ercole, *L'emigrazione italiana dall'Unità alla seconda guerra mondiale* (Bologna, 1979).

Spada, Giuseppe, *Memoria statistica e clinica degl'infermi di cholera-morbus trattati nell'ospedale di S.M. di Loreto nell'estate del 1854* (Naples, 1854).

Starr, Paul, *The Social Transformation of American Medicine* (New York, 1982).

Steel, David, 'Plague Writing from Boccaccio to Camus', *Journal of European Studies*, 11 (1981), pp. 88–110.

Stephens, Henry, *Cholera: An Analysis of its Epidemic, Endemic, and Contagious Character* (London, 1849).

Sussman, George D., 'Carriers of Cholera and Poison Rumors in France in 1832', *Societas*, 3 (1973), pp. 233–251.

Talamo, Giuseppe, *La formazione politica di Agostino Depretis* (Milan, 1970).

Talbott, John. M., *A Biographical History of Medicine* (New York, 1970).

Taylor, Philip, *The Distant Magnet: European Emigration to the U.S.A.* (London, 1971).

Thomas, Keith, *Religion and the Decline of Magic* (London, 1971).

Thomas, Louis-Vincent, *Anthropologie de la mort* (Paris, 1975).

Thompson, E. P., 'The Moral Economy of the English Crowd in the Eighteenth Century', *Past and Present*, no. 50 (February 1971), pp. 76–136.

Tomasi di Lampedusa, Giuseppe, *Il gattopardo* (Milan, 1958).

Turchi, Marino, *Sulla igiene pubblica della città di Napoli: osservazioni e proposte* (Naples, 1862).

   Sulle acque e sulle cloache della città di Napoli (Naples, 1865).

Twain, Mark, *Innocents Abroad* (Hartford, Conn., 1869).

Valeri, Nino, *Giovanni Giolitti* (Turin, 1972).

Verga, Giovanni, *Mastro-Don Gesualdo* (Milan, 1979).

Verneau, Francesco, *L'Acquedotto di Napoli. Storia e descrizione ragionata dell'Opera* (Naples, 1907).

Villari, Pasquale, *Le lettere meridionali ed altri scritti sulla questione sociale in Italia* (Turin, 1971).

Vollum, R. L., Jamison, D.G., and Cummins, C. S., *Fairbrother's Textbook of Bacteriology* (London, 1970).

Wachsmuth, I. Kaye; Blake, Paul A., and Olsvik, Ørjan, eds., *Vibrio cholerae and Cholera: Molecular to Global Perspectives* (Washington, D.C., 1994).

Wall, A.J., *Asiatic Cholera: Its History, Pathology and Modern Treatment* (London, 1893).

Warner, John Harley, *The Therapeutic Perspective: Medical Practice, Knowledge, and Identity in America, 1820–1855* (Cambridge, Mass. and London, 1986).

Webb, G.E.C., *Gypsies: The Secret People* (London, 1960).

Weber, Eugen, *France, Fin de Siècle* (Cambridge, Mass. and London, 1986).

Weber, Max, *Economy and Society: An Outline of Interpretive Sociology*, ed. Guenther Roth and Claus Wittich 3 vols. (New York, 1968).

White Mario, Jessie, *La miseria in Napoli* (Florence, 1877).

Wilson, John, *Treatment of Cholera in the Royal Hospital, Haslar, in the Months of July and August 1849* (London, 1849).

Woodward, Theodore E., 'Cholera and Bacillary Dysentery: Teachable Global Health Problems', *American Journal of Tropical Medicine and Hygiene*, 23 (1974), pp. 767–770.

Wright, Peter and Treacher, Andrew, eds., *The Problem of Medical Knowledge. Examining the Social Construction of Medicine* (Edinburgh, 1982).

Yates, Dora E., *My Gypsy Days* (London, 1953).

Ziegler, Philip, *The Black Death* (London, 1969).

Zucchi, Carlo, 'Della competenza scientifica e giuridica del medico nell'esercizio dell-'amministrazione sanitaria', *Giornale della Reale Società Italiana d'Igiene*, 8 (1886), pp. 17–59.

Index

Abignente, Giovanni 206, 211, 215
Ackerknecht, Erwin 230
Adriatic Sea 79 242
age profile of mortality from cholera: *see* cholera
Albergo dei Poveri 54, 173
algid phase of cholera 114–15, 131, 132, 133
alkalinity: and vibrio 113–14
Altona: cholera outbreak of 1892–3 130
Amore, Nicola: Mayor of Naples 13, 48, 100, 101; advocates urban renewal 196, 226–7; appeals to the Church 149, 167; assumes emergency powers 101; bans festivals 145; criticizes Naples Renewal Company 219; criticizes sanitary teams 140; defeated in elections of 1889 207–8; describes overcrowding 19; as leader of the Historical Right 46; opens Vittoria Hospital 170; orders sanitary cordon 92; posthumously honoured 220, 252; preoccupied with beggars 42; proposes the Rettifilo 185–6; receives aid from the Bank of Naples 171–2; relies on state anti-cholera measures 100; reports violence against doctors 145–6; views *risanamento* as antidote to subversion 197; warns of cholera at Toulon 64
anaemia 14
anticontagionism: *see* localism
apoplexy: as misdiagnosis for cholera 97
apparent death: and cholera 120
Apulia: and cholera-riots in 1911 309; and emigration 267–8; and epidemic of 1910 220, 233–47, 297, 302; unaffected by cholera in 1884 141
Arenaccia: 'industrial neighbourhood' of 198; as a modern slum 212; high rents in 213
Argentina: emigration to 268, 338–40; and epidemic of 1886–8 338–40; Italy bans emigration to 340–44; and Paris Sanitary

Convention 339–40; and South American Sanitary Convention 339–40, 341; spurns International Exhibitions at Rome and Turin 341, 342; as threat to the conspiracy of silence 338
Arlotta, Enrico: advocate of *risanamento* 206; alderman 206, 255; criticizes Luzzatti 295; criticizes Naples Renewal Company 219; Deputy for Naples 262; and outbreak of 1910 261–2; reports industrial accidents during *risanamento* 209
arsenal 36–7
'Association for the Interest of the Economy': as electoral association of clerico-moderates 46 7
'Association for the Protection of the Interests of the Twelfth Electoral District': protests against sanitary measures 290, 300–301, 340, 343
'Association of Progress': as electoral association of the Historical Left 46–7
Auburn: cholera outbreak at 309, 319–20
auto-experiments: and cholera 130

Bagnoli 300, 313
Bahun's valve: and enteroclysis 134, 135
banchisti 274
banking crisis: and *risanamento* 217–18
Bank of Naples: charitable role in 1884 163, 170–72; discharges pawnbroking debts 171; and emigrant remittances 274; finances Vittoria and Cotugno hospitals 170; owns urban property 50; reports on Neapolitan economy 275–6
Bardonecchia lazaretto 87
Bari 235–6, 293, 300
Barletta: and cholera riot 237, 242, 293–4; and epidemic of 1910 220, 233–45, 294
barricades: threatened in 1911 2–3, 292–4

463

bassi: rent in 34, 222; as slums 20, 47, 139, 143, 225; and spread of cholera 23; survive renewal programme 215, 220, 221–2; visited by Depretis and Umberto I 165

Baudelaire, Charles 113

Bay of Naples 11, 67, 271, 272; and epidemic of 1884 96–8, 119–20; and epidemic of 1911 353; and outbreak of 1910 259, 262–3; pollution of 30, 98, 283; *see also* Nisida lazaretto

beggars: as indication of social conditions 36; and the lottery 44; and mortality in 1884 142; as preoccupation of city council 42–3

Berlin 77, 127, 126, 129, 131, 195, 311–12; declining vulnerability to cholera 177; as symbol of medical rationalism 122, 129, 131, 133, 136

Billi, Pasquale: Deputy 94; demonstrates against the Nisida lazaretto 94

Bilson, Geoffrey 177

bingeing: and outbreak of 1910 259–60; as predisposing factor in cholera 99; as protest against health regulations 144–5

bloodletting: *see* treatment of cholera

Bolla aqueduct: contamination of 27–8, 190

boarding-houses: *see locande*

Boccaccio, Giovanni 69, 308

bonfires: as means of purifying air 27, 70, 79, 103, 139, 145, 172

Borsa del Lavoro: as labour organization 290–91; protests at sanitary neglect 265; supports ban on emigration to Argentina 343; urges general strike against sanitary measures 246–7, 290, 292–3;

Bourbon dynasty 31, 36, 40, 46, 122, 150, 169, 177, 192

Bourdelais, Patrice 117, 176, 245, 248–9

brass foundries: and spread of cholera 24; and urban pollution 24

breast-feeding: as defence against cholera 118–19

Briggs, Asa 3–5, 244, 360

Britain 1, 309; and first pandemic 21–2, 150, 151; rejects land-based quarantine in 1884 84; and White Cross Volunteers 158

bronchitis 223

Brooklyn 309; and cholera outbreak in 1911 319–20

Broussais, François 126

buckets: role in spread of cholera 22, 27, 28

Buenos Aires 268, 339–40, 343

builders: diet of 21; employed in renewal 218; injured and killed during *risanamento* 208–11; insecurity of employment 21; as profession 31; as residents of *locande* 20–22; unable to flee Barletta 240; and usury 21; as victims of cholera 22; wages and hours of 20–21, 35; *see also* workers and tradesmen

building code 199

Buonomo, Giuseppe: Professor of Medicine 52;

as representative of the medical profession 229

burial regulations: *see* cemetery

Busca: and emigration to France 65; and epidemic of 1884 88–9, 96, 164; visited by King Umberto 164

Cabrini, Angiolo: socialist Deputy 273; attacks Luzzatti 295; describes abuses of *locandieri* at expense of emigrants 273

cachexia 42

cafès: closed in epidemic of 1884 108–9

Cagliari: cholera outbreak of 1912 247, 326–7, 331–2

Calabria 267, 268: and epidemic of 1911 307, 308, 310–11; escapes cholera in 1884 141; and fear of cholera in 1884 74, 90, 177; as place of refuge in 1884 108

Calcutta 75, 353, 354

Calissano, Teobaldo: Secretary of State for the Interior 236, 293

Camorra: complicity of Bourbons and Liberals with 40–41; composition of 41–2; and control of the slaughter-house 41; and emigration 271–5; and ideology of honour 39; and illegal gambling 39–40, 44; makes elections 41, 46, 153–4; and monopoly pricing 40–42; organization of 39–42; populist rhetoric of 39; and prostitution 39–40, 287; resists sanitary measures in 1910–11 246, 289–96; threatens Henry Geddings 335–6; under attack in elections of 1910 253–7; and usury 39–40

Campania 108, 141, 249, 268, 273, 300, 328, 350

Cantani, Arnaldo: Professor of Medicine 52, 53; advocates therapeutic rationalism 129–31; directs Neapolitan cholera hospitals 129, 136, 137; employs enteroclysis and hypodermoclysis, 133–6 355–6; warns against premature burial 121

capital: shortage of 31, 36–7

Capodimonte Insane Asylum 173

carabinieri 39; clash with demonstrators in 1884 99, 146; clash with demonstrators at Taranto in 1910 293–4; enforce cholera regulations in Barletta in 1910 237–8

Carmignano aqueduct: contamination of 26–7, 190

Carmine Prison: and riot in 1884 148–9

Caro, Orazio: Director of the Office of Hygiene 225, 228–9, 242, 328; author of mendacious account of epidemic of 1910–11 250–53, 306–7, 330–31; critic of conditions at Cotugno Hospital 225; physician at Conocchia Hospital in 1884 136; supporter of Cantani and enteroclysis 136

carriers: of cholera 114

Casale, Alberto: Deputy 47; as Camorra boss 47, 274; and lawsuit against socialist paper *La Propaganda* 47, 253–7

Casale trial 253–6, 274
catgut industry 24, 103–4
Catholic Church: and accommodation with
  medical science 243; boycotts International
  Exhibitions of 1911 341; as critic of
  risanamento 200; divisions within, 50–51; and
  the Liberal state 44–5, 50–51, 166–8, 243; and
  resistance to authority in Sicily 169; and
  theology of cholera as divine punishment 74,
  113, 139, 166–9, 214
Catholic faction 46–7; holds power 253–8,
  263–5; under attack by the Popular Bloc
  254–6, 265; *see also* Girolamo Giusso,
  Francesco Del Carretto
Cavallotti, Felice 158, 159
Cavour, Camillo 166–7, 194, 360–61
Celesia: Cardinal Archbishop of Palermo 72–3,
  74
cemetery 109; burial regulations in 1884 102–3,
  120–21, 140; burial regulations in 1910 279;
  and conspiracy of silence in 1911 316; and
  fear of apparent death, 121; and first burial in
  1884 96; located at Poggioreale 36; as
  metaphor for localist theory, 188
cerebral haemorrhage 223; as misdiagnosis for
  cholera 235
cesspits: emptied as anti-cholera measure 103,
  351; prevalence of 25, 27–8, 36, 280
Chamber of Commerce, Naples 246, 286;
  protests against Luzzatti's sanitary measures
  286, 290, 292–3
chamber-pots: and spread of cholera 28
Chevalier, Louis 3–4, 176, 244, 360
Chiaia: *sezione* of Naples 11, 147, 265
children and cholera: *see* cholera
chlorotic anaemia: *see* women
cholera: and abandonment of sufferers 67; age
  profile of deaths from 116–20; algid phase of
  114–16, 125, 131, 132, 133; and assaults on
  physicians 1, 4, 67, 77–8; class profile of 15,
  141–4; and crime 70; and dietary excesses 43;
  'epidemic' and 'sporadic' 22–3, 98, 102, 190;
  and flight 1, 5, 67, 69–70, 144, 149, 160; and
  malnutrition 43; pejorative moral associations
  of 112–13; and 'premonitory diarrhoea' 43;
  reaction phase of 115–16, 125; and revival of
  religiosity 5, 67, 99; and riot 1, 67; seasonality
  of 68; and the 'Southern Question' 4–5, 154,
  192, 361–3; spread by water and food 15–16,
  26–30, 82, 83, 119; and 'stragglers' 175; and
  suicide 70–71; symptoms of 112–21; and
  threat of general strike 3, 292–4, 301, 343;
  and xenophobia 1, 149–54; *see also*
  complications of cholera, epidemic, outbreak
  of cholera, mortality from cholera, pandemic,
  substances used in treatment of cholera,
  symptoms of cholera, treatment of cholera
cholera-belt 127
cholera gravis 114, 161, 264, 356

cholera nostras 74–5, 122; as misdiagnosis of
  cholera 117–18, 338
cholera sicca 114
Church: *see* Catholic Church
Ciccotti, Ettore: advocates urban renewal 265;
  attacks Luzzatti 295; and downfall of Alberto
  Casale and Celestino Summonte 253–7;
  elected as reform candidate in 1900 254
cigars: as means of purifying air 76
Ciliento, Nicola: first verified case of cholera in
  1884, 97–8
cisterns: *see* water-tanks
Civiltà cattolica: and theology of cholera 73–4,
  243
chlamydia parasite 223
class profile of cholera victims: *see* cholera
Clavières lazaretto 87
cockroaches: prevalence of in the Lower City 19
'collapse' phase of cholera 114–15, 131, 132, 133
collapsing buildings on *risanamento* sites
  208–11
colmate 188, 217
coma: in cholera patients 116
Commissariat of Emigration 291, 322, 340
Committee for the Assistance of the Victims of
  Cholera: *see* White Cross
complications of cholera: gangrene 116;
  meningitis 116; pneumonia 116; renal failure
  116; toxaemia 116; uraemia 116; *see also*
  symptoms of cholera
concealment of cases 105, 116, 145
Conocchia Hospital: as cause of alarm 111–12,
  121; invaded by relatives of patients 146–7;
  mortality rate at 112, 161–2; opening of
  causes riot 147–8; and poisoning phobia 137,
  161–2; re-opened 102–3; as site of
  experimentation 135–6, 316; unprepared in
  1884 102, 170; visited by Archbishop
  Sanfelice 168; visited by the King 164–5
conscription 50, 266
conspiracy of silence: enforcement of 333–53;
  and epidemic of 1910–11 2–3, 6, 246–53,
  257–8, 260, 262–5, 281–5, 297–367; and
  French collusion, 33–8; ordered by Giovanni
  Giolitti 305–7, 345–52; and sanitary
  conditions 14–15; and United States collusion
  321–6, 333–7
constipation: and epidemic of 1884 170–71; and
  malnutrition 42
'Constitutional Association': as electoral
  association of the Historical Right 46–7
consumption levy: *see dazio consumo*
consumption of food: decline since unification
  42–3, 216
contagionism: and anticontagionism 67–8; and
  Catholic doctrine 169; as dominant medical
  ideology 230; and germ theory of Robert
  Koch 68; and prophylaxis against plague
  78–9; *see also* Robert Koch, localism

contagio-miasmatism: *see* localism
'contract labour': and emigration 268–9
Cooter, Roger 226
cordons sanitaires: *see* quarantine, land-based
Corfu: lazaretto at 80; as port of origin of
gypsies in Apulia 239
Cotugno Hospital: and concealment of epidemic
of 1911 311–12, 313–15, 316, 318, 353;
conditions of criticized 224–5; and epidemic
of 1910 261, 264–5, 283; feared by patients
225, 279; founded during *risanamento* 190;
and mortality in 1911 357; and patient
management in 1911 355–6
cows: *see* domestic animals
crafts: decline of 34–5; wages in 34–5; *see also*
workers and tradesmen
Crispi, Francesco 364–5
Crissolo lazaretto 87
croup: mortality in 1884 105
cuts: as mutilation of *risanamento* 215–20, 227

Darwin, Charles 77–8
D'Azeglio, Massimo 73
dazio consumo: as basis of local government
finance 37–8; and renewal of Naples 194–5;
resented by the populace 38, 50; as source of
insolvency of Naples 37–8; *see also* tax policy
of Liberal regime
De Ambris, Alceste 342
De Bonis, Teodosio: Professor of Medicine 100;
alderman responsible for health 100–101, 167;
directs anti-cholera campaign 100–104; as
follower of Pettenkofer 102, 195, 226; and
opening of the Vittoria Hospital 170; as
supporter of Cantani and enteroclysis 135–6
Defoe, Daniel 69
De Giaxa: Professor of Medicine 258; informant
for United States Public Health and Marine
Hospital Service 258, 320–21
Delaporte, François 176, 245
Del Carretto, Francesco: Mayor of Naples 253,
310, 311; conceals epidemic of 1911, 35,
311–13, 333; and elections of 1910, 23–7, 310;
minimizes outbreak of 1910 262–5; resists
sanitary measures in 1910 293; seeks foreign
investment 276–7
De Luca, Gennaro: considers poverty and
unemployment in Naples 216; industrialist
and city councillor 216; supports revolt
against sanitary measures in 1910 290, 292,
335
De Martino, Domenico: elected reform candidate
in 1900; spokesman for the *locandieri* 287–8,
290, 292
demographic panic: in France 14; in Naples 14
Department of Public Health (*Direzione
Generale della Sanità*) 238, 292; as agency of
the Ministry of the Interior 45–6, 89; compiles
secret cholera files for winter of 1910–11

297–9; directs anti-cholera campaign in 1911,
351–2; falsifies statistics for epidemic of 1911,
32–3; misleads American authorities 248; and
official account of epidemic of 1910 251;
organizes anti-cholera campaign in 1910
239–40; warns of approach of the sixth
pandemic 233
Department of State: *see* United States
Department of State
depletive therapy: *see* treatment of cholera
Depretis, Agostino: as Prime Minister 70, 90, 95,
96, 163–4, 357–8; conceives plan to renew
Naples, 15, 181, 196–7, 216, 226–7; defends
renewal bill in parliament 191–4; employs
anti-plague measures against cholera 78,
84–7, 241–2; as leader of the Historical Left
192–3; revokes anti-plague measures 89;
visits Naples in 1884 163–9
De Renzi, Errico: Professor of Medicine 52; and
age profile of cholera deaths 116–18; directs
anti-cholera campaign in Mercato in 1884
136; provides mortality statistics for 1884,
106–7; supports Cantani and enteroclysis 136
De Seta, Francesco: Prefect of Naples 262; and
fabrication of statistics, 262
De Zerbi, Rocco: Deputy 15, 157; editor of *Il
Piccolo* 157; and electoral corruption 47; leader
of the Historical Right 157; leads
demonstration against the Nisida lazaretto 94;
and mortality in Lower Naples 15; president of
the White Cross, 157–63; rapporteur of bill for
renewal of Naples 157, 194–6; supports
municipal renewal plan 207–8
dialect: as lingua franca 47, 104
diarrhoea: *see* symptoms of cholera
Dickens, Charles 17, 44
diet: of Neapolitan poor 20–21, 42–4, 222; as
predisposing factor in cholera 15–16, 170–71;
see also food
Di Fratta, Pasquale: Director of the
Commissariat of Emigration 293, 294
Di Giacomo, Salvatore 19
diphtheria: mortality in 1884, 105
Direzione Generale della Sanità: *see* Department
of Public Health
disinfectants and purifiers: aluminium chloride
103; bichloride of mercury 87; carbolic acid
17, 27, 64, 87, 103; chlorine 87; corrosive
sublimate 87, 120; sulphur 27, 70, 78–9, 87,
103, 145; tar, 70; *see also* bonfires
divination 110
doctors: hired in 1911 313; mortality of in 1884
143; standing of in Naples 51–5, 101–2,
225–30; as targets of violence 1, 77–8, 145–7,
149, 241; *see* also localism, treatment of
cholera, Arnaldo Cantani, Robert Koch, Max
von Pettenkofer, Mariano Semmola
domestic animals: and urban pollution 19–20,
23–4

domestic servants 31, 34
donkeys: *see* domestic animals
Don Marzio 264, 310
dry cupping: *see* treatment of cholera
Duomo, Via del 11, 25; and renewal of 200–202
Durey, Michael 22, 151, 176, 245
dustmen: *see* street-sweeping
dysentery 133–4

eclampsia: as cause of death 223
Egypt: and cholera epidemic of 1883 59, 75, 83,
     94, 170, 233
elderly: as residents of *locande* 20
elections: of 1874, and 'parliamentary
     revolution' 192–3; of 1900 253–4; of 1910
     253–7
electoral law of 1882: terms of 47; *see also*
     franchise
electoral reform: as threat to Catholic
     administration 256–7
eliminant therapy: *see* treatment of cholera
Ellis Island: outbreaks of cholera at 248, 286,
     318–20, 321–2, 344; and rejection of
     immigrants 274–5; vigilance redoubled in
     1911 304
embolism 135
Emmanuel, King Victor II 51
emigrant banks 274
emigrants: and cholera in 1884 64–98; and
     remittances 274, 302; as residents of *locande*
     20–21, 263, 271–5; spread cholera to the
     United States 248, 318–20; and xenophobia in
     France 65; *see also* emigration
emigration: banned by Giolitti to Argentina
     331–4; to France 64–6; and the Neapolitan
     economy, 27–77; to the New World 266–77,
     334, 338–45; and sanitary vigilance of the
     United States 248, 325, 334; as source of
     cholera in Naples in 1910 236; *see also*
     emigrants
emigration agents 268–9
emotions: as predisposing factors in cholera 104
endocarditis 223
enemas: *see* treatment of cholera
Engels, Friedrich 17
enteritis: as cause of death in 1884 105; as
     misdiagnosis for cholera 91
enteroclysis: *see* treatment of cholera, Arnaldo
     Cantani
enterotoxin 114
epidemic, cholera: of 1836–7 in Naples 15, 16,
     104, 106, 177; of 1854 in Naples 15, 16, 177; of
     1865–7 in Italy 85, 86; of 1865–7 in Naples 15,
     16, 49; of 1873 in Naples 15, 16, 49; of 1883 in
     Egypt 59, 75, 83, 94, 170, 233; of 1884 in
     Provence 59–94, 164; of 1884 in Naples 15,
     22–3, 49, 50, 99–178; of 1884–7 in Italy 85, 86;
     of 1885–6 in Sicily 169; of 1886–8 in
     Argentina 338–9; of 1892–3 in Hamburg 1,

152–3; of 1910 in Naples 15, 22–3, 233–56; of
     1911 in Italy 297–359; of 1911 in Naples 15,
     297–359; of 1911 in Sicily 247, 306; *see also*
     outbreak of cholera, pandemic
epidemic, plague: *see* plague
'European cholera': *see cholera nostras*
Evans, Richard 1, 117–20, 152–3, 177, 229–30,
     245, 248–9
eviction: as result of *risanamento* 2, 198–200;
     207–8, 211–15
'expansion neighbourhoods': erection of new
     slums in 211–13; high rents in 199–201,
     211–13; and homelessness resulting from
     risanamento 197–8; and lack economic
     infrastructure 199–201; overcrowding in
     211–13; and precedent of the Via Duomo
     201–2
expropriation of landlords: and *risanamento*
     199–201
extreme unction 109

Fabre Line 271, 287
factionalism 46–7
Faculty of Medicine of the University of Naples
     52, 157, 227–8
Fazio, Eugenio: Professor of Hygiene 15, 108;
     describes cholera in 1884 106, 107
Ferry, Jules: Prime Minister of France 63, 74
fevers 4, 14, 20; miasmatic 14; 'Naples' 14;
     pernicious 14; petecchial 14; puerperal 105;
     relapsing 4; scarlet 4; typhoidal 14; as
     symptom of reaction stage of cholera 115–16
final destination cards: as United States
     sanitary measure 304
fishermen: and cholera in 1910 at Naples 35,
     263; and cholera in Apulia in 1910 233–5; and
     cholera at La Spezia 83; as residents of the
     Santa Lucia neighbourhood 35; wages and
     living conditions of 35; *see also* workers and
     tradesmen
flagellants 110
flatulence: during epidemic of 1884 170–71
Flaubert, Gustave 113
fleas: and plague 78–83
flies: prevalence of in Lower City 19
flight: as defence against epidemic disease 5,
     69–70, 78, 143–4, 149, 241, 245; from
     Marseilles and Toulon in 1884 68–70; from
     Naples in 1884 107–9, 139, 156, 160–61; from
     La Spezia in 1884 91; from Apulia to Naples
     in 1910 240–41, 301–2; from Barletta and
     Trani in 1910 240; from Naples in 1910 242,
     263; promoted by localism 68–9, 107, 108; and
     social class 107–8
Florence: as model for urban renewal 49; as
     place of refuge in 1884 108; and preventive
     measures in 1910, 278
Foggia 237, 300; as place of refuge in 1884
     108

fondaci: demolitions of prior to *risanamento* 199; population of relocated in 1884 104; scheduled for demolition in *risanamento* 186–7, 199; survive renewal 215, 220–21, 222; visited by Depretis and Umberto I 165; as worst slums in Naples 19–20, 49, 102, 139, 143, 220

food: bean soup, in diet of the poor 21; bread, contaminated 30, cost of 34, 223, in diet of the poor; consumption of, decline since unification 42–3, 216; crabs 30, 36; fruit, condemned by authorities 144, 170–71, 172–3, consumed in protest at health regulations 144–5, cost of 34, 223, in diet of the poor 19–20, 21, 100, 222, as predisposing factor in cholera 16, 100, 170–71, price inflated by Camorra 41; macaroni, cost of 34, 222, in diet of the poor 21; meat, consumption encouraged 104, 170–71, 172–3, cost of 21, 34, missing from diet of the populace 222, price control of 104, trade controlled by Camorra 41; pizza 24, 36, 43; shellfish, consumption 30, 36, banned in 1910 and 1911 280, 293–4, 351, condemned by medical opinion 170–71, discouraged in 1884 172–3, as means of spreading cholera 30, 35, 119–20, 170–71, role in cholera outbreak of 1910 262–3; *see also* bingeing, diet

Forti Messina, Anna Lucia 177 249–50

Fortunato, Giustino 363

foundries: and arsenical poisoning 24; as factors in spread of cholera 24; and high mortality from cholera in 1884 142; as sources of pollution 24

France 1; and collusion with Italian conspiracy of silence 337–8, 343–4; and demographic panic 14; and first pandemic 82, 151; rejects land-based quarantine in 1884 84; and White Cross volunteers 158; *see also* Marseilles, Provence, Toulon.

Franchetti, Leopoldo 201

Francis-Joseph, Emperor 156

franchise: excludes women 46; restricted by property qualification 45; *see also* electoral law of 1882

fumigation 62, 70, 79, 83–4, 86, 87–8, 102–3, 140, 159, 319

Fusco, Salvatore: Deputy 161; critic of Naples Renewal Company 209–10, 219; White Cross leader 161, 209

Galasso, Giuseppe 252–3

Galen 122

galvanism: at Conocchia Hospital 136–7; as treatment for cholera at the Pharo Hospital in 1884 77

Ganges River 59, 101, 113

ganglionic nerves: considered seat of cholera 122–3

gangrene: *see* complications of cholera

Garcia, Antonio Fernandez 245

Gasperini, Prefect of Bari: suggests concealment of cholera by fictive diagnoses 235–6

gastro-enteritis: as cause of death 223; as disease of children 118, 223; as fictive diagnosis for cholera 258, 259, 264, 302, 375, 425–6; as indication of the failure of *risanamento* 265; as misdiagnosis of cholera 117–18; as pervasive summer illness 43, 116–17, 220, 265

Geddings, Henry Downes: Medical Officer at American Consulate 258; accuses Italy of deceit 258–9, 324–6; attacked as slanderer of Naples 291–2, 335; defamed by Italian authorities 335; discovers cholera in 1911 299–300; honoured by Italy 292; predicts return of cholera in 1911 297, 299–300; signatory to Paris Sanitary Convention 258; threatened by Camorra 335–6

gender and cholera: *see* cholera, women

'general sweep': *see* street-sweeping

general strike: and epidemic of 1910–11 3, 246–7, 292–3, 301, 343

Genoa: anti-plague lazaretto at 80; and emigration 237, 246, 286, 338; and epidemic of 1911 325; as rival to Naples 246, 290–93, 300–301; vulnerability to cholera 233, 246, 247; wages in 32–3

Germany 1, 84, 129, 136, 153, 267, 312; as model of preventive health 241–2; outbreak of cholera in 1905 233; rejects land-based quarantine in 1884 84; *see also* Berlin, Hamburg, Prussia

Gesù e Maria Hospital 54

Giambarba, Adolfo 186, 188, 209

Giolitti, Giovanni: Prime Minister 2, 236, 208; and electoral reform 256–7; orders ban on Italian emigration to Argentina 340–44; orders conspiracy of silence 6–7, 246–7, 301–2, 305–17, 345–59, 364–7; returns to power in 1911 296

Giusso, Girolamo: Mayor of Naples 13–14, 31–2, 48; Director of the Bank of Naples 31–2, 170; White Cross volunteer 158; critic of renewal plan 198–201, 204–6, 208

glass craft 34

goats: *see* domestic animals

gonorrhoea 275

Gramsci, Antonio 50, 45, 242; and theory of 'passive revolution' 45, 46, 50

ground-water: and localist theory of cholera 187–90

gypsies: internment of 238–40; as targets of xenophobia 1, 73, 238–40

Hamburg: and commercial pressure to conceal cholera 246; and epidemic of 1892 1, 117–18, 119, 152–4

Hapsburg Empire: and defences against plague 80–82; outbreak of cholera in 1905 233; rejects land-based quarantine in 1884 84; threat of cholera from 93

Haughwout, Frank: American Consul at Naples 32; compiles wage statistics 32–4; criticizes Town Hall as unprepared in 1884 102; accuses city of falsifying statistics 105

Haussmann, Georges 181, 184, 189, 194; *see also* 'productive spending'

hemorrhoids: as indication of malnutrition 42

Hippocrates 80, 122, 124

Historical Left: and elections of 1874 192–3; and 'parliamentary revolution' 192; and 'Southern Question' 192–3; in Naples 192

Hoffman Island 322

homelessness 42–3, 46, 222–3; as a result of *risanamento* 208, 216–17; as priority of anti-cholera campaign, 13–14

honour: as ideology of the Camorra 39

horses: *see* domestic animals

hospitals: inadequacies of 54–5; dread of in 1884 111–12, 160, 162, 147, 172; service improves 172; *see also* Conocchia, Cotugno, Maddalena, Pharo, Piedigrotta and Vittoria Hospitals.

housing: damp 19, 222; heat, absent in homes of the poor 222–3; housing code, absence of 17; and sanitary crisis in Naples 17–23; *see also* *bassi*, 'expansion neighbourhoods', *fondaci*, homelessness, *locande*.

Hugo, Victor 17

huxters: *see* pedlars

hypodermoclysis: *see* treatment of cholera

ileocolonic valve 134, 135

ileum: centre of cholera infection 113–14, 133–4

illiteracy: prevalence in Naples 20, 31, 50, 139, 153–4; among Italian emigrants to France 65, 76; among Italian emigrants to the New World 269; in the South 90, 266–7

Imbriani, Matteo Renato: city councillor and critic of *risanamento* 210

indigestion: as predisposing factor in cholera 16

Indo-China 62–3

industry: in Naples 30–35, 37, 42

influenza 15

insurrection: threatened against sanitary measures 292–3

International Exhibitions of 1911: at Rome and Turin 301–2, 307, 323, 341, 345–7; boycotted by the Catholic Church 341

International Sanitary Conference at Vienna 1874: condemns use of anti-plague measures against cholera 84

International Sanitary Conference at Rome 1885: opposes use of anti-plague measures against cholera 85

International Sanitary Convention of 1903: *see* Paris Sanitary Convention

Isernia: and cholera outbreak of 1884 92–3, 96, 98

Italian Socialist Party 252–7, 265, 291, 342–3

Jedda 59, 233

Jesuits 73–4, 243

Jews: as targets of xenophobia 73, 149, 238

Johnson, James 123

jugular vein: and bloodletting 123

Klein, Edward Emanuel 130

Knox, Philander Chase: United States Secretary of State 301–2, 321, 323, 324, 344, 351

Koch, Robert: accounts for decline of epidemics 173–4; as apologist for centralization 195, 436; condemns use of anti-plague measures against cholera 82–4; diagnostic techniques of 237, 348; directs anti-cholera measures in Prussia 241–3; discovers *vibrio cholerae* 75; and germ theory of disease 1–2, 68, 101–2, 152, 189, 230, 242–3, 279, 299, 329–30, 348; and individual prophylaxis 143–4; influences Arnaldo Cantani 129–31; and 'Koch's Postulates' 130–31; and problem of identifying final cases in an epidemic 175; and rationalist epistemology 126; and role of alcohol in epidemics 100; visits Provence in 1884 75–6; warns against tank-wells 29

Kraut, Alan 249, 259

labour: redeeming power of 196–7

Labriola, Arturo: and downfall of Alberto Casale and Celestino Summonte 253–7, 362

laissez-faire: and economy of Naples 27, 37, 45; and sanitary conditions in Naples 17, 22, 27, 50, 140, 154, 226, 295

Lancet 51–2, 124–5, 127, 129, 152, 164, 308

landlords: and mortality from cholera in 1884 143

landfills (*colmate*): and *risanamento* 188, 217

La Plata 338–43

La Propaganda: socialist newspaper 47, 257, 265, 345; and lawsuit by Alberto Casale 47, 253–6

La Spezia: epidemic of 1884 88, 90–92; epidemic of 1911 325

Latta, Thomas: and rehydration therapy 126–7

laundry trade 17; and cholera at La Spezia 95–6, 97; and cholera at Naples 97; prevalence of 24; and spread of cholera 24

lavatories 21, 23, 29

law of 15 January 1885: presented to parliament 191–5, 226–7; and *risanamento* 195, 201, 202; as a 'special law' 193, 226, 363

law of 7 July 1902: and additional funds for *risanamento* 219–20, 255

lawyers: and mortality from cholera in 1884 143

lazarettos: and cholera phobia 160–61, 237; deployed by Venice against plague 79–80; deployed against cholera in 1884 86–8; evaded by refugees from France 88–90; and plague in Mediterranean ports 80; *see also* quarantine, land-based and quarantine, maritime.

Leca, Ange-Pierre 176, 245

leeches: and eliminant treatment of cholera 123

Lefebvre, Georges 137–8

Leishman, John: United States Ambassador to Italy 301–2, 321, 322, 323; reports threats against American health officials 351; urges collusion with concealment of 1911 epidemic 322–3

Leo XIII, Pope 166–8

lepers: as scapegoats in time of plague 149

leprosy: and theology of disease 71

La Libertà 256, 257–8, 264, 310

Libyan War 307, 358

light: absence of in the Lower City 17, 19, 21–2; lack of as factor in spread of cholera 23

Lister, Joseph 133–4

Livorno: and epidemic of 1911 317, 325; and vulnerability to cholera 247

localism: and atmospheric poison 67; as basis of *risanamento* 185–90, 195, 217, 226; and cholera-germ 68; and decentralization 195, 436; dominant in French medical profession in 1884 67; dominant in Italian medical profession in 1884 102, 138–9, 229–30; and dread of hospitals 147; as instrument of power by the medical profession 226–7; in opposition to contagionism of Robert Koch 67–8; in opposition to use of anti-plague measures against cholera 82–3; and sanitary reform 68–9; and seasonality of cholera 68; and social hierarchy 226; as spur to flight 67–9; and telluric conditions 68; as theory of Max von Pettenkofer 67–9

locande: as boarding-houses for transient population 21–3; conditions of 213; cost of a room in 21–2; and emigration 20–21, 263, 271–5; emptied during epidemic of 1884 103–4, 108–9, 173; and the epidemic of 1884 22, 97–8; and the epidemic of 1910 22, 263, 263; and *laissez-faire* 22; overcrowding in 21–2; and pressure to conceal cholera 246, 285–96; prevalence of in Porto 21–2; as sanitary concern in 1910 278, 295; and spread of cholera 21–3, 97–8; survive renewal programme 220–21; and typhoid 22

lockout: threatened in epidemic of 1910–11 2–3, 246–7, 292–4, 301, 343

lodging-houses: *see locande*

Lombroso, Cesare: and phobia of gypsies 238

London 123; declining vulnerability to cholera 17; density of 17–18; population of 18, 36; unemployment in 36

Longmate, Norman 151, 176

Loreto Hospital 54, 92

lottery: and the Camorra 44; and epidemic of 1884 99–100; and poverty 44

Lower City 100, 103, 141, 143, 145–6, 154, 156–7, 160, 162, 170–71, 197– 8, 280, 284: and anti-cholera campaign of 1911 351–2; and class tensions 171; configuration of 11, 17–19, 380–81; density of population in 1912 222; mortality in 13–16; and mortality from cholera in 1884 106–7; and mortality from cholera in 1911 328–32; overpopulation in 17–19; and policy of 'thinning' the population 173; population of 11; renewal of 181–230; *see also* housing, poverty, water supply, sewers, cholera

Lucci, Arnaldo: advocate of urban renewal 265; and downfall of Alberto Casale and Celestino Summonte 253–7; socialist city councillor 253–4

Luzzatti, Luigi: Prime Minister, 6, 236, 299, 301, 357–8; and anti-gypsy terror 237–40; downfall of 246–7, 257, 285–96; and electoral reform 256–7; and epidemic of 1910 237–42, 305, 365–6; as Jewish 238; and protection of emigrants 287

lymphatic constitution: as indication of malnutrition 42

Maddalena Hospital 111, 121, 164–5; and mortality in 1884 112, 161–2; opening of causes riot 147–8; used as quarantine station in 1911 313

Madonna: cult of 109–10

Magendie, François: and rehydration therapy 126

malaria 68, 105, 125

Malatesta, Errico: as White Cross volunteer 158

malnutrition: as predisposing factor in cholera 15–16, 30–31, 43; prevalent in Naples 42–3, 49, 153–4, 222–3

Malta: and cholera epidemic of 1865 83

Mancini, Pasquale Stanislao: Foreign Minister 163–4; advocate of renewal 185–6

Mann, Thomas 113; reports conspiracy of silence in 1911 307

manure: contaminates vegetables 26; pollutes water supply 27

Manzoni, Alessandro 149, 152

Marghieri, Alberto 184; as advocate of subcontracting system 204–6; alderman responsible for public works 196; and ambition to transform the poor 197–8; believes in ineradicability of poverty 196–7; declares *risanamento* a failure 220–21; defeated in elections of 1889 207–8; rapporteur of city renewal plan 196–201

Mario, Jesse White 362

market gardening: and the recycling of waste 26; as means of spreading cholera 26, 280, 284; regulated in 1910 and 1911 280, 351

Marseilles: cholera outbreak of 1883 59–62; cholera epidemic of 1884 64–6, 96, 164; cholera outbreak of 1911 337–8, 343–4; and commercial pressure to conceal epidemics 246; lazaretto at 80; plague epidemic of 1720–22 80, 81; vulnerable to cholera 68

Martin Garcia: quarantine station at Buenos Aires 340, 341

Martinoli: Chief Engineer of the Company for the Renewal of Naples 210–11; and lethal building practices 210–11

Materdei: 'expansion neighbourhood' of 197–8

Il Mattino 19, 221–2, 272–3, 291, 310

Mayhew, Henry 17

McGrew, Roderic 116–17, 245

measles 4; endemic disease of children 116–17; mortality in 1884 105; mortality in the New World 112

Mecca 59, 73, 235

Medical Association of Venice: silenced in 1911 348–50

medical periodicals: and concealment in 1911 316–17

medico condotto: inadequate numbers of in the Mezzogiorno 46; inadequate numbers of in Naples 52–3, 101–2; lack of authority among the populace 52–3; as municipal public health doctor 46; service improved after *risanamento* 228–9

meningitis: as cause of death 223; as complication of cholera 116; as misdiagnosis of cholera 91, 302

Mercato: *sezione* of Naples 11, 15, 17, 19–20, 40, 84, 104, 106–7, 109, 110–11, 117, 121, 171, 200, 265; *see also* Lower City

mercury: and syphilis 125; and cholera: *see* substances used in treatment of cholera, treatment of cholera

messengers: and mortality from cholera in 1884 142

Messina: and plague of 1743 80

Mezzocannone, Via 215

miasmatism: *see* localism

Milan 206; expenditure on education and health 49; and growth since unification 14; and plague of 1630 149; and anti-cholera measures in 1910 278; as prototype for urban renewal 49, 181, 184, 202; size of in 1884 17, 18; and volunteers for White Cross 156; wages in 33

miracle of the blood of San Gennaro 162–3

Molfetta: and cholera riot 240–42, 293–4; and sanitary cordons 240

Moltke, S.S. 318, 319

Monnier, Marc 40

Montecalvario: *sezione* of Naples 158

Montefusco, Alfonso: author of mendacious account of cholera in 1910 257–8, 264–5, 315–16; and cholera as intoxication of the nervous system 355–6; critic of conditions at the Cotugno Hospital 225; Medical Director of Cotugno Hospital 225, 252, 257, 315; and patient management in 1911 355–7; physician at Conocchia Hospital in 1884 136; supporter of Cantani and enteroclysis 136

Morana, Giovanni Battista: Secretary of State at the Interior 85; directs Italian defense against cholera in 1884 85–9, 237, 302

Morris, R.J. 151, 176

mortality from cholera: from 1836 to 1884 in Naples 15, 16, 104–9; in 1911 in Italy, 326–33; in Paris 152; *see also under* Conocchia, Cotugno, Maddalena, Piedigrotta Hospitals, Lower City, poverty, women

'mortality bulge' in 1911 329–30

'mortality revolution' 181

mosquitoes: and terror at Toulon 71

mould 19

mourners: professional 36

mud 17; contaminates water supply 27

municipal officials: and mortality from cholera in 1884 143

Municipal Sanitary Committee 101–2, 103–4, 107, 121

Munthe, Axel 19, 362

Mussolini, Benito 359

'Naples fever' 14

Naples Renewal Company: founding of 206; and fraudulent stock issue 206–7; granted loose contract 206; and harsh treatment of tenants 211–15; monopoly power of 204–7, 215; presents misleading financial figures 218–20; Technical Committee of 207, 210–11, 215; threatens bankruptcy 215; unpopularity of 208–9, 218–20; violates building code 211–13

Naples Water Works Company Ltd. 189–90

Nardi, Achille: alderman 197–8; Camorra boss 197; supporter of *risanamento* 197–8

National Association of Medical Ethics 52

Navigazione Generale 271, 319

nephritis: as cause of death 223

nervous system: considered site of cholera infection 122–3, 136–7, 355–6, 402

New York City: and Italian immigration 268, 270–71; population density in 17–18

New York Harbor 303, 304, 309, 318–20, 321, 322; *see also* Ellis Island

Nicotera, Giovanni: Deputy for Naples 193; and *risanamento* bill 193

Nisida lazaretto: demonstration against 94; re-activated in 1883 59; as source of cholera at Naples 93–8

Nitti, Francesco Saverio 14, 267, 363; attacks Luzzatti sanitary policy 286, 295, 296, 362

notification: as requirement of the Paris
Sanitary Convention 302–3, 320, 324, 343
nurses: lack of training at the Cotugno Hospital
224, 225

Ocana, Esteban Rodriguez 245
October festival: *see ottobrate*
Office of Hygiene: directed by Orazio Caro 228,
290; founded 228; hires additional personnel
in 1911 313–14; manages anti-cholera
campaign of 1910 250–51, 277–85, 305; as
means of medicalizing population 228–9,
242–3; placed under control of Rome in 1911
305, 351
Old City: *see* Lower City
olive oil 31: export threatened by cholera in
1911 301–2
opere pie: as Catholic benevolent associations
31, 50; and medical needs of Naples 53–5; and
ownership of urban property 50
opiates: *see* substances used in treatment of
cholera
Orientale: 'expansion neighbourhood' of 198
orphans 117, 173, 312
O'Shaughnessy, William: and rehydration
therapy 126
Osservatore romano 72, 96, 111, 140–41, 200,
308, 341
Ottocalli: as an 'expansion neighbourhood' 198,
212
ottobrate: banned in 1910 280–81; as popular
festival 43; as predisposing factor for cholera
43, 119–20
Ottoman Empire: and defences against plague
81–2
outbreak of cholera: of 1886 in Naples 175–6,
178; of 1887 in Naples 175–6, 178; of 1893 in
Naples 175–6; of 1894 in Naples 175–6, 178;
of 1905 in Hapsburg Empire 233; of 1911 in
New York 249, 286, 309, 318–20, 344; of 1911
at Ellis Island 248, 286, 318–20, 321–2, 344;
see also epidemic, pandemic
overcrowding: and propagation of cholera
17–23, 173
overpopulation: *see* population of Naples

Pace Hospital 54
Pacini, Filippo 68; and apparent death in
cholera 120–21
Palermo: and cholera epidemic of 1911 247, 309,
320–21, 324–5, 327, 331–2, 354–5; and Italian
emigration 269–70, 321; lazaretto at 80; and
visit of Leonard Rogers 355–7
pallor: as indication of malnutrition 42
pandemic: first 1–2, 81–3, 114, 150–51, 241, 359;
fifth 1; sixth 2; Britain in first 21–2, 150, 151;
Estonia in first 82; France in first 151; Paris
in fifth 152–4, 243–4; Prussia in first 81–2,
150; Russia in first 81–2, 150; Russia in sixth

233–5, 238–9; Revel in first 82; Sicily in first
150; *see also* epidemic, outbreak of cholera
Paraguay 339–40
Paris: and cholera riots 151; and declining
vulnerability to cholera 177; density of 17, 18;
and fifth pandemic 152–4, 243–4; as model
for renewal of Naples 181–5, 194; and
mortality from cholera 152
Paris Clinic: as model of scientific medicine 54,
122, 129
Paris Commune of 1871: as warning to City
Hall 197
Paris Sanitary Convention of 1903 2, 281, 302–5,
318, 320–22, 324, 325, 334, 336–7, 338, 340–41
Parisi, Raffaele: Deputy Director of the White
Cross 50, 160–61; describes pervasive distrust
of officials 50
Parlati, Francesco: municipal councillor and
critic of *risanamento* 204–6, 208
parliament 45, 185; denied opportunity to
consider epidemic of 1911 311, 357–9, 366–7;
and fall of Luzzatti government 294–6; and
risanamento bill 191–6, 226–7
'parliamentary revolution' of 1876 192
'passive revolution': *see* Antonio Gramsci
Pasteur, Louis 75, 76, 152, 226
pedlars: and mortality from cholera in 1884 142;
as Neapolitan profession 31, 35–6; prevalence
of Camorra among 41–2; regulated during
epidemic of 1911 351; as residents of *locande*
20; *see also* workers and tradesmen
Pellet, Marcellin: French Consul 17; describes
Neapolitan passion for gambling 44; gives
impressions of slums 17
Pelling, Margaret 3–5, 7, 67–8, 230
Pendino: *sezione* of Naples 11, 15, 17, 28–9, 40,
101–2, 106–7, 110, 171, 200, 214, 215, 243; *see
also* Lower City
Persia 59, 233
pest-houses: *see* lazarettos
pestilence: *see* plague
Pettenkofer, Max von: as advocate of flight
68–9, 107–8; as apologist for decentralization
195, 436; condemns use of anti-plague
measures against cholera 83; hygienist at
Munich 67, 102–3, 181, 229–30; and
individual prophylaxis against cholera 144,
436; and miasmo-contagionism 67–9; *see also*
localism
Pharo Hospital, Marseilles 64, 112, 128; and
conditions during the epidemic of 1884 76–8,
137; sends volunteer nurses to Naples 158
Phoofuto, Pule 245
phylloxera 266
physicians: *see* doctors
'physiological treatment of cholera': *see*
treatment of cholera, Mariano Semmola
Pian di Latte lazaretto 87–8
Piattamola lazaretto 87

Il Piccolo 67, 157, 163, 208
Piccolo San Bernardo lazaretto 87
Piedigrotta Hospital: as cholera hospital 111,
  164–5; mortality rate in 1884 112, 162;
  opening of as occasion for riot 147–8
pilgrims: as scapegoats for plague 149; and
  spread of cholera 235
Pilgrims' Hospital 54–5
Pius IX, Pope 166–7
Pius X, Pope 341
pizza 24, 36, 43
plague: compared with cholera 109, 149–53,
  176–7; development of defensive measures
  against 78–81; epidemic at Marseilles in 1720
  80, 81; epidemic at Messina in 1743 80; and
  the International Sanitary Convention of 1903
  302–3; mortality from 112–13, 176–7; and
  theology of disease 71–2; *see also* fleas, rats
pneumonia: as complication of cholera 116; as
  cause of death 223; and rejection of
  immigrants by the United States 275
Poggioreale: cemetery of 36, 279; location of
  Vittoria and Cotugno Hospitals 170, 190; site
  of the Cholera Cemetery in 1884 103, 120; site
  of the Neapolitan slaughter-house 41; suburb
  of Naples 41
poisoning hysteria 149–54, 242; in Italy in 1884
  89–90, 138–41, 168, 407; in Italy in 1910 241,
  252–3; in Provence in 1884 77–8; in the
  United States in 1911 309, 357
Pollitzer, R.: and anti-gypsy mythology 239; and
  misleading statistics for 1911 250
Ponte Rossi: 'expansion neighbourhood' of 198
'Popular Bloc': and elections of 1910 253–7, 310,
  323, 345
population of Naples: in 1836–73 16; in 1884 18;
  density in 1884 18; growth since unification
  14; in 1910 220
port: declines after unification 36–7; dependent
  on emigration 270–72; idle during epidemic of
  1884 109; idle during outbreak of 1910 285–6,
  288–9; as sanitary risk factor 191
porters 34; and mortality from cholera in 1884
  142; as Neapolitan profession 31, 34;
  prevalence of Camorra among 42
Portici: as site of market gardening 26
Porto: *sezione* of Naples 11, 15, 16, 17, 19, 21–3,
  93, 96, 97–9, 104, 106–7, 110, 145, 158, 161,
  171, 200, 214, 215, 243, 265, 287, 290–92; *see
  also* Lower City
Posillipo Hill: as place of refuge in 1884 108
post-mortem muscular twitching: and dread of
  cholera 120
poultry: *see* domestic animals
Poveglia lazaretto 93
poverty: ignored by *risanamento* planners
  196–201; and mortality in 1884 141–4; as
  predisposing factor in cholera 15–16;
  prevalence of in Naples 30–44; prevents

measures of individual prophylaxis 143–4;
  remains prevalent after rebuilding 211–15,
  221–5
premature burial: and cholera 120–21
'premonitory diarrhoea': as warning sign of
  cholera 43, 388
prepaid tickets: and emigration 268–9
press: fails to report epidemic of 1911 307–11;
  secretly financed by Ministry of the Interior
  347–8
Prisco, Giuseppe: Cardinal Archbishop of
  Naples 281
prisons: conditions in 148–9; riots in 1884
  148–9; thinned out in 1884 104
'Problem of Naples': and cholera 4–5, 192,
  361–3; *see also* 'Southern Question'
processions: and the epidemic of 1884 99, 110,
  145, 168
'productive spending': as financial justification
  for *risanamento* 194–5; invoked by Georges
  Haussmann 194–5; invoked by Camillo
  Cavour 194
La Propaganda: and lawsuit of Alberto Casale
  47, 253–5; as Neapolitan socialist newspaper
  47, 261, 310
prostitution: and the Camorra 40, 274, 287; as
  indication of poverty 36
protection racket: and the Camorra 39–40
Provence: and cholera epidemic of 1884 59–98,
  107, 121, 137, 164, 241; and Italian emigration
  64–6, 160; and plague epidemic of 1720–22 81
Prussia: and first cholera pandemic 81–2, 150
ptyalism 125
pulse: of cholera patients 114–15
Punjab, the 59, 233
Public Security Law of 1889 239
purging: *see* symptoms of cholera
putrefaction: as only certain sign of death 121;
  of unburied bodies of cholera victims 109

quarantine, land-based 78–98; adopted by Italy
  in 1884 84–98, 303; condemned by Third and
  Fourth International Sanitary Conferences 84,
  85; creates terror 89–91; as defence against
  plague 78–81; deployed by Hapsburg,
  Hohenzollern and Romanov autocracies
  against cholera 81–2; fails against cholera in
  Egypt in 1883 83; fails against cholera in
  Malta in 1865 83; as means of spreading
  cholera 83–4; as model for anti-cholera
  measures in first pandemic 81–3; regarded as
  useless against cholera by French Academy
  82; regarded as useless against cholera by the
  international medical community 82–3;
  rejected against cholera by Britain 82;
  discourages sanitary reform, 84; rejected in
  Western Europe in 1884 84–5, 151–2; rejected
  by Paris Sanitary Convention 303–4; *see also*
  lazarettos.

quarantine, maritime: as defence against plague 78–81; deployed in 1884 93–8; and Paris Sanitary Conference 246–7, 302–6; employed by the United States in 1911 303–4, 321, 336, 347; employed by Argentina in 1911 339–42
Quarantine Regulations of the United States 304
Quarcino lazaretto 87
'Question of Naples': *see* 'Problem of Naples'

radicals: *see* Popular Bloc
rag trade: as means of spreading cholera 15–16, 24, 263, 351
Raineri, Giovanni: Minister of Agriculture, Industry and Commerce 299; produces misleading cholera statistics 299, 331–2
rationalism: and therapeutics of cholera 122, 129–36
rats: as carriers of plague 80; prevalence of in Lower City 19, 220;
Raulot, Jean-Yves 117, 176, 248–9
Ravicini, Serafino: Inspector-General of Public Health 237; and cholera epidemic of 1910 237–8
reaction phase of cholera: *see* cholera
Red Cross 158
Regina Margherita: 'expansion neighbourhood' of 198
Reggio Calabria 90, 301
rehydration therapy: *see* treatment of cholera
religiosity, popular: revival of in epidemic of 1884 99–100, 109–10, 160, 162–3
renal failure: as complication of cholera 116
rent: cost of, 34, 39, 222; in 'expansion neighbourhoods' after *risanamento* 199–200, 211–14; rises after unification 38–9; as source of poverty 38–9, 42, 50
republicans: *see* Popular Bloc
restaurants: in epidemic of 1884 108–9
'resurrection men' 151
Rettifilo 165, 185–7, 215–16, 220–21, 227
Revel: and the first cholera pandemic 82
'rice-water stools': *see* symptoms of cholera
rickets 14
ringworm 275
riots: and cholera 149–50, 244–5; absence of during fifth pandemic at Hamburg and Paris 152–4; in Apulia and Latium in 1911 309; at Carmine and San Francesco prisons in 1884 148–9; and cholera epidemic of 1910 1, 237, 242, 245–6; feared by rulers of Naples 31; and first pandemic in Britain 151; and first pandemic in Europe 359; and opening of Maddalena and Piedigrotta Hospitals in 1884 147–8; against sanitary cordons at La Spezia 91–2; at Taranto in 1910 293–4
risanamento 181–230; and cholera, direct influence of 1884 epidemic 181; collapse of buildings 208–11; and Cotugno Hospital 190; and cuts, effects of 215–20; demolition of

slums 187; engineering plans 186–8; eviction of the poor 198–207; failure of 215–25, 281–5; financial provisions for 191–201; hygienic purpose of 185–6; landfills 187–8; and localist theory, influence of 184–90, 195, 226; and medical profession, 225–30; models for 49, 181, 184, 192, 202; and overcrowding, elimination of 187, 211–12; Paris as a precedent for 181–5, 194; and political conflict in 1910 253–8; reassuring mythology of 243–5, 250–53, 281–2; and the Rettifilo 186–7; sanitary code 188; Serino aqueduct 189–90, 214, 220, 226, 250, 295; sewers 188–9; subsoil, purification of 186–90; sunlight, role of 186, 211; and University of Naples 227–8; ventilation, role of 186, 211, 214; *see also* Naples Renewal Company
Risorgimento 36–7, 40, 42–6, 50, 51–2, 54, 72, 73, 166–7, 191, 194, 301–2, 345–6, 360–61, 362
Rodinò, Giulio: alderman and Director of the Department of Health 229, 250, 255–6, 280, 328; author of mendacious account of epidemic of 1910–11 250–52, 305, 315
Rogers, Leonard: banned from Italian mainland hospitals 353, 354–7; and epidemic of 1911 at Palermo 353–7; and rehydration therapy 126, 353–7
Roma 141, 262, 265, 277, 310–11, 345
Romano, Rosa: last cholera victim of 1884 104
Rome: and cholera outbreak in 1911 337; density of 18; and flood of 1882 as precedent for financing *risanamento* 192; as place of refuge in 1884 108; population of 18; as prototype of urban renewal 202; and *risanamento*, 192; as rival to Naples 37; threatened by outbreak of 1910 260; and visit of Leonard Rogers 354–5
Rosenberg, Charles 3–4, 176–7, 244, 245
Royal Hygiene Society 46, 97, 258, 317, 346
Royal Neapolitan Academy of Medicine and Surgery 52, 139, 317, 174
rubber teat: and cholera among infants 118–20
Russia 1, 59, 65; experiments in treatment of cholera 356; and first pandemic 81–2, 150; and sixth pandemic 233–5, 238–9, 309

Saigon 62, 63
sailors: and cholera at Toulon 62–3, 66
Saint Anne: cult of 109–10
Saint Nicholas of Bari 239
Salerno: as place of refuge in 1884 108
Salvemini, Gaetano 365
San Bernardo lazaretto 87
San Carlo all'Arena: *sezione* of Naples 107, 133; flight from 107–8; and mortality from cholera in 1884 107
San Dalmazzo lazaretto 87

San Donato, Gennaro Di: Mayor of Naples 14–15, 48; critic of Depretis 192–3; denounces immobilism of City Hall 49–50; helps to draft bill for *risanamento* 193; leader of the Historical Left 48

San Efremo: 'expansion neighbourhood' 198

San Eligio Hospital 54

Sanfelice, Guglielmo, Archbishop of Naples: and acceptance of medical science 145–6; compared with Archbishop Celesia of Palermo 73–4, 147; and miracle of the blood 141–2; and reconciliation with the modern world 145; supports authorities during epidemic of 1884 145–7, 150, 166–9, 214; and theology of cholera 73; visits Conocchia Hospital 168

San Ferdinando: *sezione* of Naples 265

San Francesco Prison: and riot in 1884 148

San Gennaro: cult and miracle of 162–3, 169; feast of 259–60; patron saint of Naples 109–10, 166, 169

San Giuliano, Antonio Di: Foreign Minister 293, 321, 323; and ban on emigration to Argentina 340–41; and insalubrity of *locande* 272; seeks American support to conceal epidemic of 1911 321–2; urges deportation of Henry Geddings 335; urges policy of concealment 349

San Giuseppe: *sezione* of Naples 11

sanitary blockade: *see* quarantine, land-based

sanitary commissioners: stationed on emigrant ships to United States 321–2; stationed on emigrant ships to Argentina 339–41

sanitary cordons: *see* quarantine, land-based

San Lorenzo: *sezione* of Naples 11

Sampiero, S.S.: first ship to dock at Nisida 94

Santa Brigida: neighbourhood of 193–4; renewal of 193–4, 213

Santa Fé: province of 268

Santa Lucia: neighbourhood of fishermen 35; renewal of 193–4, 213, 214, 215

Santa Maria della Vita Hospital 54

Santoliquido, Rocco: Director-General of Public Health 235, 293–4; directs concealment of cholera 306, 348–9; reports riots in 1910 261; veteran of epidemic of 1884 235

Sardinia: avoids cholera in 1884 141; and falsification of statistics 327; and quarantine in 1884 86; and outbreak of 1912 247, 306, 327; threatened by outbreak in Apulia 236

Saredo, Giuseppe: and Camorra control of municipal slaughter-house 41, 42; as critic of local health administration policies health 49, 53; as critic of contract with Naples Renewal Company 206; as critic of *risanamento* 211–15, 219–20, 253; and downfall of Liberal administration of Naples 254; and effects of tax system on Naples 38

Saredo Report: *see* Giuseppe Saredo

Sarthe, S.S.: and outbreak of cholera at Toulon 62–3, 74, 75

scarification: as treatment for cholera 125

scirocco: prevailing wind of Naples 102, 174, 175, 186, 190

scurvy 14

seamstresses 34

Sebeto River: and market gardening 26; pollution of 26, 283; as municipal boundary 147; role in epidemic of 1911 351

Semmola, Mariano: Professor of Medicine 52, 53; advocate of therapeutic minimalism 129, 131–3, 135, 136; alarmed at building accidents during renewal 208–9; city councillor 208–9; editor of *La medicina contemporanea* 129; Medical Director of the White Cross 137; and nervous aetiology of cholera 355–6; and 'physiological treatment' of cholera 133, 136; taken ill with cholera 144

senile marasmus 223

septicaemia 127, 354

Serao, Matilde 16, 362; author of *Il paese di Cuccagna* 44; and the 'bowels of Naples' 16; describes Neapolitan passion for gambling 44; regards renewal programme as a betrayal 220

Serino aqueduct 189–90, 202, 243–4, 257–8, 278, 284, 313, 336

sewage farming: *see* market gardening

sewer system of Naples 16, 29–30, 284

sexual impotence: and cholera phobia 138

sheep: *see* domestic animals

Sicily: and emigration 267, 268; and epidemic of 1885–6 169; and epidemic of 1911 247, 306; escapes cholera in 1884 141; and fear of cholera in 1884 74, 90, 177; and first pandemic 150; and quarantine in 1884 86; threatened by outbreak in Apulia 236

silk craft 34

slaughter-house: Camorra control of 41

smallpox 4; endemic in Naples 116–17; mortality in Naples in 1884 105; mortality in the New World 112; and social class 15

snow: as evidence of concealment in 1911 317–18, 438

Snow, John: and aetiology of cholera 23, 144; and public health policies 195; and role of lodging-houses in cholera 21–2

Società Operaia 287; and anti-cholera prophylaxis 177–8; merges with the White Cross 157, 159; organizes volunteers in 1884 156–7

soldiers: as means of spreading cholera 59, 83–4, 89, 92–3; mortality from cholera in 1884 89, 143–4, 371

Sonnino, Sidney 201, 345, 347; condemns conspiracy of silence 345

soup kitchens: and anti-cholera campaign of 1884 104–5, 172–3; and anti-cholera campaign in 1910 294; and anti-cholera campaign of 1911 305–6; established by private charity 170, 171
South American Sanitary Convention of 1904 339, 341
'Southern Question': and cholera 5, 154, 361–2; Naples as a symbol of 31; and rise of the Historical Left 192–3
Spain: and cholera epidemic of 1884 84
'sporadic' cholera 22–3, 98, 102, 190
Staten Island 309, 319–20
Stella: *sezione* of 170
stralci 215–20, 227
street-sweeping: as factor in insalubrity of Naples 23–6; intensified during epidemic of 1884 103; intensified during epidemic of 1911 351; organization of in Naples 24–6
Striano, Carmine 274, 287, 288, 292
subcontracting system: and favouritism 219–20; and *risanamento* 204–6; and substandard building 208–11
subsoil: considered source of cholera 102, 107, 154; contamination of 14, 28, 29–30, 101, 102, 103, 190; to be purified by *risanamento* 186–90; *see also* localism
substances used in treatment of cholera: acetate of lead 126; alcohol 126, 356; ammonia 126; ammonio-citrate of iron 125; arsenic 109, 125; boric acid 134; caffeine 356; calomel 123, 124, 125, 356; camphor 126, 356; capsicum 126; carbolic acid 133–6; carbonate of soda 133; castor oil 123, 125; chalk 126; colocynth 123; copper sulphate 126; croton oil 123; ether 126; hydrocyanic acid 126; iodine 134, 356; ipecacuanha 123; laudanum 77, 126, 133; milk 126; morphine 77, 126; musk 126; mustard 123; oxygen 77, 135, 356; phosphorus 125; potassium permanganate 134; prussic acid 125, 128; quinine 136; salicylic acid 134; salt water 123; sodium chloride 132; strychnine 125, 128, 137, 356; sulfuric acid 134; tannic acid 134; tartar emetic 123, 125; thymol 135; zinc 123
Sue, Eugène 17
Suez Canal 62
suffocation 115–16, 356
suffrage: *see* franchise
suicide: and cholera, 112, 70–71; and mortality in 1884 105, 107
Summonte, Celestino: Mayor of Naples and camorrista 219–20; downfall of 253–4
sweat: role in spreading cholera 174
sympathetic nerves: considered seat of cholera 122–3
symptoms of cholera: asphyxia 115–16, 356; blood pressure 115; chills 115; cramp 76–7, 115, 354; diarrhoea 76–7, 114–15, 122–3, 354,

355–6; dizziness 115; fever 115–16; hiccoughs 115; nausea 115; pulse rate 114–15; 'rice water stools' 23, 114; temperature 144–5; thirst 115; *see also* complications of cholera
syphilis 68; and deportation of immigrants from the United States 275; mortality in 1884 105; positive associations of 113; prevalent in Naples 14; treatment by mercury 125;

Taragona: cholera outbreak of 1911 344
Taranto: insurrection of 1910 293–4
tax policy of Liberal regime: as source of impoverishment 30, 37, 46, 65, 192; *see also dazio consumo*
terror and cholera: and age profile of victims 116–20, 139–40; and cholera hospitals 76–7; and Christian theology 71–4; and class profile of victims 138–44; emerges in 1884 66–78; and land-based quarantine 83, 89–92; and municipal prophylactic measures 138–41; and post-mortem muscular twitching 120; and premature burial 120–21; and symptomatology of cholera 112–21; and treatment 121–38; *see also* poisoning hysteria.
theology of cholera: *see* Catholic Church
therapeutic minimalism: *see* treatment of cholera, Mariano Semmola
thirst: as symptom of cholera 115
Thomas, Keith 151
Toledo, Via 25, 32, 48, 158, 334
Tomasi di Lampedusa, Giuseppe 52
Tonkin 62, 74, 235
Torre Annunziata 298, 332–3
Toulon 90, 91; and epidemic of 1884 62–78, 86, 88, 96, 101, 164
tourism: threatened by cholera in 1911 235, 301–2, 307, 322, 341, 343, 349, 353
trachoma: and deportation of immigrants from Ellis Island 275; prevalence in Naples 223
Trani: and cholera riot 242; and epidemic of 1910 220, 233
Transatlantica Steamship Company 290, 291
transfusions: and treatment of cholera, 126, 128
treatment of cholera 121–38; alterative therapy 125; astringent system 125, 126, 131; blisters 124; cauterization 124, 125; cold-water system 127, 405–6; counter-irritation 125; by dry cupping 123; depletive therapy 122–5, 353–4, 403–4; by enteroclysis and hypodermoclysis 133–5; and 'etiological treatment' 356; by galvanism 77, 127, 136–7; inhalation therapy 127; and leeches 123; at Naples in 1911 355–7; by plugging the bowel 127; rehydration therapy 126–7, 353–4; by 'remedial injury' 125; by sedatives 126; by stimulants 126; sweating treatment 123; and therapeutic minimalism 128–9, 131–2; by transfusion 126; by venesection 123–6, 128; *see also* substances used in treatment of cholera

tuberculosis 4, 14, 220; as cause of death 223; and deportation of emigrants from the United States 275; as endemic disease 116–17; and mortality in 1884 107; and mortality in Italy 102–3; positive associations of 112–13; prevalent in Naples 14, 220; and social class 15

Turati, Filippo 273, 295

Turchi, Marino 52, 174, 361

Turin 206; expenditure on welfare in 49; growth of since unification 14; population in 1884 18; and preventive measures against cholera in 1910, 278; as prototype of urban renewal 202; wages in 32–3

typhoid 4, 14, 15, 22, 220; as endemic disease 116–17, 220; and mortality in 1884 105

typhus 4

Twain, Mark 15, 17–18, 221

Umberto I, Corso 165, 185–7, 215–16, 220–21, 227

Umberto I, King 122, 181; conceives plan to renew Naples 165, 216; inaugurates renewal 207; visits Busca in 1884 164; visits Naples in 1884 163–9, 172

unemployment 36, 39–40; and recession after 1907 277–8, 290

unification of Italy: *see* Risorgimento

'United Associations': and elections of 1910 256

United States: collusion with Italian conspiracy of silence 321–6, 333–7; and conflicts in time of cholera 245; and Italian immigration 236, 246, 249, 266–77; and outbreak of 1911 248, 249, 286, 309, 318–20, 344, and return migration 288; as signatory of International Sanitary Convention of 1903 302–5, 318, 324; *see also* United States Public Health and Marine Hospital Service, Henry Downes Geddings

United States Department of State 105; and collusion with conspiracy of silence 321–4; reports on conditions of labour in Europe 32–6

United States Public Health and Marine Hospital Service: and anti-cholera measures in 1911 303–4, 321–2; and epidemic of 1910 248, 258–9, 286; and epidemic of 1911 300, 318–21, 340; issues final destination cards 304; misled by Italy 250, 259, 286, 324–5; opposes collusion with policy of concealment 334; protests at Italian concealment 320, 324–5, 334; *see also* Henry Downes Geddings

University of Naples: and benefits of *risanamento* 227–8; and the medical profession 52, 139, 144, 157

untori: *see* poisoning hysteria

Upper City: configuration of 11, 380–81; mortality in 15; social composition of 24, 26, 49, 32, 162; water supply of 26

uraemia: as complication of cholera 116

urban renewal: *see risanamento*

Uruguay 339–40, 341

usury 21, 32, 40

Varignano lazaretto: as probable source of cholera at La Spezia 93–6

Vasto: 'expansion neighbourhood' of 198

venesection: and eliminant treatment of cholera 123, 124–6, 128

Venice 233; and anti-plague measures 79–80; and cholera outbreak of 1911 309, 327, 332, 348–50, 355; population of in 1884 17, 18

Ventimiglia 87–8

Verbicaro: and cholera epidemic of 1911 307, 308, 310–11

Verga, Giovanni 113, 150

vermin: prevalence of in the Lower City 19, 21

Vibrio cholerae: as pathogenic agent of cholera 16, 22, 26 , 59, 76, 78, 83, 87, 89, 98, 100, 104, 113, 114, 121, 129, 130, 133, 134, 174, 233, 234, 240, 249, 280, 283–4, 303

Vicaria: *sezione* of Naples 11, 15, 17, 106–7, 110, 148, 171, 214, 251, 252, 263; *see also* Lower City

Victor Emanuel II, King 166–7

Victoria, Queen 156

vigilantes: employed to locate cholera sufferers 237–8

Villari, Pasquale 362

Vittoria Hospital: as basis for Cotugno Hospital 170–71, 190; as cholera hospital 111, 224; founded with funds from Bank of Naples 170 71

Vomero 158; 'expansion neighbourhood' of 198; as place of refuge in 1884 108

vomiting: as symptom of cholera 114–15, 123, 126

wages: of Italian farm workers 267; of Neapolitan builders 20–21; of Neapolitan workers 32–5, 222

Warner, John Harley 122, 128

washerwomen: *see* women

water supply of Naples 26–9, 101, 119; contamination of Bolla and Carmignano aqueducts 26–8; contamination of water-tanks 27–8, 259; contamination of wells 28–9, 49, 98, 259, 284

water-closets: absence of in Naples 21, 23, 29

water-tanks: contamination of in Lower Naples 27–8; in Upper Naples 26

weather: and epidemic of 1884 174, 175; and outbreak of 1910 259, 283–4

wells: contamination of 20, 24, 28–9, 49, 98, 259, 284; sealed during epidemic of 1884 100, 173; and spread of cholera in 1884 98; and spread of cholera in 1910 259; sealed in 1911 351

West Bengal 59, 265

White Cross 111, 137, 155–63; distributes rations and supplies 161; international membership of 158; military discipline of 138; political and social composition of 158; role of in reducing cholera phobia 159–63; and unpaid status of volunteers 160; treats patients in homes 159

White Star Line 271

William I, Emperor 156

wine: adulteration of 49, 104; consumption of in October festivities 43; cost of 34, 196; drunk by visitors 11; export threatened by cholera in 1911 301–2; exported via Naples until unification 31; as predisposing factor in the spread of cholera 43, 100, 119–20; role in the epidemic of 1884 99–100, 175

women: and amenorrhoea 42; and breast-feeding 118–19; as builders 34; and chlorotic anaemia 42; and cholera phobia 138; as domestic servants 34; excluded from franchise 46–7; as homeworkers 143; and hospitalization 141; and job segregation 33, 143; as laundresses 24, 36, 95–6; and Loreto and Pace hospitals 54–5; medicalized by the Office of Hygiene 228; and menstrual irregularities resulting from cholera phobia 138; and mortality from cholera in 1884 143; and opposition to municipal sanitary measures 141; and predisposition to cholera in laundry trade 24, 95–6; and prostitution 36, 40; and puerperal fever 105; as sellers of

wicker chairs and matches 36; and school demonstration in 1884 99; soup kitchens for 150; as tobacco factory operatives 33; unemployment of 36; wages and employment of 32–4, 36; as White Cross volunteers 158

wool: exported via Naples until unification 31; craft 34

workers and tradesmen: bakers, 34, 142; blacksmiths 34; builders 20–22, 31, 208–11, 240; butchers 24, 31, 41, 42; cabmen 34, 41, 42; charcoal burners 142; clerks 143; cobblers 34; day labourers 143; dockers 41, 42; fishermen 35, 83, 233–5, 263; fishmongers 24; gardeners 34; gravediggers 140–41; hairdressers 142; hatters 34; joiners 34; kiln-men 142; manual labourers 143; newspaper vendors 35–6; pedlars 20, 31, 35–6, 41–2, 351; porters 31, 34, 42, 142; ragpickers 24, 142, 263; shopkeepers 143; street-sweepers 23–6, 351; stretcher-bearers 109, 145–6; tailors 34; tanners 34; town criers 109; *see also* doctors, nurses, women

World Health Organization: and anti-gypsy mythology 239; and misleading statistics for 1911 250

Wyman, Walter: Surgeon-General of the United States 236, 248, 297, 318, 320, 335, 344–5

xenophobia: *see* Jews, gypsies

Zola, Emile 17